W9-BJJ-673

INTRODUCTION TO NEUROGENIC COMMUNICATION DISORDERS

INTRODUCTION TO NEUROGENIC COMMUNICATION DISORDERS

Edition 6

Robert H. Brookshire, PhD, CCC/SP
Professor Emeritus, Department of Communication Disorders
University of Minnesota
Minneapolis, Minnesota

with 174 illustrations

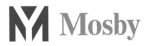 Mosby

An Affiliate of Elsevier Science

St. Louis London Philadelphia Sydney Toronto

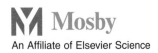

An Affiliate of Elsevier Science

11830 Westline Industrial Drive
St. Louis, Missouri 63146

SIXTH EDITION

Introduction to Neurogenic Communication Disorders   0-323-01686-3

Copyright © 2003, Mosby, Inc. All rights reserved.

No part of this publication may be reproduced, stored in a retrieval system, or transmitted in any form or by any means, electronic, mechanical, photocopying, recording, or otherwise, without prior permission of the publisher.

Some material was previously published.

Notice

Speech Pathology is an ever-changing field. Standard safety precautions must be followed, but as new research and clinical experience broaden our knowledge, changes in treatment and drug therapy may become necessary or appropriate. Readers are advised to check the most current product information provided by the manufacturer of each drug to be administered to verify the recommended dose, the method and duration of administration, and contraindications. It is the responsibility of the licensed prescriber, relying on experience and knowledge of the patient, to determine dosages and the best treatment for each individual patient. Neither the publisher nor the editor assumes any liability for any injury and/or damage to persons or property arising from this publication.

The Publisher

Previous editions copyrighted 1997, 1992.

Library of Congress Cataloging-in-Publication Data
Brookshire, Robert H.
    Introduction to Neurogenic Communication Disorders / Robert H. Brookshire.—6th ed.
        p. cm.
    Includes bibliographical references and index.
    ISBN 0-323-01686-3 (alk. paper)
    1. Communicative disorders. I. Title.
RC423 .B74 2002
616.85'52—dc21   2002067153

Acquisitions Editor: Kellie White
Developmental Editor: Christie Hart
Associate Developmental Editor: Jennifer Watrous
Publishing Services Manager: Pat Joiner
Project Manager: Rachel E. Dowell
Designer: Mark A. Oberkrom

GW/QWF

Printed in the United States of America

Last digit is the print number: 9 8 7 6 5 4 3 2 1

For Lisa

The autumn wind touches the mountain _____
The spring leaf falls to earth

Foreword

The remarkable capacity of humans to communicate emerged in a gradual, evolutionary way. Today it explodes on the scene during the early years of life. As normal communicators, we benefit from the reliability and adaptability conferred by evolution. We could be reminded daily—if we stopped to think about it—of the crucial roles that speech, language, and communication ability play in our social, emotional, intellectual, and working lives.

Of course, we usually don't stop to think about it. Communication is so much a part of our "selves" that the wonder of it becomes apparent only when we choose to study it. Readers of this book probably already have a better sense than most of the complexity of the processes that make us normal speakers, listeners, readers, writers, and communicators.

Most of you have chosen to embark on an effort to learn about what happens when—because of neurologic disease—the ability to communicate becomes impaired. Such impairments seem to insult and diminish the accomplishments of evolution. Fortunately, neurologic disease does not happen to an entire species. Unfortunately, it does happen to people, often in ways that disable, handicap, and devastate. It is one of life's paradoxes that our speech and language ability permits us to study the effects of its destruction and then share that knowledge with others. Such study should be conducted with a keen awareness that our "subjects" deserve our commitment to use what we learn from them both responsibly and productively.

Don't misinterpret the word *introduction* in the title of this book. The contents herein represent more than a handshake. The text provides a solid foundation in the neurology of communication, as well as the causes, symptoms, diagnosis, and management of the most frequently encountered neurologic communication disorders. Serious students will leave this book prepared to study the disorders in greater depth. Aspiring clinicians will leave it prepared to develop the skills necessary to work with people whose lives are affected by the disorders.

Many texts about neurogenic communication disorders have come and gone over the years. Some texts became extinct because of limited substance, some because they failed to communicate their content effectively, and some because their content no longer reflected current knowledge, thinking, or practice. This sixth edition of *Introduction to Neurogenic Communication Disorders* has come to life because it reflects the evolution of several things. First, the assessment, diagnosis, understanding, and management of neurogenic communication disorders and their causes have changed in subtle to dramatic ways. Those changes are reflected in these pages.

Second, the range of communication disorders to which we must attend has broadened. When the first edition of this text was published, clinicians were "up to speed" if they knew something about aphasia, dysarthria, and apraxia of speech. We now appreciate, by virtue of their increasing prevalence and careful clinical observation and research, that right hemisphere lesions, traumatic brain injury, and dementia can affect communication in ways that often are not captured by our concepts of aphasia and motor speech disorders. Those changes are also reflected in these pages. Finally, Dr. Brookshire's very special talents as a clinician, researcher, and teacher have evolved. No book reaches a second, let alone a sixth edition, without its author having gotten something right the first time and then building on it in a way that keeps the ever-evolving needs of its readers in mind. The content of this book reflects what a recognized expert believes are the core of "facts" and concepts necessary to a foundation

for understanding neurogenic communication disorders. You should also know that you will be learning from someone whose clarity of thought and expression have been, for many years, greatly respected and admired by his colleagues and appreciated by his students.

Be assured that the organization, style, and clarity of this book will meet your needs if you are coming to this complex subject for the first time. I suspect this book also will become a friend and valuable resource to those of you who already have or will develop a lasting interest in neurogenic communication disorders. It almost certainly will contribute to your own evolution as students, teachers, researchers, or clinicians.

Joseph R. Duffy, PhD
Head, Division & Section of Speech Pathology
Department of Neurology
Mayo Clinic
Rochester, Minnesota

Preface

I have written this book to provide its readers with a general understanding of neurogenic communication disorders—their causes, symptoms, typical course, treatment, and outcome. I have tried to be practical about what I have included in this book. I have tried to include material that I believe to be both important and useful to those who are beginning their study of neurogenic communication disorders. My decisions regarding what to include and what to leave out no doubt reflect my personal biases about who, how, and why we treat. It also reflects my experiences in thirty-some years of teaching university students about neurogenic communication disorders and my sense of what has seemed important to them.

I have not tried to identify all areas of controversy, and sometimes I may have presented my own opinions as facts. One fact, I think, is inescapable—that even such seeming facts as the pyramidal system and apraxia of speech are in one sense matters of opinion or convenient fictions. What passes for "fact" in the scientific and clinical literature about neurogenic communication disorders (and in the literature relating to many other areas of knowledge as well) is in truth opinion, intuition, or someone's best guess about what seems true. The content of this book represents my best guess about what is likely to prove true over time, and I hope that I have guessed right more often than not.

I believe that clinical competence comes as much (or more) from one's development of intuitions based on regularities observed across patients than from reading the literature. I also believe that treatment of neurogenic communication disorders combines *art* and *science,* and that many empirically verified facts may prove trivial or irrelevant to helping the neurologically compromised adult become a better communicator.

This book is neither a training manual nor a catalog of techniques. Reading it will not make the reader competent to evaluate, diagnose, or treat patients with neurogenic communication disorders. No book or collection of books can do that. Clinical competence comes from blending knowledge acquired from clinical and scientific literature, supervised clinical training, and independent clinical experience. This book will, I hope, help the student get started on the road to clinical competence by providing a basic understanding of what neurogenic communication disorders are, what the individuals who have them are like, and how neurogenic communication disorders may be measured and treated.

Now for an editorial note. The word "aphasic" is an adjective, and not a noun. I strongly believe that using the word "aphasic" as a noun, as in

"Wernicke's aphasics" depersonalizes those for whom we provide services, in addition to being stylistically deplorable. Therefore readers will not find me referring to "aphasics" in this book, and I trust that readers will, in their own writing, speech, and professional activities, focus on the person and not the condition.

THOUGHT QUESTIONS

I have included a few Thought Questions at the end of each chapter. In them I have tried to present situations such as those clinicians may encounter in the course of their work with individuals who may have neurogenic communication disorders. Responding to the thought questions will require that the reader combine factual knowledge with logic and intuition to arrive at reasonable responses. There are no *correct answers* to most of the thought questions, and my responses represent my *best guesses* and are not necessarily the only reasonable responses. I believe that the process by which readers arrive at their responses to the thought questions is more important than the responses themselves, provided that the responses are logically consistent and are based on reasonable interpretations of relevant information. I trust that readers will be challenged and perhaps entertained as they respond to the thought questions, and that doing so helps them to practice and sharpen their clinical thinking.

Robert H. Brookshire

Acknowledgments

Few of the ideas in this book are truly my own. The influence of colleagues, students, and the patients I have known and worked with permeates the contents. Without them, this book would not exist.

My special thanks:

- To Linda Nicholas for her continuing support, tolerance, and understanding while this edition was a work in progress.
- To Christie Hart, Jennifer Watrous, and Kellie White, my editors at Elsevier Science, for their professionalism, patience, impeccable advice, and unwavering good humor during the preparation of this book for publication.
- To Keith Roberts and the Graphic World crew for their keenness of eye, attention to detail, and concern for quality during final editing and page layout.
- To Mary Kennedy, PhD, for her insightful review of material related to right-hemisphere syndrome and traumatic brain injury.
- To O.M. Reinmuth, MD, for his meticulous review of material related to neurology.
- To Jeanne Robertson, whose drawings illustrate key concepts with elegance and clarity.
- To the friends, colleagues, and patients who have made my professional life rewarding, challenging, and a never-ending source of education and enlightenment.

Robert H. Brookshire

Contents

Neuroanatomy and Neuropathology

As its title suggests, this book is about neurogenic communication disorders. The prefix *neuro-* in *neurogenic* means *related to nerves or the nervous system*. The suffix *-genic* in *neurogenic* means *resulting from* or *caused by*. Phrased in everyday language, therefore, this book is about communication disorders caused by pathology in the human nervous system.

Neurogenic communication disorders in adults encompass a variety of specific abnormalities, all caused by nervous system pathology:

- Aphasia—characterized by impaired comprehension and production of language, usually caused by pathology affecting the language-competent half of the brain.
- Right-hemisphere syndrome—characterized by impaired comprehension and production of abstract information and impaired appreciation of visuospatial relationships, usually caused by pathology affecting the non-language-competent half of the brain.

- Traumatic brain injury syndrome—characterized by impaired attention and memory, impaired appreciation of abstract information, and altered interpersonal behavior, usually caused by diffuse brain pathology.
- Dementia—characterized by memory impairments, personality changes, and altered behavior, usually caused by pathology affecting brain regions related to memory, attention, and affect.
- Dysarthria—characterized by impaired speech production, usually caused by pathology affecting nerves controlling the muscles involved in speech or by pathology affecting the speech muscles themselves.

Neurogenic communication disorders are an important consequence of nervous system abnormalities. Their features, severity, and outcome reflect the location, magnitude, and nature of the abnormality. Consequently, clinicians who wish to assess, diagnose, and treat neurogenic commu-

1

nication disorders must have at least rudimentary knowledge of the human nervous system and what can go wrong with it. The intent of this chapter is to provide that knowledge. This chapter begins by describing the anatomy of the parts of the nervous system likely to be affected when neurogenic communication disorders appear. Then it describes some of the major pathologic processes that underlie the most common neurogenic communication disorders.

Unfortunately for those learning neuroanatomy, the human nervous system contains a confusing array of parts; almost every part has several different names, and most of the parts are convenient fictions invented by humans to make it easier to describe, analyze, draw, and communicate about the nervous system. The proliferation of names for parts of the nervous system began in the 19th century, when many investigators were studying the nervous system, when communication among investigators was slow and inefficient, and when there was a tendency for explorers of the nervous system—like explorers of the planet—to name things they discovered after themselves.

Eventually, practitioners began to call for more descriptive names because the old names were difficult to remember and most of the parts of the nervous system already had been named, so the new people couldn't name things after themselves. Nevertheless, there still remains some gratification to be had from attaching a name to something, even if that something already has a name. Thus, the proliferation of names has not completely stopped, although it has slowed to a crawl.

Many names for parts of the nervous system seem obscure today, and some have lost currency and perhaps should be abandoned. However, many names and the concepts that underlie them are traditional despite their scientific faults and need to be understood for purposes of communicating with other professionals.

In this chapter, I will give the most common multiple names when I describe a part of the nervous system. Thereafter I will use the most descriptive and therefore the easiest-to-remember names.

THE HUMAN NERVOUS SYSTEM
Cellular Structures

Glial cells and *neurons* (nerve cells) make up most of the cellular structure of the central nervous system. Glial cells are the bricks and mortar of the brain. They support and separate neurons and nerve fiber tracts and are thought to serve other functions such as regulating fluid levels in nervous system tissues, removing foreign substances from nervous system tissues, and participating in brain metabolism.

All nervous system activity begins with nerve cells, or neurons (Figure 1-1). The activity of pools of neurons distributed throughout the nervous system leads to sensation, perception, discrimination, emotion, behavior, and the actions of muscles, organs, and glands. All neurons have the same general structure, although they differ widely in size and shape. A typical neuron has a cell body from which project small hairlike structures called *dendrites* and a longer, thicker tubular structure called an *axon*. Dendrites receive information (in the form of chemical and electrical changes) from other neurons and transmit the information to the cell body. Axons carry information away from the cell body to other neurons via their dendrites. Most neurons are *multipolar*, meaning that there are many dendrites projecting from the cell body. Some neurons are *unipolar* (have only one dendrite) or *bipolar* (have two dendrites). Neuronal cell bodies come in various sizes. The largest are about 20 times the size of the smallest (Nolte, 1993). Axons differ in length and diameter. Most are only a few millimeters long, but some, such as those that connect neurons in the cerebral cortex to neurons in the lower spinal cord, are several feet long. Longer axons tend to be larger in diameter. The diameters of the longest axons in the human nervous system

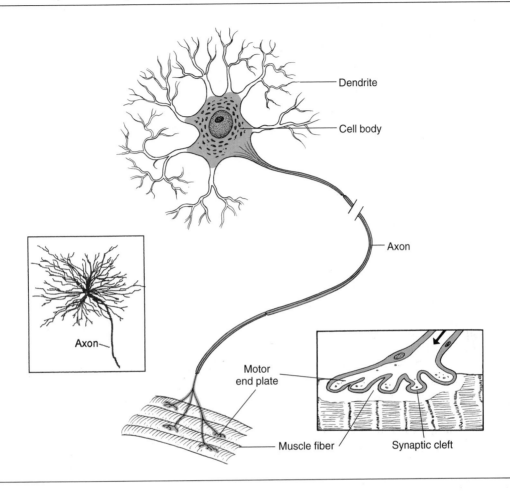

Figure 1-1 ■ **A simplified drawing of a motor neuron, showing the cell body, axon, and myoneural (muscle–nerve) junction. A motor end plate (the junction between a neuron and a muscle fiber) is shown on the lower right. The insert on the left shows a tracing of a real spinal motor neuron to show the complexity of dendritic structures relative to the simplified drawings provided in most textbooks.**

are about 20 times the diameter of the smallest. Larger-diameter axons conduct information faster than smaller-diameter axons. Axons with the smallest diameters conduct information at about 1 meter per second, whereas axons with the largest diameters conduct information at up to 120 meters per second. Some axons (mostly the longer, thicker ones) are covered with a thin layer of a white fatty substance called *myelin*. Myelin provides electrical insulation for nerve axons, much like the coatings on electrical

wires, and allows axons to conduct information at higher rates.

Some neurologic diseases (e.g., multiple sclerosis) are characterized by degeneration and loss of the myelin from neuron axons. Loss of myelin causes weakness and impaired control of muscles served by the affected neurons.

The point at which the axon of one neuron encounters a dendrite of another is called a *synapse*. The tiny space between an axon and a dendrite is called the *synaptic cleft*. Transmission of nerve impulses across the synaptic cleft is a chemical process. A chemical transmitter substance is released by the axon and drifts across the synaptic cleft, where it stimulates the dendrite of a second neuron. The stimulation causes a change in the second dendrite's electric charge. This change (if it is especially strong, or if it is combined with the response of other stimulated dendrites), causes the second neuron to fire, sending a signal down its axon to stimulate the dendrites of yet another neuron.

Neurons may be categorized according to their function. *Sensory neurons* either respond directly to stimulation (such as touch or temperature) or receive input from sensory receptor cells (such as those in the retina or inner ear). *Motor neurons* connect to muscles and glands. *Interneurons* connect other neurons. Interneurons far outnumber motor and sensory neurons; more than 99% of human neurons are interneurons (Nolte, 1993). (And sensory neurons outnumber motor neurons by about 4 or 5 to 1.)

Anatomists customarily divide central nervous system tissues into *gray matter* and *white matter*. Gray matter is composed primarily of neuronal cell bodies, dendrites, and glial cells. Collections of functionally related nerve cells within gray matter are called *nuclei*. Nuclei are differentiated from surrounding tissue by cell type, cell density, and function (e.g., the nucleus ambiguus, which sends motor fibers to the pharynx and larynx and plays an important part in swallowing).

> Living gray matter is actually pink because of its rich blood supply. When it loses its blood supply it turns gray. Anatomists call it gray matter because it is gray when it arrives at their dissecting tables.

White matter is composed primarily of myelinated axons. White matter is white because the myelin around the axons is white. Collections of axons within the white matter may be called by various names, the most common of which is *tract*. The names of many tracts provide information about their origin and destination (e.g., the *corticospinal tract*, which begins in the cerebral cortex and ends in the spinal cord, and a personal favorite, the *habenulointerpeduncular tract*, which extends from the habenula to the interpeduncular nucleus).

Topography of the Human Nervous System

From the 1800s to the present, most of those who have described the human nervous system divide it into two parts: the *central nervous system* and the *peripheral nervous system*. The central nervous system lies within the skull and vertebrae. It includes the *brain*, the *brain stem*, the *cerebellum*, and the *spinal cord*. The central nervous system allows us to perceive and discriminate sensory stimuli and express emotions, keeps processes such as respiration and heartbeat going, organizes and regulates behavior, and permits us to engage in mental pursuits such as thinking, remembering, and understanding this sentence.

Most of the *peripheral nervous system* lies outside the skull and vertebrae. Neuroanatomists often divide it into two functional systems—the *somatic nervous system* and the *autonomic nervous system*. The somatic nervous system enables us to perceive sensory stimuli and carry on volitional motor activity. The autonomic nervous system is a self-regulating system that controls the glands and the operations of vital functions such as breathing, heartbeat, and blood pressure.

The Protective Envelope

The central nervous system is fragile but well protected from injury by a covering of bone, membranes, and fluid. The skull and vertebrae provide a durable external envelope. Strong membranes anchor the brain and spinal cord to the skull and the vertebrae. A layer of fluid cushions the central nervous system and provides a buoyant medium to minimize displacement of central nervous system tissues by abrupt movements of the head and body.

Skull The *skull* encloses and protects the brain, brain stem, and cerebellum. Human skulls are roughly symmetric, although one half usually is slightly larger than the other. The human skull is made up of eight plates, joined together to form a continuous surface (Figure 1-2). The plates of an infant's skull are less firmly joined than those of an adult's, making the infant's skull pliable and elastic (a characteristic for which mothers in childbirth have cause to be thankful). Skull elasticity diminishes across the life span. An 80-year-old person who falls and strikes his or her head is much more likely than a 20-year-old to receive a skull fracture. The adult human skull is thin in the front and on the sides (3 to 5 mm)

and thick in the back (15 to 20 mm). Blows to the front of the head are more likely to cause skull fracture than blows to the back of the head.

> That human skulls are thicker in back than in front may be at least partially a result of natural selection. A person who falls backward is more likely to strike his head than a person who falls forward because the person who falls forward can break the fall by extending hands and arms. Those whose skulls were thin in back may have been less likely to survive the perils of prehistoric times than those whose skulls were thick in back.

The space inside the skull is called the *cranial vault*. The ceiling and walls of the cranial vault are smooth, but the floor is irregular, with numerous depressions, openings, partitions, and

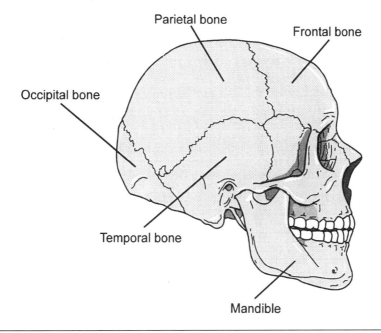

Figure 1-2 ■ **A lateral view of the human skull. The four bony plates on each side of the skull are called, reading counterclockwise, the frontal bone, the parietal bone, the occipital bone, and the temporal bone.**

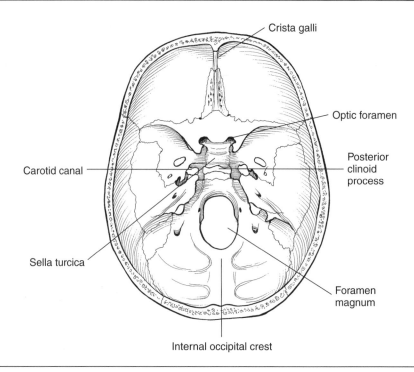

Crista galli

Optic foramen

Posterior clinoid process

Carotid canal

Sella turcica

Foramen magnum

Internal occipital crest

Figure 1-3 ■ **The floor of the cranial vault. The crista galli, the posterior clinoid process, and the sella turcica are three of several ridges and projections that arise from the floor of the cranial vault.**

ridges giving it a craggy appearance (Figure 1-3). The large opening in the base of the cranial vault is called the *foramen magnum* (great opening). It is the opening through which the brain stem passes on its way to the spinal cord.

Foramen comes from a Latin word meaning "aperture." In anatomy a foramen is an aperture or opening in tissue or bones.

Vertebrae The *vertebrae* are bony structures that support and protect the spinal cord. There are 33 vertebrae, and neuroanatomists typically divide them into 5 categories. The uppermost 7 are called *cervical vertebrae,* the next 12 are called *thoracic vertebrae,* the next 5 are called *lumbar vertebrae,* the next 5 are called *sacral*

vertebrae, and the lowest 4 are called *coccygeal vertebrae* (Figure 1-4). The 5 sacral and the 4 coccygeal vertebrae are fused into two larger structures, the *sacrum* and the *coccyx,* respectively.

Sacrum comes from Latin and means, roughly, "sacred bone." Coccyx comes from Greek, and means "cuckoo," or more likely "cuckoo's beak."

The vertebrae are separated by disks of cartilage and are held together and in alignment by muscles, tendons, and ligaments. The lower vertebrae are larger than those at the top, giving them greater weightbearing capacity and helping them resist twisting forces, which tend to converge in the lower back. Down the center of the chain of vertebrae is a roughly circular opening through

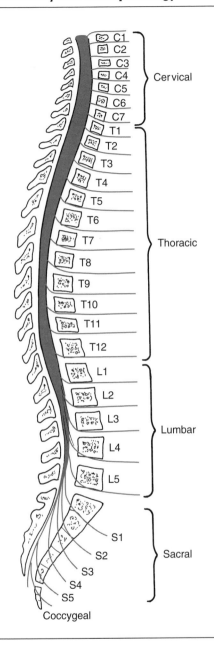

C1
C2
C3
C4   Cervical
C5
C6
C7
T1
T2
T3
T4
T5
T6
T7   Thoracic
T8
T9
T10
T11
T12
L1
L2
L3
L4   Lumbar
L5

S1
S2   Sacral
S3
S4
S5
Coccygeal

Figure 1-4 ■ **The human spine, showing the division of vertebrae into cervical, thoracic, lumbar, sacral, and coccygeal groups.**

which the spinal cord passes. Notches between the vertebrae provide spaces through which nerves and blood vessels pass. These notches are called the *intervertebral foramina.*

Pathologic changes in the vertebrae or the intervertebral discs may create pressure on nerves and blood vessels, causing neurologic symptoms (pain, loss of sensation, weakness, paralysis). Patients with spinal nerve or blood vessel compression make up a significant part of most neurosurgeon's caseloads, and decompression of spinal nerves and blood vessels is a common neurosurgical procedure.

Meninges Three membranes, called *meninges,* enclose the central nervous system (the brain, brain stem, cerebellum, and spinal cord). The outer membrane is called the *dura mater.* The middle membrane is called the *arachnoid,* and the inner membrane is called the *pia mater* (Figure 1-5). Because the meninges help to *cushion* the central nervous system, the mnemonic *PAD* (for *p*ia, *a*rachnoid, and *d*ura) may help the reader keep them in order.

The *dura mater* is a tough (*dur*able), slightly elastic membrane that encloses the brain and spinal cord and lines the inner surface of the skull. In the skull the outer surface of the dura mater adheres to the inner surface of the cranial vault, and the inner surface of the dura mater is attached to the arachnoid. The dura mater has two layers. In most of the dura mater the two layers are fused, but in the *dural venous sinuses* the two layers separate to form a complex system of cavities and channels. The venous sinuses

Sinus is from a Latin word meaning *cavity* or *channel.* In anatomy sinus means a groove, hollow, or cavity, often for the storage or transport of fluids such as blood.

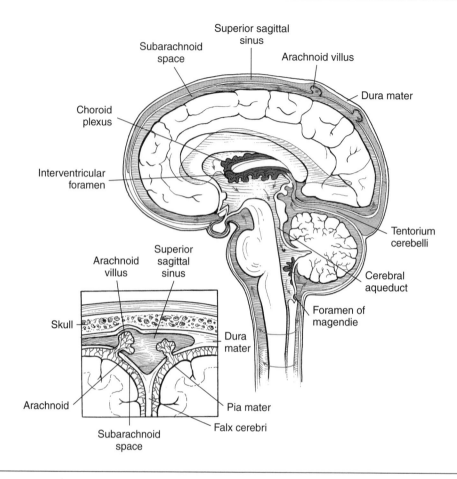

Figure 1-5 ■ The meninges and related structures. Cerebrospinal fluid (CSF) circulates throughout the ventricles and subarachnoid space. Its direction of flow is indicated by arrows. CSF is passed into the blood via the arachnoid villi, which protrude into the venous sinuses.

collect venous blood flowing down from the brain and discharge it into the internal jugular vein for return to the heart and lungs. Some of the venous sinuses are shown in Figure 1-6.

Rigid sheets of dura mater extend into the cranial vault in several places, dividing it into compartments (Figure 1-6) and providing support for the brain, brain stem, and cerebellum. The largest of these dural sheets are called the *falx cerebri* and the *tentorium cerebelli.* The *falx cerebri* is a long, crescent-shaped band of dura mater that protrudes downward along the

midline of the skull from front to back, dividing the cranial vault into two side-by-side compartments. The *tentorium cerebelli* is a dome-shaped sheet of dura mater protruding forward horizontally from the back of the cranial vault, creating two compartments, one above the other. The brain occupies the upper compartment, and the cerebellum occupies the lower one.

The *arachnoid* is a cobweb-like sheet of tissue sandwiched between the dura mater and the pia mater. The arachnoid contains no blood vessels and does not conform closely to the con-

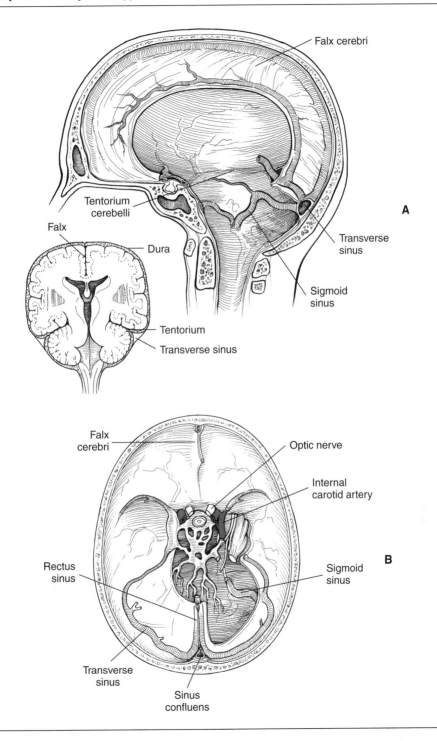

Figure 1-6 ■ A, Dural projections. B, Major venous sinuses. The venous sinuses are cavities between sheets of dura mater into which arterial blood passes on its way back to the heart.

> Ordinarily there is no space on either side of the dura mater, but in some pathology fluid may accumulate between the dura mater and the skull or between the dura mater and the arachnoid. The most frequent source of such accumulation is bleeding from the blood vessels on the surface of the dura mater.

tours of the underlying tissues, creating a space (the *subarachnoid space)* between the arachnoid and the pia mater. The subarachnoid space is filled with *cerebrospinal fluid* (CSF), a clear, colorless fluid that cushions and protects the central nervous system against trauma, provides a pathway for metabolic and nutritional compounds to reach the central nervous system, and (perhaps) provides a medium for transport of waste products away from the central nervous system. At the base of the brain there are several large spaces between the arachnoid and the pia mater. These spaces are filled with CSF (like the rest of the subarachnoid space) and are called *subarachnoid cisterns.*

> *Arachnoid* comes from the Greek *arachne,* which means *spider* or *cobweb. Cistern* is a generic name for cavities or spaces for the storage of fluids.

The arachnoid protrudes into the venous sinuses at many places. These protrusions are called *arachnoid villi* (Figure 1-5). The arachnoid villi provide sites at which excess cerebrospinal fluid is absorbed and removed from the subarachnoid space.

The pia mater is a fragile membrane that adheres tightly to the brain's surface, following the contours of the brain. On the outer surface of the pia mater, in the space between the pia mater and the arachnoid, are many veins and arteries. Numerous blood vessels cross the space between the pia mater and the arachnoid, and the pia mater is connected to the arachnoid by thin filaments of tissue.

> *Pia* is from a Latin word meaning *tender* (appropriate here because the pia mater is a fragile membrane, easily torn or cut).

GENERAL CONCEPTS 1-1

- *Neurons* (nerve cells) are the basic units of the nervous system.
- Neurons receive input via *dendrites* and transmit output via *axons.*
- *Nerve fiber tracts* form the white matter in the nervous system. They are made up of bundled axons and are white because the myelin covering of the axons is white.
- The human *central nervous system* consists of the *brain, brain stem, cerebellum,* and *spinal cord.* It is enclosed within the *skull* and *vertebrae.*
- The *peripheral nervous system* lies outside the skull and vertebrae. It consists of *cranial nerves* and *spinal nerves.*
- Three membranes surround the human central nervous system. They are called *meninges.* The *dura mater* is the outer membrane, the *arachnoid* is the middle membrane, and the *pia mater* is the inner membrane.
- Rigid sheets of dura mater divide the skull into compartments. Two important dural partitions are the *falx cerebri,* which crosses front to back high on the midline of the cranial vault, and the *tentorium cerebelli,* which crosses transversely above the cerebellum and below the posterior base of the brain.
- *Cerebrospinal fluid* (CSF), a clear, colorless fluid, surrounds the human central nervous system and fills the subarachnoid space.

Structure of the Central Nervous System

The central nervous system is shaped somewhat like a tree. The spinal cord forms the trunk. Above the spinal cord the central nervous system broadens gradually into the canopy-like top formed by the brain hemispheres. As the central nervous system progresses upward from the spinal cord to the brain hemispheres, structures progress from phylogenetically more primitive to phylogenetically more advanced.

For descriptive purposes the central nervous system is divided into five segments. They are the *spinal cord,* situated in the torso; the *brain stem,* perched atop the spinal cord; the *cerebellum,* which reposes behind the brain stem and below the brain hemispheres; the *diencephalon,* which is buried deep within the brain hemispheres; and the *cerebrum,* represented by the brain hemispheres, ensconced at the top. Neuroanatomists often lump the cerebrum and diencephalon together and call the lump the *brain.*

Brain The brain is the largest member of the central nervous system family. It is a gelatinous mass of nerve cells and supportive tissue floating in cerebrospinal fluid. An average human brain weighs about 3 pounds and is about three-fourths water. Because of its great water content, the brain is soft and mushy. If a human brain is removed from its skull, its supporting membranes, and its flotation system, it slowly collapses into a shapeless lump.

The one-fourth of the brain that is not water is made up of glial cells, neurons, and connective tissue. Glial cells support and separate nerve fiber tracts. Glial cells are 5 to 10 times more numerous than neurons and account for about half of the brain's solid mass. Even so, the brain contains more than 10 billion neurons (which means 50 billion to 100 billion glial cells). The brain is a big spender. It contains only about 2% of total body mass, but receives 20% of cardiac output and consumes 25% of the oxygen used by the body. The brain is not thrifty. It has no metabolic or oxygen reserves and is completely dependent on a constant supply of oxygen and nutrients. If the brain's blood supply is cut off for more than about 10 seconds the brain's owner loses consciousness, and after about 20 seconds the brain's electrical activity stops. If blood supply to the brain is interrupted for more than 2 or 3 minutes, permanent brain damage is almost certain.

Cerebrum The cerebrum contains about three-fourths of the nervous system's mass. The cerebrum is divided into two halves, or *hemispheres,* by a deep fissure (the *longitudinal cerebral fissure).* The longitudinal cerebral fissure sometimes is called the *interhemispheric fissure* or the *superior longitudinal fissure.* (It seems to be a rule that the more prominent a fissure is, the more names it gets.) The *falx cerebri* lies within the longitudinal cerebral fissure for most of the fissure's length.

The surface of the hemispheres is covered by a layer of *cortex,* which is pink and rich in nerve cells and blood vessels. The cortex is crisscrossed by a network of convolutions, making the brain look something like the surface of a pecan. The convolutions (ridges) are called *gyri,* and the depressions (valleys) are called *sulci.* Very deep sulci sometimes are called *fissures.*

Gyrus (singular for *gyri*) is from a Greek word meaning *circle. Sulcus* (singular for *sulci*) is from a Latin word meaning *furrow* or *ditch.*

Two prominent fissures appear on the lateral surface of each brain hemisphere. One courses down the lateral surface of each hemisphere, dividing the cortical surface into roughly equal anterior and posterior regions (Figure 1-7). This fissure is called the *central fissure, fissure of Rolando,* or the *central sulcus.* The other prominent fissure traverses the lateral surface of each hemisphere from front to back. This fissure is called the *lateral cerebral fissure* or *fissure of Sylvius* (Figure 1-7); sometimes it is called the *frontotemporoparietal fissure,* after the parts of the brain surface that surround it. The *calcarine fissure* is a less prominent groove inside the longitudinal cerebral fissure at the back of the brain. (Note that this short, less prominent fissure gets only one name.)

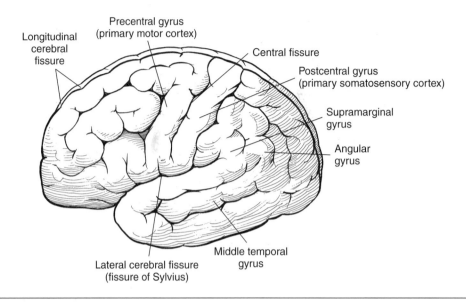

Longitudinal cerebral fissure

Precentral gyrus (primary motor cortex)

Central fissure

Postcentral gyrus (primary somatosensory cortex)

Supramarginal gyrus

Angular gyrus

Middle temporal gyrus

Lateral cerebral fissure (fissure of Sylvius)

Figure 1-7 ■ Prominent gyri and sulci on the surface of the human brain. The left brain hemisphere is shown. The gyri and sulci on the surface of the right hemisphere are essentially mirror images of those on the surface of the left hemisphere. There is considerable variability across brains in the location, shape, and prominence of the landmarks, sometimes making them difficult to identify.

The left and right hemispheres of the human brain are structurally similar, but not identical. Right-handed adults' left hemispheres tend to be slightly larger than their right hemispheres, and their left-hemisphere lateral fissure tends to be slightly longer than the one in their right hemisphere (von Bonin, 1962). However, right-handers' parietal lobes go the opposite direction—their right-hemisphere parietal lobe is larger than their left-hemisphere parietal lobe (Rubens, 1977). In spite of their structural similarity, the two hemispheres are in many respects functionally specialized, with different functions represented in each hemisphere.

Traditionally each hemisphere has been divided into four *lobes*—the *frontal lobe,* the *parietal lobe,* the *occipital lobe,* and the *temporal lobe*—named after the parts of the skull that cover them (Figure 1-8). The lobes are topographic conventions and do not reflect differences in the structure or functions of the brain; although dif-

ferent brain regions differ in structure and function, the structural and functional differences do not correspond to the boundaries of the lobes.

The *frontal lobes,* as their name implies, are at the front of the brain. The cortex in the frontal lobes accounts for about one-third of all the cortex in the brain. The lateral cerebral (Sylvian) fissure marks the lower boundary for each frontal lobe, and the central (Rolandic) fissure marks the posterior boundary.

The *parietal lobes* lie behind the central fissure and above the lateral fissure in each hemisphere. The posterior boundary of each parietal lobe is an imaginary line an inch or two forward from the *occipital pole* (farthest back point in the hemisphere).

The *occipital lobes* form the posterior part of each hemisphere. They extend from the imaginary line forming the posterior boundary of the parietal lobe to the longitudinal cerebral fissure at the occipital pole.

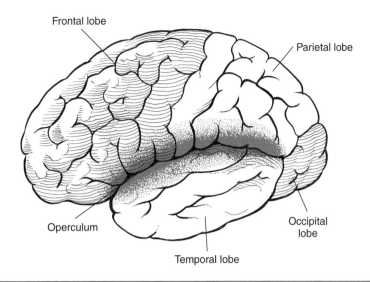

Figure 1-8 ■ **Lobes of the brain. Much of the occipital lobe is hidden from view within the longitudinal cerebral fissure. The lobes are arbitrary divisions and do not represent either architectural or functional differences.**

The *temporal lobe* makes up approximately the bottom one-third of each hemisphere. The lateral cerebral fissure marks its upper boundary, and its lower boundary is on the underside of the hemisphere, near the midline. Its posterior boundary is the imaginary line marking the anterior boundary of the occipital lobe.

The *insula* is a patch of cortex folded into the lateral cerebral fissure. It is hidden from view by folds of the frontal, parietal, and temporal lobes. The insula is sometimes called the *island of Reil*. The folds of cortex that conceal the insula are called the *operculum.*

> *Operculum* is from a Latin word meaning *cover* or *lid*—in this case the cortex that folds over and covers the insula.

Cerebral Ventricles Four fluid-filled cavities, called *cerebral ventricles,* lie deep within the brain. The ventricles are connected by narrow passageways and are filled with CSF. There are two crescent-shaped *lateral ventricles,* one in each hemisphere (Figure 1-9). They are the largest ventricles and are roughly symmetric. The *third ventricle* is an irregularly-shaped disk-like cavity standing on edge on the midline beneath the lateral ventricles. The *fourth ventricle* is a narrow tubular cavity extending downward through the brain stem, ending at an opening into the subarachnoid space (Figures 1-5, 1-9).

Each lateral ventricle is connected to the third ventricle by an *intraventricular foramen (foramen of Munro).* The third ventricle is connected to the fourth ventricle by the *cerebral aqueduct (aqueduct of Sylvius).* The ventricles

> As noted earlier, a foramen is an aperture or opening. In physiology an aqueduct is a tube or channel. Aqueducts are tubular; foramina are not.

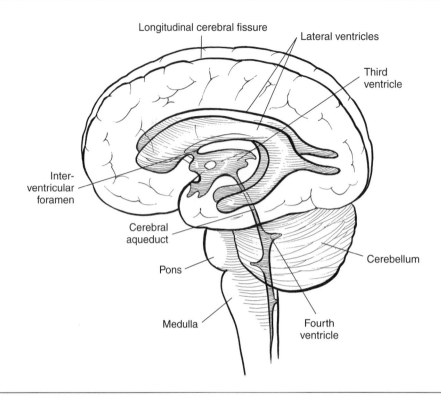

Figure 1-9 ■ **Cerebral ventricles. The ventricles form a fluid-filled space in the center of the brain and brain stem. One lateral ventricle is located deep within each brain hemisphere. The third and fourth ventricles are located on the midline. Most of the fourth ventricle is in the brain stem.**

hold about 15% of the cerebrospinal fluid in the central nervous system, and the subarachnoid space holds the remaining 85%.

The ventricles contain the *choroid plexus,* a spongy mass of vascular tissue that is the body's primary producer of cerebrospinal fluid. (A small amount of cerebrospinal fluid is produced by cells on the surface of the brain.) Cerebrospinal fluid circulates throughout the central nervous system. It flows from the lateral ventricles to the third ventricle through the intraventricular foramina and from the third ventricle to the fourth ventricle by way of the cerebral aqueduct (Figure 1-9). It passes from the fourth ventricle into the subarachnoid space through the *median aperture* (or *foramen of Magendi*) and the (two) *lateral apertures* (*foramina of*

Luschka). From there it circulates either upward around the brain hemispheres or downward around the spinal cord. Eventually it is resorbed into the blood through the arachnoid villi. In healthy adults the cerebrospinal fluid is completely replaced approximately every 8 hours.

Changes in the chemical composition of cerebrospinal fluid may indicate neurologic disease. For example, the presence of blood cells in the cerebrospinal fluid suggests bleeding into the subarachnoid space, and reduced glucose levels suggest bacterial infection (the bacteria consume the glucose).

Diencephalon The diencephalon is located deep in the substance of the brain, at the top of the brain stem. The *thalamus* and the *basal ganglia*—structures that play important roles in movement and sensation—are located in the diencephalon.

Diencephalon is from Greek, and means, literally, *through-brain. Thalamus* comes from a Latin word meaning *little nut.*

The *thalamus* consists of a pair of egg-shaped nuclei, one on each side of the third ventricle (Figure 1-10). The thalamus is a major relay center for motor information coming down from the motor cortex and for sensory information going up to the sensory cortex. The thalamus receives input from many sources (the cerebellum, the basal ganglia, other subcortical regions, and the brain stem) and its fibers project to much of the cortex.

Because of its major role as a relay center for information going to the cortex, the thalamus is thought to play a part in regulating the overall electrical activity of the cortex. Many sensory pathways synapse at the thalamus, and perhaps because of this, the thalamus plays an important part in maintaining consciousness, alertness, and attention.

The *basal ganglia* consist of several nuclei adjacent to the thalamus, deep in the substance of the brain (see Figure 1-10). The number of basal ganglia varies somewhat, depending on who is writing about them. Most writers include the *caudate nucleus,* the *putamen,* and the *globus pallidus* in the basal ganglia. Some add the *subthalamic nucleus* and the *substantia nigra.* To make things even more complicated, the putamen and the globus pallidus often are lumped together and named the *lenticular nucleus.* The lenticular nucleus (putamen and globus pallidus) is separated from the thalamus, and the caudate nucleus is separated from the lenticular nucleus by a band of nerve fibers called the internal capsule (described later).

The *subthalamic nucleus,* as the name implies, is located just beneath the thalamus, and the *substantia nigra* is just beneath the subthalamic nucleus. The precise functions of the subthalamic nucleus and the substantia nigra are unknown, although their numerous connections to the other basal ganglia suggest that they collaborate with them in important ways. The substantia nigra, as the name implies, is darkly colored.

Degeneration (and fading) of the substantia nigra is seen frequently in *Parkinson's disease.*

The basal ganglia receive input from multiple sites in the cortex (almost all in the frontal lobe) and send (or relay) information, via the thalamus, to the cortex. The basal ganglia control major muscle groups in the trunk and limbs to produce the postural adjustments necessary for dealing with shifts in body weight and to compensate for inertial forces accompanying movement. Damage in the basal ganglia causes a variety of problems with movement and sensation, depending on the location of the damage, but most are characterized by loss of voluntary movements and the appearance of involuntary movements.

Brain Stem The brain stem provides the communicative and structural link between the brain and the spinal cord, although structurally it is simply a continuation of the spinal cord. The *cranial nerves,* which serve the muscles and sensory receptors of the head, originate here. The brain stem also serves as the only pathway by which motor nerve fiber tracts from the brain reach the spinal cord and as the only pathway by which sensory nerve fiber tracts from the periphery reach the brain. For this reason, damage in the brain stem often has important effects on motor and sensory functions.

Brain stem structures regulate some aspects of breathing and heart rate and play a role in

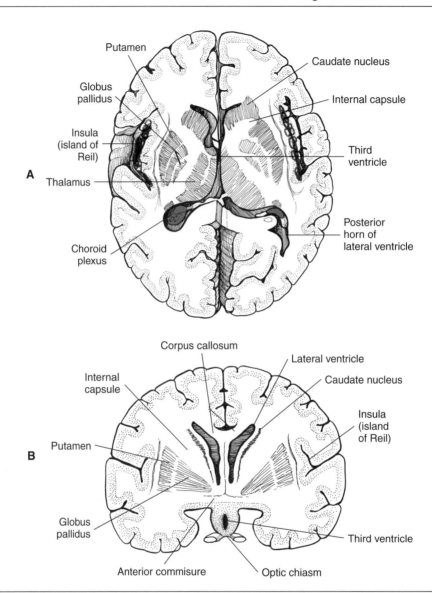

Figure 1-10 ■ **Basal ganglia and related structures. A, The brain has been cut on a horizontal plane at about the middle of the third ventricle. B, The brain has been cut on a vertical plane just anterior to the thalamus. The corpus callosum (B) is the major interhemispheric nerve fiber tract. It forms the roof of the lateral ventricles. The anterior commissure is a minor interhemispheric fiber tract. (See also Figure 1-13.)**

integrating complex motor activity. Some brain stem structures help to regulate a person's overall level of consciousness, primarily by means of the *reticular formation,* in the brain stem's central core. Because structures in and just above the brain stem control many of the body's vital functions (e.g., breathing, heart rate, and temperature regulation) brain stem injuries may have disastrous, even fatal, results.

For descriptive purposes anatomists divide the brain stem into three parts—the *midbrain* (upper), the *pons* (middle), and the *medulla* (lower). The *midbrain* (mesencephalon) connects the brain stem with the cerebral hemispheres (via the *cerebral peduncles*). Cranial nerves 3 and 4 (which connect to muscles that move the eyes) originate in the midbrain.

> The word *peduncle* comes from a Latin word meaning *foot. Pedestrian* and *pedal* are more common descendants of that Latin word. In neuroanatomy *peduncle* refers to various stem-like or stalk-like connecting structures in the brain.

The midbrain merges into the *pons* at the level of the cerebellum. The pons is identified easily by a prominent forward bulge in the brain stem. The pons contains several nuclei involved in hearing and balance, plus the nuclei of three cranial nerves (5, 6, and 7). Pontine damage typically produces paralysis of muscles responsible for moving the eyes horizontally, but large lesions in the anterior pons may cause *locked-in syndrome,* in which patients are conscious but cannot talk and are quadriplegic (all limbs are paralyzed). These patients may communicate only by eye blinks or by moving the eyes vertically.

The *medulla* is a tapered section of the brain stem connecting the pons and the spinal cord. The medulla contains the nuclei for five cranial nerves (8 through 12) as well as several nuclei concerned with balance and hearing. Nerve fiber tracts for volitional movement cross from one side of the central nervous system to the other in the medulla. The point at which they cross is called the point of *decussation.* Medullary damage typically causes combinations of vertigo (dizziness), paralysis of muscles in the throat and larynx, and various combinations of sensory loss in the limbs and sometimes the face.

Cerebellum The cerebellum lies just behind the pons and medulla (see Figure 1-9) and looks much like a miniature brain. It has two hemispheres, each with an outer layer of gray matter, the *cerebellar cortex.* The cerebellum does not initiate movements, but coordinates and modulates movements initiated elsewhere (primarily by the motor cortex). The cerebellum plays a major role in regulating the rate, range, direction, and force of movements. Cerebellar damage causes clumsy movements—a condition called ataxia.

Spinal Cord The spinal cord in a normal adult is about 18 inches long. It extends from the first cervical vertebra to the first lumbar vertebra, and from there it continues downward as a fine bundle of nerve fibers, which reminded Andreas Laurentius, a 17th-century German physiologist, of a horse's tail. Accordingly he named the bundle the *cauda equina* (Latin for *horse's tail*), an appellation that has continued to this day.

The spinal cord has an outer layer of *white matter* and a central core of *gray matter* (Figure 1-11). In cross-section, the gray matter resembles a butterfly. The white matter contains ascending and descending nerve fiber tracts. The gray matter contains motor and sensory neurons. The motor neurons are located primarily in the *anterior horns* of the central gray matter, and most sensory neurons are located in the *posterior horns* (Figure 1-11). The spinal cord is connected to muscles and sensory receptors by *spinal nerves.* Motor neurons in the anterior horns connect with muscles via *efferent spinal nerves,* and sensory receptors in the body's periphery connect to sensory neurons in the posterior horns via *afferent spinal nerves.*

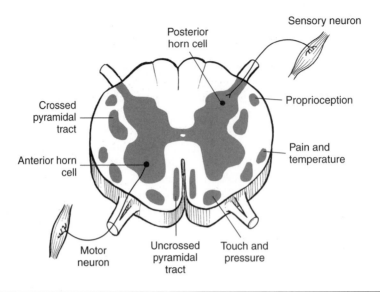

Figure 1-11 ■ **Cross-section of the human spinal cord showing motor and sensory fiber tracts. The posterior columns (which contain the posterior horn cells) primarily serve sensory functions, and the anterior columns (which contain the anterior horn cells) primarily serve motor functions.**

GENERAL CONCEPTS 1-2

- The human brain is divided into two *hemispheres,* which are structurally similar but functionally different.
- The brain is covered by a thin layer of gray matter called *cerebral cortex.* The cerebral cortex is rich in nerve cells and is crisscrossed by ridges (*gyri*) and grooves (*sulci*).
- Deep sulci are called *fissures.* Two prominent fissures on the human brain are the *central fissure* (fissure of Rolando) and the *lateral cerebral fissure* (fissure of Sylvius).
- The surface of each hemisphere traditionally is divided into four lobes—the *frontal* lobe, the *parietal* lobe, the *occipital* lobe, and the *temporal* lobe, named after the parts of the skull that overlie them.
- The *cerebral ventricles* are cavities within the brain, filled with CSF. There are two *lateral ventricles,* one *third ventricle,* and one *fourth ventricle.* They are interconnected by *foramina* (openings) and an *aqueduct* (tubular channel).

- The diencephalon contains the *thalamus* and *basal ganglia.* The thalamus and basal ganglia modulate, integrate, and regulate motor output and sensory input.
- The brain stem (*midbrain, pons,* and *medulla*) serves as a conduit for all motor output from the central nervous system to the peripheral nervous system and for all sensory input from the peripheral nervous system to the central nervous system.
- The *nuclei* of most cranial nerves are located in the brain stem, as are centers that control vital functions such as respiration and heart rate.
- The *cerebellum* is located behind the brain stem. It resembles a miniature brain and is responsible for controlling the rate, force, direction, and amplitude of volitional movements.
- Most spinal cord motor neurons (*anterior horn cells*) are located in the anterior horns of the spinal cord central gray matter. Most spinal cord sensory neurons (*posterior horn cells*) are located in the posterior horns of the spinal cord central gray matter.

Fiber Tracts in the Central Nervous System

Communication among parts of the central nervous system depends on bundles of nerve axons arranged into nerve fiber tracts. (As noted earlier, these tracts form the *white matter* of the nervous system.) Neuroanatomists have divided central nervous system nerve fiber tracts into three major categories—*projection fibers, commissural fibers,* and *association fibers.*

Projection fibers are the long-distance carriers of the central nervous system. They carry information from the brain to the brain stem and spinal cord or from peripheral sensory nerves to the brain via the spinal cord.

Projection fibers that carry command and control signals from the brain to muscles and glands are called *efferent (motor) projection fibers.* They originate at neurons in the motor and premotor cortex and progress down through the brain, converging to pass through the basal ganglia to the brain stem and spinal cord to synapse with cranial nerves and spinal nerves.

Projection fibers carrying sensory information from receptors in the periphery to the brain are called *afferent (sensory) projection fibers.* The sensory process begins in sensory receptor cells scattered throughout the peripheral nervous system. These receptor cells convey sensory information to the spinal cord or brain stem via peripheral sensory nerves, which synapse with neurons in the spinal cord and brain stem.

> I know of no great mnemonic for remembering *efferent* versus *afferent.* It may help to remember that in the alphabet *a* precedes *e* and that sensations (*a*fferent) often precede responses (*e*fferent).

As the axons of these spinal and cranial neurons travel upward through the spinal cord and brain stem they form a compact and dense band of fibers until they reach the level of the thalamus and the basal ganglia. As they pass between the thalamus and the basal ganglia the fiber tracts become known as the *internal capsule.* From the internal capsule they fan out to destinations in the cortex, primarily in the postcentral gyrus and other parts of the parietal lobe.

> The term *capsule,* as in *internal capsule,* is misleading. In ordinary use the word denotes enclosure or case. As used here it denotes a horizontal slice of the motor and sensory fibers passing between the brain and lower centers taken at the level of the thalamus and basal ganglia. The label *capsule* apparently comes from early dissections, wherein the dense white matter and membrane-like appearance of the nerve fibers, compared with the gray matter of the basal ganglia and thalamus, suggested a capsular structure.

Motor Pathways from the Brain to the Spinal Cord Several fiber tracts descend from the brain, midbrain, and brain stem, eventually synapsing with motor neurons at lower levels. The *corticospinal* tract begins in the cerebral cortex and connects with motor neurons in the spinal cord. These spinal motor neurons control muscles responsible for volitional movement of the trunk and limbs. The *corticobulbar tract* begins in the cerebral cortex and connects with motor neurons in the brain stem. These brain stem motor neurons are responsible for volitional movement of muscles of the head and neck. The *vestibulospinal tract* begins in the brain stem and connects with spinal-cord motor neurons that control muscles responsible for quick movements in response to sudden changes in body position such as occurs in loss of balance or falling. The *descending autonomic tract* begins at structures deep within the brain and connects with motor neurons in the brain stem and spinal cord. These motor neurons are responsible for modulating autonomic functions such as heart rate and blood pressure.

Sensory Pathways from the Spinal Cord to the Brain The sensory pathways in the spinal cord are complex and are the scourge of medical students who must learn them. The pathway for *pain and temperature* ascends in the lateral spinal cord to the thalamus and parietal lobe (see Figure 1-11). It is a crossed pathway, which crosses where the peripheral nerve enters the central nervous system. The pathway for *proprioception* (the ability to tell the position of the head and limbs without seeing them) and *stereognosis* (the ability to identify objects by touch) ascends through the dorsal (posterior) spinal cord to the cerebellum and the postcentral gyrus in the parietal lobe. This pathway is also a crossed pathway, but it ascends on the ipsilateral side of the spinal cord and crosses in the brain stem. The pathway for *light touch* ascends in the ventral (anterior) spinal cord to the brain stem and parietal lobe. This pathway contains both uncrossed fibers and fibers that cross at the brain stem.

> The complexity of spinal cord sensory pathways, although the bane of students who must learn them, is a blessing for neurologists who must deduce what is wrong with patients with sensory abnormalities. A neurologist often can identify the location (and sometimes the nature) of spinal cord abnormality by noting how pain and temperature sense, proprioception, and stereognosis are affected in various parts of the body.

Reflex Arc Some reflexive motor responses are accomplished at the level of the lower motor neuron. This reflexive activity is accomplished by the *reflex arc,* which permits rapid movements without the participation of higher neural systems. The reflex arc has five parts—a *sensory receptor,* an *afferent (sensory) neuron,* an *interneuron,* a *motor neuron,* and an *effector* (usually a muscle) (Figure 1-12). Stimulation of the sensory receptor generates an electrical sig-

nal, which is transmitted by the afferent neuron to the interneuron in the posterior column of the spinal cord. The interneuron transmits the impulse to the motor neuron in the anterior column of the spinal cord. The motor neuron activates a muscle or gland. Because they are executed at the level of the spinal cord, reflexes permit very quick but indiscriminate responses to stimulation. Consequently, many of these reflexes serve protective functions (e.g., the sneeze, cough, and eye-blink reflexes).

Commissures Commissural fiber tracts (commissures) are the regional carriers of the central nervous system. They provide communicative links between the brain hemispheres. There are three commissures—the *corpus callosum,* the *anterior commissure,* and the *posterior commissure* (Figure 1-13).

The *corpus callosum* is by far the largest and most important commissure. Besides providing the primary pathway for interhemispheric communication, it provides the major structural bridge between the hemispheres and forms much of the roof of the lateral ventricles. The corpus callosum is crescent-shaped, with the open side of the crescent facing down. The anterior third of the corpus callosum is called the *genu,* the central third is called the *rostrum* or *body,* and the posterior third is called the *splenium.* Nerve fibers crossing through the corpus callosum are spatially arranged to minimize their length; fibers crossing through the genu (the front portion) connect cortical regions of the anterior frontal lobes, fibers crossing through the rostrum (the middle) connect cortical regions of the posterior frontal and the anterior parietal lobes, and fibers crossing through the splenium (the back portion) connect cortical regions of the posterior parietal and occipital lobes. Damage to the corpus callosum interrupts communication between the hemispheres, giving rise to a variety of signs and symptoms, depending on the location of the damage.

The *anterior commissure* crosses the midline deep within the brain near the thalamus. The *posterior commissure* crosses just below the

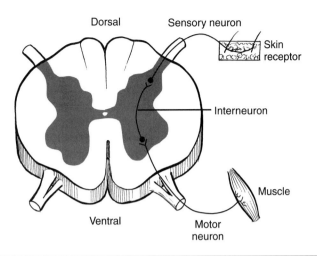

Figure 1-12 ■ **Reflex arc. Stimulation of a sensory nerve is transmitted to a motor nerve via an interneuron, making possible rapid responses to stimuli (usually painful ones) without participation of higher centers in the nervous system.**

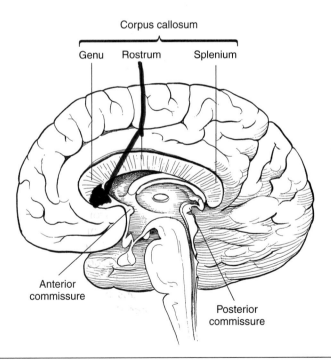

Figure 1-13 ■ **Interhemispheric fiber tracts (commissures) of the human brain. The brain hemispheres have been cut apart at the superior longitudinal fissure, and the cut ends of nerve fibers making up the corpus callosum, anterior commissure, and posterior commissure are visible.**

posterior end of the corpus callosum. The anterior and posterior commissures are much smaller than the corpus callosum, and their importance for interhemispheric communication is debated. Given that the anterior commissure and the posterior commissure together are about 1/100th the size of the corpus callosum, it is very likely that the corpus callosum is the major player in interhemispheric communication.

Association Fibers Association fibers are the local carriers in the central nervous system. They connect cortical areas within a hemisphere. If the cortical areas are close together (in the same lobe) the association fibers connecting them are called simply *association fibers*. If the cortical areas are farther apart (in different lobes) the association fibers connecting them get a shorter but harder-to-remember name. The name is *fasciculus,* the plural of which is *fasciculi.* Fasciculi are bundles of nerve fibers con-

> *Fasciculus* comes from a Latin word for *bundle. Fascist* comes from that same word.

necting nonadjacent regions within a hemisphere. However, they never cross the midline. If they did, they would be called commissures.

Neuroanatomists have described three major fasciculi in the human brain—the *uncinate fasciculus,* the *cingulum,* and the *arcuate fasciculus* (Figure 1-14). The uncinate fasciculus is a direct pathway connecting the inferior frontal lobe with the anterior temporal lobe in each hemisphere. The cingulum runs along the top of the corpus callosum and connects deep regions of the frontal and parietal lobes with deep regions of the temporal lobe and midbrain in each hemisphere. The uncinate fasciculus and the cingulum apparently play no major part in speech and language. This is not the case for the arcuate fasciculus, sometimes called the *superior longitudinal fasciculus* (Figure 1-14). It is a crescent-shaped fiber tract that connects posterior and central regions of the temporal lobe in each hemisphere with posterior and inferior regions of the frontal lobe. From its origin in the temporal lobe it sweeps around the back of the lateral fissure, about an inch below the cortex. Then it curves forward and downward to the

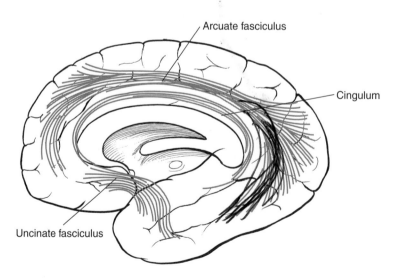

Arcuate fasciculus

Cingulum

Uncinate fasciculus

Figure 1-14 ▪ **Major fasciculi in the human brain. The arcuate fasciculus is believed to play an important part in many speech and language processes.**

frontal lobe. As we shall see, the arcuate fasciculus plays a central role in some models of how the brain deals with language.

GENERAL CONCEPTS 1-3

- *Projection fiber tracts* carry information from motor neurons in the brain to neurons in the brain stem or spinal cord (*efferent projection fibers*) or from sensory neurons in the peripheral nervous system to the brain (*afferent projection fibers*).
- The *corticospinal tract* connects motor neurons in the brain cortex with motor neurons in the spinal cord.
- The *corticobulbar tract* connects motor neurons in the brain cortex with motor neurons in the brain stem.
- Sensory pathways in the spinal cord are complex. They ascend in various regions of the spinal cord; some cross, some do not cross, and those that cross do so at various levels in the spinal cord.
- Some protective reflexes (e.g., sneeze, eye blink) are accomplished within the spinal cord, by *reflex arcs.*
- The *internal capsule* is a segment of efferent and afferent projection fiber tracts at the level of the thalamus and basal ganglia.
- *Commissural fiber tracts* cross between the brain hemispheres. The *corpus callosum* is the primary commissural fiber tract. The *anterior commissure* and the *posterior commissure* are minor ones.
- *Association fiber tracts* connect regions within a brain hemisphere. Shorter tracts (within a lobe) are called *association fibers.* Longer tracts (connecting regions in different lobes) are called *fasciculi.*
- The *arcuate fasciculus* connects regions in the temporal lobes with regions in the frontal lobes. It is important for some neurophysiologic explanations of language.

Blood Supply to the Brain

As mentioned previously, the brain is a major consumer of oxygen and glucose, both of which get to the brain by way of the blood. At any given time, about 25% of all the blood in the body is in the brain. Because the brain is such a massive consumer of oxygen and glucose, and because it has no significant reserves, cutting off the brain's blood supply usually has catastrophic consequences. Consequently, it is not surprising that interrupted blood supply is a common cause of brain injury.

The mechanical process of getting blood to the brain begins at the heart, which provides the pumping pressure to push the blood through the arteries. The heart pumps oxygenated blood into the *aorta,* the major artery from the heart. From the aorta the blood is distributed to two *subclavian arteries*—one on each side of the body. Each subclavian artery then branches off into a *common carotid artery.* The common carotid arteries ascend into the neck where they each divide into an *internal carotid artery* and an *external carotid artery.* (This is going to be complicated. Figure 1-15 may help.) The external carotid artery heads off for the face, and we can ignore it from here on. The internal carotid arteries proceed upward toward the brain on each side of the neck, near the surface, just behind the angle of the jaw. The carotid arteries eventually connect to opposite sides of the *circle of Willis.*

> If you place your open hand on your neck under the angle of your jaw, you should feel a relatively strong pulse at about your middle or ring finger. That pulse comes from your internal carotid artery.

Now let's return to the subclavian arteries and follow them to where each branches into a *vertebral artery* (one on each side). The vertebral arteries follow the anterior surface of the medulla upward until they join together (*anastomose*) at the base of the pons to form the *basilar artery.* The basilar artery continues upward along the midline of the pons and even-

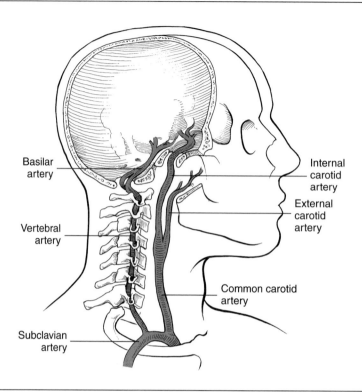

Figure 1-15 ■ **How blood gets to the brain. The subclavian arteries branch off from the aorta, which is the major artery from the heart. The common carotid arteries branch off from the subclavian arteries. Each common carotid artery eventually divides into an external and an internal carotid artery. The external carotid arteries supply blood to the face, and the internal carotid arteries supply the central regions of the brain. The vertebral arteries also branch off the subclavian artery. They supply posterior regions of the brain via the basilar artery.**

tually connects into the posterior part of the *circle of Willis.*

The circle of Willis is a heptagonal set of arteries centered at the base of the brain (Figure 1-16). Three pairs of cerebral arteries branch upward from the circle of Willis—two *anterior cerebral arteries,* two *middle cerebral arteries,* and two *posterior cerebral arteries.* (One artery of each pair is in each hemisphere; Figure 1-17.) The anterior cerebral arteries supply the upper and anterior regions of the frontal lobes and the corpus callosum. The middle cerebral arteries have fan-shaped distributions and supply most of the lateral surfaces of the brain hemispheres,

plus the thalamus and basal ganglia. The posterior cerebral arteries supply blood to the occipital lobes and the lower parts of the temporal lobe.

As mentioned earlier, the internal carotid arteries and the basilar artery all connect to the underside of the circle of Willis. For this reason the circle of Willis provides a common pathway connecting the three major feeder arteries (the two carotid arteries and the basilar artery) to the six cerebral arteries. Because the cerebral arteries all have access, via the circle of Willis, to the blood supplied by each of the feeder arteries, if one feeder artery is blocked, the other two feeders still may provide enough blood to main-

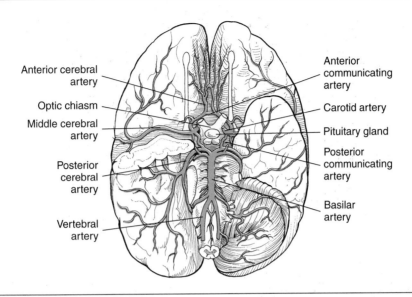

Figure 1-16 ■ **How blood is distributed to the brain by the circle of Willis. Occlusions below the circle of Willis may not cause as much damage as occlusions above the circle of Willis because the circle of Willis provides a common pathway for blood coming from the three major feeder arteries (two internal carotid arteries and the basilar artery) to the cerebral arteries that branch off the top of the circle of Willis.**

tain blood supply to the cerebral arteries. However, this safety valve function works only when blockage is *below* the circle of Willis. Occlusion of a cerebral artery above the circle of Willis almost inevitably causes brain damage because the cerebral arteries share no common source once they leave the circle of Willis.

The compensation provided by the circle of Willis may be less than one might expect because occlusion of a feeder artery is most common in patients with generalized vascular disease, which compromises blood flow through the entire arterial system. For these patients collateral flow from the other feeder arteries also is likely to be compromised by the vascular disease. Furthermore, the cerebral arteries and the arteries in the circle of Willis may themselves be narrowed or occluded by the disease.

The amount of brain tissue affected by occlusion of a cerebral artery depends on where in the artery the occlusion occurs. Occlusions in the trunk or a main branch of a cerebral artery affect large regions of the brain, whereas occlusions in peripheral branches affect smaller regions. Furthermore, the distributions of the cerebral arteries overlap slightly at their boundaries so that occlusions at the periphery of an artery's distribution may not cause as much brain damage as one might expect because of collateral blood supply from an adjacent artery. These areas of overlapping blood supply are called *watershed* areas (Figure 1-17).

GENERAL CONCEPTS 1-4

- Two *vertebral arteries* and two *internal carotid arteries* supply blood to the brain. The *basilar artery* connects the vertebral arteries to the *circle of Willis.*
- The circle of Willis is a ring-shaped set of arter-

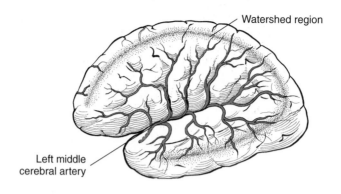

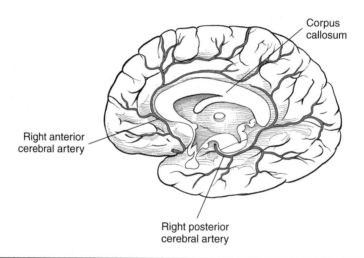

Figure 1-17 ■ **Distributions of the cerebral arteries. The watershed region is where the distributions of the cerebral arteries overlap. Occlusions in the watershed region may have relatively small effects on cerebral functions because of collateral circulation from the neighboring artery.**

ies at the base of the brain. It connects the basilar artery and the carotid arteries to the *cerebral arteries,* which supply blood to the brain hemispheres.

- The circle of Willis may help to mitigate the effects of occlusion of a feeder artery below the circle of Willis by making it possible for blood supplied by other feeder arteries to reach the cerebral arteries.
- Three pairs of cerebral arteries supply blood to the brain hemispheres. The *anterior cerebral artery* supplies the upper and anterior frontal lobes and the anterior corpus callosum. The *middle cerebral artery* supplies the posterior frontal lobe, most of the parietal and temporal lobes, plus the thalamus and basal ganglia. The *posterior cerebral artery* supplies the occipital lobe and the inferior temporal lobe.
- Occlusions of the main branch of a cerebral artery are more serious than occlusions in *watershed regions* (where the distributions of the cerebral arteries overlap).

Now we will leave the central nervous system and explore the *peripheral nervous system,* which connects the central nervous system to the world outside.

Peripheral Nervous System

The peripheral nervous system serves as a conduit for sensory information from the body's sensory receptors to the central nervous system and for transmission of motor commands from the central nervous system to the muscles. Its major components are the *cranial nerves* and the *spinal nerves.*

Cranial Nerves The *cranial nerves* control muscles in the head and neck and carry sensory information from sensory receptors in the head and neck to the central nervous system. Most cranial nerves synapse with the central nervous system in the midbrain, pons, and medulla.

> Cranial nerves 1 (olfactory) and 2 (optic) are sensory tracts that project directly into the brain above the level of the brain stem. Therefore they probably ought to be considered parts of the central nervous system. However, they were called cranial nerves in the 19th century, and the custom persists.

Twelve cranial nerves lie on each side of the central nervous system midline. Each cranial nerve controls muscle groups on its side of the midline or receives sensory input from receptors on its side of the midline. Traditionally the 12 paired cranial nerves are labeled, from top to bottom, with the Roman numerals I through XII. This labeling system apparently began with Galen, a Roman physician who died about 200 AD. Contemporary writers (including this one) sometimes substitute Arabic numerals for Roman numerals.

Each cranial nerve has a name. Some are descriptive—such as *optic* (1), *olfactory* (2), and *facial* (7)—and some are cryptic—such as *trigeminal* (5) and *vagus* (10). Some serve only motor functions (3, 4, 6, 11, 12), some serve only sensory functions (1, 2, 8), and the rest serve both motor and sensory functions. The cranial nerves, their names, their motor or sensory functions, and where they connect with the central nervous system are summarized in Table 1-1. Several mnemonic devices (most scatologic) have been devised by students who must memorize the cranial nerves and their names. The following socially acceptable but not very literary mnemonic is passed along:

On old Olympus's towering tops,
a Finn and German vend at hops.

Calling the accessory nerve the *spinal accessory* nerve makes the mnemonic slightly more literary:

On old Olympus's towering tops,
a Finn and German vend some hops.

Table 1-1 shows how these mnemonic devices work.

Spinal Nerves The *spinal nerves* provide motor input to and gather sensory information from viscera, blood vessels, glands, and muscles below the level of the head and neck. Each spinal nerve synapses with neurons in the spinal cord. There are 31 pairs of spinal nerves, divided into five categories (from top to bottom)—*cervical* (8 pairs), *thoracic* (12 pairs), *lumbar* (5 pairs), *sacral* (5 pairs), and *coccygeal* (1 pair; Figure 1-18). Each spinal nerve has a posterior *dorsal root* (sensory) and an anterior *ventral root* (motor), arising from the posterior and anterior columns of the spinal cord respectively (see page 17). For this reason, spinal sensory neurons are called posterior horn cells and spinal motor neurons are called *anterior horn cells.* The anterior and posterior spinal columns sometimes are called the anterior and posterior *horns.*

> The names of the cranial and spinal nerves often are abbreviated. *C3* stands for the third cervical nerve, *T4* for the fourth thoracic nerve, and so on (Figure 1-18).

T A B L E 1 - 1				
The cranial nerves				
Nerve	**Name**	**Type***	**Function**	**Mnemonic**
1	Olfactory	S	Smell, taste	On
2	Optic	S	Vision	old
3	Oculomotor	M	Eye and eyelid movement	Olympus's
4	Trochlear	M	Eye movement	towering
5	Trigeminal	S,M	Sensation from face; motor to masseters, palate, pharynx	tops,
6	Abducens	M	Eye movement	a
7	Facial	S,M	Sensation from anterior tongue; motor to facial muscles	Finn
8	Vestibular	S	Balance, hearing	and
9	Glossopharyngeal	S,M	Sensation from posterior tongue, soft palate, pharynx; motor to pharynx	German
10	Vagus	S,M	Motor to larynx, pharynx, viscera; sensation from viscera	vend
11	Accessory (spinal accessory)	M	Motor to larynx, chest, shoulder	at (some)
12	Hypoglossal	M	Motor to tongue	hops.

*S, sensory; M, motor.

GENERAL CONCEPTS 1-5

- Cranial nerves and spinal nerves are parts of the *peripheral nervous system.*
- Cranial nerves serve structures in the head and neck. Spinal nerves serve structures in the torso and limbs.
- Most cranial nerves arise from nuclei in the brain stem. Spinal nerves arise from nerve cell bodies in the central gray matter of the spinal cord. Each spinal nerve has an *anterior motor* (efferent) branch and a *posterior sensory* (afferent) branch.

Central Nervous System Functional Anatomy

Functional Anatomy of the Cerebral Cortex Neuroanatomists typically divide the cortex of the human brain into two major functional categories—*primary cortex* and *associa-*

tion cortex. Primary cortex is responsible for specific motor or sensory functions. Association cortex is responsible for combining, refining, interpreting, and elaborating crude sensory information coming from primary cortical sensory areas and for organizing and planning action sequences for the primary motor cortex. Association cortex interprets sensory information and plans motor activity.

Primary Cortex The first region of primary cortex to be identified according to its functional responsibility was the *primary motor cortex.* It is a narrow strip of cortex located immediately in front of the central fissure in each hemisphere, corresponding roughly to the area of the precentral gyrus. The nerve cells in the primary motor cortex are responsible for initiating and controlling voluntary and precise skilled movements of skeletal muscles *contralateral* to (on the opposite side of the body from) the primary motor cortex. The left-hemisphere primary motor cortex controls muscles on the right side of the body and vice versa.

The *primary somatosensory cortex* lies just behind the central fissure in each hemisphere, corresponding roughly to the area of the post-central gyrus. The primary somatosensory cortex is responsible for *somesthetic* (skin, muscle, joint, and tendon) sensation from the contralateral side of the body. (Gross perception of pain, temperature, and light touch are not the exclusive responsibility of this strip of cortex. Lower structures in the brain also mediate these perceptions.)

> Some contemporary neurophysiologists (such as Nolte, 1993) combine the motor and somatosensory cortex into a single *sensorimotor cortex,* apparently to illustrate the important role somatosensory information plays in regulation and control of movement. For simplicity's sake I have elected to remain with the traditional division of precentral and postcentral cortex. However, the reader should keep in mind that the somatosensory cortex plays an important role in regulating and controlling almost all volitional movement.

The *primary auditory cortex* is located on the upper surface of the temporal lobe, on the lower lip of the lateral fissure, corresponding roughly to the transverse temporal gyrus (better known as the *gyrus of Heschl*). The auditory cortex in each hemisphere receives input from both ears, and together they are responsible for hearing.

The *primary visual cortex* is located in the occipital lobe, surrounding the calcarine fissure, and is responsible for vision. Each visual cortex receives half the visual input from each eye.

The *primary olfactory cortex* is located in the posterior inferior frontal lobe and insula and is responsible for our sense of smell. Figure 1-19 shows the location of these functional areas.

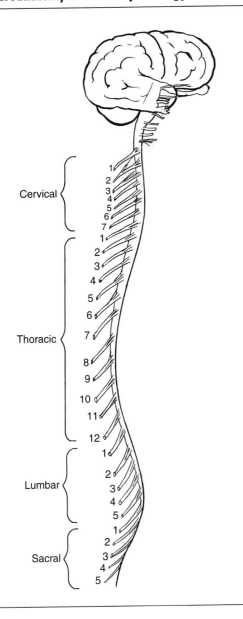

Figure 1-18 ▪ Human central nervous system, showing the vertical location of cranial and spinal nerves and the division of spinal nerves into cervical, thoracic, lumbar, and sacral nerves.

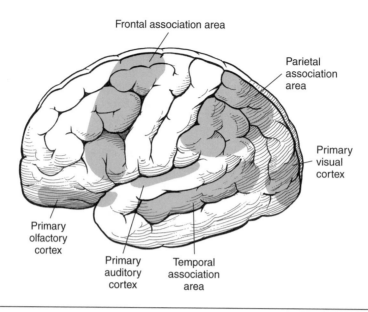

Figure 1-19 ■ Association areas and primary auditory, visual, and olfactory cortex of the human brain. The association areas, like the lobes, represent arbitrary divisions. No differences in brain architecture mark these divisions, and their size and location vary, depending on who is drawing the picture. The right hemisphere contains mirror-image representations of these cortical areas.

The regions of primary cortex are organized so that sensation from the surface of the body, input from the visual fields, or auditory frequencies are projected onto their respective cortical regions in topographic arrays, with point-to-point connections between the cortex and tactile receptors in the skin, visual receptors in the eyes, and auditory receptors in the cochlea. (The olfactory cortex seems not to be arranged topographically.)

Stimulating primary motor cortex produces gross unrefined movements of major muscle groups, sometimes associated with primitive movement sequences such as licking, chewing, or swallowing. Stimulating primary somatosensory cortex produces gross unrefined sensations such as numbness, tingling, or electric-shock–like sensations. Stimulating the olfactory cortex typically produces sensations of peculiar odors and tastes. Stimulating the visual cortex typically produces an experience of light flashes. Stimulating the auditory cortex typically pro-

duces buzzing or roaring sensations. Damage to primary motor or sensory cortex impairs the motor or sensory functions previously served by the destroyed cortex.

Association Cortex Several association areas in the human brain have been described in the literature, of which four are most relevant to neurogenic communication disorders (see Figure 1-19).

1. The *frontal association cortex* is a strip of cortex just in front of the primary motor cortex. Sometimes the frontal association cortex is called the *premotor cortex.* It plays an important part in planning and initiating complex volitional movements.

2. The *parietal association cortex* participates in processing of tactile information and seems to be responsible for position sense, visuospatial processing, and awareness of extrapersonal space.

3. The *temporal association cortex* is important for discriminating and processing auditory

information and for many language-related processes.

4. The *parieto-occipital association cortex* is important for discriminating and processing visual information. The parieto-occipital association cortex participates in many of the precise visual processes involved in reading.

Stimulation of association cortex usually causes combinations of sensory phenomena (usually unpleasant) and primitive movements of muscle groups (e.g., eye closure, twisting of the body, or limb contraction). Destruction of association cortex usually does not cause specific motor or sensory deficits but creates impaired discrimination, recognition, or comprehension of categories of stimuli, depending on which region of association cortex has been destroyed. For example, destruction of temporal association cortex may prevent a person from recognizing the significance of sounds, although the person's perception of the sounds is intact.

Functional Anatomy of the Lobes of the Brain

Frontal Lobes The frontal lobes are intimately involved in planning and executing volitional behavior. The primary motor cortex in the posterior frontal lobes is responsible for initiating complex volitional movements. The premotor cortex, just in front of the primary motor cortex and sometimes called the *frontal association area*, is responsible for planning sequential volitional movements (see Figure 1-19). The anterior frontal lobes regulate general activity levels and play a role in formulating intentions, plans, and patterns for volitional behavior.

Damage to the primary motor cortex causes weakness or paralysis of muscle groups on the contralateral side of the body. Damage to the premotor cortex causes disruption of complex volitional movement sequences. Damage to the anterior frontal lobes may cause a variety of impairments, including disturbed affect, attentional impairments, and difficulties initiating and maintaining behavior. Whether the left and right anterior frontal lobes serve different cognitive

or behavioral functions is not well understood, in part because unilateral damage to otherwise normal frontal lobes is relatively rare (Gainotti, 1991). Consequently, the two frontal lobes usually are lumped together when anterior frontal lobe syndromes are described.

Parietal Lobes The parietal lobes are important for perception, integration, and mediation of touch, body awareness, and visuospatial information. The primary sensory cortex, responsible for somesthetic sensation, forms the anterior margin of the parietal lobe, and the strip of cortex just behind it appears to be important for interpretation of somesthetic sensory information. Damage in this strip of cortex sometimes causes a (contralateral) phenomenon called *tactile agnosia* (or *astereognosis*), in which a person is unable to recognize objects by touch, despite intact tactile perception. Damage in the association cortex in either parietal lobe typically disturbs position sense and causes various visuospatial impairments, in which the patient has difficulty drawing or copying geometric designs, discriminating complex visual stimuli, and appreciating spatial relationships, including attention to locations in extrapersonal space.

Temporal Lobes The temporal lobes are important for perception and processing of auditory stimuli. The primary auditory cortices are located in the upper temporal lobes, and auditory and auditory-visual association areas are found in the mid-temporal and posterior temporal regions, respectively. The anterior temporal lobes appear to be important in pitch discrimination and for separating an auditory signal from a noise background, as when one engages in conversation at a cocktail party. The association cortex in the left temporal lobe is important for comprehension of verbal material, both spoken and written, and for language processes involving semantics and syntax. The right temporal lobe appears to be important for interpretation of complex nonverbal visual stimuli and for recognition and comprehension of nonverbal sounds, including receptive components of music. Damage in temporal association cortex sometimes causes *audi-*

tory agnosia (inability to recognize familiar sounds, although hearing is intact).

Occipital Lobes The occipital lobes contain the primary visual cortex and the visual association areas. Destruction of visual cortex in either hemisphere causes blindness in regions of the contralateral visual fields. Damage in association cortex adjacent to the visual cortex in either hemisphere typically causes *visual agnosia* (inability to recognize visually-presented familiar stimuli, although visual perception is adequate) and distorted visual perceptions. Damage in visual association cortex in the left hemisphere usually causes severe reading impairment. Bilateral destruction of the visual cortex results in a phenomenon called *cortical blindness.* Patients who are cortically blind have extreme difficulty discriminating visual shapes and patterns, but they remain sensitive to light and dark. In some cases perception of simple visual stimuli may be preserved, although the patient usually has difficulty reporting them or incorporating them into other mental activity.

GENERAL CONCEPTS 1-6

- The primary olfactory cortex is in the inferior frontal lobes.
- The *primary motor cortex* of each hemisphere is responsible for skilled volitional movement of *contralateral* muscle groups. Neurons in the left motor cortex connect with muscles on the right side of the body and vice versa.
- The *premotor cortex,* just in front of the primary motor cortex in each hemisphere, is a strip of association cortex responsible for organizing and planning complex volitional movements.
- The *primary sensory cortex* in the anterior parietal lobe of each brain hemisphere is responsible for contralateral skin, muscle, joint, and tendon sensation.
- The *parietal association cortex* is responsible for position sense and for interpreting tactile and visuospatial information.
- The *primary auditory cortices* are in the upper temporal lobes. The *temporal associa-*

tion cortices are responsible for interpreting auditory information.

- Association cortex in the left temporal lobe is responsible for many language-related processes.
- Association cortex in the right temporal lobe is responsible for interpreting nonverbal auditory information, including receptive aspects of music.
- The *primary visual cortex* is in the posterior occipital lobe. The *parieto-occipital region* is responsible for interpreting complex visual stimuli. The left hemisphere parieto-occipital region is important for visual processes involved in reading.

Functional Anatomy of the Motor System
Normal motor performance depends on the integrated activity of three systems—the pyramidal system, the vestibular-reticular system, and the extrapyramidal system. Damage within any one system produces characteristic impairment of motor performance that often points to the location and sometimes to the nature of the damage.

Pyramidal System The pyramidal system is responsible for initiating most, if not all, skilled volitional movement. The pyramidal system originates at pyramidal neurons in the cerebral cortex. (They are called pyramidal neurons because they have pyramidal shapes.) The axons of the pyramidal neurons converge into a dense band of nerve fibers that descends through the internal capsule to neurons in the brain stem and spinal cord.

The pyramidal system is a *direct system. Direct* means that the only synapses in the pyramidal system are where cortical neurons connect with neurons in the brain stem or spinal cord. (Consequently some of the axons in the pyramidal system are from 2 to 3 feet long. The longest axons are those that synapse with the lowermost spinal nerves.) The smaller the number of synapses in a neural circuit, the faster is the circuit's response time. Pyramidal circuits, being single-synapse circuits, have especially quick response times.

The motor neurons in the pyramidal system (the *corticobulbar* and *corticospinal* tracts) are called *upper motor neurons*. The cell bodies of upper motor neurons are located in and near the primary motor cortex. The axons of upper motor neurons pass through the midbrain, brain stem, and spinal cord to synapse with the cell bodies of motor neurons in the brain stem and spinal cord (called *lower motor neurons*). The lower motor neurons synapse with muscles at specialized junctions called *motor endplates*.

> The pyramidal system fibers that connect with neurons in the brain stem are called the *corticobulbar tract,* and the fibers that connect with neurons in the spinal cord are called the *corticospinal tract*. In total, the fiber tracts of the pyramidal system are called *projection fiber tracts*.

Neurons in the primary motor cortex collaborate to produce skilled volitional movements. The neurons in the primary motor cortex are arranged topographically so that a functional map of the motor cortex can be created, showing which cortical areas are responsible for volitional movements of given muscle groups. Such a map, sometimes called a *homunculus* (little man), is shown in Figure 1-20.

> The word "homunculus" dates from the 16th and 17th century, when it referred to an exceedingly minute human body which was thought to inhabit each sperm cell. Development of the embryo and subsequent growth from infant to adult was believed to represent the growth of the homunculus.

It can be seen in Figure 1-20 that cortical responsibility for muscle groups is arranged in upside-down fashion on the motor cortex. Motor cortex for the foot and toes is located at the top

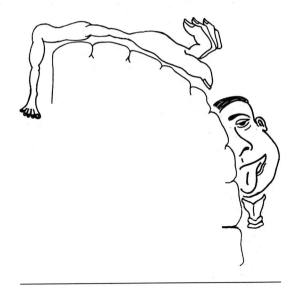

Figure 1-20 ■ A "homunculus" representing the allocation of motor function in the motor cortex. The size of the body part portrayed in the figure represents the amount of cortex devoted to innervation of the muscles in that body part.

of the primary motor cortex, and representation for the knee, hip, shoulder, elbow, wrist, hand, and face progresses laterally and downward. The representation of the body in Figure 1-20 looks odd because the size of a body part in the figure represents the amount of motor cortex assigned to various muscle groups. The differences in cortical representation shown in Figure 1-20 relate in a general way to the precision of movement required from muscle groups. The hand, mouth, tongue, larynx, and lips are allocated large amounts of motor cortex relative to the trunk, legs, and upper arms because the muscles of the hand, mouth, tongue, larynx, and lips are called on to perform more diverse, intricate, and pre-

> Remember that neurons in the left motor cortex control muscles on the right side of the body and vice versa.

cise movements than the muscles of the trunk, legs, and upper arms.

The *primary somatosensory cortex* is not part of the pyramidal system. However, it is described here because of its location near the primary motor cortex, its topographic similarity to the motor cortex, and its importance to skilled movement. The primary somatosensory cortex is located just behind the central fissure. It is topographically arranged as a mirror image of the motor cortex. Sensation from the face is represented at the lower (lateral) end of the sensory cortex, and sensation from the foot is represented at the top, inside the superior longitudinal fissure.

Vestibular-Reticular System The vestibular-reticular system (also not part of the pyramidal system, but related to it) is responsible for balance and orientation of the body in space and for maintaining general states of attention and alertness. It is made up of neurons scattered throughout the brain stem and cerebellum. Like pyramidal system neurons, the neurons in the vestibular-reticular system synapse with lower motor neurons. Unlike the pyramidal system, the vestibular-reticular system is not under volitional control—its functions are largely automatic and preprogrammed. Some writers combine the vestibular-reticular system with the extrapyramidal system. Although they have structural similarities, they apparently serve different functions, so they are described separately here.

The Extrapyramidal System The extrapyramidal system is a diffuse system of subcortical structures and pathways. It arises from diverse locations in the central nervous system (primarily the basal ganglia) and projects to cranial and spinal nerves. (According to some neuroanatomists, "extrapyramidal" is synonymous with "basal ganglia.") The extrapyramidal system is phylogenetically older than the pyramidal system, and it is an *indirect* system, which means that it is made up of networks of neurons, with chains of neurons and multiple synapses between the origin and destination of any extrapyramidal system pathway. The extrapyramidal system does not initiate movements but adjusts muscle tone and posture concurrent with volitional movements. Damage in the extrapyramidal system causes distortion or abolition of volitional movements and the appearance of involuntary movements.

Because the paths of the pyramidal, vestibular-reticular, and extrapyramidal systems are common throughout much of their course, an injury that affects one usually affects all three. Therefore we commonly see combinations of pyramidal, extrapyramidal, and sometimes vestibular signs when any of the divisions is damaged.

Because of its diffuseness, some writers dismiss the concept of the extrapyramidal system as a convenient fiction without neuroarchitectural validity. (The same could be said about many other conventional physiologic divisions.) Some neuroanatomists argue that the concept of the extrapyramidal system should be abandoned, and some contemporary descriptions of the nervous system do not mention it. However, the demise of the extrapyramidal system seems likely to be a slow one because it has a long history and it provides "a convenient shorthand for two broad classes of motor disorders" (Nolte, 1993).

How the Nervous System Produces Volitional Movement

The process by which the nervous system produces volitional movement is complex and not completely understood. It is clear that several subsystems participate in all but the simplest movements. The following greatly simplified scenario should provide a general sense of the process by which the nervous system moves from intention to accomplishment.

Activation of cortical regions in the anterior frontal lobes prepares the motor system for movement. The premotor cortex creates a set of neurally coded instructions for the intended movement sequence and transmits the instructions to the primary motor cortex. The primary motor cortex sends the command and control information necessary to execute the plan downward via the pyramidal tract to the cranial nerves (via the corticobulbar tract) and spinal nerves (via the corticospinal tract). The vestibular nuclei, midbrain, and reticular formation adjust balance and posture before and during the movement. The cerebellum modulates the rate, force, and direction of the movement. The extrapyramidal system adjusts muscle tone and posture to make the movement smooth and continuous.

GENERAL CONCEPTS 1-7

- The *pyramidal system* is responsible for skilled volitional movement. The pyramidal system begins with neurons in the primary motor cortex (*upper motor neurons*) whose axons synapse with neurons in the brain stem (*corticobulbar tracts*) and spinal cord (*corticospinal tracts*).

- Neurons in cranial nerves and spinal nerves are called *lower motor neurons.* Neurons in the motor cortex are called *upper motor neurons.*

- Muscle groups are represented in the primary motor cortex in topographic arrays. Motor neurons for the face, larynx, and head are represented in the upper part of the primary motor cortex, and motor neurons for the leg and foot are represented at the lower end.

- The amount of cortical representation for a muscle group reflects the precision and complexity of movements performed by the muscle group.

- The *vestibular-reticular system* is a self-regulating system that maintains balance, orientation of the body in space, and general levels of alertness and arousal.

- The *extrapyramidal system* is a diffuse system of subcortical structures and nerve fiber tracts. Its primary function is that of adjusting skeletal muscles concurrent with volitional movement.

- Damage in the extrapyramidal system disrupts or abolishes volitional movements and causes nonvolitional movements to appear.

NEUROLOGIC CAUSES OF ADULT COMMUNICATION DISORDERS

This section describes some major neurologic causes of adult language disorders, primarily aphasia (in which comprehension and production of spoken and written verbal materials is compromised), and the pragmatic communicative impairments exhibited by some adults with right-hemisphere damage. It will not deal with the neurologic causes of dysarthria (speech impairments caused by nervous system damage) or traumatic brain injury (linguistic and cognitive impairments following traumatic injury to the nervous system, usually caused by blows to the head). The neuropathology of dysarthria and traumatic brain injury are addressed in subsequent chapters.

Stroke

Stroke is a generic term for a disturbance of brain function caused by vascular disruptions (loss of blood supply or bleeding). A more technical term for stroke is cerebrovascular accident (CVA). During the past decade public information campaigns have substituted the label *brain attack* for stroke and cerebrovascular accident. The appellation brain attack was adopted because of its resemblance to heart attack, presumably to reinforce the public's awareness of the need for immediate medical attention when symptoms of a stroke are experienced. Symptoms are abrupt and include:

- Weakness or numbness on one side of the body
- Impairment of vision, especially in one eye
- Difficulty speaking or understanding speech
- Episodes of dizziness or falls
- Severe headache, especially with any of the other symptoms

Stroke is the third leading cause of death in the United States. Each year about 500,000 U.S. residents experience strokes, and about 150,000 die as a consequence of a stroke. In any given year there are approximately 2 million survivors of stroke in the United States (Caplan, 1988). About 80% of stroke patients survive for at least 1 month after their stroke, but only about one third are alive 10 years later. Of those who survive a stroke, about 85% are able to return to their prestroke living environment, usually with some level of persisting impairment, whereas 15% are sufficiently impaired to require institutional care (Greenberg, Aminoff, and Simon, 1993).

The brain is remarkably intolerant of sudden changes in its oxygen and glucose supply. The onset of communicative disorders following strokes is almost always dramatic, with symptoms developing rapidly and becoming maximally expressed within a few minutes to a few hours. During the first few days after a stroke, parts of the brain that are not actually damaged or destroyed may be functionally impaired, unless the stroke is a very small one. Consequently, major strokes often yield a pattern in which there is immediate general disruption of cerebral functions, gradually resolving to more limited (*focal*) disruption of specific processes, depending on what parts of the brain have been permanently damaged.

Strokes can be *ischemic* (a term that means *deprived of blood*) or *hemorrhagic* (a term that means *caused by bleeding*), although the occurrence of ischemic stroke is far higher (80% ischemic vs. 20% hemorrhagic strokes). Ischemic stroke (sometimes called *occlusive* stroke) occurs when an artery is blocked and part of the central nervous system loses its blood supply. If the occlusion lasts more than a few (3 to 5) minutes, death (*necrosis*) of central nervous system tissue is likely. The medical term for death of tissue caused by loss of blood supply is *infarct.*

Ischemic Stroke Ischemic strokes can be either *thrombotic* or *embolic.* In *thrombotic strokes* (cerebral thrombosis), an artery is gradually occluded by a plug of material accumulating at a fixed location within the artery. In *embolic strokes,* an artery is suddenly occluded by material that moves through the vascular system and blocks the artery.

Thrombotic Stroke Most cerebral thromboses occur in the large arteries supplying blood to the brain (internal carotid arteries, vertebral arteries, and the basilar artery). Thromboses are uncommon in smaller arteries. (Arteries become smaller in diameter as they get farther from the heart until they become capillaries, after which the venous system begins.) A thrombosis typically begins in an area of increased turbulence, which means that thromboses favor locations at which arteries change direction or divide (at *bends* and *bifurcations*). Debris in the bloodstream tends to accumulate at these locations, just as it does in river bends and junctions. In rivers, the debris may include driftwood, cola bottles, and overturned canoes. In arteries the debris consists mainly of fatty substances (lipids) and fibrous material, which accumulate on the lining of the artery. These accumulations are called *atherosclerotic plaque.* The turbulence and increased velocity of the blood flowing through the narrowed artery abrade and roughen the inner lining of the artery. Plaque forms at these roughened areas and gradually thickens over the course of years, until it may eventually fill the *lumen* (space within the artery).

Atherosclerotic comes from a combination of Greek words meaning *paste* (athero-) and *hard* (sclero-). *Plaque* comes from a French word meaning *plate* or *slab.*

As the size of the lumen diminishes (a condition called *stenosis*), the volume of blood flowing through the narrowed artery decreases (although its velocity increases—the Bernoulli effect). Sometimes the plaque in the arterial wall cracks or ulcerates. Then blood platelets and fibrin (a protein found in blood) adhere to the ulceration, accelerating clot development. The clot eventually may occlude the artery, or parts of the clot may break off and become *emboli* traveling through the vascular system, eventually occluding smaller vessels downstream from the original clot.

Embolic Stroke In embolic strokes (cerebral embolism), an artery is occluded by a fragment of material that travels through the circulatory system until it reaches a blood vessel smaller than its own diameter, where it lodges, occluding the artery. The material in the embolus may be a blood clot that has broken loose from its site of formation, a fragment of arterial lining, a piece of atherosclerotic plaque, tissue from a tumor, a clump of bacteria, or other solids that may move through the arteries. The most frequent sources of emboli are fragments from thromboses in the heart, followed by fragments of atherosclerotic plaque from an artery. Patients with atrial fibrillation ("heart palpitations") are particularly susceptible to cerebral embolism because the lack of strong atrial contraction promotes pooling and clotting of blood in the left atrium, which then embolizes.

Determining whether the cause of a particular event is thrombotic or embolic is difficult, so the diagnostician may hedge by referring to ischemic incidents as *thromboembolic* events. However, thrombotic and embolic events differ in their progression. Because embolic strokes are a consequence of sudden blockage of an artery, their symptoms usually are maximally expressed within a few minutes. Thrombotic strokes, because they arise from slowly developing occlusion of an artery, tend to develop in an irregular, stepwise manner, sometimes preceded by transient periods of ischemia.

Transient Interruptions of Cerebral Blood Supply Many stroke patients have a history of *transient ischemic attacks* (TIAs), which are temporary (less than 24 hours, and usually less than 30 minutes) disruptions of cerebral circulation causing rapidly developing episodes of sensory disturbance, limb weakness, slurred speech, visual anomalies, dizziness, confusion, mild aphasia, or other symptoms that resolve completely. Most transient ischemic attacks are thought to be caused by small emboli that temporarily occlude an artery, then break up or dissolve. Transient ischemic attacks sometimes occur when a stationary thrombus has nearly, but not completely, occluded an artery. When an artery is nearly occluded, otherwise insignificant decrements in blood pressure may be sufficient to interrupt blood flow through the artery, causing a transient ischemic attack. They occasionally (but rarely) may be caused by *cerebral vasospasm* of a nearly occluded artery, in which the muscles of the arterial wall contract, narrowing the lumen and compromising blood flow.

Transient interruptions of blood supply to the brain that last more than 24 hours but completely resolve within a few days sometimes are called *reversible ischemic neurologic deficits* (RINDs). Interruptions of blood supply to the brain that last more than 24 hours but leave minor deficits after a few days sometimes are called *partially reversible ischemic neurologic deficits* (PRINDs). The general public, many physicians, and some neurologists forego these categorizations and call any transient episode of sensory disruption, weakness, slurred speech, visual anomalies, dizziness, confusion, or aphasia caused by temporary interruption of blood supply to the brain a *small stroke.*

Transient ischemic attacks and wholly or partially reversible ischemic neurologic deficits are manifestations of cerebrovascular disease. Consequently, their occurrence often presages a full-blown stroke. According to Greenberg, Aminoff, and Simon (1993), about one-third of patients who have transient ischemic attacks or RINDs will, within 5 years, have a stroke that leaves them with permanent neurologic deficits.

Hypoperfusion Insufficient blood supply to the brain and brain stem sometimes may be caused by *hypoperfusion,* in which the brain's blood supply is compromised not by occlusion of arteries but by insufficient blood volume. Insufficient blood volume is most commonly caused by massive bleeding elsewhere in the body or by insufficient cardiac pumping capacity (usually from heart disease). The pattern of cerebral damage caused by hypoperfusion is different from that caused by occlusion. Occlusions usually cause localized regions of dense neuron loss in brain tissue supplied by the affected artery or branch. Hypoperfusion usually causes diffuse and less dense damage in the watershed regions (border zones) of the cortex supplied by the artery or branch. This is because the blood, under low pressure, tends not to penetrate into the border zones, where vessel diameters are small and flow resistance is high. Although hypoperfusion causes cerebral ischemia, it is a not a stroke, and, unlike ischemic strokes, it usually has a gradual onset, rather than a sudden one. Because it is a cause of cerebral ischemia (albeit a minor one), it is discussed in this context.

General Effects of Ischemic Stroke Rubens (1977) and Keefe (1995) have described some of the physiologic changes that take place following major ischemic strokes. Within the first few hours after the stroke, neurons deprived of blood supply die. Brain tissue swells in and around the area damaged by the stroke. If the damaged area is large, the swelling may raise intracranial pressure and cause displacement of brain tissue remote from the site of the stroke. Blood flow to both hemispheres diminishes. Neurotransmitters are released, not only in the brain substance in and around the stroke, but throughout the brain and into the CSF. Their presence upsets neuronal metabolism and perhaps contributes to reduced cerebral blood flow. Neurons in undamaged parts of the brain that connect with destroyed neurons degenerate because of the lost connections (*transneural degeneration*). Surviving neurons that have lost some but not all of their input from neurons in the damaged region become hypersensitive to residual input from the damaged region (*denervation hypersensitivity*).

The phenomenon of *diaschisis* also plays a role in the impairments seen immediately after stroke. In diaschisis brain function is disrupted in regions distant from the site of injury but connected to it by neuronal pathways. For many years diaschisis was an unproven phenomenon, but studies with positron emission tomography (PET) have confirmed that destruction of brain tissue in one area is followed by reductions in cerebral metabolism in other areas, primarily those that have substantial neuronal connections to the damaged area (Metter and others, 1983, 1984).

Brain swelling, reduction in cerebral blood flow, neurotransmitter release, transneural degeneration, denervation hypersensitivity, and diaschisis, individually or in combination, create diffuse impairment of brain functions, behavior, and mental status, which gradually resolves over time. In the first hours and days after the patient's stroke, the symptoms generated by this diffuse impairment are superimposed on the more focal symptoms caused by death of tissue at the site of the stroke. As time passes, cerebral swelling diminishes, cerebral blood flow to undamaged tissue is restored, and neurotransmitters released as a consequence of the injury are resorbed. Diaschisis slowly resolves. Axons of neurons in brain tissue near the infarct establish new connections with neurons that have lost direct connections with the infarcted area (*collateral sprouting*). As these physiologic repairs take place, the patient's condition gradually improves, with diffuse impairment of behavior and mental status resolving to a more specific (*focal*) collection of symptoms reflecting the permanent loss of neurons in the infarcted area.

Often it is difficult to predict a patient's eventual neurologic recovery (and their residual level of impairment) during the first few days after a stroke because the permanent effects of the tissue destruction caused by the stroke are masked by the stroke's temporary effects on brain chemistry and function. Consequently, clinicians often delay making predictions about a patient's eventual level of recovery until these temporary effects have diminished (usually within 2 weeks to a month).

Hemorrhagic Strokes Hemorrhagic strokes (cerebral hemorrhages) are caused by rupture of a cerebral blood vessel. They may be caused by weakness of a vessel wall, by traumatic injury to a vessel, or (rarely) by extreme fluctuations in blood pressure. Hemorrhages from the blood vessels of the meninges or on the surface of the brain are called *extracerebral hemorrhages* because the bleeding is outside the brain. Hemorrhages within the brain or brain stem are called *intracerebral hemorrhages* because the bleeding is within the brain substance.

Extracerebral Hemorrhage   To complicate matters further, extracerebral hemorrhages can be subclassified as *subarachnoid, subdural,* or *epidural* hemorrhages, depending on where the blood accumulates. If the bleeding is beneath the arachnoid, between the arachnoid and the pia mater, it is called a *subarachnoid hemorrhage.* Subarachnoid hemorrhages are the most common extracerebral hemorrhages. If the bleeding is beneath the dura mater, it is called a *subdural hemorrhage,* and if it is above the dura mater, between the dura mater and the skull, it is called an *epidural hemorrhage.*

Hemorrhages involving the dura mater, whether subdural or epidural, usually are caused by traumatic head injuries in which dural blood vessels are torn or lacerated. *Subarachnoid hemorrhages* usually are caused by leaking or ruptured blood vessels on the surface of the brain, brain stem, or cerebellum. Such leaks often come from *aneurysms.*

Aneurysms are pouches formed in weakened arterial walls. Blood pressure within the artery causes the weakened section of the arterial wall to stretch, much like an inflating balloon. The resulting malformations are sometimes called *berry aneurysms* or *saccular aneurysms* because of their berry-like or sack-like appearance (Figure 1-21). The stretched arterial walls within aneurysms are thin, weak, and susceptible to rupture.

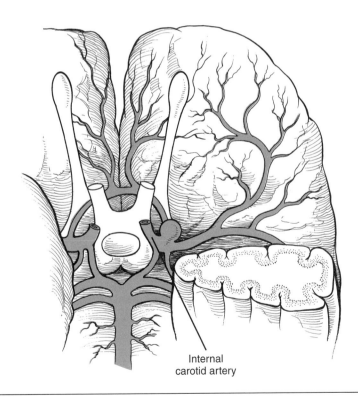

Internal
carotid artery

Figure 1-21 ■ **"Berry" aneurysm on the left anterior communicating artery in the circle of Willis. Aneurysms are most common in the arteries at the base of the brain.**

About half of all berry aneurysms occur in the arteries at the base of the brain (in the vertebral arteries, basilar artery, internal carotid arteries, and the circle of Willis). Almost all of the others occur in the anterior and middle cerebral arteries. Very few (2% to 3%) occur in the posterior cerebral artery. If an aneurysm is detected before it ruptures, it may be surgically repaired by clamping or tying off the neck of the aneurysm, by wrapping the aneurysm, or by tying off the artery that supplies blood to the aneurysm. Sometimes aneurysms that are leaking but have not ruptured can be repaired, but when an aneurysm ruptures, repair often is impossible. Ruptured aneurysms cause bleeding into the subarachnoid space with substantial risk of death or irreversible brain damage.

Some subarachnoid hemorrhages arise from *arteriovenous malformations* (AVMs). Arteriovenous malformations are collections of dilated, thin-walled veins connected to a tangled mass of equally thin-walled arteries (Figure 1-22). They occur in all parts of the brain, brain stem, and spinal cord, but most large ones develop deep in the cerebral hemispheres. As is true for aneurysms, the vessel walls in arteriovenous malformations usually are weak and susceptible to hemorrhage. Almost all arteriovenous malformations are present at birth and become larger with the passage of time. When arteriovenous malformations become large, they may cause headaches and other central nervous system symptoms. If they are identified before massive bleeding occurs, they may be surgically excised or the blood vessels that connect to the malformation may be tied off or plugged. According to Adams and Victor (1981) the risk of bleeding from AVMs is about 1% to 2% per year, which suggests that a patient with an AVM is unlikely to reach the age of 60 or 70 without a hemorrhage.

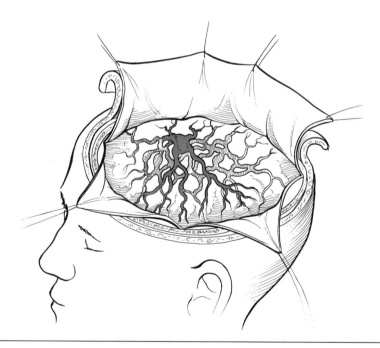

Figure 1-22 ■ **Arteriovenous malformation (AVM). AVMs are tangled masses of arteries and veins that gradually increase in size over time. The greatest risk to patients with AVMs is rupture and subsequent hemorrhage.**

Intracerebral Hemorrhage Almost all *intracerebral hemorrhages* (about 90%) occur in patients with high blood pressure (*hypertension*). The most obvious reason for this relationship is the pressure on arterial walls caused by hypertension. A less obvious reason is that chronic hypertension leads to degenerative changes in the small penetrating arteries deep in the brain, weakening them and creating *microaneurysms.* These microaneurysms are vulnerable to rupture, with consequent leakage of blood into the brain. This leakage often causes the brain to swell, exerting pressure on adjacent vessels, which then rupture, leading to a cascading series of events in which the hemorrhage grows by displacing adjacent brain tissue and stretching and tearing small blood vessels in the vicinity. The most common sites for intracerebral hemorrhages are the small penetrating arteries in and around the thalamus and basal ganglia, but intracerebral hemorrhages also occur in the brain stem (especially the pons) and the cerebellum.

Intracerebral hemorrhages dissect brain matter along white matter tracts but tend not to destroy the tracts themselves. An intracerebral hemorrhage eventually may decompress itself by bleeding into the ventricles or subarachnoid space. Because of their location—usually deep in the brain—most intracerebral hemorrhages are not surgically repairable, and surgery usually is attempted only if the bleeding is life threatening and the hemorrhage is accessible. Medical management usually includes reducing blood pressure, maintaining adequate respiration, and regulating fluid intake.

Recovery from Ischemic and Hemorrhagic Strokes Ischemic and hemorrhagic strokes have different courses of recovery. The *pattern* of recovery depends largely on whether the stroke is ischemic or hemorrhagic, and the *eventual level* of recovery depends largely on the amount of brain tissue destroyed and the location of the destruction.

Neurologic recovery from *ischemic strokes* is greatest in the first week or two and diminishes over time, until the patient's condition stabilizes (Figure 1-23).

Recovery from ischemic strokes is greatest for patients in the middle severity ranges. Patients who remain severely impaired when the acute effects of the stroke have dissipated (2 to 4 weeks poststroke) usually have large regions of tissue destruction in the brain and are likely to remain severely impaired after the transient effects of the stoke have resolved. Patients with extremely mild impairments in the first days and weeks poststroke also may show little neurologic recovery because they have little room to recover—small amounts of improvement bring them back to (or near) their premorbid levels.

How long it takes for recovery from ischemic strokes to be completed has not been specified. The most dramatic neurologic recovery takes place in the first 2 to 4 weeks poststroke. Most recovery of language takes place within the first 3 months post onset (Culton, 1969; Sarno and Levita, 1971), and neurologic recovery is essentially complete by 6 months post onset (Basso,

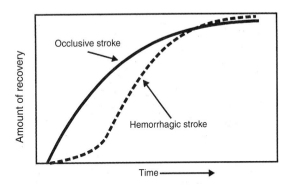

Figure 1-23 ■ **General course of neurologic recovery from stroke. The graph represents the average pattern of recovery for groups of patients. The recovery of individual patients often differs from the group average. These patterns are based primarily on clinical experience and anecdotal evidence because there is little empirical evidence documenting patterns of neurologic recovery for groups of patients with occlusive or hemorrhagic strokes.**

Capitani, and Vignolo, 1979), although some slow neurologic recovery may continue for additional months or years (Caplan, 1993).

Neurologic recovery from *hemorrhagic strokes* usually follows a different course from that for occlusive strokes. Patients with hemorrhagic strokes often show little improvement for the first 4 to 8 weeks post onset, followed by a period of rapid recovery (see Figure 1-23). Recovery then slows and stabilizes, usually at a level above that for occlusive stroke patients with equivalent deficits at onset. Most patients with hemorrhagic strokes, like those with ischemic strokes, essentially have completed their neurologic recovery by 6 months post onset.

That hemorrhages do not destroy white matter (nerve fiber tracts), whereas occlusive strokes do destroy them, may explain why patients with hemorrhages tend to experience better recovery than patients with occlusive strokes.

GENERAL CONCEPTS 1-8

- *Stroke* is a label for loss of blood supply to the brain. Strokes may be caused by *occlusion* of a cerebral artery (*thrombosis, embolus*) or by hemorrhage (*bleeding*).
- *Thromboses* are slow accumulations of material within an artery, causing its gradual occlusion.
- *Emboli* are fragments of material that travel through cerebral arteries and lodge in a branch that is smaller than the embolus.
- Symptoms of thrombotic strokes tend to develop gradually over hours to days, often in stepwise fashion. Symptoms of embolic strokes tend to appear suddenly with maximal symptoms within a few minutes.
- Many strokes are preceded by transient episodes of sensory disturbance, weakness, slurred speech, or other symptoms, most of which resolve within minutes to hours. *Transient ischemic attacks* are the most common of these transient episodes.

- Low blood volume or low blood pressure may lead to *hypoperfusion,* in which blood does not penetrate into small-diameter arteries in border zones of arterial supply.
- Major strokes usually are followed by temporary (days to weeks) disruption of cerebral function, caused by *brain swelling, neurotransmitter release, diminished cerebral blood flow, transneural degeneration, denervation hypersensitivity,* and *diaschisis.* The diffuse effects of these processes eventually resolve, leaving the patient with residual focal impairments.
- *Extracerebral hemorrhages* may be *epidural* (between the dura mater and the skull), *subdural* (between the dura mater and the arachnoid), or *subarachnoid* (between the arachnoid and the pia mater).
- Subarachnoid hemorrhages usually come from ruptured *aneurysms* (weakened balloon-like pouches in cerebral artery walls). Some come from *arteriovenous malformations* (tangled masses of thin-walled cerebral arteries and veins).
- Most intracerebral hemorrhages occur in people with high blood pressure. Most are caused by a combination of increased arterial pressure and the formation of *microaneurysms* on penetrating cerebral arteries deep within the brain hemispheres.
- Recovery from ischemic strokes tends to be most rapid in the first days and weeks post-stroke with gradual slowing of recovery thereafter. Recovery from hemorrhagic strokes often is slow during the first 4 to 8 weeks post-stroke, followed by a period of rapid recovery, which then slows and stabilizes.
- Recovery from either ischemic or hemorrhagic strokes is essentially complete by 6 months post-stroke.

Other Neurologic Causes of Communication Disorders

Most of the other neurologic conditions that may cause communicative impairments are insidious, rather than abrupt, in onset (excluding traumatic brain injury, discussed later in this book).

Insidious neurologic conditions make their presence known slowly, over a long interval, sometimes with intermittent periods of stabilization or even remission, until the patient receives treatment, becomes incapacitated, or dies.

The major insidious conditions that affect the central nervous system include:

- Intracranial tumors
- Hydrocephalus
- Infections and toxins
- Nutritional and metabolic disorders

Any of these conditions can cause impaired communication. However, when impaired communication is caused by these conditions, dementia or personality disruptions usually accompany the communication impairment. Insidious conditions usually do not have a clearly definable time of onset, and patients often do not see their physician when the first symptoms appear because the symptoms are mild and appear innocuous. Consequently, the pathologic condition may be advanced when the patient first seeks medical attention. In some cases delay may have no significant consequences, but in other cases (such as with an intracerebral tumor) delay may have serious, and sometimes disastrous, results.

Intracranial Tumors Tumors growing within the cranial vault may be either *primary* (originating there) or *secondary* (originating elsewhere and migrating to intracranial locations). The process by which a tumor appears at a secondary site in the body is called *metastasis,* and such tumors are called *metastatic tumors.*

Primary intracranial tumors most often are found in the cerebrum and the cerebellum. They occur at all ages but are most common in adults from 25 to 50 years old. The causes of most primary intracranial tumors remain a mystery. Some appear to be related to previous injuries, and there is a tendency for some kinds of intracranial tumors to occur in families.

Intracranial tumors, whether primary or secondary, have similar effects on the central nervous system. The tissue around the tumor swells. This swelling is one of the major causes of observable symptoms in patients with cerebral tumors. If the tumor exerts pressure on circumscribed areas of the brain or brain stem, localized symptoms (motor impairments, sensory loss) may follow. If the tumor causes general swelling of the brain and brain stem, then widespread symptoms of cerebral dysfunction related to pressure and displacement of brain tissue are likely. It is common to see localized symptoms in the early stages of tumor growth, with increasing and more generalized dysfunction as tumor growth and swelling of brain tissue cause intracranial pressure to increase.

When cerebral swelling is severe, *herniation* may occur. Large masses in the brain hemispheres (or smaller ones in the brain stem) may force the brain stem downward through the foramen magnum or may squeeze parts of the brain against dural projections such as the falx cerebri or the tentorium, causing compression, shearing, and bleeding of brain tissues. Pang (1989) describes four major types of herniation.

Subfalcine herniation is the most common and least ominous. It occurs when one brain hemisphere is pushed against the falx cerebri, the rigid sheet of dura mater that projects downward into the superior longitudinal fissure (Figure 1-24, *B*). Subfalcine herniation does not always generate focal neurologic symptoms, unless the anterior cerebral artery is compressed, in which case the patient may complain of numbness and weakness in the contralateral leg.

Lateral transtentorial herniation usually occurs as a consequence of masses in the temporal lobe. The mesial surface of the temporal lobe is squeezed against the tentorium, the rigid sheet of dura mater that separates the space occupied by the brain from that occupied by the cerebellum (Figure 1-24, *C*). The herniation creates pressure on CN 3, causing ipsilateral pupillary dilation. The pressure also forces the brain substance downward into the foramen magnum, stretching tissues and blood vessels at the base of the brain and in the brain stem. The resulting brain stem ischemia may lead to coma and, if brain stem hemorrhages occur, to irreversible coma or death.

Central transtentorial herniation is caused by swelling near the apex of the brain or in the frontal lobes. The brain mass is pushed against the tentorium and downward into the foramen magnum. As in lateral transtentorial herniation, structures and blood vessels at the base of the brain and in the midbrain are stretched and distorted, with consequent impairment of vital functions. Irreversible coma or death are common consequences.

Tonsillar herniation is caused by swelling in the cerebellum, pons, or medulla. The cerebellar tonsils (hence the name *tonsillar*) are extruded through the foramen magnum, where they exert pressure on the medulla (Figure 1-24, *D*). The brain stem is displaced downward, with consequent shearing and distortion. Respiration is compromised, heart rate decreases, blood pressure rapidly increases, and coma soon follows.

The overall course of patients with intracranial tumors is one of deterioration. In the early stages, when intracranial pressure is low, the patient may complain of nonspecific alterations in mental function such as forgetfulness, lack of initiative, drowsiness, blurred or double vision, lightheadedness, or vertigo. About one-third of patients report headaches early in the course of tumor development. Such headaches can take several forms, but most are not affected by analgesics. Vomiting sometimes occurs in the early stages of tumor growth, and seizures often are seen throughout the course of tumor growth when the tumor is within the brain substance.

Patients who have tumors and elevated intracranial pressure almost always exhibit cognitive impairments, are lethargic, and may be stuporous. In most cases, these patients report unremitting bifrontal and bioccipital headaches that are not affected by analgesics and are present day and night. Vomiting frequently occurs, and the patient may be unsteady and generally clumsy.

The number of symptoms generated by a tumor and the rate at which symptoms progress is determined by the *size, rate of growth,* and *location* of the tumor. Large tumors generate more extreme symptoms. Faster-growing tumors produce symptoms more quickly than slower-growing ones because the brain adapts to slowly developing masses better than faster developing ones. If a slowly growing tumor is located in or near areas that serve important functions (sensory and motor cortex, brain stem), a relatively small tumor may generate major symptoms quickly. If the tumor is located in a "silent" area of the brain, it may grow to surprising volume before generating observable symptoms.

Different kinds of intracranial tumors have different rates of growth and differ in malignancy. *Gliomas* are the most common intracranial tumors. Gliomas can be divided into several subtypes, but the two most important ones are *astrocytoma* and *glioblastoma multiforme.* Astrocytomas are the most common and the most benign (nonmalignant) of the gliomas. They usually grow slowly, and symptom development may span 5 or 6 years. Postoperative survival of 10 or more years is common. In some cases, astrocytomas may be removed completely, in which case the patient is considered cured. However, even benign astrocytomas can cause substantial neurologic impairments, or even kill the patient, if the tumor is strategically located (e.g., in the brain stem).

Glioblastoma multiforme is the next most common glioma. It is also one of the most malignant and rapidly growing of all intracranial tumors. Symptoms typically develop during a period of 3 months to 1 year, and the average postsurgical survival is only about 6 to 9 months.

Meningiomas are relatively common tumors, and as the name implies, they arise from the meninges. They are among the most benign of all intracranial tumors because they are slow growing, are well-defined, and do not usually invade the brain substance. For this reason they often can be completely removed. The symptoms of meningiomas are slow to develop because they are slow growing. However, when symptoms do appear, meningiomas are among the most localizable of intracranial tumors because they generate pressure at specific places on the cortex, and they rarely cause general increases in intracranial pressure.

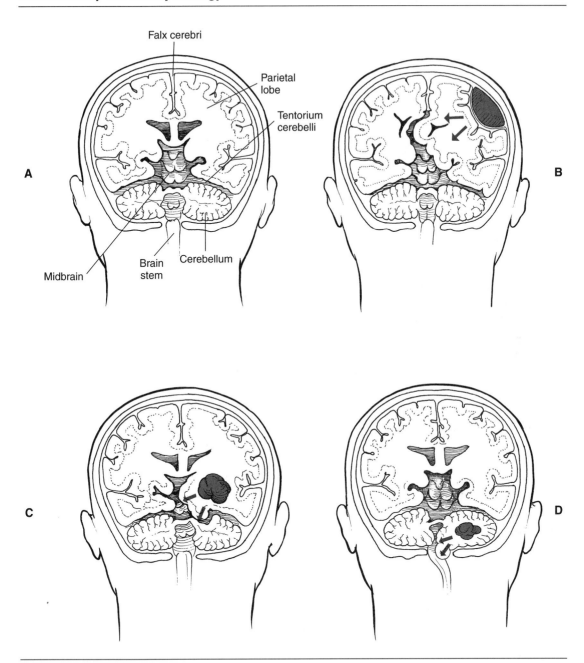

Figure 1-24 ■ **Examples of herniation syndromes. A, Cross-section of a normal brain and skull. B, Displacement of brain tissue caused by a mass above the right parietal lobe, which pushes adjacent regions of the right hemisphere under the falx cerebri (*subfalcine herniation*). C, Displacement of the mesial temporal lobe around the tentorium cerebelli by a mass in the temporal lobe (*transtentorial herniation*). D, Displacement of the right cerebellar tonsil downward into the foramen magnum by a mass in the right cerebellar hemisphere (*tonsillar herniation*).**

Secondary intracranial tumors (metastatic carcinomas) are tumors that form from cancerous cells that have migrated (usually through the bloodstream) from the primary tumor site to the brain, where they settle and grow. The primary sources for metastatic carcinoma of the brain are, in decreasing order of frequency, the breast, the lungs, and the pharynx and larynx. Metastatic carcinomas of the brain usually are grossly well-defined, but multiple sites of metastasis within the brain are common. Metastatic tumors usually cause substantial local swelling around the tumor site. The prognosis for most metastatic brain tumor patients is poor. The average survival after diagnosis of metastatic brain tumor is 2 to 6 months.

Hydrocephalus Hydrocephalus refers to a condition in which the cerebral ventricles are enlarged, either as a result of increased pressure within the ventricles or as a result of brain atrophy (shrinkage). *Obstructive hydrocephalus* is caused by obstruction of the intraventricular passageways through which CSF circulates. The obstruction blocks the flow of CSF from the ventricles into the subarachnoid space. Sometimes obstructions are caused by material circulating in the CSF (plugs of bacteria, bits of floating tissue), but more often they are caused by swelling of nearby brain tissue.

The most frequent site of obstruction is the *cerebral aqueduct,* which connects the third and fourth ventricles. The cerebral aqueduct is the longest and narrowest of the passageways between the ventricles and consequently is the most susceptible to obstruction, usually because of swelling of adjacent brain tissues or displacement of brain tissue by tumors. Because cerebrospinal fluid is formed in the cerebral ventricles, anything that blocks the exit of cerebrospinal fluid from the ventricles causes the pressure within the ventricles to rise. As the pressure rises the ventricles enlarge, the brain is compressed against the skull, and the patient becomes mentally dulled, lethargic, and hyporesponsive.

The primary medical treatment for obstructive hydrocephalus is *intraventricular shunt.* A cannula (hollow needle connected to a small flexible tube) is passed through the brain into the ventricles. Excess cerebrospinal fluid is then forced (by intraventricular pressure) through the shunt, decreasing the pressure within the ventricles. The tube may be passed into the neck or the abdominal cavity, where the excess fluid is allowed to drip away. The patient's response to shunt placement usually is dramatic, with few long-term residual deficits, unless intracranial pressure has reached exceptionally high levels or has continued for weeks or months.

Nonobstructive hydrocephalus is a generic label for several other conditions that cause ventricular enlargement. One of the most common causes of nonobstructive hydrocephalus is cerebral atrophy. Nonobstructive hydrocephalus is not accompanied by elevated intracranial pressure.

Infections The central nervous system ordinarily is strongly resistant to bacterial or viral infection, but such infections sometimes occur. The major bacterial infections are *bacterial meningitis* and *brain abscess.* In *bacterial meningitis,* the pia mater, arachnoid, and the cerebrospinal fluid become infected with bacteria, causing inflammation, swelling, and fluid exudate from the meninges. The patient becomes feverish, chilled, and lethargic and complains of headache, drowsiness, and stiff neck. If the infection is severe, the patient may progress into coma. Bacterial meningitis exacerbates quickly and can be fatal if not promptly treated. The standard treatment is antibiotic medications, which usually cure the infection, although neurologic sequelae may persist.

Brain abscess is caused by introduction of bacteria, fungus, or parasites into brain tissues from a primary infection site elsewhere in the body. Transmission may be through the blood or by migration through tissues. In about 40% of cases, the primary source of infection is the nasal sinuses, middle ear, or mastoid cells. In about 30% of cases the source is the lungs or cardiovascular tissue. Symptom development in brain abscess is slower than symptom development in bacterial meningitis, and brain abscesses tend to generate localized symptoms (such as visual anomalies or sensory loss) rather than the generalized symptoms of meningitis. However, patients with brain abscess—like those with meningitis—complain of fever, chills, headache, lethargy, and drowsiness. The usual treatment is surgical drainage of the abscess in combination with antibiotic medication. Recovery usually is dramatic, although the patient may be left with chronic deficits related to destruction of brain tissue by the abscess.

Numerous viruses may infect the central nervous system. The two major sources of central nervous system viral infections are general infections, such as mumps or measles, and viruses transmitted by insect or animal bites, such as equine encephalitis or rabies. The progression of viral infections depends on the virus. Sometimes (as in viral meningitis), symptoms develop quickly, followed by gradual improvement. Sometimes symptoms develop slowly, followed by gradual improvement (e.g., when the body's immune system successfully eliminates the infection). Sometimes (as in acquired immunodeficiency syndrome—AIDS), symptoms develop slowly and continue to worsen, usually ending in death. In some cases (as in rabies) symptoms develop quickly and dramatically, invariably ending in death. A few antiviral medications that are not toxic to the body have been developed and may be of benefit. Otherwise, treatment of viral infections is palliative—directed toward maintaining the patient's vital functions, providing adequate nutrition, and regulating fluid balance, to help the patient's natural defenses rid the body of the virus.

Toxemia Toxemia is caused by introduction into the nervous system of substances that inflame or poison nerve tissue. Toxemia may be caused by drug overdoses, drug interactions, bacterial toxins (tetanus, botulism, diphtheria), or heavy metal poisoning (lead, mercury). The course of heavy metal or chemical poisoning (such as may occur in occupational exposure to the compounds) is usually one of decreasing mentation and increasing lethargy, with motor or sensory disruptions generally occurring only in advanced stages of poisoning. Poisoning with bacterial toxins usually follows a more acute course, with symptoms developing quickly, followed by slow recovery, unless the poisoning ends in death. Treatment usually is directed toward removal of the source of the toxin and, sometimes, purging the system of the toxin.

Metabolic Disorders Metabolic disorders are common causes of central nervous system dysfunction but, like other insidious processes, rarely cause isolated communication disorders. Severe hypoglycemia may cause deterioration of cerebral function, leading to confusion, stupor, or coma. Thyroid disorders may generate central nervous system symptoms (apathy, confusion, and intellectual deterioration). Treatment of metabolic disorders usually involves correcting or compensating for the metabolic imbalance, and central nervous system symptoms usually regress or resolve when the metabolic disturbance is corrected.

Nutritional Disorders Although rare in the United States, nutritional disorders sometimes cause central nervous system dysfunction and occasionally may generate communicative impairments. One classic nutritional deficiency syndrome is *Wernicke's encephalopathy,* caused by thiamine deficiency and usually associated with alcoholism. The primary symptoms of Wernicke's encephalopathy are paralysis of some of the muscles that move the eyes; clumsy, staggering gait; and mental confusion. Other vitamin deficiencies, including deficiencies in vitamin B_{12} and nicotinic acid, may cause variable neurologic symptoms. Neurologic syndromes associated with vitamin or mineral excess also may be seen (e.g., overdosage of vitamin A). In the case of nutritional deficiencies, treatment usually involves replenishment of the deficient compound by medication, together with dietary adjustment; in the case of vitamin or mineral excess, treatment is directed toward reducing the patient's intake of those compounds.

GENERAL CONCEPTS 1-9

- Intracranial tumors cause displacement of cerebral tissue. Some also destroy cerebral tissue.
- When displacement of cerebral tissues is severe, *herniation* may occur. In herniation,

brain tissue is pressed against or pushed across rigid partitions such as the falx cerebri or through apertures such as the foramen magnum.

- Subfalcine herniation (a brain hemisphere is pressed against the falx cerebri) is the least dangerous form of herniation. Transtentorial herniation (the brain is pushed downward against the tentorium cerebelli) and tonsillar herniation (the cerebellum and brain stem are pushed downward through the foramen magnum) are much more dangerous because of risk to brain stem structures that control vital functions such as respiration and heartbeat.

- Meningiomas and astrocytomas are relatively benign (nonmalignant) cerebral tumors. Glioblastoma multiforme is among the most dangerous (malignant).

- Obstructive hydrocephalus (enlarged cerebral ventricles) usually is caused by blockage in the cerebral aqueduct, which connects the third ventricle to the fourth ventricle. Obstructive hydrocephalus raises intracranial pressure and may displace brain tissue.

- Nonobstructive hydrocephalus is not caused by blockage of CSF transit in the ventricular system. It does not increase intracranial pressure.

- Bacterial or viral infections, toxemia, metabolic disorders, or nutritional disorders sometimes cause neurogenic communication disorders as part of a larger complex of behavioral and cognitive decline. Medical treatment usually resolves these conditions, together with any associated speech, language, or cognitive impairments.

THOUGHT QUESTIONS

Question 1-1 Mr. Johnson is a 72-year-old right-handed man who has just suffered a thrombotic stroke in the posterior branch of the middle cerebral artery. Mrs. Redmond is a 53-year-old right-handed woman who has just suffered a thrombotic stroke in the posterior watershed region of her left middle cerebral artery. Describe the probable nature and magnitude of their impairments, and describe any differences

that you might expect in their neurologic recovery.

Question 1-2 Mr. Carillo arrives in the emergency room complaining of double vision, slurred speech, weakness in his left arm, back pain, and a severe headache. He states that he has been in good health for the last several years except for mild hypertension, for which he takes medications, and he denies previous episodes suggestive of neurologic problems. He states that he works as a mechanic in a local garage and that his symptoms began shortly before lunchtime. He denies falling or any workplace accidents. He states that the back pain began as he was helping a co-worker move a heavy transmission, but that he noticed no other symptoms at that time. At lunch about an hour later his head began to ache. He finished his lunch but noticed left-arm weakness as he began work. His headache became progressively worse, and he notified his supervisor, who brought him to the emergency room. What happened to create Mr. Carillo's symptoms?

Question 1-3 Patients who are experiencing subfalcine herniation often complain of weakness and sensory loss in one leg. Why does this symptom appear? Which leg will be affected?

Question 1-4 Harry Lang, age 46, appeared at his dentist's office (Dr. Payne) complaining of increased sensitivity to heat and cold in his left upper molars. He reported that he had had some sensitivity to heat and cold in the affected teeth for many months, but that within the past day the sensitivity had suddenly increased to the point that either hot or cold substances touching the teeth caused sudden, stabbing pain that radiated from his jaw up into his left cheek. "It feels like someone ran a red-hot poker up inside my head," he explained. Harry's dentist checked Harry's teeth and found moderate abrasion at and above the gum line in the affected teeth. He explained to Harry that the abraded areas probably permitted heat and cold to reach the nerves within the teeth, and recommended that Harry switch to a toothpaste for sensitive teeth. Harry switched to the recommended toothpaste, but his symptoms persisted. He called his dentist, who told Harry, "Well, I guess you'll just have to live with it." Harry decided to see Dr. Luck, another dentist. Harry described his symptoms to Dr. Luck, and after examining Harry, Dr. Luck recommended that Harry see a neurologist. Why do you think Dr. Luck made that recommendation?

Question 1-5 There is an interesting difference between the United States and England in the laterality of Bell's palsy (paralysis of muscles on one side of the face, caused by inflammation or damage in the facial nerve—CN 7). In the United States Bell's palsy affects the left side of the face significantly more often than it affects the right side of the face. In England Bell's palsy affects the right side of the face significantly more often than it affects the left side of the face. What might explain this puzzling phenomenon?

2

Neurologic Assessment

Most patients with neurogenic communication disorders are examined by a physician (usually a neurologist) before they arrive at the speech-language pathologist's door. The physician's report of the examination provides important information about the origin, nature, and potential course of the neurologic problems underlying the patient's communication disorders. The neurologist's report of the examination of the patient is an important part of the patient's medical record. This chapter provides an overview of how the neurologist goes about examining a patient and the kinds of information the neurologist gathers in the examination.

The neurologist typically begins by interviewing the patient and family members to find out what brought the patient to the neurologist's attention, how the symptoms first expressed themselves, and how they changed over time. Then the neurologist evaluates the patient's motor, sensory, and mental status. Finally, the neurologist may or-der laboratory tests or imaging studies to answer unresolved questions about the nature and severity of the patient's nervous system pathology.

> One could substitute "speech-language pathologist" for "neurologist" in the preceding paragraph because the diagnostic routine for neurogenic communication disorders follows the same format. Substituting "tests of communicative ability" for "laboratory tests" makes the paragraph fit the speech-language pathologist's typical diagnostic routine.

THE INTERVIEW AND PHYSICAL EXAMINATION
Symptom Development

Many diseases and pathologic processes exhibit characteristic progressions of symptom development that point toward a diagnosis. Gradual and uninterrupted development of symptoms over months to years may suggest a slowly progressive degenerative disease such as Huntington's chorea or a slowly growing tumor. Rapid and uninterrupted development of symptoms over days to weeks may suggest an infection, a rapidly growing tumor, or a rapidly progressive degenerative disease such as amyotrophic lateral sclerosis. Rapid development of symptoms over minutes to hours suggests occlusive vascular disease of large arteries. Gradual development of symptoms over months or years with periods of remission ranging from weeks to months suggests occlusive vascular disease of small arteries or a slowly developing degenerative disease such as multiple sclerosis (Figure 2-1).

Family History

Some neurologic diseases are hereditary or familial. (*Hereditary* diseases have a definite genetic inheritance pattern; *familial* diseases have a greater than expected occurrence in families but do not exhibit a definite inheritance pattern.) Several progressive neurologic diseases are hereditary (e.g., Huntington's disease, myotonic dystrophy, Friedreich's ataxia). Some dementing illnesses and some forms of epilepsy may be familial. When a disease is hereditary and the inheritance pattern is known, the family history and the patient's complaints may lead directly to a diagnosis. When a disease is known to exhibit familial patterns, the history may point

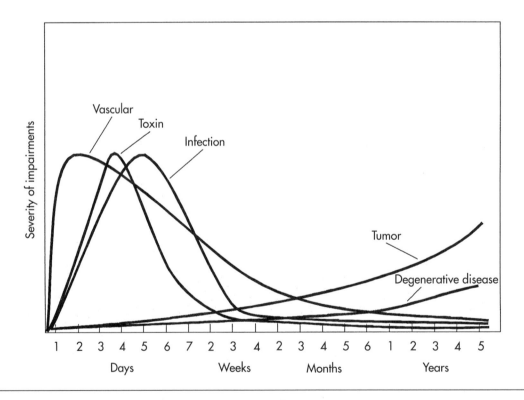

Figure 2-1 ■ Progression of symptoms in major categories of neurologic disease. The curves represent overall trends. Specific diseases within a category may differ somewhat from the trend for the category in which the disease is located. For example, multiple sclerosis is a degenerative disease with an overall pattern of gradual increasing severity, but there are periods of exacerbation and remission within this overall pattern.

to a probable diagnosis, in which case the patient's symptoms and the results of the neurologic examination and laboratory tests serve primarily to confirm or refute the diagnosis.

THE NEUROLOGIC EXAMINATION

In the neurologic examination the neurologist systematically evaluates the function of each part of the nervous system. The neurologist assimilates, integrates, and analyzes information from the patient's medical history, the patient's current symptoms and complaints, and the neurologic examination to arrive at a diagnosis of the nature and location of nervous system pathology. There is no standard neurologic examination, and different neurologists go about the examination in different ways, but all cover the major components of the nervous system—the motor system, the sensory system, equilibrium, and consciousness and mentation. Most begin with assessment of the motor and sensory functions served by the cranial nerves.

The Cranial Nerves

History and Current Complaints Patients with pathology affecting cranial nerves or the sensory branches of mixed cranial nerves typically complain of diminished or distorted sensation. Some patients report sensory hallucinations in the modality of the affected cranial nerve. Patients with pathology affecting motor branches of cranial nerves complain of diminished strength or paralysis (sometimes called *palsy*) of the muscles served by the nerve. Cranial nerve or cranial nerve nucleus pathology creates motor and sensory deficits on the same side of the body as the damaged nerve or nucleus. When the pathology lies in fibers connecting the cranial nerve or its nucleus to the brain (the corticobulbar tract), motor and sensory impairments are contralateral to the damaged nerve fibers.

Testing Cranial Nerve Function The neurologist typically begins examination of the cranial nerves at the top, with CN 1, and works

A general rule: central nervous system damage to motor or sensory nerves above the medulla (where pyramidal fibers decussate) causes impairment on the side of the body contralateral to the damage. Central nervous system damage to motor or sensory nerves below the medulla causes impairment on the same side of the body as the damage.

down to CN 12. The neurologist may forego evaluation of the *olfactory nerve* (CN 1) in routine neurologic examinations unless there is reason to believe that the olfactory nerve has been injured. Injury to the olfactory nerve causes loss of the sense of smell (*anosmia*). If the neurologist suspects olfactory nerve injury, he or she tests its function by asking the patient to identify odors such as cloves, peppermint, coffee, or tobacco.

Most injuries to the olfactory nerve are caused by traumatic injuries, especially falls in which the back of the head strikes a hard surface. The impact stretches and shears the olfactory nerves. The patient loses the sense of smell and also loses appreciation of complex taste sensations, which depend on olfaction. The patient retains perception of elementary taste sensations—sweet, sour, salty, and bitter—which depend on sensory receptors on the tongue. Occasionally a frontal lobe tumor may press on the olfactory bulb and cause loss of the sense of smell.

The *optic nerve* (CN 2) carries visual information from the eyes to the visual cortex. Pathology affecting the optic nerve may cause loss of visual acuity, blindness in portions of the visual field, and (sometimes) impairment of color vision, especially red and green. Sensory information transmitted by the optic nerve serves to elicit the *pupillary light reflex* (constriction of the pupil when a bright light is shined on the eye). The muscles that accomplish the pupillary reflex are innervated by CN 3.

The neurologist evaluates the function of the optic nerve by testing the patient's visual acuity, color vision (sometimes), and visual fields (see p. 59). The neurologist also estimates the size of the patient's pupils, notes whether they are equal or unequal in size, and tests their responsiveness to light (the pupillary reflex).

The neurologist uses an ophthalmoscope to evaluate the condition of the optic disk (a yellowish, oval region of the retina located at the back of the eyeball). Examining the optic disc provides information about a variety of conditions, most of which do not involve the optic nerve. Optic disk swelling (*papilledema*) may suggest increased intracranial pressure, local inflammation, or an ischemic condition. Fading (*pallor*) of the optic disk and impaired visual acuity or visual field blindness may suggest inflammation, nutritional deficiency, degenerative disease, or optic atrophy, as in optic nerve compression.

Next the neurologist tests cranial nerves that innervate the external muscles of the eyes (the muscles are called, collectively, the *extraocular muscles*). The extraocular muscles are served by three cranial nerves—the *oculomotor* nerve (CN 3), the *trochlear* nerve (CN 4), and the *abducens* nerve (CN 6). The extraocular muscles act together to move the eyes laterally and vertically and to keep the eyes fixated on the same spatial location. At rest, equal and opposing actions of the extraocular muscles (six for each eye) keep the eyes in midline position, looking straight ahead. When the eyes move, the extraocular muscles act together to keep the eyes moving in synchrony.

When the function of an extraocular muscle is disrupted (a condition called *ophthalmoplegia*), the eye served by the affected muscle cannot be moved in the direction of the muscle and may, at rest, deviate in the opposite direction because of the unopposed action of the other extraocular muscles. Patients with extraocular muscle weakness or paralysis often complain of double vision (*diplopia*) because the affected

eye is not looking in the same direction as the unaffected eye. The diplopia often disappears when the patient looks in the direction in which the affected eye deviates because that brings the two eyes into alignment.

Injury to the oculomotor nerve (CN 3) causes the eyelid on the affected side to droop (*ptosis*) because the muscles that raise the eyelid are paralyzed. Oculomotor nerve injury also causes chronic downward and outward deviation of the affected eye because the muscles that rotate the eye upward and inward (the medial rectus, superior rectus, inferior oblique muscles) are paralyzed and do not counteract the action of the lateral rectus muscle, which is innervated by the abducens nerve (CN 6). Patients with oculomotor nerve injury often experience diplopia except when looking downward and outward (when both the affected and unaffected eye are looking in the same direction). The oculomotor nerve innervates the muscle that changes the pupillary opening. Consequently, injury to the oculomotor nerve disrupts the pupillary light reflex and the pupillary accommodation reflex (constriction of the pupils when the eyes converge to focus on a near object).

Injury to the trochlear nerve (CN 4) paralyzes the muscle that moves the eye downward (the superior oblique muscle), causing chronic upward and outward deviation of the affected eye because of the unopposed action of the other extraocular muscles. The patient experiences diplopia when looking down because the affected eye cannot follow the unaffected eye downward. Patients with trochlear nerve injury often have trouble descending stairs because of this diplopia. Some learn to tilt their head down and away from the side of the affected eye, thereby bringing the eyes into alignment and eliminating diplopia.

Injury to the abducens nerve (CN 6) paralyzes the lateral rectus muscle, causing inability to rotate the eye outward. The affected eye deviates inward at rest because of the unopposed action of the other extraocular muscles. The patient experiences diplopia when looking toward

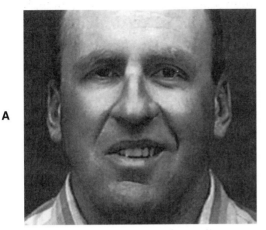
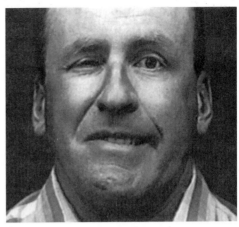

A

B

Figure 2-4 ▪ Patient with right-side facial weakness caused by pathology affecting the right-side facial nerve (CN 7). A, The man is spontaneously smiling. He has slight droop on the right side of his mouth. B, Patient is volitionally retracting his lips. The muscular effort expended in retracting his lips on the right causes his right eye to close. (From Duffy, J.R. [1995]. *Motor speech disorders: substrates, differential diagnosis, and management.* St. Louis: Mosby.)

7th nerve palsy). The neurologist checks for facial nerve damage by asking the patient to wrinkle the forehead, close and open the eyes, pucker, smile, and perform other movements of the facial muscles both passively and against resistance. If the results of the motor examination suggest cranial nerve pathology, the neurologist may test taste sensation in the anterior part of the patient's tongue.

Next the neurologist tests the function of the *acoustic-vestibular* nerve (CN 8). The acoustic (cochlear) branch of CN 8 provides the pathway by which auditory information reaches the brain, and the vestibular branch serves balance and position sense. The neurologist tests the acoustic branch by assessing the patient's hearing acuity for whispered speech, ticking clocks or watches, and the sounds made by tuning forks (which are used to test both air-conduction and bone-conduction hearing). If the patient complains of vertigo, the neurologist may assess the function of the vestibular branch of CN 8 by *caloric testing,* in which water is injected into the ear canal and the appearance of

nystagmus is monitored. Normally, nystagmus appears within about 20 seconds after the water enters the ear canal. If the vestibular branch of CN 8 is compromised, nystagmus may fail to appear, appear later than usual, or disappear earlier than usual.

The neurologic examination becomes more relevant to communication as the neurologist moves on to examine the *glossopharyngeal* nerve (CN 9) and the *vagus* nerve (CN 10). The neurologist tests the sensory functions of the hypoglossal and vagus nerves by evaluating the patient's sensitivity to touch on the posterior wall of the pharynx and the presence of a gag or swallowing reflex when the posterior tongue and

When the glossopharyngeal nerve is affected by pathology, the vagus and the accessory nerves also usually are affected because they travel through the same small opening in the skull. They are tested together because they share control of some muscle groups.

pharynx are stimulated. Diminished or abolished sensation in the posterior pharyngeal wall and diminished or absent gag and swallow reflexes implicate the sensory divisions of CN 9 and CN 10.

Loss of taste sensation in the posterior third of the tongue and loss of the gag reflex implicate the sensory branch of the glossopharyngeal nerve (CN 9). (The sensory branch of the vagus nerve, which is CN 10, carries sensations from the abdominal viscera.) The neurologist evaluates the motor function of CN 9 and CN 10 by asking the patient to swallow and by observing the position of the velum (soft palate). Injury to the hypoglossal nerve causes the midline of the velum to be displaced toward the side away from the injured nerve both at rest and when the patient phonates (because of the unopposed action of the contralateral muscles). Injury to the vagus nerve causes widespread dysfunction of muscles of the soft palate, pharynx, and larynx. Damage to the recurrent laryngeal nerve, which arises from the vagus nerve, causes weakness or paralysis of the ipsilateral vocal fold.

Perception of sweet, sour, salty, and bitter tastes depend on sensory receptors (*taste buds*) in the tongue. The facial nerve (CN 7) innervates taste buds in the anterior two-thirds of the tongue and permits perception of sweet, salty, and sour tastes. The glossopharyngeal nerve (CN 9) innervates taste buds in the posterior one-third of the tongue and permits perception of bitter tastes. A few taste buds are scattered throughout the oral cavity and pharynx. Patients with facial nerve (CN 7) or glossopharyngeal nerve (CN 9) pathology often lose these aspects of taste sensation on one side of the tongue.

The *spinal accessory* nerve (CN 11) controls muscles of the neck and shoulders. The neurologist tests the spinal accessory nerve by assessing the patient's ability to turn the head, to resist the neurologist's attempts to rotate the patient's head, to shrug the shoulders, and to elevate the shoulders against resistance. Injury to CN 11 causes the patient's shoulder on the affected side to droop, interferes with arm movements above the shoulders on the affected side, and interferes with head turning toward the side opposite that of the injured nerve (the head is rotated to the *right* with the *left* sternomastoid muscle).

The *hypoglossal nerve* (CN 12) provides motor input to tongue muscles that protrude the tongue, retract the tongue, and curl the tongue into a convex shape. The neurologist evaluates the function of the hypoglossal nerve by testing the patient's ability to protrude the tongue and move it from side to side, both freely and against resistance. Injury to CN 12 causes the patient's tongue to deviate toward the side of the injured cranial nerve on protrusion. This happens because the muscles that pull the tongue forward on the side of the injured cranial nerve are weak or paralyzed. Injury to CN 12 also prevents the patient from volitionally moving the tongue to the corner of the mouth on the side of the injured nerve and prevents the patient from pushing his or her tongue into the cheek on the affected side (because the muscles that pull the tongue toward that side are weak or paralyzed).

Speech-language pathologists often carry out similar evaluations of cranial nerve function with patients who have speech impairments caused by weakness, paralysis, or incoordination of muscle groups involved in speech.

The neurologist's active testing of muscle strength and movement during evaluation of cranial nerve functions is accompanied by observation of muscles at rest to look for signs of involuntary movements (*fasciculations, fibrillations*) and *atrophy* (wasting away), all of which are signs of compromised innervation. These phenomena are discussed later in this chapter.

Assessing Visual Fields As noted previously, the neurologist's examination of CN 2 (the optic nerve) usually includes assessment of the patient's visual fields. The presence of visual field blindness suggests damage in an optic nerve, the optic tract, or the visual cortex.

> The nerve fibers serving vision are called the *optic nerve* between the eye and the optic chiasm and the *optic tract* from the optic chiasm to the visual cortex. The optic nerve is outside the brain proper, and the optic tract is within the brain substance.

The nature of a patient's visual field blindness provides the neurologist with important clues about the location of the neurologic damage causing the blindness. This is true because of how the human visual system is arranged. In the human visual system, fibers from the right side of each retina project to the visual cortex in the right hemisphere, and fibers from the left side of each retina cross the midline (at the *optic chiasm*) and project to the visual cortex in the left hemisphere (Figure 2-5).

Because light rays travel in straight lines, light rays that pass through the pupils from the right side of visual space strike the left side of each retina (see Figure 2-5). For the same reason, light rays passing through the pupils from the left side of visual space strike the right side of each retina. Information from right-side visual space stimulates optic nerve fibers that innervate the left side of each retina. These optic nerve fibers transmit the information to the visual cortex in the left hemisphere via the optic tract (see Figure 2-5). Information from the left side of visual space stimulates optic nerve fibers that innervate the right side of each retina. These optic nerve fibers transmit the information to the visual cortex in the right hemisphere via the optic tract (see Figure 2-5). In summary:

- Information from right-side visual space goes to the left side of each retina.

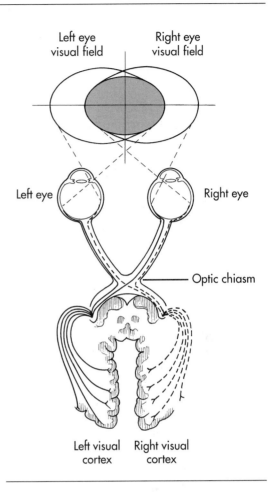

Figure 2-5 ■ **The human visual system. Each hemisphere receives visual input from contralateral visual space. Visual fibers from the nasal (inner) half of the retina in each eye cross at the optic chiasm and project to visual cortex in the contralateral hemisphere. Visual fibers from the temporal (outer) half of each retina do not cross and project to visual cortex in the ipsilateral hemisphere.**

- The left side of each retina connects to visual cortex in the left hemisphere.
- Therefore, information from right-side visual space goes to the left hemisphere.
- Information from left-side visual space goes to the right side of each retina.

- The right side of each retina connects to visual cortex in the right hemisphere.
- Therefore, information from left-side visual space goes to the right hemisphere.

To test a patient's visual fields, the neurologist covers one of the patient's eyes and asks the patient to look straight ahead while the neurologist introduces visual stimuli (usually the neurologist's wiggling index finger) into various locations in the patient's field of vision. Patients with blindness in parts of the visual field do not report stimuli when they are presented in the affected regions of the visual field. Blindness in certain regions of a patient's visual field may suggest (or confirm) the location of the lesion (or lesions) responsible for the patient's deficits.

If a lesion destroys one optic nerve (Figure 2-6, *A*), the patient is blind in that eye. If a lesion destroys the crossing fibers at the optic chiasm (Figure 2-6, *B*), the patient exhibits *bitemporal hemianopia* (blindness in the lateral visual fields for both eyes) because the fibers that transmit visual information from lateral visual space in both eye fields are destroyed. Bitemporal hemianopia is a rare phenomenon, most frequently caused by tumors that press on the optic chiasm.

If a lesion destroys the optic tract posterior to the optic chiasm (Figure 2-6, *C*), the patient is blind in the contralateral visual half-field. Such blindness is called *homonymous hemianopia* (or *hemianopsia*) and occurs following deep lesions in the temporoparietal region. Destruction of the visual cortex in one hemisphere (Figure 2-6, *D*) also causes contralateral homonymous hemianopia.

> *Homonymous* means that the same part of the visual field is affected in each eye. *Hemianopia* means literally "half vision."

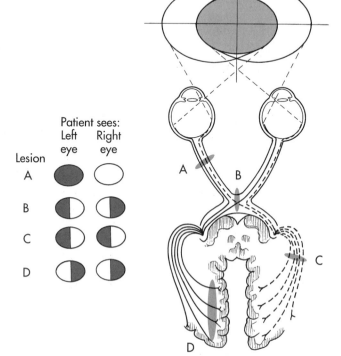

Figure 2-6 ■ **How damage in the human visual system affects vision. A,** Lesions in the optic nerve cause blindness in the eye served by the nerve. **B,** Lesions that destroy the optic chiasm cause loss of vision in both lateral eye fields because they destroy the crossing fibers from the nasal half of the retina in each eye. **C** and **D,** Lesions posterior to the optic chiasm cause contralateral visual field blindness because they interrupt the fibers from the nasal half of the retina in the contralateral eye and the fibers from the temporal half of the retina in the ipsilateral eye.

Sometimes visual field blindness affects less than half of a visual field. Such partial blindness is called *quadrantanopia* (quadrantic hemianopia). Technically, quadrantanopia means that vision in one-fourth of the visual field is lost, but in practice this label is applied to blindness affecting anywhere from about one-third of the visual field to patches comprising one-eighth of the visual field or less. Quadrantanopia typically is caused by damage in the upper or lower optic radiations on their way to the visual cortex. Lesions in the inferior parietal lobe may damage the upper optic radiations and cause blindness in the lower quadrant of the contralateral visual field. Lesions in the temporal lobe may damage the lower optic radiations and cause blindness in the upper quadrant of the contralateral visual field. (Inferiorly placed lesions posterior to the optic chiasm produce contralateral superior quadrant blindness and vice versa.)

> A general principal: lesions posterior to the optic chiasm cause contralateral visual field blindness, and lesions anterior to the optic chiasm cause ipsilateral visual field blindness. Lesions high in the optic radiations produce blindness in the inferior regions of the visual fields, and lesions low in the optic radiations produce blindness in the superior regions of the visual fields.

A neurologist who is uncertain about the presence or extent of a patient's visual field blindness may refer the patient for a specialized test called *perimetry,* in which the patient's visual fields are tested with a specialized instrument called a *perimeter.* In perimetry, small visual stimuli (dots, points of light) are moved through the patient's visual fields in semicircular paths, and the locations at which the patient sees or does not see the stimuli are recorded. Perimetry yields a graphic depiction of the patient's intact and deficient visual fields. Some examples of perimetry plots are provided in Figure 2-7.

A phenomenon called *macular sparing* is common in visual field blindness. The macula is a small circular area near the center of the retina. It is the area of greatest visual acuity. In macular sparing, vision in the center of the visual field for a hemianopic eye (that part of the visual field served by the macula) is spared.

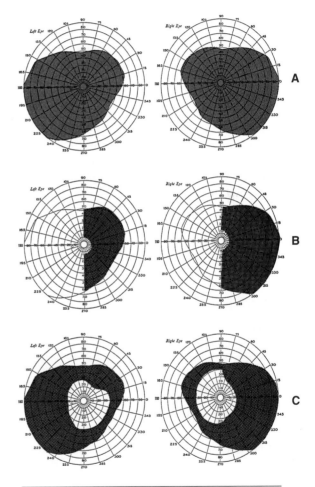

Figure 2-7 ■ **Examples of three perimetry plots. A, Normal visual fields. The lightly shaded areas show the area of vision for each eye. B, Right homonymous hemianopia (blindness in the right visual field of both eyes). The dark areas show the area of blindness for each eye. C, Bitemporal hemianopia (blindness in the lateral visual fields of both eyes).**

Macular sparing is common in hemianopia caused by posterior cerebral artery occlusions wherein the visual cortex in the occipital lobe is damaged. Macular sparing occurs for two reasons. First, a large area of visual cortex is devoted to the macula, relative to the peripheral retina. Second, the distributions of the posterior cerebral artery and the middle cerebral artery overlap near the cortical area assigned to the macula, making collateral blood supply available to this region of cortex. If the optic tract or the visual cortex is destroyed completely, macular sparing does not occur.

Patients with visual field blindness often mistakenly conclude that they have lost vision in the eye on the side of the vision loss, assuming—logically but erroneously—that the right eye sees everything to the right of the midline and that the left eye sees everything to the left of the midline.

> Rosalina Vasquez, who is 62 years old, arrived at her ophthalmologist's office and stated, "I can't see out of my left eye. It started 3 days ago." As part of his examination of Ms. Vasquez, the ophthalmologist assessed her visual fields and found evidence of left homonymous hemianopia. He referred Ms. Vasquez to a neurologist, who confirmed the presence of left hemianopia but also found signs of weakness in her left arm and leg. Subsequent brain imaging tests revealed evidence of a stroke in Ms. Vasquez's right temporal lobe.

Bilateral destruction of the visual cortex causes *cortical blindness*. Patients who are cortically blind cannot discriminate shapes and patterns, but may be sensitive to light and dark. Sometimes the cortically blind patient's perception of simple visual stimuli may be preserved, although the patient usually has difficulty reporting them or incorporating them into mental activity. Occasionally patients with cortical blindness may claim that they can see, producing elaborate confabulations when asked to describe their surroundings. This condition is called *Anton's syndrome*, or *visual anosognosia* (*anosognosia* means *denial of illness*).

When confronted with evidence that he could not see, one 45-year-old cortically blind patient responded, "Well, it's no wonder that I can't see what color your shirt is in such poor light. Take me outside where the light's better, and I'll tell you what color it is."

GENERAL CONCEPTS 2-1

- The pattern of symptom development and the patient's family history often provide information that leads the neurologist toward a diagnosis of the patient's neurologic impairments.
- The neurologist's assessment of cranial nerve functions is an important part of the neurologic examination. The neurologist typically begins the examination with CN 1 and progresses to CN 12.
- The neurologist tests the function of cranial sensory nerves by assessing the patient's perception of visual and auditory stimuli and the patient's sensitivity to touch, pain, and temperature in the face, scalp, and oral structures.
- The neurologist tests the function of cranial motor nerves by testing the integrity of the pupillary, corneal, and jaw-jerk reflexes; by assessing the range of movement of the extraocular muscles; and by assessing the strength and range of movement of the muscles of facial expression, velum, tongue, jaw, neck, and shoulders.
- The neurologist supplements active testing of cranial nerve function with observation of muscles at rest to detect signs of atrophy or involuntary movements.
- Injury to the optic nerve or optic tract produces characteristic patterns of blindness that affect various portions of the patient's visual fields, depending on the location of the injury.
- Injury to the optic nerve (anterior to the optic chiasm) causes blindness in the eye on the side of injury.
- Destruction of one optic tract (posterior to the optic chiasm) causes blindness in the vi-

sual field contralateral to the side of injury (*homonymous hemianopia*).

- Destruction of lower optic radiations causes blindness in the upper part of the contralateral visual field. Destruction of upper optic radiations causes blindness in the lower part of the contralateral visual field (*quadrantanopia*).
- Bilateral destruction of the visual cortex causes *cortical blindness.*

Evaluating the Motor System

History and Current Complaints The patient's description of problems with movement and control help the neurologist to determine the potential involvement of the motor cortex, neural pathways, the cerebellum, the extrapyramidal system, or nerve–muscle junctions—information that subsequently can be embellished by the neurologic examination. Patients with damage in upper motor neurons or the motor cortex usually complain of generalized weakness on one side of the body or of arm, hand, finger, or leg weakness. Patients with leg weakness often report episodes of falling. Patients with cerebellar damage complain more of clumsiness than of weakness—such as slurred speech, clumsiness of the arm, hand, and fingers, and/or leg and foot on both sides of the body. Patients with damage in the basal ganglia typically complain of stiffness, difficulty initiating movement, and tremor of the hands and fingers. Patients with lower motor neuron damage typically complain of weakness in muscles innervated by the damaged cranial or spinal nerves. Patients with disturbances of nerve–muscle transmission usually complain of excessive fatigue, double vision, slurred speech, or a combination of such symptoms.

Evaluating Movement At the beginning of the examination, the neurologist watches the patient enter the room and sit down. The neurologist observes the patient's general appearance, posture, gait, and behavior, and notes characteristics that may suggest abnormalities in the patient's motor system—stooped or slumping posture; slow, effortful, or clumsy movements; diminished spontaneous movement or its converse; hyperactivity; evidence of muscle atrophy (wasting away); and the presence of abnormal movements or unintentional movements. Following this period of observation (which usually takes only a few minutes and may be completed during the interview) the neurologist evaluates the patient's motor system during movement. During this part of the examination, the neurologist systematically evaluates the patient's *reflexes, muscle tone, muscle strength,* and the range over which the patient's muscles can be stretched or flexed (*range of movement*).

Evaluating Reflexes Nervous system pathology may abolish, diminish, or exaggerate reflexes that normally are present and may cause the appearance of abnormal reflexes that should not be present in adults. The neurologist evaluates both *superficial* and *deep* (tendon) reflexes, comparing the presence and magnitude of reflexes on one side of the body to those on the other side. The presence and magnitude of reflexes usually is quantified with a rating scale such as the following:

0	Absent
1+	Diminished
2+	Normal
3+	Brisk (faster, greater amplitude)
4+	Clonus (rhythmic contraction, relaxation)

Superficial reflexes are elicited by stroking, touching, or brushing the surface of body parts. Normal superficial reflexes include the *gag reflex* (gagging or retching when the back of the tongue or the oropharynx is stimulated), the *swallow reflex* (initiation of swallowing when the back of the tongue and pharyngeal walls are stimulated), the *corneal reflex* (blinking when something touches the cornea), and the *plantar flexor reflex* (bending downward of the toes when the sole of the foot is stroked).

Pathologic superficial reflexes include the *plantar extensor (Babinski) reflex,* the *palmar (grasp) reflex,* and the *sucking reflex.* The plantar extensor reflex is elicited by forcefully stroking the sole of the foot, at which time the toes bend upward and fan out, in contrast with the (normal) plantar flexor reflex, in which the toes bend downward and do not fan. The palmar (grasp) reflex is elicited by stroking the palm, which causes the hand to close involuntarily. If the grasp reflex is strong, the patient may be unable voluntarily to release objects held in the affected hand (such as the neurologist's jacket). The sucking reflex, as its name implies, consists of reflexive sucking movements elicited by touching or stroking the patient's lips. Pathologic superficial reflexes sometimes are called *primitive reflexes,* in part because many of them are present in infants and disappear as the infant matures.

Deep reflexes (sometimes called *tendon reflexes* or *deep tendon reflexes*) are elicited by tapping or suddenly stretching muscles or tendons, causing brief contraction of the muscle whose tendon is tapped or stretched. Perhaps the best-known tendon reflex is the *patellar reflex* or knee-jerk reflex, elicited by tapping the patellar tendon, just below the kneecap. Tendon reflexes may be *exaggerated, diminished,* or *absent* (a condition called *areflexia*).

Exaggerated reflexes, either alone or in combination with the appearance of pathologic reflexes, suggests damage in contralateral upper motor neurons (*corticobulbar* and *corticospinal tracts*). The damage releases the reflexes from the inhibitory control ordinarily maintained by the cortex and midbrain structures. Diminished or absent reflexes suggest damage in the peripheral nervous system (lower motor neurons, sensory fibers, the reflex arc) or the muscles themselves.

Evaluating Muscle Tone and Range of Movement The neurologist evaluates *muscle tone* (the tension remaining in a muscle or muscle group when it is voluntarily relaxed) by squeezing individual muscles, moving the patient's limbs while the patient neither assists nor resists the movement (*passive movement*), and sometimes by shaking one or more limbs. The neurologist evaluates *range of movement* by moving each limb through its full range while the patient keeps the muscles relaxed, noting any resistance to movement or the patient's complaints of pain during movement.

Increased resistance to passive movement is called *hypertonia.* There are two major categories of hypertonia—*spasticity* and *rigidity.* In *spasticity* the muscles of the limb are tense, hard, and resist stretching. Spastic muscles are more resistant to fast stretch than to slow stretch. If the examiner begins to move a limb slowly, the limb moves with little resistance. If the examiner abruptly increases the rate at which the limb is moved, the limb's resistance to movement also increases abruptly. This phenomenon is called the *spastic catch.* Spastic muscles are most resistant to movement as passive movement begins. Their resistance diminishes as the limb is moved at a constant rate through its range. This is called the *clasp-knife phenomenon* (which only readers who have used clasp knives may appreciate). Tendon reflexes are intensified by spasticity. Spasticity almost always is caused by a contralateral upper motor neuron lesion, either in the motor cortex or in corticospinal or corticobulbar tracts.

In *rigidity* the relaxed limb evenly resists movement in any direction. The source of the rigidity is increased resting tone of the muscles. Rigid muscles are hard and resist both active and passive movement. Rigidity affects flexor muscles more than extensor muscles, pulling the patient into a stooped posture. Tendon reflexes are not accentuated by rigidity, and their amplitude may be diminished by the patient's increased muscle tone. If rigidity affects the facial muscles, the patient exhibits an unchanging, expressionless, mask-like countenance (called *masked facies*), which is a prominent feature of advanced Parkinson's disease. Rigidity is a prominent characteristic of many extrapyramidal diseases, including Parkinson's disease.

Decreased resistance to passive movement is called *hypotonia* or *flaccidity.* When shaken, flaccid limbs flop to and fro (the *rag doll* phenomenon). Flaccid muscles provide little or no resistance to passive movement. Limbs with flaccid muscles often can be hyperextended. Tendon reflexes usually are diminished by hypotonia. Diminished muscle tone arises from many diseases affecting the nervous system or muscles, so the presence of hypotonia does not in itself point to a specific disease. However, hypotonia of muscles within the distribution of a specific cranial nerve or spinal nerve almost always signifies damage to the nerve or its nucleus (lower motor neuron).

Evaluating Muscle Strength The neurologist assesses the strength of the patient's muscles by asking the patient to move them, freely and against resistance, and to maintain their contraction against pressure exerted by the neurologist. The strength of muscle groups usually is quantified on a 6-point (0–5) scale recommended by the Medical Research Council:

5 Normal strength
4 Active movement against resistance and gravity
3 Active movement against gravity but not resistance
2 Active movement only when gravity is eliminated
1 Flicker or trace of contraction
0 No contraction.

Muscle weakness can be caused by damage in the brain, in the brain stem, in the spinal cord, in the extrapyramidal system, in the neuromuscular junction, or in the muscles themselves. Damage in the brain, brain stem, or spinal cord above the level at which corticobulbar or corticospinal fibers decussate (damage in upper motor neurons) causes motor impairments on the contralateral side of the body. Usually numerous muscle groups or all the muscles on one side of the body are affected, and the affected muscles are spastic.

Damage in cranial nerves or spinal nerves (lower motor neurons) typically produces hypotonia and weakness or flaccid paralysis on the same side as the affected nerves. For example, damage to cranial nerve 7 (the facial nerve) causes flaccid paralysis in the muscles of the lower face on the same side as the nerve damage, but the muscles of the lower face on the other side are unaffected. See Table 2-2 for a summary of differences in neurologic signs between upper motor neuron pathology and lower motor neuron pathology.

When pathology is caused by diseases that affect the muscles (*myopathy*) or the neuromuscular junctions, there usually is no right–left division between affected and unaffected muscles. Instead, the patient exhibits general weakness or weakness of large muscle groups in which the weakness is not related to the midline of the

---

T A B L E   2 - 2

Differences in neurologic signs between upper motor neuron pathology and lower motor neuron pathology

	Lower motor neuron	Upper motor neuron
Weakness, paralysis	Flaccid	Spastic
Atrophy	Present*	Absent†
Tendon reflexes	Diminished or absent	Increased
Pathologic reflexes‡	Absent	Present
Fasciculations, fibrillations	Often present	Absent

*Muscle atrophy develops over time and may not be obvious in early stages.
†Muscle atrophy sometimes develops because of prolonged disuse, but muscles remain spastic.
‡Plantar extensor (Babinski) reflex, grasp reflex, sucking reflex, and so on.

body. (The muscles in the upper limbs may be weaker than those in the lower limbs, or distal muscles in the hands and feet may be affected more than proximal muscles, and so forth.)

> In general, motor impairments that respect the midline of the body (affecting only muscles on one side of the midline) suggest nervous system damage, rather than damage to muscles themselves. Central nervous system damage typically causes motor impairments contralateral to the damage, and peripheral nervous system damage typically causes motor impairments ipsilateral to the damage.

Paralysis or severe weakness of one limb is called monoplegia. Paralysis of both limbs on the same side is called *hemiplegia.* Paralysis of both legs is called *paraplegia,* and paralysis of all four limbs is called *quadriplegia.* The suffix denoting weakness is *paresis.* Substituting *paresis* for *plegia* provides equivalent terminology denoting limb weakness (monoparesis, hemiparesis, paraparesis, and quadriparesis).

> Paraplegia and quadriplegia almost always are caused by spinal cord pathology (trauma, infection, vascular accidents). Paraplegia is caused by pathology affecting the lumbar–sacral spine, and quadriplegia is caused by pathology affecting the cervical spine. Monoplegia usually is caused by upper motor neuron damage, but occasionally results from focal spinal cord pathology. Hemiplegia almost always is caused by upper motor neuron damage.

Evaluating Volitional Movements The neurologist evaluates the *speed, accuracy,* and *coordination* of the patient's volitional movements. *Slowness of volitional movements* can come from many sources. Common nervous system sources include lower motor neuron disease (flaccidity), upper motor neuron disease (spasticity), extrapyramidal disease (rigidity), and peripheral myopathy (weakness). *Diminished accuracy* of volitional movements (in the absence of deficits in strength or sensation that compromise movement accuracy) usually suggests damage in the cerebellum or the extrapyramidal system. Besides producing overall slowing of volitional movements, extrapyramidal damage frequently produces involuntary movements called *dyskinesia.* These involuntary movements are superimposed on (and sometimes replace) volitional movements. The form of the involuntary movements often provides helpful clues regarding the part of the nervous system that has been damaged.

Tremor is a pattern of cyclic, small-amplitude, involuntary movements primarily affecting the arms, legs, and head. Distal muscles (those farthest from the trunk) are more likely to exhibit tremor than proximal muscles (those nearest the trunk). Some tremor is present in normal muscles (called *benign* or *physiological* tremor) but is so slight that it is not usually visible. Pathologic tremor may appear in relaxed muscles (*resting tremor*), during certain postures (*postural tremor*), or only during movement (*intention tremor*). *Resting tremor* is a characteristic sign of Parkinson's disease. It often begins in the patient's hand or foot and over the years gradually spreads to other muscle groups, causing rhythmic flexion and extension of the fingers, hands, feet, or both. When it affects the fingers, the thumb and fingers characteristically are flexed and thumbtips rub against fingertips, giving the tremor its characteristic *pill-rolling* quality.

Chorea (from the Greek word for *dance*) refers to quick, forceful, and abrupt involuntary movements (*choreiform movements*) that disappear during sleep. When chorea is mild, patients may appear persistently restless, and their choreiform movements may resemble clumsy volitional movements. At rest, the muscles of patients with chorea tend to be hypotonic, but muscle strength usually is normal. However, sustained muscle contraction may be interrupted by involuntary movements, leading to a phenomenon called *milkmaid's grasp,* when hand muscles are affected.

> Some patients with chorea attempt to disguise the choreiform movements by incorporating them into voluntary movements. However, the strategy usually fails because the combination of voluntary and involuntary movements usually appears grotesque and exaggerated.

Ballism (or *hemiballism* if it affects only one side of the body) is an extreme form of chorea. In ballism, the involuntary limb movements are violent and the limbs are flung wildly about, creating risk of injury to the patient's limbs and to anyone who may be nearby. Like other varieties of pathologic movements, choreiform movements disappear during sleep. Chorea often is a manifestation of hereditary neurologic disease, but sometimes appears as a consequence of anoxia, brain hemorrhage, toxemia, cerebrovascular disorders, or damage in the extrapyramidal system. Its presence suggests damage in the basal ganglia or other parts of the extrapyramidal system.

Athetosis refers to a condition in which resting muscle groups are disturbed by slow, writhing, sinuous movements that increase with emotional tension and disappear during sleep. Athetosis is especially prominent in the proximal limb muscles and neck muscles. Athetoid movements are involuntary, purposeless, and often appear to flow from one muscle group to another. Athetoid movements often are associated with chorea, in which case the disorder may be called *choreoathetosis.* Athetosis often is caused by birth trauma or anoxia that causes damage in the basal ganglia or extrapyramidal system.

> *Athetosis* is from a Greek word meaning *without position or place.*

Dystonia is a condition in which muscle groups (especially those in the limbs and neck) maintain abnormal involuntary contractions or postures over long durations. Because the contractions persist, and because they often cause gross postural deformation, dystonia is sometimes called *torsion spasm.* In its less severe forms, dystonia may resemble athetosis, and the terms are sometimes used interchangeably. Dystonia is caused by damage in the basal ganglia or other parts of the extrapyramidal system. Dystonia often is inherited, but may occur in conjunction with acquired neurologic diseases. It sometimes occurs as a consequence of prolonged medication (or overmedication) with various psychoactive drugs (such as tranquilizers) or drugs for the control of Parkinson's disease (such as levodopa).

In *myoclonus,* individual muscle groups contract in short irregular bursts, causing abrupt, brief, twitching movements of the muscle group. The contractions may range from nearly imperceptible movements of a single muscle group to overt movements involving multiple muscle groups, which cause overt movement of limb, neck, or facial muscles. Myoclonic movements typically are irregular in duration and rate and are most easily observed when the affected muscles are at rest. Persisting myoclonus occurs in epilepsy, dementia, and some cerebellar disorders. Occasional episodes of myoclonus sometimes occur in persons with no detectable nervous system disease (a jumping leg, the whole-body jerk of light sleep).

Fasciculations are fine, rapid, irregular, twitching movements caused by contractions of groups of muscle fibers. The contractions are not large enough to cause overt limb, head, or facial movements, but are observable as dimpling or rippling of the skin over the fasciculating muscle fibers. The presence of fasciculations in combination with weakness, muscle atrophy, or both suggests damage in lower motor neurons (spinal nerves or anterior horn cells in the spinal cord, cranial nerves or cranial nerve nuclei in the brain stem). Transient fasciculations often are experienced by normal persons and, when not accompanied by muscle weakness or atrophy, are not considered a sign of nervous system pathology.

Fibrillations are contractions of a single muscle fiber or a small group of fibers. They are too small to be seen but are measurable with sensitive instruments. Like fasciculations, they may signify damage in lower motor neurons, and like fasciculations, they often occur in persons without nervous system *pathology*.

Persistent fasciculations or persistent fibrillations usually are signs of lower motor neuron (cranial nerve or spinal nerve) pathology. They often are the first signs of lower motor neuron disease.

Tics (sometimes called *habit spasms*) are stereotypic repetitive movements such as blinking, coughing, clearing the throat, or sniffing that appear when the individual is nervous or under stress. Tics can be volitionally inhibited, but when the individual's attention is no longer focused on the tic, they reappear. Tics have no known relationship to nervous system pathology. The characteristics of abnormal movements and their common sources are summarized in Table 2-3.

Central nervous system pathology sometimes causes clumsiness or incoordination of volitional movements in the presence of normal muscle strength—a condition called *ataxia*. Several forms of ataxia have been described in the neurology literature, but by far the most frequently occurring is *cerebellar ataxia* (caused, not surprisingly, by cerebellar damage). In cerebellar ataxia the average speed and velocity of ataxic movements may be normal, but acceleration at the beginning of movements is slowed and braking at the end of movements lags, causing overshoot of the target. If an ataxic patient is asked to hold a limb in position against resistance and the resistance is abruptly removed, the ataxic patient

characteristically is unable to relax the muscles quickly, and the limb swings uncontrollably in the direction of the previous resistance (the *rebound* phenomenon).

Complex volitional movements or movements requiring rapid changes in direction are the most dramatically affected by ataxia. Complex movements often are broken down into a succession of small individual movements with a jerky, segmented quality (called *decomposition of movement*). Rapid alternating movements—such as alternately turning the hands palm up, then palm down—are slow and awkward, and their range and force are distorted (*dysmetria*). Volitional limb movements often are compromised by a slow, coarse tremor, which appears as a rhythmic oscillation at right angles to the direction of the movement.

Ataxia comes from Greek and means, literally, *out of order.*

Evaluating Gait If a patient can stand and walk, observation of the patient's standing and walking often provides screening information that may help the neurologist determine the nature and location of a patient's nervous system pathology.

Patients with *unilateral corticospinal damage* (hemiplegia, severe hemiparesis) walk with what is called *circumducted gait*—the patient tilts toward the nonaffected side and swings the paralyzed leg out and forward from the hip without flexing the knee (this movement is called *circumduction* of the leg). The patient's spastic arm is flexed and held close to the body. Patients with mild hemiparesis may swing the affected leg normally, but drag the foot because of weakness in the muscles that lift the leg. (These patients often become regular customers at a shoe repair shop because the shoe on the affected side wears excessively.)

Patients with *lower motor neuron disease* or *peripheral myopathy* may have difficulty standing

T A B L E   2 - 3

Characteristics and common causes of abnormal movements. Tremor, chorea, athetosis, dystonia, and myoclonus usually are associated with extrapyramidal system pathology. Fasciculations and fibrillations usually are associated with lower motor neuron (cranial nerve, spinal nerve) pathology.

Disorder	Characteristics	Frequent causes
Intention tremor	Slow (3-5 cycles per second). Appears during volitional movement or is accentuated by it.	Cerebellar pathology. Sometimes toxicity, medications.
Resting tremor	Moderate rate (4-6 cycles per second). Present when muscles are at rest; diminishes or disappears during volitional movements.	Extrapyramidal disease, especially Parkinson's disease. Sometimes heavy-metal poisoning.
Chorea	Quick, irregular muscle contractions occurring involuntarily and unpredictably in different muscle groups.	Basal ganglia or extrapyramidal pathology caused by hereditary diseases, drug toxicity, anoxia, cerebrovascular disorders.
Athetosis	Slow, sinuous, writhing movements. May move from muscle group to muscle group. Increase with emotional tension. Disappear during sleep.	Pathology affecting basal ganglia and extrapyramidal system. Drug toxicity, anoxia.
Dystonia	Sustained involuntary contractions of muscle groups, often causing postural distortion (torsion spasm).	Pathology affecting basal ganglia and extrapyramidal system. Drug toxicity, anoxia.
Myoclonus	Abrupt, rapid, nonrhythmic twitching movements of individual muscle groups. Often large enough to cause movements of limbs or other body parts.	Occasionally occurs in healthy persons. Extrapyramidal disease, metabolic disorders, infectious disease.
Fasciculations	Rapid, irregular, small, twitching movements of small groups of muscle fibers. Do not cause overt movement but can be seen by dimpling or rippling of skin over affected muscles.	Occasional fasciculations are common in healthy persons. Chronic fasciculations may be caused by degenerative diseases of anterior horn cells, spinal nerve compression, peripheral nerve disease.
Fibrillations	Microscopic contractions of small groups of muscle fibers.	Occasional fibrillations are common in healthy persons. Chronic fibrillations may be caused by primary muscle disease, anterior horn cell disease, spinal nerve disease.
Tics (habit spasms)	Stereotypic behaviors (e.g., blinking, coughing, throat clearing) appearing when the individual is under stress.	Not known to be related to nervous system pathology.

and may be unable to maintain erect posture if leg and hip muscles are affected. If the muscles in the front of the lower leg are affected, the patient may exhibit *foot drop,* in which the toes hang down as the foot is lifted, leading the patient to lift the leg abnormally high to allow the toes to clear the ground (*steppage gait*). If the patient's trunk and hip muscles are involved, the patient may exhibit *waddling gait,* caused by tipping the pelvis toward the non-weightbearing side.

> Patients with impaired position sense in the legs also may exhibit steppage gait. They lift their feet higher than necessary because they cannot tell how far their foot is lifted. However, their toes do not dangle as they step.

Patients with *extrapyramidal damage* may exhibit disruptions in sitting and standing posture and in walking because of dyskinesia. Patients with *chorea,* if they can walk at all, do so in irregular fashion, their progress interrupted by sudden dipping and lurching produced by irregular and involuntary contractions in legs and trunk muscles.

> The irregular dipping and lurching walking style of patients with chorea sometimes resembles the movements in some forms of dance, leading some practitioners to label it *dancing gait.*

Patients with *athetosis* and some patients with *dystonia* may have difficulty maintaining erect posture because of slow, sinuous, and writhing movements of the arms and legs. (Patients with severe athetosis or dystonia usually cannot stand or walk unaided.) Patients with *Parkinson's disease* assume a stooped, forward-leaning posture on standing and, when asked to walk, often experience difficulty starting and stopping. The patient with Parkinson's disease

typically shuffles for a few steps before making more normal, but still shortened, strides. Occasionally the Parkinson's patient's steps become very short and rapid, until the patient is nearly running in tiny shuffling steps (called *festinating gait*).

Patients with *cerebellar disease* who can walk typically do so with a broadbased stance with feet wide apart. Their steps are clumsy and irregular both in length and rhythm, and they lurch from side to side. They turn with difficulty and have a tendency to fall to one side. Walking heel-to-toe is extremely difficult and usually impossible for these patients.

> Because the clumsy, staggering gait of patients with cerebellar disease resembles that of intoxicated people, they are sometimes mistakenly thought to be intoxicated by those they meet in public.

GENERAL CONCEPTS 2-2

- The neurologist evaluates the integrity of the patient's motor system by evaluating *reflexes, muscle tone, muscle strength,* and *range of movement.*
- Exaggerated reflexes or the appearance of primitive reflexes suggest damage in *upper motor neurons* (corticobulbar or corticospinal tracts). Diminished reflexes suggest damage in *lower motor neurons* (cranial nerves, spinal nerves).
- *Muscle spasticity* suggests injury to upper motor neurons. *Muscle flaccidity* suggests injury to lower motor neurons, neuromuscular junctions, or the muscles themselves. *Muscle rigidity* suggests injury to the extrapyramidal system.
- Injury to upper motor neurons *above the medulla* (where upper motor neurons decussate) causes *contralateral muscle weakness* and *exaggerated reflexes.* Injury to upper motor neurons in the *brain stem or spinal cord* (after decussation) causes *same-side muscle weakness* and *exaggerated reflexes.*

- Injury to *lower motor neurons* (cranial nerves, spinal nerves, and their nuclei) causes *same-side muscle weakness* and *diminished reflexes.*
- *Extrapyramidal damage* often produces *involuntary movements* (dyskinesia).
- *Tremor* is characterized by rhythmic, small-amplitude movements. Resting tremor is a sign of Parkinson's disease.
- *Chorea* is characterized by quick, forceful, and abrupt involuntary movements.
- *Athetosis* is characterized by slow, writhing, sinuous involuntary movements.
- *Dystonia* is characterized by prolonged involuntary contractions of muscle groups.
- In *myoclonus* individual muscles contract in short, irregular bursts.
- *Fasciculations* are fine, rapid, irregular, visible contractions of small groups of muscle fibers.
- *Fibrillations* are irregular contractions of individual muscle fibers or small groups of fibers that are too small to be seen.
- *Cerebellar injury* often causes disruptions in the force, velocity, and targeting of movements (*ataxia*) causing jerky, segmented movements (*decomposition of movement*).
- Patients with hemiplegia or severe hemiparesis often walk with *circumducted gait.* Patients with lower motor neuron disease or peripheral myopathy often walk with *steppage gait* or *waddling gait.* When patients with dyskinesia walk, their progress is interrupted by involuntary movements. Patients with Parkinson's disease often walk with *festinating gait.*

Evaluating Somesthetic Sensation

History and Current Complaints Patients with pathology in the regions serving somesthetic (bodily) sensation may complain of *pain, numbness,* or *abnormal sensations.* Of the three, pain usually poses the most difficult diagnostic problem. Pain is one of the body's responses to tissue damage. It is an important symptom in many diseases, not only those involving the nervous system. However, not all pain is a sign of disease, and not all pain is a consequence of tissue damage (e.g., the pain associated with muscle cramps, intestinal gas pains, and most headaches).

The patient's history usually provides the neurologist with clues to the cause of the pain, and the neurologic examination defines the extent to which the pain is caused by nervous system involvement. Knowing what relieves or exacerbates the pain may help the neurologist determine its source. When pain is exacerbated with movement or effort, or if it changes with changes in posture, its source may be mechanical (compression of nerves, inflammation of joints). If the pain is unaffected by movement, effort, or posture, its source may be inflammation of peripheral nerves or lesions affecting sensory pathways in the central nervous system.

Other kinds of unusual sensations also give the neurologist clues to the location and nature of nervous system pathology. Numbness or loss of sensitivity usually points to damage in cranial nerves, spinal nerves, or sensory nerve fiber tracts. Abnormal sensitivity to stimulation (called *hyperesthesia*) or abnormal sensation in the absence of stimulation (e.g., tingling or burning—called *paresthesia)* suggests a disturbance in the peripheral nerves or central sensory pathways. Sensory loss in an entire limb or on one side of the body suggests damage in ascending spinal cord tracts or the sensory cortex (complete loss is called *anesthesia;* partial loss is called *hypesthesia*). Patterns of sensory loss that are inconsistent with what the neurologist knows about the sensory system may suggest a functional, rather than an organic, cause.

Examining Somesthesis The neurologist assesses the patient's somatic sensation by systematic stimulation of sensory receptors. Sensory abnormalities may affect *deep sensation* (from the muscles, tendons, and joints), *superficial sensation* (from the skin), or both. *Deep sensation* includes *joint sense* (the ability to tell the position of the limbs without seeing them) and *sensitivity to vibration. Superficial sensation* includes the perception of *light touch, superficial pain* (pinprick), and *temperature.* Evaluation of these categories of sensation helps the neurologist diagnose pathology affecting the spinal cord. The categories of sensations affected by spinal cord pathology and the parts of the body exhibiting sensory disruption permit the neurologist to predict the level within the spinal cord at which the pathology exists (spinal cord lesions typically produce sensory deficits below the level of the lesion) and to determine if the lesion affects the front, back, middle, or sides of the spinal cord.

Fortunately complete transection of the spinal cord (Figure 2-8) is rare; it is usually the result of traumatic injury. Patients who suffer

spinal cord transection lose all sensation below the level of the transection, are paralyzed in all muscles served by spinal nerves below the level of the transection, and lose bowel and bladder reflexes (these reflexes usually eventually return).

The posterior columns of the spinal cord, which travel up the back of the spinal cord at the midline, carry "well-localized sensations of fine touch, vibration, two-point discrimination, and proprioception (position sense) from skin and joints" (Waxman, 2000). However, some tactile information travels by other pathways. Pathology affecting the posterior half of the spinal cord, including the posterior columns (Figure 2-8), causes impairment of precise tactile sensation (crude tactile sensation remains) plus impairment of vibration and joint sense on both

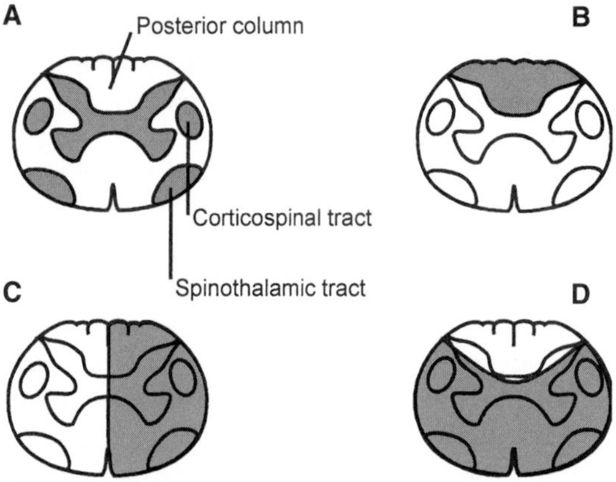

Figure 2-8 ■ **Three spinal cord pathology syndromes. A,** Cross-section of normal spinal cord. **B,** *Posterior column syndrome* causes loss of precise tactile sensation, plus vibration and joint sense. Pain and temperature sensation are spared. **C,** *Hemitransection syndrome (Brown-Sequard syndrome)* causes ipsilateral loss of precise tactile sensation, vibration, and joint sense, plus contralateral loss of pain and temperature sensation. **D,** *Anterior myelopathy* causes loss of pain and temperature sensation and subtle impairment of light touch on both sides of the body. Precise tactile sensation, vibration, and joint sense are preserved. Spastic paraplegia occurs below the level of spinal cord pathology.

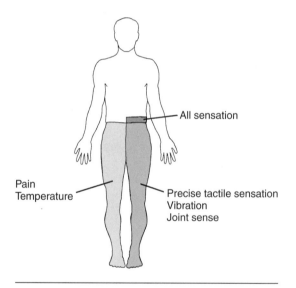

Figure 2-9 ■ **Brown-Sequard (hemitransection) syndrome.** Pain and temperature sensations are lost contralateral to the side of spinal cord injury, and precise tactile sensation, vibration, and joint sense are lost ipsilateral to the side of spinal cord injury. All ipsilateral sensation is lost at the level of the injury, caused by destruction of all sensory fibers entering the spinal cord at that level. Ipsilateral muscles below the level of spinal cord injury are paralyzed.

sides of the body. Pain and temperature sensation are unaffected.

The spinothalamic tracts, which travel up the sides of the spinal cord (one on each side), carry pain and temperature sensations and some light touch sensation. Pathology affecting one side of the spinal cord (*hemitransection syndrome, or Brown-Sequard syndrome;* in Figure 2-8) causes loss of sensation relative to the midline of the body. Precise tactile sensation, vibration, and joint sense are lost at and below the level of the injury ipsilateral to the spinal cord pathology (the posterior columns travel up the spinal cord on the same side as the spinal nerves that connect into them). Pain and temperature sense are lost at and below the level of the injury contralateral to the spinal cord pathology. (Sensory nerves that join the spinothalamic tracts cross the spinal cord and connect into the contralateral spinothalamic tract at approximately the level at which the nerves enter the spinal cord.) The sensory impairments are accompanied by spastic hemiplegia of muscles served by spinal nerves at and below the level of the hemitransection because of destruction of one corticospinal tract (Figure 2-9).

> Sometimes a neurosurgeon will cut nerve fibers in a patient's spinothalamic tract to relieve intractable pain—an operation called cordotomy. The patient also loses temperature sensation below the level of the cordotomy.

Pathology affecting the anterior spinal cord (*anterior myelopathy*) causes loss of pain and temperature sensation and subtle impairment of light touch on both sides of the body, attributable to transection of both spinothalamic tracts. Precise tactile sensation, vibration, and joint sense (conveyed by posterior columns) are preserved. The sensory impairments are accompanied by paralysis of muscles on both sides of the body, at and below the level of the spinal cord pathology, because of damage to both cortico-

spinal tracts (see Figure 2-8). Anterior myelopathy most often is associated with occlusion of the anterior spinal artery, which supplies the anterior two-thirds of the spinal cord.

Regional loss of superficial sensation, rather than loss on one side of the body or loss below a given level of the spinal cord, suggests damage either in cranial nerves or spinal nerves. Knowing the usual distribution of sensory regions for the cranial and spinal nerves (the regions are called *dermatomes*) helps the neurologist decide which cranial or spinal nerves are affected (Figure 2-10). When the area of sensory impairment matches the dermatome for a cranial nerve or a spinal nerve, the neurologist can conclude that the patient's neuropathology involves that cranial nerve or spinal nerve.

> When the sensory fibers of a cranial nerve or a spinal nerve are destroyed, all skin sensation is lost in the central part of the sensory field for the damaged nerve, but some sensation usually remains at the periphery because of overlap with adjacent sensory nerves.

The neurologist may simultaneously stimulate two symmetric points on the body (e.g., simultaneously touch the right forearm and the left forearm) to detect slight impairments in sensory function (a procedure called *double simultaneous stimulation*). If sensory function on one side is compromised, the patient reports only the stimulus on the less impaired side. Inability to detect stimulation on the impaired side during double simultaneous stimulation is called *extinction* and typically is associated with cortical lesions.

Some patients lose the ability to identify objects by touch and palpation although their superficial sensation is unimpaired. They report light touch and pinprick without error, yet cannot identify common objects (such as a comb or a key) when the objects are placed, out of sight, in either hand. Such problems in recognition of

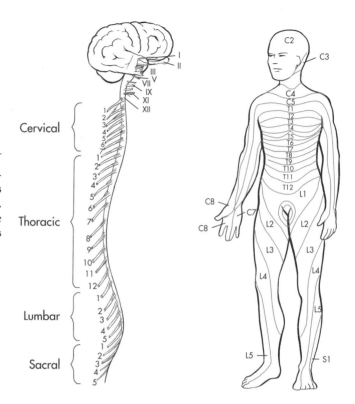

Figure 2-10 ■ **Pattern of skin sensa-**
tion on the human body as it relates
to cranial nerves and spinal nerves.
Each cranial nerve and spinal nerve
serves a specific region (these regions
are called *dermatomes*).

objects by touch are called *astereognosis.*
Astereognosis usually is caused by damage in
the sensory cortex of the contralateral parietal
lobe or adjacent regions.

> *Stereo* is from Greek. One of its meanings is
> *three-dimensional. Gnosis* also is from Greek.
> It translates as *knowledge.*

Evaluating Equilibrium

History and Current Complaints Patients
with impairments of equilibrium usually complain of feeling dizzy or light-headed or report
subjective illusions of movement or changes in
position. When a patient complains of *dizziness,*
the neurologist is likely to ask questions to find
out what the patient means by dizziness. Some
patients may be referring to *vertigo*—the sensa-

tion that the body or the environment is moving
(usually rotating) when it is not. Vertigo usually
is caused by problems in the inner ear, the
vestibular branch of the acoustic nerve (CN 8),
or the brain stem. The presence of persisting or
recurring vertigo may suggest involvement of
the vestibular system or, less frequently, the
brain stem and/or cerebellum. Severe vertigo
with sudden onset often is a result of vascular
problems in the brain stem or cerebellum.
Episodic vertigo may be caused by transient insufficiency of cerebral blood flow or may reflect
Meniere's disease (increased pressure in inner
ear structures that play a role in equilibrium).
Progressive vertigo may be caused by toxicity,
some vitamin deficiencies, or degenerative neurologic disease. Except for mild cases, attacks of
true vertigo are most often accompanied by
nausea, vomiting, pallor, and sweating, and any
head movement increases the severity of the at-

tack. Most patients with true vertigo quickly learn that they must remain immobile during an attack.

Some patients may complain of light-headedness, faintness, or giddiness. Such sensations sometimes are experienced by normal healthy individuals, in which case they may be related to anxiety, hyperventilation, sudden changes in head position, or other transitory conditions.

Evaluating Stance, Gait, and Nystagmus
The patient's *stance, gait,* and *nystagmus* often provide clues that point toward the source of a patient's problems with equilibrium. Patients with disequilibrium typically stand with feet wide apart. When asked to stand with feet together, they are reluctant to do so and may be unwilling or unable to bring their feet completely together. Patients whose disequilibrium is caused by loss of proprioceptive feedback from the legs and feet usually can compensate for the loss by relying on visual input to maintain their balance. When these patients close their eyes, they become increasingly unsteady and may fall (*Romberg's sign*). Patients whose disequilibrium is caused by cerebellar pathology are unsteady with eyes open or closed, although the unsteadiness is worse when they close their eyes.

Patients with disequilibrium typically walk with a wide-based gait. When a patient's disequilibrium is caused by loss of proprioceptive feedback, the patient is likely to walk with *steppage gait* (see "Evaluating Gait" earlier in this chapter). Patients with vestibular disease and patients with loss of proprioceptive feedback usually walk better when provided support (a cane or the examiner's arm), and both do much worse when walking in the dark or with eyes closed. Having patients with disequilibrium walk with feet close together or with heel to toe along a straight line always exaggerates their symptoms.

Nystagmus (abnormal and involuntary oscillation of the eyes, either at rest or when tracking a visual target) commonly is seen in patients with vestibular disorders. *Caloric testing,* in which cold and/or warm water is introduced into the ear canal, often produces characteristic patterns of nystagmus in patients with vestibular pathology. The relationships between the nature of a patient's nystagmus and the nervous system pathology that causes it are too complex to be dealt with here, but these relationships often point directly to the site of the patient's nervous system pathology.

Evaluating Consciousness and Mentation

History and Current Complaints Changes in consciousness or mentation may be caused by a great variety of diseases and pathologic states. In general, changes in mentation or consciousness implicate the brain hemispheres and, to a somewhat lesser extent, the brain stem. Such changes may be experienced by patients with cerebrovascular disease, head injury, alcohol or drug abuse, central nervous system infections, brain tumors, brain abscesses, metabolic disturbances, nutritional deficiencies, dementing illness, and several other diseases and conditions. Consequently, changes in consciousness or mentation, by themselves, rarely point unequivocally to a diagnosis, but when combined with information from the history and neurologic examination, they may point toward a diagnosis with relative certainty. The neurologist may summarize the assessment of a patient's consciousness and mentation by assigning one of several labels that signify, in a general sense, the nature of the patient's condition.

Confusion Patients with confusion (*delirium, acute confusional state*) usually have normal or slightly lowered overall levels of consciousness, but are impaired in their orientation to the environment (where they are, what day it is, and so on). Confused patients' attention spans are short, their memory for recent events is poor, and they cannot think clearly. Acute confusional states are transitory, but a period of confusion may evolve to a more circumscribed but longer-lasting syndrome. For example, a stroke patient may exhibit confusion immediately following the stroke, with the confusion gradually clearing, leaving the patient not confused but aphasic.

• *Lethargy* or *somnolence*. Lethargic or somnolent patients are drowsy, fall asleep at inappropriate times, sleep longer than usual, and are difficult to awaken. Lethargy and somnolence may be transitory and separated by periods of normal alertness and attention, or they may be progressive, ending in coma and death. Confusional states and lethargy come from a variety of causes, including drug or alcohol intoxication or withdrawal, endocrine disturbances, nutritional disorders, infections, cerebrovascular disorders, head trauma, and psychiatric illness.

• *Syncope.* Syncope (fainting spells) denotes transitory loss of consciousness caused by reduced blood supply to the brain. Syncopal episodes usually are accompanied by autonomic irregularities—rapid respiration; rapid and feeble pulse; pallor; perspiration; and cold, clammy skin. Syncope may be caused by diminished cardiac output, abnormally low blood pressure, dehydration, drugs, or stress and anxiety.

• *Fugue state.* Fugue state is a temporary disturbance of consciousness, lasting from a few minutes to several days. During a fugue state the patient engages in normal activities of daily life. However, the patient does not later remember the events or activities that took place during the fugue state. Fugue states are seen in combination with psychiatric illness and (rarely) as a consequence of epilepsy.

• *Amnesia.* Amnesia denotes complete loss of memory for a limited interval. Amnesic patients usually are aware of, and distressed by, the missing memories. Amnesic states are often present in psychiatric illness and are a frequent consequence of traumatic brain injury.

Although *epileptic seizures* include loss of consciousness, they are more dramatic and somewhat better understood, and their relationship to nervous system pathology is more straightforward than the changes in consciousness and mentation described above. Seizures are caused by abnormal patterns of neuronal discharge in the brain. These discharges interfere with normal brain activity and may cause periods of depressed mental function, confusion, uncontrollable muscle contraction and relaxation, and usually loss of consciousness.

Seizures usually signify pathology in the brain hemispheres. Seizures sometimes follow brain injury, alcohol or drug withdrawal, central nervous system infections, hypoglycemia (abnormally low blood sugar), or other diseases. Seizure-like phenomena sometimes occur as a consequence of psychiatric conditions (pseudo-seizures).

Seizures have been divided into two major categories, reflecting differences in what happens to the patient during the seizure:

• *Generalized seizures* are seizures in which the patient loses consciousness. In *tonic-clonic seizures* (sometimes called *grand mal seizures* or *convulsions*) there is massive discharge of neurons in the brain, causing contraction of almost all the muscles of the body, followed by a series of intermittent *clonic jerks.* Tonic-clonic seizures last from 1 to 3 minutes on the average and are never remembered by the patient (perhaps because the patient loses consciousness). In *absence* seizures (formerly called *petit mal* seizures), the loss of consciousness lasts only a few seconds, and the patient usually does not fall. The patient may stare, stop moving and talking, drop things, or move the head and limbs aimlessly and involuntarily.

• *Partial seizures* (sometimes called focal seizures) are seizures in which there is localized discharge of neurons in the brain, with the pattern of discharge varying widely across patients. The patient who experiences a partial seizure usually experiences clonic movements of individual muscle groups but does not lose consciousness, although typically there is some clouding of consciousness and disruption of mental activity. Partial seizures may last for a few seconds to several minutes or even (rarely) hours. The magnitude of the seizure activity is related to how much of the brain is involved in the neuronal discharge. Partial seizures suggest localized areas of abnormal discharge, and generalized seizures suggest that major portions of both brain hemispheres are involved.

Occasionally an individual goes into a state of unremitting seizure activity or experiences a chain of seizures that occurs so frequently that the patient does not regain consciousness in the intervals between seizures. This condition is called *status epilepticus* and is a medical emergency, demanding preservation of the patient's airway and administration of intravenous antiseizure medications.

Evaluating Mental Status Standard neurologic examinations usually provide for rudimentary assessment of the patient's *level of consciousness, attention and concentration, orientation and memory, mood and behavior, thought content,* and *language and speech.* In the neurologist's report of the neurologic examination, the neurologist typically comments on the patient's *level of arousal* (e.g., awake and alert, lethargic, somnolent, stuporous, or comatose) and the patient's *responsiveness to stimulation* (e.g., responsive, unresponsive, appropriate, inappropriate). The neurologist describes the patient's *attention and concentration* in terms of the patient's performance in tasks requiring low levels of mental effort, such as counting backward or reciting the alphabet backward. The neurologist describes patients' *orientation* in terms of their answers to questions about themselves (*person*); where they are (*place*); and day, date, and time of day (*time*). If the patient is considered oriented to person, place, and time, the neurologist's report may describe the patient as *oriented X3.*

The neurologist's report also addresses the patient's *mood and behavior* (e.g., apathetic, elated, depressed, stable, variable). The neurologist describes the patient's *thought content* in terms of its appropriateness and rationality and whether hallucinations or delusions are present. The neurologist tests the patient's *memory* by asking the patient to recall short lists of numbers or words. The neurologist evaluates the patient's *language and speech* by asking the patient to carry out simple spoken commands, repeat words and phrases, name pictures or objects, read words and sentences, and write words and short sentences.

Several more or less standardized screening tests of mental status have been published. One of the most widely used by neurologists is the *Mini Mental State Examination* (MMSE) (Folstein, Folstein, & McHugh, 1975). The MMSE takes from 5 to 10 minutes to administer and contains 11 items to screen *orientation* to time and present location, *immediate memory* for a 3-word list, *attention* (counting backward by 7 or spelling a word backward), object *naming,* phrase *repetition, comprehension* of spoken instructions, *writing* a sentence, and *copying* a geometric figure. Normal adults typically score from 25 to 30 points (of a possible 30). Scores below 25 usually are considered an indication of compromised mental status.

Teng and Chui (1987) published a revision of the MMSE (the *Modified Mini-Mental State Examination: 3MS*) to sample a broader range of performance across a wider range of difficulty and to provide more sensitive scoring than provided for in the MMSE. The 3MS adds four items to the MMSE (*date and place of birth, naming four-legged animals, similarities, delayed recall*) and broadens the range of scores to 0 to 100 by providing scaled scores for original MMSE items and adding scores for the new items. Tombaugh, McDowell, Kristjansson, and Hubley (1996) reported that the MMSE and the 3MS yield comparable results, but that inclusion of a verbal fluency item (*four-legged animals*) in the 3MS increased test sensitivity. Table 2-4 gives examples of items that may be included in screening tests of mental status.

GENERAL CONCEPTS 2-3

- A standard neurologic examination includes evaluation of *deep sensation* (joint sense, deep pain sensation, sensitivity to vibration) and *superficial sensation* (light touch, superficial pain, temperature).
- The distributions of sensory regions for cranial and spinal nerves are called *dermatomes.*
- *Double simultaneous stimulation* may reveal slight impairments in sensory function.
- *Confusion* (delirium, acute confusional state), *lethargy* (somnolence), *syncope,* and *fugue state* represent disturbances of consciousness and mentation. *Amnesia* represents loss of memory for a limited time.
- *Seizures* are caused by abnormal patterns of neuronal discharge in the brain. In *general-ized seizures* and *absence seizures* the patient loses consciousness. In *partial seizures* the patient does not lose consciousness.
- A neurologist's assessment of a patient's mental status usually includes assessment of the patient's *level of consciousness, attention and concentration, orientation and memory, mood and behavior, thought content,* and *language and speech.* The assessment often is conducted using a standard screening test such as the *Mini Mental State Examination.*

LABORATORY TESTS

Laboratory tests provide information about the patient that cannot be obtained from the interview and the physical examination. In addition to standard laboratory tests such as analysis of blood and urine, the neurologist may order special tests to aid in the diagnosis of the patient's neurologic disorder.

TABLE 2-4

Examples of items typically included in screening tests of mental status

Orientation to self	Where were you born? What is the date of your birth?
Orientation to time	What year is it now? What is today's date? What day of the week is it? What time is it right now?
Orientation to place	What state are we in? What city are we in? What is the name of this place? Are we in a (hospital, school, home . . .)?
Memory	Recalling a list of words (typically three words; tested immediately and after one or more intervening tasks).
Attention, concentration	Counting backward from 20. Saying the alphabet backward. Spelling a word backward.
Mental flexibility	Making similarities (e.g., How are a table and a chair alike?).
Naming	Confrontation naming (common objects). Categorical naming (e.g., four-legged animals, articles of clothing).
Repetition	Repeating a word and phrase.
Auditory comprehension	Following sequential commands (e.g., Take this paper in your left hand, fold it in half, and give it to me).
Reading comprehension	Following printed instructions (e.g., Close your eyes. Make a fist.)
Writing	Writing to dictation (e.g., Write on this paper, "I would like to go out.")
Visuospatial ability	Copying simple geometric forms.

Radiologic Imaging Studies

In radiologic imaging studies x-rays are passed through body tissues onto a sheet of photographic film to create a negative image of internal structures. The x-rays pass readily through low-density tissues but are blocked by dense tissues such as bone. Low-density tissues appear as dark areas on the x-ray plate, and higher-density tissues appear as lighter images. Sometimes fluid containing a substance that blocks x-rays (called *contrast medium*) may be injected into internal structures (such as veins or arteries) that ordinarily would not appear on an x-ray image. The images obtained from such tests are said to be *contrast enhanced.*

Standard x-ray images of the skull, spine, or both may provide useful information regarding the probable causes of a patient's symptoms. X-ray images of the skull (skull films) may show fractures, abnormal deposits, or abnormal calcification of structures within the skull (Figure 2-11). X-ray images of the spine (spine films) may provide evidence of congenital deformities, fractures, displacement of intervertebral discs,

degenerative changes, or tumors involving the vertebrae and spinal cord (Figure 2-12).

Cerebral angiography (sometimes called *cerebral arteriography*) is a method by which the veins and arteries of the brain and brain stem can be visualized (Figure 2-13). In this procedure, a contrast medium is injected into one of the arteries supplying blood to the brain (usually a carotid artery, but occasionally a vertebral artery), and a sequence of x-ray images of the head is taken. The contrast medium fills the injected artery and its branches and eventually makes its way into the cerebral veins, so that when the sequential x-ray plates are developed the physician can visualize the rate of circulation through the larger cerebral vessels. (Angiograms do not show the smallest vessels.)

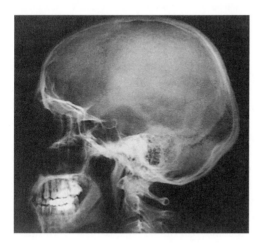

Figure 2-11 ■ **X-ray image of a normal adult skull.** (From Ballinger, P.W. [1995]. *Merrill's atlas of radiographic positions and radiologic procedures,* [8th ed.]. St. Louis: Mosby.)

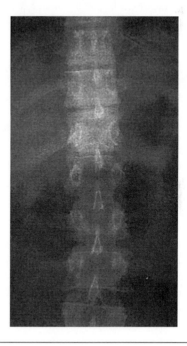

Figure 2-12 ■ **X-ray image of a normal human spine (thoracic and lumbar regions).**

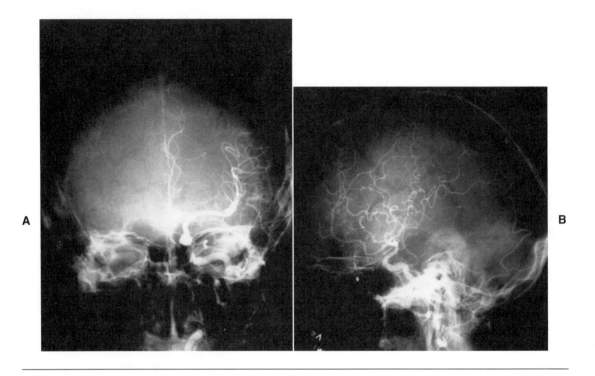

Figure 2-13 ■ **Normal cerebral angiogram. The image on the left (A) is taken from the front of the head. The anterior cerebral artery proceeds upward on the midline, and the middle cerebral artery proceeds laterally and upward on the right side of the image. The image on the right (B) is taken from the side of the head. The middle cerebral artery and portions of the posterior cerebral artery can be seen. The carotid artery is visible in both views.**

Angiograms are useful in detecting occlusions of arteries or their branches because occluded vessels do not fill with contrast medium and are not visible on angiography. Blood vessels that are narrowed but not occluded (a condition called *stenosis)* fill slowly. Slow filling of vessels is detected by evaluating the progress of the contrast medium through the blood vessels from the beginning to the end of the series of x-ray plates. Angiography may show the presence of space-occupying lesions such as tumors or abscesses if the lesion displaces cerebral blood vessels from their customary locations.

A recently developed procedure, called *digital-subtraction angiography,* provides improved image quality and lessens the amount of contrast medium that must be injected into the vascular system. Digital-subtraction angiography uses a computer-averaging technique, in which the signals from nonvascular structures are deleted from the image, yielding an enhanced image of vascular structures (Figure 2-14).

Myelograms, like arteriograms, involve injection of radio-opaque fluid into the central nervous system, but in myelography the fluid is injected into the subarachnoid space around the spinal cord. After the fluid is injected, one or more x-ray images of the spine are taken (Figure 2-15). Myelograms permit visualization of the subarachnoid space surrounding the spinal cord and permit indirect visualization of the spinal cord and spinal nerves, which are silhouetted against the

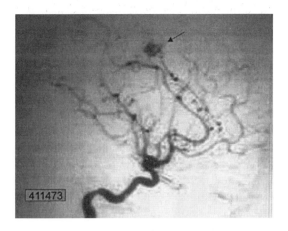

Figure 2-14 ■ **Digital-subtraction angiogram. The middle cerebral artery in the right hemisphere is shown. The angiogram indicates the presence of a vascular malformation in the upper posterior frontal lobe (*arrow*).**

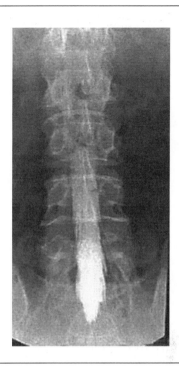

Figure 2-15 ■ **Myelogram of a normal human spine (lumbar and sacral regions). The bright region represents contrast material injected into the space surrounding the spinal cord.**

contrast medium. Myelograms are useful in diagnosing spinal cord or spinal nerve compression, structural abnormalities of the spine, and tumors or deformities of the spinal cord or spinal nerve roots. However, computerized tomography (CT) or magnetic resonance imaging (MRI) scanning of the spine often provides a simpler and less invasive procedure for obtaining the information provided by myelography.

> The neurologist may detect signs of carotid artery stenosis during the physical examination of the patient by putting a stethoscope over the carotid artery and listening to the sound of the blood moving through the artery. Blood moving through a narrowed artery creates an abnormal rushing sound, which can be heard through a stethoscope.

Computerized tomography (also called *CAT scanning*, for *computerized axial tomography*) uses a computer to process and analyze information. In CT scanning the patient is placed in

the center of a circular arrangement of x-ray generators and detectors, which rotate axially around the patient. X-rays pass through the parts of the patient's body being scanned and are picked up by detectors on the other side of the circle. The signals from the detectors are passed on to a computer, which analyzes them and generates photograph-like images that represent cross-sections of the body (Figure 2-16). The scanner moves up or down the body in regular steps so that a series of images representing consecutive "slices" of the body are obtained.

The combination of a narrow beam of x-rays, sensitive detectors, and computer enhancement of signals in CT scanning permit visualization of soft tissues not visible on standard x-ray images. In many instances CT scanning has replaced other tests because it provides better visualiza-

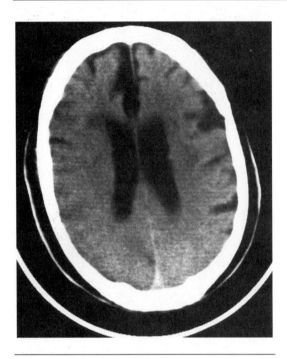

Figure 2-16 ■ CT scan of a patient with a long history of neurologic problems. The lateral ventricles (butterfly-shaped dark areas in center) are enlarged and the sulci are widened, suggesting atrophy of brain tissues. Dark areas in the anterior left hemisphere near the midline and in the lateral aspect of the right frontal lobe suggest regions of tissue destruction, probably by strokes.

tion of internal structures with less risk to the patient. The primary drawback of CT scanning is that it exposes the patient to radiation. Consequently, CT scans are not a routine part of the neurologic examination. Within the past decade several imaging procedures that do not require that the patient be exposed to radiation have been developed. They are described below.

Nonradiologic Imaging Studies

B-mode carotid imaging (sometimes called *echo arteriography*) is a noninvasive technique for visualizing superficial (extracranial) blood vessels with ultrasound. It is used to study the carotid arteries in the neck. A transducer that emits high-frequency sound waves is placed against the neck over the carotid artery. The sound waves are transmitted into the neck, where some are reflected back, depending on the acoustic absorption characteristics of the tissues beneath the transmitter. A detector picks up the reflected sound waves, and a computer analyzes the variations in the waves and generates an image of the tissues scanned. Echo arteriograms are most useful for detecting stenosis or ulceration in the carotid arteries, although they cannot reliably differentiate between severe stenosis and complete occlusion.

Transcranial Doppler ultrasound is an experimental noninvasive technique for measuring blood pressure and flow in the cerebral arteries. High-frequency sound waves are transmitted into the head by a probe attached to a computer. The computer manipulates the characteristics of the sound waves to target a particular blood vessel. If the blood within the vessel is moving, the frequency of the reflected sound waves is altered in a predictable way (the *Doppler effect*). A detector picks up the reflected sound waves and passes them to the computer. The computer analyzes changes in the frequency of the reflected waves and generates a graphic image representing blood pressure and flow within the artery.

> The Doppler effect is experienced in everyday life when a rapidly moving vehicle passes a bystander with horn or siren blaring. As the vehicle passes by, the pitch of the sound made by the horn or siren drops. This happens because the movement of the vehicle away from the listener adds to the distance between the cycles of the sound wave at the listener's ear, lowering its perceived frequency.

Magnetic resonance imaging (MRI) is a recently-developed technique that generates photograph-like images that look somewhat like the images generated by CT scans. However,

MRI scanning has two important advantages over CT scanning: it does not expose the patient to radiation, and it usually provides images with greater detail than those from CT scanning. Magnetic resonance imaging depends on the fact that the nuclei of hydrogen atoms behave somewhat like small bar magnets, so that if they are placed in a strong magnetic field, they orient themselves in the same direction, in line with the magnetic field. In MRI the body part to be imaged is placed within such a magnetic field. Then, when the hydrogen nuclei in the body tissues have aligned themselves with the magnetic field, a short pulse of electromagnetic energy is introduced into the field, causing the hydrogen nuclei to be momentarily deflected from alignment. As the nuclei swing back into alignment with the magnetic field, they emit miniscule electromagnetic signals. A set of detectors measures these signals and sends them to a computer, which constructs a photograph-like image from the signals (Figure 2-17).

In MRI scanning, as in CT scanning, the detectors are moved in steps along the axis of the body to yield images representing consecutive layers or "slices" of the body parts scanned. MRI is sensitive to differences in the chemical composition of tissues, whereas CT scanning is sensitive to differences in the density of tissues. For this reason, MRI can show differences between tissues that have similar density but different chemical composition, such as gray matter and white matter in the brain—differences that cannot be seen in CT scans.

MRI scanning is superior to CT scanning for imaging the temporal lobes, brain stem, cerebellum, and spinal cord. MRI scanning is better than CT scanning for detecting arteriovenous malformations and aneurysms. As mentioned above, MRI requires no radiation, and so far there is no evidence that the magnetic fields used in MRI are a risk to patients. However, because of the magnetic field, MRI cannot be used when patients have metal (pins, plates, pacemakers) in their body. MRI scans take a long time, and the patient must remain motionless in a noisy, con-

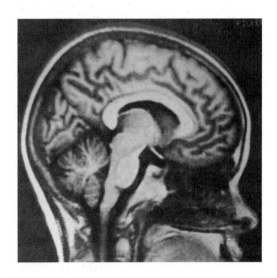

Figure 2-17 ■ **Magnetic resonance image of the head. This image shows a vertical "slice" at the midline of the brain. The brain hemisphere, cerebellum, corpus callosum, and brain stem are clearly visible.** (From Oldendorf, W., & Oldendorf, W., Jr. [1991]. *MRI primer.* Philadelphia: Lippincott-Raven.)

fining space, sometimes leading to claustrophobia and blurring of the MRI image because of patient movement (*movement artifacts*).

Regional cerebral blood flow measurement (rCBF) is a procedure for estimating blood flow in various brain regions. Because cerebral blood flow and cerebral metabolism usually are related, rCBF provides indirect estimates of regional cerebral metabolism, rather than static images of structures. rCBF can be measured in several ways, most of which require introduction into the blood of compounds, that emit small amounts of radioactivity. The compounds are administered either directly by injection of a liquid or indirectly by having the patient breathe air containing small amounts of a slightly radioactive gas, which eventually is absorbed into the blood. When the radioactive compound reaches the brain, specialized scanners detect the subatomic particles (photons, positrons) emitted by the radioactive compound, convert these events into electrical signals, and send the signals to a computer, which analyzes them and generates an image representing the blood flow in various brain regions. rCBF studies are useful in detecting vasospasm following hemorrhages and can provide information about compensatory blood flow in patients with documented cerebrovascular lesions.

Positron emission tomography (PET) also measures the metabolic activity of regions of the brain. The patient is given a solution of metabolically-active material (usually glucose) tagged with a positron-emitting isotope (oxygen, fluorine, carbon, or nitrogen). The glucose eventually makes its way to the brain, where it is metabolized. The glucose and the isotope concentrate at areas of high metabolism (which are the areas of greatest neural activity and greatest blood flow). The positrons

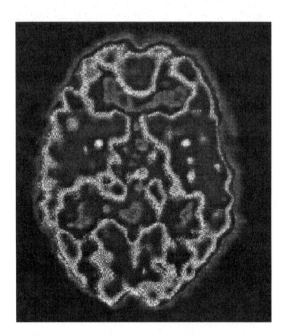

Figure 2-18 ■ **Positron emission tomography (PET) scan of a normal adult's brain in a resting state. Variations in shading represent different levels of metabolic activity. The images generated by PET scanners are in color, and different colors represent different levels of metabolic activity.**

emitted by the isotope are sensed by a set of detectors, the signals are amplified and sent to a computer, and the computer processes them to generate an image representing the regional metabolic activity of the brain (Figure 2-18).

PET scanning is at this time primarily a research tool. PET scans are expensive (the scanning facility requires a cyclotron, plus physicists and chemists to prepare the isotope). PET scanners currently are found only in institutions with large medical research operations. PET can provide estimates of regional cerebral blood flow and also may permit visualization of hypofunction in brain regions in which blood flow is not compromised and in which no structural damage is visible on standard CT scans (Metter, Riege, Hanson & associates, 1984; Metter, Riege, Hanson & associates, 1983).

Electrophysiologic Studies

Several diagnostic procedures yield recordings of the electrical activity in various parts of the nervous system. In these procedures, electrodes are placed at strategic locations to monitor the electrical activity in adjacent tissue. This low-voltage activity is amplified and sent to a recording device (usually a pen on a moving strip of graph paper), which generates a visual representation of the activity.

The *electroencephalogram* (EEG) yields a graphic record of the electrical activity of the cerebral cortex. It is obtained by placing an array of recording electrodes on the scalp. The electrodes detect the tiny electrical signals generated by the brain cortex. These signals are amplified until they are capable of operating pens that write the signals out on a moving strip of paper. The activity from a number of electrodes is traced on the paper so that tracings of the electrical activity at several cortical locations (usually 16) are obtained. The amplitude and pattern of the waveforms in the tracings, together with the location of anomalous patterns of activity, permit the neurologist to make inferences about what is happening physiologically in the patient's brain.

Localized brain lesions often cause *focal disturbances* in the EEG record in the vicinity of the lesion. The disturbance usually takes the form of aberrations in rhythm and amplitude (Figure 2-19). General disturbances of brain function usually cause general abnormalities in the EEG record across all recording sites. EEG recording is particularly useful for detecting and localizing seizure activity. In some cases, the EEG may help to distinguish between cortical and subcortical lesions in patients with overt neurologic signs of stroke. (If the EEG record from a stroke patient is normal, the stroke is likely to be subcortical; if the EEG is abnormal, the stroke is likely to be cortical.) When a patient is in deep coma, EEG recordings may be used to estimate the severity of brain injury and predict whether or not the patient will return to consciousness.

An adaptation of EEG recording, called *measurement of evoked cortical potentials,* sometimes is called *evoked response testing.* When evoked cortical potentials are measured, the patient is placed in a quiet, dark room with recording electrodes on the patient's scalp. When the patient's EEG has stabilized, tactile, auditory, or visual stimuli are presented, and the electrical activity of the cortex is measured from the electrodes. The signals from the electrodes are averaged by a computer across several stimulations. The computer calculates the cortical activity occurring within each of many time intervals following each stimulus. Changes in activity that regularly follow each stimulus are added together, and irregular (random) changes are ignored. A graphic printout of the averaged waveform attributable to stimulation then is generated. Alterations of computed waveforms for the *visual evoked response* (generated by visual stimulation), *brain stem evoked response* (generated by auditory stimulation), and *somatosensory evoked response* (generated by weak electrical stimulation of peripheral sensory nerves) suggest damage to the central nervous system conduction pathways serving those sensory modalities—damage that may not be detectable by clinical neurologic examination.

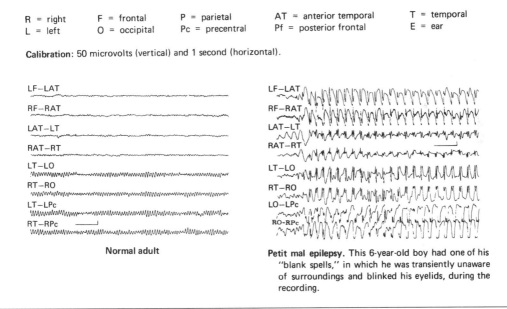

R = right   F = frontal   P = parietal   AT = anterior temporal   T = temporal
L = left   O = occipital   Pc = precentral   Pf = posterior frontal   E = ear

Calibration: 50 microvolts (vertical) and 1 second (horizontal).

Normal adult

Petit mal epilepsy. This 6-year-old boy had one of his "blank spells," in which he was transiently unaware of surroundings and blinked his eyelids, during the recording.

Figure 2-19 ■ **Examples of normal and abnormal electroencephalography (EEG) recordings. On the left is a recording from an adult with no EEG abnormalities. On the right is a recording from a patient with petit mal epilepsy, showing general disruption of cortical activity.** (From Waxman, S. [2000]. *Correlative neuroanatomy* [24th ed.]. New York: McGraw-Hill.)

In *electromyography* fine needle electrodes are inserted into muscles to record their electrical activity. Relaxed muscles normally produce no spontaneous electrical activity, but when muscles contract they produce bursts of electrical activity that are fairly predictable in terms of their amplitude, frequency, duration, and pattern. Spontaneous discharges in resting muscles (fibrillations, fasciculations) may indicate peripheral nerve disease. Other variations in amplitude, frequency, duration, or pattern may indicate disease in anterior horn cells, neuromuscular junctions, or the muscles themselves.

Nerve conduction studies are performed when peripheral neuropathy is suspected. In nerve conduction studies a nerve fiber (either motor or sensory) is stimulated at one point, and the response is measured at another point along the fiber. The time between the stimulation and the response is called the *nerve conduction velocity.* Variations in nerve conduction velocities sometimes are helpful in diagnosing the nature and extent of peripheral nerve damage.

Tests Involving Analysis of Body Tissue or Fluids

Sometimes diagnosis of the nature of nervous system pathology requires laboratory analysis of a sample of nervous system tissue or fluids. A *lumbar puncture* (sometimes called *spinal tap*) may be performed if the neurologist suspects infection or hemorrhage in the patient's central nervous system. A hypodermic needle is inserted between the vertebrae in the lower spine, below the level of the spinal cord, and a sample of cerebrospinal fluid (CSF) is taken for analysis. When the needle is inserted, the pressure with which the fluid flows into the syringe is measured. Increased pressure may suggest blockage in the circulation of CSF, the presence of space-occupying pathology such as a tumor or abscess, or swelling of brain tissue.

The CSF is analyzed for the presence of cells, bacteria, parasites, or viruses, and the chemical composition of the CSF is determined, including the amount of glucose and protein in the fluid. The presence of red blood cells or a yellowish color (*xanthochromia*) are signs of bleeding into the ventricles, meningeal spaces, or spinal cord. The presence of bacteria, parasites, or viruses proves infection with those agents. Increased protein content may suggest meningeal inflammation, a tumor, or obstructions within the spinal canal. CSF glucose levels often are lowered by bacterial infections.

Biopsies (removing a sample of tissue for laboratory analysis) may be performed when less invasive procedures do not yield a definite diagnosis. Most biopsies of nervous system tissue are *needle biopsies* (sometimes called *aspiration biopsies*), in which a hollow needle is inserted into the tissue of interest and a small amount of tissue is removed by applying suction to the needle. Sometimes *open biopsies,* in which samples of tissue are surgically excised, may be performed if the tissue is accessible to the surgeon's scalpel.

Biopsy of brain tissue sometimes is ordered to determine the nature of brain tumors, to identify the nature of infectious agents (as in brain abscess), or to permit diagnosis of certain degenerative diseases. *Muscle biopsy* may be ordered to determine if muscle weakness is caused by neuropathy or by disease of the muscle itself. *Biopsy of nerve tissue* occasionally may be ordered to determine the underlying nature of peripheral neurologic disease. *Biopsy of an artery* may be ordered to identify inflammatory or degenerative diseases involving the arterial system. Biopsies are among the least frequently ordered laboratory tests ordered by neurologists and are ordered only when less invasive procedures have failed to yield a diagnosis.

RECORDING THE RESULTS OF THE NEUROLOGIC EXAMINATION

The neurologist records the results of the neurologic examination in the patient's medical record, where it usually is the first entry in the daily record of the patient's care. The neurologist's report of the examination usually ends with a *problem list,* in which the patient's current significant medical problems are recorded. The neurologist's report of the neurologic examination and the problem list provide important information for others involved in the patient's care. An example of a neurologist's report for a patient with right hemiplegia and aphasia follows.

Report of Neurologic Examination

The patient was seen in the emergency room following reported sudden onset of right-side muscle weakness and slurred speech approximately 2 hours prior to my examination. The patient was alert and cooperative, but his speech was grossly distorted and limited to single words. Observation indicated apparent right hemiparesis and paralysis of lower facial muscles on the right. Neurologic examination of the patient yielded the following results.

Cranial Nerves

Olfactory: Not tested.

Optic: The optic discs were flat, with no evidence of exudates or hemorrhages. Venous pulsations were visible and retinal vessels were grossly normal. The macular area appeared normal, with perhaps some age-related minimal degenerative changes.

Oculomotor, trochlear, abducens: The pupils were round, equal, and responsive to light and accommodation. The extraocular muscle movements were intact. No nystagmus was observed. Visual fields were normal.

Trigeminal: The patient's jaw opened on the midline but deviated to the right when opened against resistance. Masseter muscle strength was moderately decreased on the right. Corneal reflexes were brisk and equal. Upper facial sensation was intact to pinprick and light touch. Lower facial sensation was intact on the left and moderately diminished on the right.

Facial: No ptosis was observed. Forehead wrinkling appeared normal on both sides. There was mild to moderate facial droop on right, and the right side of the patient's mouth did not retract on smile or showing teeth.

Acoustic: Hearing appeared intact to watch ticking at 3 feet. Bone conduction was not tested.

Glossopharyngeal, vagus: The patient's gag reflex was strong and prompt. The patient's soft palate was lower on the right on passive observation. On phonation the palate elevated on the left, but not the right side.

Spinal accessory: Strength of the sternocleidomastoid and trapezius muscles was slightly diminished on the right.

Hypoglossal: The tongue deviated to the right on protrusion. Right-to-left movement was normal to left and restricted to right. No tremor, fasciculations, or atrophy was noted.

Motor and Coordination

The patient was unable to stand or walk. Finger-to-finger, finger-to-nose, and rapid alternating movements on the left were within normal limits. The patient was not tested on right because of paralysis. Strength was normal on left and diminished on right (contraction but no movement, upper and lower R extremities). Spasticity and exaggerated reflexes were present on the right but not on the left. Plantar extensor reflex was elicited on the right but not on the left. No tremor, involuntary movements, fasciculations, or atrophy were observed. Biceps, triceps, brachioradialis, and ankle jerks were normal on the left and exaggerated on the right (3+), but without sustained clonus.

Sensation

Light touch, pinprick, vibration, and position sense were intact on the left. Light touch and pinprick were diminished on the right. Vibration and position sense were intact on right.

Vascular

Carotid pulses present bilaterally. Bruit present on left but not on right.

Impression

Stroke in anterior zone of left middle cerebral artery, probably thromboembolic.

Problem List

1. Right hemiplegia
2. Aphasia: nonfluent, severe

Plan

1. Rule out hemorrhage (CT scan, MRI).
2. Medications: anticoagulate if thrombotic or embolic. Dilantin 100 mg t.i.d.

Continued

Report of Neurologic Examination—cont'd

Plan—cont'd

3. Baseline measures of speech, language, mentation. Speech therapy consult.
4. Begin rehabilitation program. Physical and occupational therapist consults.

GENERAL CONCEPTS 2-4

* *Cerebral angiography* (*arteriography*) is an x-ray procedure that provides visualization of cerebral veins and arteries. Angiography is useful for detecting narrowing or occlusions of arteries.
* Myelography is an x-ray procedure that provides visualization of the spinal cord and surrounding space. Myelography is useful for detecting structural changes in the spinal cord or spinal nerve roots.
* *Computerized tomography* (CT) scanning is an x-ray procedure that produces computer-generated photograph-like images of cross-sectional "slices" of internal structures based on their resistance to the passage of x-rays.
* *Echo arteriography* and *transcranial Doppler ultrasound* yield computer-generated images of cerebral blood vessels derived from high-frequency sound waves transmitted into the head and neck.
* *Magnetic resonance imaging* (MRI) produces computer-generated photograph-like images of cross-sectional "slices" of internal structures by placing them in a strong magnetic field and introducing a burst of electromagnetic energy. MRI images reflect the chemical composition of tissues (particularly their water content).
* *Regional cerebral blood flow measurement* (rCBF) measures blood flow in various brain regions, thereby indirectly measuring brain metabolism in those regions.
* *Positron emission tomography* (PET) produces computer-generated images of cross-sectional "slices" of internal tissues, which reflect the metabolism taking place in various brain regions. PET requires the ingestion of mildly radioactive material by the patient.
* *Electroencephalography* (EEG) produces a graphic record of the electrical activity of the cerebral cortex. EEG recording is very useful for detecting and localizing seizure activity.
* *Electromyography* produces a record of the electrical activity in muscles. Electromyography is useful in diagnosing diseases of peripheral nerves, neuromuscular junctions, or muscles.
* *Nerve conduction studies* measure the speed of neural transmission. They are useful in diagnosing pathology affecting peripheral nerves.
* In *lumbar puncture* (spinal tap) a sample of cerebrospinal fluid is removed to analyze it for the presence of blood cells or infectious organisms and to detect abnormal levels of glucose and proteins, all of which are signs of central nervous system pathology.
* *Biopsy* (removal of tissue for laboratory analysis) may be performed when less invasive procedures do not yield a diagnosis.

THOUGHT QUESTIONS

Question 2-1 A 74-year-old man with a 20-year history of heart disease and two previous myocardial infarcts (heart attacks) is brought to a hospital emergency room with a sudden onset of slurred speech and right-side limb weakness. The neurologist who evaluates the patient in the emergency room makes the following observations:

* Moderate right hemiparesis, arm greater than leg
* Fluent aphasia, consistent with Wernicke's aphasia
* Left homonymous hemianopia

What do you think caused the patient's current problems? Do you see a potential connection between the patient's medical history and his current problems? Where do you think the damage in the patient's central nervous system is? Are the neurologist's observations what you would expect? If not, why not?

Question 2-2 A neurologist is administering a mental status examination to a patient with a suspected left-hemisphere stroke. The mental status examination has a memory test in which the examiner tells the patient three words that the patient is to repeat immediately and again later in the examination.

Examiner: "Here are three words. I want you to say them back to me. Remember the words because I will ask you for them later in this examination. The words are *watch, pen,* and *key.* Now say them back to me."

Patient: "Flimmer, kidder, kadder."

Examiner: "No, listen. Here they are again—*watch, pen, key.*"

Patient: "Kalder, kammer, mander."

What do you think may account for this patient's performance on this test? Suggest a way in which the neurologist might test this patient's memory for the three words.

Question 2-3 A neurologist examines a patient who says she has sensory loss on the left side of her body. She states that the sensory loss was present when she woke several days ago and has remained essentially unchanged since that time. During the examination the patient consistently fails to report touch, pinprick, heat, or cold in all regions to the left of her body's midline. The neurologists tests the patient's sense of vibration by placing a vibrating tuning fork on bony structures on both sides of the midline of the patient's body. The patient consistently reports the vibration on the right of the midline, but does not report it at any point to the left of midline. The patient's muscle strength and coordination are normal on both sides of her body, and the remainder of the neurologic examination is within normal limits. The neurologist concludes her report of this patient's neurologic examination with, "The symptoms reported by this patient are not consistent with an organic etiology. Additional testing should seek to rule out a psychogenic origin."

What led the neurologist to her conclusion?

Question 2-4 Patients with cerebellar pathology (ataxia), patients with loss of sensation and position sense in the legs, and patients with vestibular abnormalities all typically stand with feet wide apart and become unsteady and may fall if forced to stand with feet close together. A neurologist who examines a patient with such a pattern of behavior may ask the patient to stand with feet close together with eyes open and then with eyes closed.

What information might the neurologist gain by asking such a patient to close his or her eyes?

Question 2-5 Fred Smith, a 33-year-old man, was brought by a friend to a Maine emergency room one midsummer evening. Fred was pale and weak, and his breathing was rapid and shallow. He complained of "feeling strange" and of "feeling so weak I can hardly walk." Fred reported that he had been feeling fine until about an hour ago, when he began to feel "weak and shaky."

Questioning by the physician revealed that Fred and his friend had spent the day at a beach cottage, where they had spent most of the day lying in the sun drinking beer and eating Mexican food from a local restaurant. On returning to the cottage, Fred had had another beer and had eaten several oysters on the half-shell while his friend was in the shower. By the time the friend came out of the shower Fred had begun to feel unwell and weak. Fred's feelings of weakness increased rapidly, and he and his friend agreed that Fred should receive medical attention. Fred's friend drove him to the emergency room at the local medical center.

The physician's examination revealed moderate weakness and sensory loss in Fred's arms, legs, torso, and face. Fred's temperature was normal, but his breathing was rapid and shallow, and his heart rate was accelerated. The physician's screening assessment of Fred's speech, language, memory, and intellect revealed no apparent impairments of those functions.

Are Fred's symptoms likely to be caused by a neurologic problem? If so, what part of Fred's nervous system do you think is responsible for Fred's symptoms? Does this scenario suggest a possible cause for Fred's symptoms?

Assessing Adults Who Have Neurogenic Communication Impairments

Adults who have neurogenic communication impairments provide perpetual fascination and ongoing challenge for speech-language pathologists concerned with assessment, diagnosis, and treatment of brain-injured adults' communication impairments. The fascination comes from the seemingly endless array of signs, symptoms, and syndromes exhibited by these patients. Part of the challenge comes from organizing, refining, interpreting, and drawing conclusions from complex, confusing, and sometimes contradictory information to arrive at a diagnosis and formulate a plan of care. Challenge also comes from the behavioral, cognitive, and emotional consequences of brain injury. These consequences affect how brain-injured patients respond to unusual, unexpected, or demanding situations, such as interviews with strangers in white coats or tests with unfamiliar or difficult materials.

THE PROCESS OF ASSESSMENT AND DIAGNOSIS

Novice clinicians can be intimidated by the complexity of neurologic communication disorders and the seeming impossibility of making sense of a sometimes bewildering array of signs and symptoms. Watching a skilled clinician evaluate a patient who has a neurogenic communication disorder can be a mystifying experience for the novice. He or she watches the clinician take the patient through an array of tests that share no discernable common purpose, terminate some tests before completion, modify others without apparent reason, improvise new tests on the spot, and eventually arrive at a diagnosis of the patient's communication disorder, offer a prognosis, and decide about the advisability and nature of treatment.

According to *Stedman's Medical Dictionary,* a *symptom* is "any morbid phenomenon or departure from normal in function, appearance, or sensation, experienced by the patient and indicative of disease." A *sign* is "any abnormality discoverable by the physician at his examination of the patient." A *syndrome* is "a concurrence of symptoms." Symptoms are subjective data reported by the patient; signs are objective data observed by the physician. Syndromes represent inferences made by an examiner, based on patterns of signs and symptoms.

The skilled clinician's idiosyncratic approach to assessment comes from training and clinical experience. The skilled clinician is familiar with the signs, symptoms, and usual course of many neurogenic communication disorders, making them adept at synthesizing test results and patient behaviors into a pattern that points to a syndrome or a diagnostic category. When a skilled clinician recognizes an emerging pattern of test results, they deviate from their generic test routine to focus on tests that add depth and detail to the pattern. Each test result that fits the expected pattern increases the clinician's confidence that the patient's signs and symptoms represent the syndrome, whereas conflicting information moves the clinician toward an alternative diagnosis.

Skilled clinicians use their clinical knowledge without consciously thinking about it, and they cannot verbalize much of what they know. Add to that the likelihood that much of what they do is based as much on intuition as on rules or principles, and it is not surprising that clinical methods are learned as much (or more) by observation, practice, and imitation as by direct instruction.

Although (to use a cliché) there really is no substitute for experience, there are some general principles that govern the collection and analysis of clinical data. These principles relate, in a general way, to the well-known *scientific method,* formalized by John Dewey in the 1930s and repackaged by numerous authors for clinical purposes. The new package is called the *clinical method.*

> The solution of any clinical problem is reached by a series of inferences and deductions—each an attempt to explain an item in the history of an illness or a physical finding. Diagnosis is the mental act of integrating all the interpretations and selecting the *one* explanation most compatible with all the facts of clinical observation. (Adams & Victor, 1981, p. 3)

Practitioners using the clinical method usually employ a seven-step procedure to guide their clinical decision-making:

1. Gather information about the patient's impairments from the referral, the history, and examination of the patient.
2. Evaluate the patient's subjective reports (symptoms) and the objective test results (signs) to determine which symptoms and signs are relevant to the patient's current problems and to the practitioner's plan of care.

3. Determine if a distinctive cluster of symptoms and signs, representing a *syndrome,* exists.

4. Look for correlations among symptoms and signs to identify the parts of the body or the underlying physical or mental processes responsible for the observed symptoms and signs.

5. If the patient's symptoms and signs represent a syndrome for which information about the course and eventual outcome of the patient's condition are available, decide on a prognosis.

6. Use information from the patient's history, examination of the patient, and knowledge of the patient's life situation to formulate a conclusion about the degree to which the patient's condition affects the patient's daily life competence and independence.

7. Use the entire corpus of information about the patient, plus other relevant sources of information (such as clinical experience and the clinical and scientific literature), to estimate the potential effects of treatment and, if treatment is indicated, the nature of an optimal treatment program.

The clinical method encompasses two primary activities—assimilation of information and clinical decision-making. Clinical experience helps a skilled clinician sort through an abundance of facts about a patient (that the patient is male, is 55 years old, is hypertensive, has a rash on his chest, complains of numbness on the right side of his face, is missing his left index finger, and misarticulates consonant sounds) and select those that are relevant to the clinician's purpose. As each fact about the patient becomes evident, the clinician evaluates it for its meaning and relates it to other facts about the patient. This process continues until the clinician is satisfied that he or she understands the nature of the patient's problems, at which time the clinician might apply a diagnostic label and shift attention to arriving at a prognosis and making decisions about management.

A clinician who uses the clinical method gathers facts from the history, the medical record, the interview with the patient and family members, and the results of testing. With each new fact the clinician looks for relationships that might suggest a diagnosis. As additional facts become known the clinician evaluates the consistency of the new facts with the working diagnosis. When new facts suggest that the working diagnosis is no longer valid, the clinician considers alternative diagnoses and may change tests or examination procedures to gather facts that are relevant to the new diagnosis. When alternative explanations for the pattern of facts have been eliminated, the clinician settles on the diagnosis most compatible with the facts of the history, the interview, and the examination.

Harvey and associates (1988, p. 2) summarize the principles of the clinical method:

- The collection and analysis of clinical information are essentially the application of the scientific method to the solution of a clinical problem.

- These methods can be taught and learned; it is not an art in which one is either gifted or not. Proficiency can be improved by consciously considering the meaning of each piece of information as it is received.

- The process is rapidly iterative. The cycle is repeated within the time interval of asking a few questions or making physical observations. This explains the mystery of why the novice fails to ask the key question or seek the key physical finding.

- The process is an ongoing one. There are no irrefutable hypotheses, only unrefuted hypotheses. In clinical terms, the physician should not arrive at a diagnosis and abandon any further consideration of alternative explanations. He must remain alert for information that does not fit with his current hypothesis and for sources of new information that might make him alter his considerations. When uncertain, he should continue to seek ways of testing the tentative diagnosis.

- Consideration of a diagnosis that can neither be confirmed nor excluded fails to advance the decision-making process. Such a diagnosis is directly parallel to a scientific hypothesis that cannot be tested.

- Finally, clinical problem-solving is as sensitive to flawed or missing information as are scientific experiments. A major difference lies in the fact that clinical decisions must often be made on what is acknowledged to be incomplete evidence.

SOURCES OF INFORMATION
ABOUT THE PATIENT
The Referral

Patients with neurogenic communication disorders usually arrive at the speech-language pathologist's office by way of a physician's referral. The physician recruits specialists into the patient's program of care by means of *consultation requests* (sometimes called *referrals*). The information included in the consultation request provides the speech-language pathologist with a sense of the patient and a general idea of what the referring physician would like the speech-language pathologist to do. Consultation requests:

- Identify the patient (name, birth date, Social Security number, and such).
- Tell where the patient is located (hospital ward, service, unit).
- Tell what the physician would like from the consultant.
- Give the referring physician's name (and sometimes their phone or pager numbers).
- Provide space for the consultant's response.

Consultation requests span a wide range of completeness, accuracy, and legibility. The good ones are legibly written, describe the patient's

---

The advent of computerized consultation and referral procedures has had a major positive side effect, in that consultation requests are typed into a central computer and printed out on a consultation request form. Consequently, those receiving the request no longer are burdened with deciphering the scrawl of handwritten requests. Unfortunately, computerized referrals have had little effect on the arcane and nonstandard abbreviations and terms used by some physicians, nor have they had any measurable salutary effects on their spelling, clarity of style, and literary merit.

---

major current problems, provide a diagnosis (sometimes provisional), and include a brief statement of the services requested. Most contain numerous abbreviations, both standard and nonstandard, and many are telegraphic.

Figure 3-1 gives an example of a consultation request as it might be received by a speech-language pathologist. The shaded areas contain information provided by the physician.

The consultation request was sent from Dr. Ericsson, a fictional neurologist on a neurology ward, and concerns a fictional patient named Arthur Shaw. The provisional diagnosis suggests that Mr. Shaw has had a stroke (cerebrovascular accident) involving the left middle cerebral artery and that he exhibits severe aphasia. The physician has left it to the speech-language pathologist to decide where to see the patient. The "Reason for Request" section, when decoded, yields the following information about Mr. Shaw:

> Mr. Shaw is a 55-year-old right-handed male, who yesterday had a stroke in his left middle cerebral artery. He has right arm and right leg weakness and appears globally aphasic. He has a history of diabetes mellitus and hypertension.

Consultation requests such as this provide the speech-language pathologist with an important first look at the patient, the patient's history, the nature and severity of the patient's neurologic impairments, and (sometimes) the probable future course of the patient's condition. By making inferences from the information in the consultation request, the speech-language pathologist may develop an impression of the patient that goes well beyond the sketchy information provided. Consider the consultation request for Mr. Shaw. The information therein suggests several hypotheses about Mr. Shaw, his communication impairments, and his life situation:

- Mr. Shaw is right-handed and has damage in the distribution of the left middle cerebral artery. Therefore he is very likely to be aphasic—a hypothesis supported by the neurologist's description.

Medical Record	Consultation Request/Referral	
To: Speech Pathology	**From:** Ward 2N Neurology	**Date:** 8/12/00 14:36

Provisional Diagnosis: LMCA CVA, global aphasia

Requested by: Ericsson, G. 4498	**Place:** Consultant's choice	**Urgency:** Routine

Reason for Request: 55 y/o R-H M 1 day s/p recent L MCA CVA. RUE, RLE weakn. Globally aphasic. Hx DM, HTN. Pls eval pt's sp & lang & make recs.

Consultation Report

Signature and Title:		Date:

ID #:	Organization/Service:	Reg #:	Ward:

Patient Identification: Shaw, Arthur 5/17/45 503-42-9680 2K435-32-NEU	**SF 522 5/98** **Consultation Request**

Figure 3-1 ■ **Consultation request for Mr. Shaw. The shaded areas contain information provided by the referring physician.**

- Mr. Shaw is weak, but not paralyzed, on his right side. This suggests that the stroke was not a massive one affecting the entire left hemisphere. Consequently he is not likely to be globally aphasic, as the neurologist's description indicates.

- Mr. Shaw's stroke is very recent. Therefore the next few weeks should be a period of rapid spontaneous recovery.

- Mr. Shaw is 55 years old. He probably was employed when he had his stroke. His stroke may have important financial consequences for Mr. Shaw and his family.

- Mr. Shaw is diabetic and hypertensive— medical problems that could complicate his physical recovery.

- Mr. Shaw is currently on a neurology ward. The average length of stay on neurology wards (and other acute-care wards) is only a few days. This may affect how much testing, family education, and counseling the speech-language pathologist can accomplish before discharge.

- Mr. Shaw and his family are likely to be in the initial stages of coming to grips with the effects of the stroke on Mr. Shaw and family members. They will need education, support, and reassurance to deal with what has happened and to plan for the future.

Sometimes patients with severe Broca's or Wernicke's aphasia are reported by physicians to be globally aphasic because they appear to comprehend little or nothing and produce little if any intelligible speech. Physicians sometimes call patients with severe Broca's aphasia *globally aphasic* because their inability to talk makes testing of comprehension (which usually is relatively good) difficult. Physicians sometimes call patients with severe Wernicke's aphasia *globally aphasic* because their severe comprehension impairments and vague, empty, and circumlocutory speech give an impression of globally impaired language. Globally aphasic patients usually are paralyzed on one side. That Mr. Shaw is weak but not paralyzed on his right side suggests that he may not be globally aphasic.

This referral shows how information contained in a consultation request permits the speech-language pathologist to make inferences that go well beyond the explicit information in the consultation request. Inference-making is in many ways an idiosyncratic process that depends on experience, knowledge, and talent for making inferences. What a clinician infers from a consultation request may be idiosyncratic, but the information supporting the inferences is fairly consistent. The *source of the consultation* often has implications for a patient's probable length of stay, a patient's physical and medical condition, and the speech-language pathologist's role in the patient's care.

Patients in *intensive care units* (ICUs) are likely to be weak, seriously ill, or comatose. Some may have tracheotomies (openings into the trachea to provide an alternative airway or to facilitate treatment of respiratory impairments). Patients in intensive care units are confined to bed, usually with feeding, medication, or drainage tubes or monitoring equipment attached. Patients in intensive care units usually remain there only until their medical condition stabilizes and they no longer need intensive around-the-clock monitoring and care, although a few seriously ill patients may remain there for several weeks. When they leave the ICU, most are transferred to a *medical-surgical ward.* Patients in intensive care units usually are referred to a speech-language pathologist because they cannot communicate basic needs or because they have known or suspected swallowing impairments. The speech-language pathologist's typical role with these patients is to establish a system by which the patient can communicate basic needs to unit personnel, to evaluate the patient's swallowing, or both.

Most patients on medical-surgical wards (including neurology wards, which are a subcategory of medical wards) are discharged within 3 to 5 days, although some with serious illnesses or those recovering from major surgery may stay longer. Patients on medical-surgical wards usually have acute or evolving medical problems (e.g., recent stroke, pneumonia, or recent surgery). Most can get out of bed and many are ambulatory, although some may require a cane, crutches, a walker, or a wheelchair to get around.

> The primary meaning of ambulatory is "capable of walking about." Its secondary meaning is "not confined to bed." I use the word in the latter sense.

Patients on medical-surgical wards are referred to speech-language pathologists for many reasons—to request an opinion regarding the presence and severity of a communication or swallowing impairment; to request assessment of a patient's speech, language, and cognitive status; to request an opinion regarding the potential benefits of treatment; or to get help in resolving a diagnostic question. The emphasis in referrals from medical-surgical wards tends toward assessment and diagnosis—patients usually are discharged before treatment of their communication impairments becomes an important part of their overall plan of care.

Patients on *rehabilitation wards* usually stay for several weeks. Few are acutely ill and almost all are ambulatory, although most get around with the help of canes, crutches, a walker or a wheelchair. Most receive occupational, physical, and/or recreational therapy and sometimes other therapies while they are on the ward. Consequently, the speech-language pathologist is likely to serve on a treatment team with the patient's physician and rehabilitation therapists. Because of their relatively long stays, patients on rehabilitation wards usually can get a good start on treatment of their communication impairments before they leave the hospital.

Patients in *extended care centers* usually stay for weeks or months. Almost all are ambulatory. Few are acutely ill, but most have chronic medical problems (e.g., stroke-related impairments or pulmonary disease) and some may be receiving continuing treatment for chronic disease (e.g., kidney dialysis, radiation therapy, or chemother-

apy). The speech-language pathologist's focus for these patients is likely to be treatment, although some patients may require only an assessment and diagnostic workup.

Most *outpatients* seen in speech-language pathology clinics are individuals who have been discharged from the hospital but need continuing treatment for communication impairments. Most are ambulatory. Not many are acutely ill, but many have chronic low-level medical problems such as diabetes, cardiovascular disease, or pulmonary disease. Some may have degenerative disease such as multiple sclerosis or cerebellar degeneration. Some may be recovering from strokes, other neurologic incidents, or surgery. Physicians refer outpatients to speech-language pathology for many reasons, but most frequently they wish to know the cause and nature of a patient's communication impairments, to know if treatment of a patient's communication impairments is appropriate, or both.

Another source of clues to the patient's communication history and potential communicative needs is the *demographic information* about the patient provided in the referral. The patient's *age* may indicate whether the patient is working or retired and whether dependent children live at home. Disability of younger patients who are below retirement age is likely to have important financial consequences for the patient and family. As a patient's age increases, so does the probability that the patient's spouse will be medically or physically impaired, compromising the spouse's ability to care for the patient. As a patient's age increases, the greater the probability that the patient does not have a living spouse, the greater the probability that the burden of care will fall on children or other relatives, and the greater probability that the patient will be placed in an extended care facility on discharge from the medical center. Finally, as age increases, physical resilience diminishes and the likelihood of complicating medical conditions increases.

The *medical diagnosis* often supports inferences about and the nature and severity of the patient's impairments and the patient's potential for recovery by suggesting the cause, location, and extent of a patient's nervous system injury. Stroke, traumatic brain injury, and degenerative disease lead to different predictions concerning the pattern and degree of recovery. Damage in the brain hemispheres is likely to compromise higher mental processes (language and cognition). Brain stem damage is likely to compromise motor and sensory functions, but spare higher mental processes. The extent of a patient's nervous system pathology usually is directly related to the number and severity of the patient's symptoms, and, in a less direct way, to the eventual outcome of treatment. For example, massive damage in the central zone of the language-dominant hemisphere causes more profound language impairment than does damage localized within an outlying region of the cortex.

The *services requested* specify the role of the speech-language pathologist in the patient's care. A physician may refer a patient with progressive neurologic disease and ask the speech-language pathologist to establish baseline measures of speech and language against which the progression of the patient's disease may be measured. A physician may refer a patient with a questionable neurologic diagnosis and ask the speech-language pathologist to administer tests to help clarify the diagnosis. A physician may refer an aphasic patient whose competence to make financial and legal decisions is questionable and ask the speech-language pathologist to evaluate the degree to which the patient's communicative and cognitive impairments affect the patient's financial and legal competence. Some consultation requests are generic in what they ask for (e.g., assessment or treatment of the patient's communication impairments) and leave the specifics to the speech-language pathologist.

Occasionally a consultation request will focus on one aspect of a patient's care but neglect other aspects of care to which the speech-language pathologist may contribute. For example, a patient with a brain stem stroke may be referred for evaluation of the patient's swallowing with no mention of coexisting dysarthria. The speech-language pathologist who knows that dysarthria is a common consequence of brain stem injuries may suggest extending the evaluation to include speech as well as swallowing.

> Clinicians always must recognize that the patient's physician retains primary responsibility for the patient's overall plan of care. Changes or additions to the plan of care prescribed by the physician may be made only with the physician's knowledge and consent.

The Medical Record

The medical record is a legal document that provides a complete record of the patient's medical care. Medical records are divided into sections, with different kinds of information in each section. How medical records are divided depends to some extent on the medical facility in which the record is located, but most resemble the arrangement described in the following sections. The speech-language pathologist reviews the medical record and extracts information relating to the patient's potential communication impairments. This information is summarized in freehand or, more often, on a form for that purpose.

Patient Identification The patient identification section usually is at the bottom of each page in the record and includes the patient's name, date of birth, Social Security number, and ward. It also may contain other information about the patient, such as home telephone number and diagnostic or other codes.

Personal History The patient's personal history contains demographic information about the patient (occupation, marital status, children, where the patient lives and with whom, vocation, and work history). Information about the patient's emotional and social history also may appear here—for example, the presence of previous or current emotional or personal problems, the nature of the patient's relationships with others, and whether the patient has a history of alcoholism or other substance abuse. In Figure 3-2

Personal History: Mr. Shaw is a 55-y/o accountant (college grad). Married, with two children; son 28, daughter 24, neither living at home. Wife (Florence) is a secondary-school teacher. Nonsmoker x 10 yrs. Occasional social ETOH—non-abuser. Both parents deceased (mid-80s), apparently of natural causes. Employed at time of apparent neurologic incident.

Medical History: Past medical history includes adult-onset diabetes mellitus diagnosed in 1991, hypertension diagnosed 1993, and a possible TIA in March of last year. The patient's wife reports that at the time of the apparent TIA they were watching television when the patient became confused, did not answer questions, and seemed not to understand. The patient's symptoms apparently cleared in an hour or two, and they did not seek medical advice or assistance. Medications on admission include tolbutamide 500 mg twice a day, chlorothiazide 500 mg twice a day, which apparently control the patient's hypertension and diabetes, and occasionally aspirin.

Background: The patient was accompanied to this medical center by his wife, who provided this information. The patient apparently was in good health until this apparent neurologic event, which occurred at approximately 0815 hrs this day. The patient was getting dressed for work when he experienced a sudden onset of speech difficulties and leg weakness. The patient did not vomit, lose consciousness, or report double vision, nausea or vertigo. He arrived at the emergency room at this medical center at 0905 hrs. The neurologic examination began at approximately 0920 hrs.

Habits: The patient is an ex-smoker (0.5 ppd x 10 years) and has not smoked for approximately the past 10 years. The patient apparently drinks three or four glasses of wine per week and other alcoholic drinks occasionally but his wife reports that he has never been a heavy drinker.

Physical Examination: The patient looks his stated age and is in no apparent distress. He appears alert and is oriented x 3. **Vital signs:** Blood pressure 162/89, pulse 72, temperature 98.6, respiration 18. **HEENT exam:** No signs of trauma or deformation. Moist mucous membranes. Neck negative for lymphadenopathy or thyromegaly. No carotid bruit. **Cardiovascular exam:** Normal S1, S2, without gallop or murmurs. **Lungs:** clear to auscultation. **Abdomen:** soft and nontender. No organomegaly or palpable masses. **Lower extremities:** no pedal edema.

Neurologic Examination: The patient is globally aphasic. Listening comprehension evaluation showed that he is able to follow very simple commands like "close your eyes" or "open your mouth." He is unable to give yes-no answers to questions. He is a little bit confused as to right/left commands. He is unable to do complex commands. Reading evaluation showed the patient unable to identify a letter. He had paraphasic errors in single-word identification (example: "wrisp" for "wrist"). The patient was unable to follow commands on reading because of inability to comprehend. Expression evaluation showed that the patient was unable to read a narrative. He was unable to repeat "no ifs, ands, or buts." He was also unable to name objects like watch or pin. **Cranial nerve examination:** It was difficult to examine the patient's visual acuity because of his aphasia. Acuity appears within normal limits, but the patient exhibits a questionable right-sided field cut. Funduscopic examination showed no evidence of papilledema. His pupils are 3 to 4 mm bilaterally, round, equal, and reactive to light and accomodation. He had intact extraocular movements. His corneal reflexes are present bilaterally. His jaw jerk was +1. He had symmetrical nasolabial folds and wrinkles. His tongue is midline and so is his uvula. He has symmetrical gag reflex bilaterally. He has symmetrical strength in his shoulders bilaterally.

Motor examination: The patient has no pronator drift and no involuntary movements. His muscle tone is normal bilaterally. His strength appears 5/5 on the left and 4/5 in the right upper extremity and 3/5 in the right lower extremity. Grasp reflex on right. He had external rotation in his right lower extremity. His coordination exam was unremarkable for dysmetria. Deep tendon reflexes are +2 on the left and +3 on the right, except +1 in both ankles. Plantar reflex on right. **Sensory examination:** Impossible to establish accurately because of patient's aphasia. However, the patient withdraws both lower and upper extremities to pinprick stimuli. **Gait:** The patient walks slowly, but with symmetrical arm swings bilaterally. Mild dragging of right foot.

Problem List:
1. Probable LH stroke
2. Aphasia
3. Hypertension
4. Adult-onset diabetes mellitus

(Signed)

G. Ericsson

G. Ericsson, M.D.

Date: 8/11/00

Patient ID
  Shaw, Arthur 5/17/45
  503-42-9680
  2K435-32 NEU

Figure 3-2 ■ **Report of the neurologist's examination of Mr. Shaw.**

the neurologist has summarized Mr. Shaw's personal history at the beginning of the neurologic examination.

Medical History The medical history usually comes from a physician who interviews the patient and summarizes the interview in the patient's medical record, sometimes adding information from previous medical records. The medical history describes the patient's previous illnesses, injuries, or medical conditions and current disabilities and complaints. The physician documents past signs, symptoms, and diagnoses, such as strokes, disorientation, confusion, slurred speech, loss of consciousness, or seizures, and lists chronic medical conditions such as diabetes, vascular disease, heart disease, pulmonary disease, hearing loss, and visual problems.

Figure 3-2 shows the neurologist's summary of Mr. Shaw's medical history, which is a characteristic one for stroke patients. Diabetes and hypertension each increase the risk of stroke, and when they appear in combination, the risk is greater than when either appears separately. Mrs. Shaw's description of the March 1999 incident, when combined with his diabetes and hypertension, suggests the occurrence of a transient ischemic attack.

The events that brought Mr. Shaw to the hospital (see Figure 3-2, *Background*) also are characteristic of stroke, and their nature and progression suggest an occlusive stroke rather than a brain hemorrhage. Occlusive strokes tend to occur early in the day and are not strongly related to physical exertion; symptoms usually increase gradually, often in a step-wise manner. Hemorrhagic strokes tend to occur during physical exertion, and symptom development usually is rapid and accompanied by headache, nausea, and sometimes vomiting. Mr. Shaw's past history of smoking and his moderate alcohol consumption are unlikely to have much to do with the cause of his current symptoms.

Physical and Neurologic Examination

The results of the physician's examination of the patient (including the neurologic examination) are reported here. The physician's report of the examination usually ends with a *problem list*, in which relevant preexisting and current symptoms and complaints are summarized.

The neurologist's report of Mr. Shaw's physical and neurologic examination (see Figure 3-2) follows the standard format. It begins with the neurologist's observations of Mr. Shaw's appearance, mood, and orientation (*oriented x3* means oriented to *person, place,* and *time*). The report continues with a summary of Mr. Shaw's physical examination. Mr. Shaw's *vital signs* are within normal limits, except for slightly elevated blood pressure. The remainder of the physical examination is generally unremarkable. (*Lymphadenopathy* means "enlarged lymph glands." *Thyromegaly* means "enlarged thyroid gland." *Bruit* is the rushing sound blood makes in a constricted or roughened artery—in this case the carotid artery in the neck. S_1, S_2, *gallop,* and *murmur* are heart sounds. *Auscultation* means "listening to the sounds of various body structures"—usually by means of a stethoscope. *Organomegaly* means "enlarged organs." *Palpable* means "detectable by touch." *Pedal edema* means "swelling of feet or ankles.")

The neurologist's description of Mr. Shaw's speech and comprehension suggests that Mr. Shaw is aphasic with severely impaired comprehension. Because little information about Mr. Shaw's speech is provided, it is not clear from the neurologist's report whether Mr. Shaw is truly globally aphasic or has severe Wernicke's aphasia.

The neurologist's examination of Mr. Shaw's cranial nerve functions follows the standard top-down format, beginning with visual acuity (CN 2) and moving on to eye movements and pupillary responses (CN 3, 4, 6); face (CN 5, 7); tongue, larynx, and pharynx (CN 9, 10, 12); and neck and shoulders (CN 11). The vestibular-acoustic branch of CN 7, concerned with balance and hearing, often is tested indirectly by observing the patient's response to spoken questions and instructions during the examination and by observing the patient's balance during tests involving standing and walking. The results of testing Mr. Shaw's cranial nerves do not suggest cranial nerve damage, but indicate damage in the posterior left hemisphere. (Symmetric nasolabial folds and wrinkles suggest no significant upper motor neuron damage in corticobulbar tracts serving the lower face, which in turn suggests no major frontal lobe involvement and slightly diminishes the probability that Mr. Shaw is globally aphasic.) The neurologist reports a slightly diminished jaw-jerk reflex—of minor significance given the negative results of other cranial nerve functions.

The neurologist's omission of CN 1 testing (smell, taste) is typical. CN 1 rarely is tested in routine neurologic examinations unless the neurologist has reason to suspect a pathologic condition in the olfactory nerve or olfactory cortex.

The neurologist's examination of Mr. Shaw's motor functions reveals slight weakness on Mr. Shaw's right side (with his leg somewhat weaker than his arm), brisk reflexes on his right side (but diminished in both ankles), a grasp reflex in his right hand, and a probable plantar extensor (Babinski) reflex in his right foot. These findings are consistent with damage affecting Mr. Shaw's left-side corticospinal tract. That Mr. Shaw's weakness is not severe is consistent with posterior brain damage, which spares the majority of corticospinal fibers.

A *grasp reflex* is an involuntary closing of the hand when the patient's palm is stroked. It is a sign of upper motor neuron damage in the contralateral corticospinal tract. *Pronator drift* is a sign of muscle weakness. It is seen when the patient is asked to hold his or her arms out straight in front, palms up, with eyes closed. Weakness in the arm muscles causes the weak arm to rotate toward a more natural palms-down position, and sometimes the weak arm sags in response to the pull of gravity. Mild weakness in leg muscles sometimes causes the leg to rotate outward, especially when the patient is lying down.

The neurologist's examination of Mr. Shaw's somesthetic sensory functions and gait are generally unremarkable, except for a slight right foot drag, which is consistent with the motor examination. Overall, the neurologic examination suggests that Mr. Shaw has had a stroke involving the posterior left hemisphere, with possible scattered damage extending into the frontal lobe. The most probable communication diagnosis appears to be one of Wernicke's aphasia—not global aphasia.

Doctor's Orders

Doctor's orders are written by the patient's primary physician (and sometimes by other patient-care personnel) to stipulate how the patient is to be cared for, including medications, special precautions, tests and consultations, diet, monitoring of fluid or caloric intake, rehabilitation services, and other important aspects of the patient's care. Each order is signed by the person writing it, and the person who carries the order out initials it and writes the time at which it was carried out. Information from this section of the medical record adds to the speech-language pathologist's sense of the plan of care. The speech-language pathologist will wish to know what laboratory tests have been ordered, what medications have been prescribed, whether diet modifications or restrictions have been ordered, whether other therapies such as physical therapy or occupational therapy have been ordered, and what other specialists have been consulted. This information alerts the speech-language pathologist to the need for collaboration with others involved in the patient's care, and, in the case of other therapies, alerts the speech-language pathologist to the need for coordinating the patient's speech clinic appointments with others.

Figure 3-3 shows the neurologist's orders for the period immediately following Mr. Shaw's admission to the neurology ward. The first order is for a computerized tomography (CT) scan of Mr. Shaw's head to rule out cerebral hemorrhage as the cause of his neurologic deficits. Head CT

MEDICAL RECORD	DOCTOR'S ORDERS

DATE AND TIME	PROB. NO.	ORDERS	NURSE'S INITIALS
8/11/00 1035	1	**Lab:** Head CT with contrast. R/O hemorrhage vs occlusion Ericsson	JAN 1045
8/11/00 1035	1	**Lab:** ECG. 55-y/o male with probable CVA, aphasia. Ericsson	JAN 1045
8/11/00 1035	1	Activity: Up in chair as tolerated. Ericsson	JAN 1045
8/11/00 1035	3, 4	Meds: chlorothiazide 0.5g. b.i.d. tolbutamide 0.5g. b.i.d. Ericsson	JAN 1055
8/11/00 1035	1,3	Diet: Low fat, no added salt. Ericsson	JAN 1055
8/11/00 1035	1	**Lab:** coag time, sed rate. Ericsson	JAN 1100
8/12/00 0905	1	**Lab:** Carotid u/s. R/O stenosis Ericsson	JAN 0930
8/12/00 1420	2	Speech Pathology consult: 55 y/o R-H M 1 day s/p L MCA CVA. RUE, RLE weakn. Globally aphas. Hx DM, HTN. Pls eval pt's spch & lang & make recs. Ericsson	MRB 1435
8/12/00 1420	1, 2	Social work consult: 55 y/o M 1 day s/p L MCA CVA. Globally aphasic. Pls assist with d/c planning. Ericsson	MRB 1440
8/12/00 1420	1	Rehab consult: 55 y/o M 1 day s/p L MCA CVA. Globally aphasic. RUE, RLE weakness. Pls assess and make rec's. Ericsson	JAN 1440
8/12/00 1600	1	Activity: No restrictions on ward. Pt. not to leave ward w/o supervision. Ericsson	JAN 1620
8/12/00 1600	1	**Lab:** serum triglycerides, cholesterol. Ericsson	MRB 1620

Patient Identification:
Shaw, Arthur 5/17/45
503-42-9680
2K435-32 NEU

DOCTOR'S ORDERS

Figure 3-3 ■ **Excerpts from the physician's orders for Mr. Shaw's care.**

scans are one of the first laboratory tests ordered for patients with probable strokes because the medical treatment of hemorrhagic strokes is markedly different from that of occlusive strokes. Treatment of occlusive strokes often entails administration of blood thinners (anticoagulants), and blood thinners worsen hemorrhagic strokes. Consequently, ruling out cerebral hemorrhage is a critical concern in the early phase of treatment. The next order is for an electrocardiogram, perhaps to rule out coronary artery disease or atrial fibrillations as a source of emboli.

> *Atrial fibrillations* are irregularities in the heartbeat in which the normal rhythmic contractions of heart muscles are replaced by rapid and irregular contractions. The rapid and irregular contractions can cause blood clots or fragments of tissue to break loose and travel through the bloodstream.

The next order gives permission for Mr. Shaw to be out of bed and sitting in a chair, but not to walk unassisted—a routine precaution for patients in the first day or two post-stroke. The next order prescribes continuation of the medications Mr. Shaw has been taking for his hypertension and diabetes. The neurologist prescribes a standard low-fat, low-salt diet. (In most medical facilities a dietician sees all newly admitted patients and recommends diets to meet their nutritional and hydration needs.)

The last order on Day 1 is for laboratory tests of coagulation time and sedimentation rate, which reflect the time it takes Mr. Shaw's blood to clot. Shorter-than-normal coagulation time and faster-than-normal sedimentation rate suggest a greater risk of blood clots in the vascular system and may be an indication that anticoagulant therapy is needed.

On Day 2 the neurologist orders a carotid ultrasound to determine if Mr. Shaw has stenosis (narrowing) of his carotid arteries. The order suggests that the neurologist is moving toward a diagnosis of occlusive stroke, rather than hem-

orrhagic stroke. Neurologists often order carotid ultrasound tests early in the care of patients with suspected occlusive strokes. If the results show stenosis, the probability that the patient's stroke is occlusive increases. If the stenosis is severe, the neurologist may order a follow-up cerebral angiogram to get a more precise indication of the location, severity, and nature of the stenosis than can be ascertained from the somewhat fuzzy image provided by the carotid ultrasound.

The neurologist also orders referrals to speech pathology, social work, and rehabilitation medicine and amends his previous day's order to permit Mr. Shaw to move about the ward without assistance, probably in response to the neurologist's observations and those of ward personnel that walking poses no risk to Mr. Shaw. Finally, the neurologist orders laboratory analysis of a sample of Mr. Shaw's blood to determine if the level of fatty compounds that play a part in atherosclerosis is elevated.

Progress Notes

Progress notes are written by patient-care personnel to provide a chronologic record of the patient's physical, behavioral, and mental status during hospitalization. The admitting physician usually writes the first progress note, which includes a brief description of the patient, a summary of the patient's history, and a concise summary of the significant aspects of the physical and neurologic examination. The physician's initial progress note usually ends with the physician's conclusions about diagnostic issues and the plan for the immediate future care of the patient. Day-to-day changes in the patient's behavior or condition routinely are described in progress notes, and the results of assessments (including the speech-language pathologist's assessment of communication) are recorded in the progress notes.

Entries in the progress notes by physicians, nurses, ward personnel, and other specialists provide information about the patient's alertness, orientation, and mood as well as the patient's responses to caregivers and behavior toward other patients on the ward and may indicate whether the patient can walk, dress, bathe, and accomplish other activities of daily living. Reports from specialists such as psychologists, social workers, and physical therapists provide the speech-language pathologist with insights into aspects of the patient's condition not covered by the physical and neurologic examination, and reading the specialists' goals and objectives helps the speech-language pathologist get a sense of their plans for the patient's care. If the patient is evaluated or treated by other services such as occupational therapy, physical therapy, psychologic counseling, vocational counseling, or social work, their reports and comments may be found in the progress notes. The physician's interpretations of laboratory tests also may be found there.

Figure 3-4 gives a page of progress notes from Mr. Shaw's medical record. The first entry is the neurologist's admitting note. A summary of the findings of the neurologic examination follows. The A/P (assessment/plan) section describes the neurologist's diagnostic hunches and plans for the patient's care. From the neurologist's plans for carotid ultrasound and magnetic resonance imaging (MRI) angiogram, it appears that he or she suspects an occlusive stroke, but has decided not to anticoagulate Mr. Shaw (probably because he or she wants to see the results of the CT scan first). If the CT shows no hemorrhage, the neurologist plans to administer anticoagulant medications. Finally, the neurologist plans to include rehabilitation medicine, speech pathology, social work, and ophthalmology in Mr. Shaw's care, no doubt to deal with his weakness, aphasia, post-hospital placement, and potential visual field blindness, respectively.

The progress notes continue with several entries by nursing personnel, which give a picture of Mr. Shaw as ambulatory, alert, and oriented, but with significant communication impairments. Several comments suggest that Mr. Shaw is aphasic, with significant problems in understanding what others say ("understanding seems to be a major problem," "tends to ramble," "doesn't appear frustrated or even acknowledge the com-munication block," "doesn't always get what you say"). However, he appears to be pleasant, cooperative, and helpful, suggesting that behavioral abnormalities are unlikely to be a major management issue. The last entry is by the speech-language pathologist, who acknowledges receipt of the consultation request, gives her initial impressions, and directs those reading the progress note to a language screening assessment reported elsewhere in the progress notes.

Laboratory Reports

Most medical records have a separate section for laboratory reports. Results of tests such as blood tests, CT scans, and electroencephalogram reports are found here. The speech-language pathologist reviews this section of the medical record to discover what laboratory tests have been ordered and to note the results of the completed tests, paying particular attention to the results of CT and MRI scans, angiograms, cerebrospinal fluid cultures, and any other tests that reflect the status of the patient's nervous system and thus have implications for the patient's communication impairments.

Figures 3-5 and 3-6 contain examples of two reports that may be found in the *laboratory reports* section of a medical record. Figure 3-5 shows the neuroradiologist's report of a head CT scan performed on Mr. Shaw. It suggests that Mr. Shaw has had an occlusive stroke in the white matter beneath the left temporo-parietal cortex and that the stroke extends into the cortex. The stroke apparently was caused by occlusion in the posterior distribution of the middle cerebral artery. Importantly, there is no evidence of a hemorrhagic stroke.

Figure 3-6 shows the radiologist's report of Mr. Shaw's carotid ultrasound test. It indicates that Mr. Shaw has thickening of the arterial walls and atherosclerotic plaque distributed throughout both carotid arteries. Neither Mr. Shaw's left nor his right common carotid arteries are narrowed significantly, but both internal carotid arteries show significant stenosis, with the right artery more so than the left. Mr. Shaw's left ex-

MEDICAL RECORD	PROGRESS NOTES

Date, Time	Note
8/11/00 1015	Neurology Admit Note: 55-y/o man s/p L MCA stroke 8/11/00 approx. 8:15 a.m. Pt apparently in good health previously. Sudden onset RUE, RLE weakness, slurred speech. Brought to MC by wife. No apparent preceding symptoms or headache. **PMH:** AODM, x 5 yrs. HTN x 3 yrs. Poss. TIA 3/99. **PE:** BP 162/89. P 72. T 98.6 R 18. Lungs clear. Neck supple, Mental Status: Pt awake & responsive, though inappropriate. Responds "I'm fine." Cannot give name or repeat. Follows midline commands -- close eyes, open mouth. Cannot follow complex commands. CN: EOM full, no nystagmus. Pupils equal, reactive. Face symmetric. Tongue midline. Palate midline, elevates symmetrically. Motor. Unable fo follow specific commands. Appears to give normal resistance in arms and legs. Can walk with support. R leg externally rotated when lying. Inc. grasp, plantar on R. Coordination: able to follow and locate moving target. **A/P:** Pt presents with acute alteration in language and comprehension. Also subtle signs of motor deficit on R. Obtain CT or MRI to r/o bleed. Stroke vs TIA most likely diagnosis. Obtain carotid ultrasound for risk factors. Consider MRI angiogram for vascular abnormalities. No clear indication for anticoagulation. Consider ASA or ticlopidine if CT shows no bleed. Will consult rehab, spch, sw, opth. *G. Ericsson*
8/11/00 1105	**Nursing Admission Note**. Pt. alert, oriented in no apparent distress. Wife present, participated in orientation to ward. Pt. is responsive to stimulation, but unable to respond with appropriate answers. Can transfer from bed to chair w/o assistance. Sits upright w/o tipping. Walks with assistance, but seems to have no problems with strength, balance, judgment. No signs of confusion. Continent x2. May need assistance with ADLs for a few days. Not an apparent fall risk. Patient can talk, but doesn't always make sense. Can say name, "I'm fine," "o.k." etc. Understanding seems to be a major problem. *J Nelson*
8/11/00 1245	**Nursing note.** Pt. alert, oriented. Pleasant & cooperative. Tends to ramble. Needs to be kept on one subject as much as possible. Wife came in with pt. Very concerned. Needs reassurance, support. *J Nelson*
8/11/00 1500	**Nursing note.** Pt. ambulating w/o assistance. Had late lunch. Appetite good. Pleasant and helpful. Offers no complaints. *M Benson*
8/11/00 1805	**Nursing note.** Patient seems to have severe receptive and expressive communication probs. Doesn't appear frustrated or even acknowledge the communication block. Needs seem to be met. No problems with ADLs. *M Benson*
8/11/00 2200	**Nursing note.** Pt sleeping calmly. No apparent prob's. *G Taylor*
8/12/00 0610	**Nursing note.** Slept all night. No complaints. Awake and alert. Carried out ADLs w/o assistance. Doesn't always get what you say. Sometimes helps to repeat, remind pt. of topic. *L Smith*
8/12/00 1000	**Speech-Language Pathology Note:** Consultation request received. Pt. seen briefly @ bedside. Impression: moderate-severe Wernicke's aphasia. Full report to follow. *G. Becker* SPEECH-LANGUAGE PATHOLOGIST

Patient ID
  Shaw, Arthur 5/17/45
  503-42-9680
  2K435-32 NEU

MEDICAL RECORD

PROGRESS NOTES

Figure 3-4 ■ Series of progress notes from Mr. Shaw's medical record. The notes are not necessarily continuous. Ordinarily several notes would be entered on a patient's first day on the ward.

MEDICAL RECORD

RADIOGRAPHIC REPORT

NAME: Shaw, Arthur   **WARD:** 2N, Neuro
ID#: 503 42 9680   **REQ. M.D.:** Ericsson
AGE: 55   **CASE #:** 3937

DATE OF EXAMINATION: August 12, 2000: 1433
EXAMINATION: CT HEAD WITH CONTRAST

Clinical History:
55-year old male with suspected LH stroke 8/11/00. Rule out hemorrhage.

Comparisons: There are no previous studies available for comparison.

Findings: Enhanced CT scan of the head. A new area of decreased attenuation in the left temporo-parietal white matter and extending into the overlying cortex consistent with a new occlusive infarct. No evidence of hemorrhage. The ventricles are in a midline position without evidence of mass effect.

Impressions: New area of infarction in the left temporo-parietal region consistent with occlusion of posterior branch of left middle cerebral artery. See above findings.

Films were read by: *Mary C. Richman*

Mary C. Richman, M.D., Neuroradiologist

Figure 3-5 ■ CT scan report from Mr. Shaw's medical record.

---

ternal carotid artery also may be narrowed, as indicated by increased blood velocities during the systolic phase of Mr. Shaw's heartbeat.

Figure 3-7 shows how a speech-language pathologist transfers information from Mr. Shaw's medical record to a form used in a speech-language pathology clinic. The form includes personal information about Mr. Shaw, labels his communication disorder, and summarizes the information from Mr. Shaw's medical record. The information in this form provides a quick reference for speech pathology clinic personnel who may be involved in Mr. Shaw's care

and serves as a record of Mr. Shaw's medical history and current problems, should that information be needed in the future if his medical records are not readily available.

The speech-language pathologist's review of a patient's medical record provides information about the patient's medical and neurologic problems, the patient's potential communication impairments, and the patient's behavioral and emotional state. This information helps the speech-language pathologist formulate a plan for assessing the patient's language and communication. The impressions gleaned from the patient's med-

MEDICAL RECORD

RADIOGRAPHIC REPORT

NAME: Shaw, Arthur
ID#: 503 42 9680
AGE: 55

WARD: 2N, Neuro
REQ. M.D.: Ericsson
CASE #: 2302

DATE OF EXAMINATION: August 13, 2000: 0803
EXAMINATION: NON-INVASIVE CAROTID W IMAGING

Clinical History:
55-year old male with suspected LH stroke 8/11/00. Rule out carotid stenosis.

Comparisons: There are no previous studies available for comparison.

Findings: Intimal thickening and focal areas of soft plaque are identified throughout both carotid systems.

The right common carotid artery has no associated hemodynamically significant stenosis. The right internal carotid artery has increased peak systolic velocities of 160 cm per second. This is consistent with a severe stenosis (60% to 79%) of the right internal carotid artery. The right external carotid artery demonstrates no hemodynamically significant stenosis.

The left common carotid demonstrates no associated hemodynamically significant stenosis. The left internal carotid artery has slightly increased peak systolic velocities of 130 to 140 cm per second with a diastolic velocity of 40 cm per second. This is consistent with a mild to moderate stenosis (20 to 59%) of the left internal carotid artery. There are increased peak systolic velocities in the left external carotid artery consistent with an underlying stenosis.

Impressions:
1. Severe stenosis (60 to 79%) of the right internal carotid artery.
2. Mild to moderate stenosis (20 to 59%) of the left internal carotid artery.
3. Increased peak systolic velocities of left external carotid artery consistent with underlying stenosis.
4. Right vertebral artery not visualized on this examination.

Films were read by: *Warren E Davies*

　　　　Warren E. Davies, M.D., Radiologist

Figure 3-6 ■ Report of a carotid ultrasound test from Mr. Shaw's medical record.

ical record will be firmed up by an interview with the patient and assessment of the patient's language and communication. Then the speech-language pathologist will write a response to the consultation request. The speech-language pathol-

ogist's response to the neurologist's consultation request for Mr. Shaw is shown in Figure 3-8.

The speech-language pathologist's response to the consultation request follows a common format. It begins with subjective observations,

SPEECH PATHOLOGY SERVICE

Patient Information

Patient Name: Shaw, Arthur	**Soc Sec Number:** 503 42 9680	**Referral Date:** 8/12/00
Home Address:	**Occupation:** Accountant	**Physician:** Ericsson 4498
6877 Lakeview Court	**Marital Status:** M (Florence)	**Med Diagnoses:**
Riverview, MN 55444-1212	**Education:** College (B.A.)	L MCA CVA, aphasia
Birthdate: *5/17/45*	**Home Phone:** 612/ 555-9888	
Referring Ward: 2N (Neuro)	**Referring Service:** Neurology	**SPS File #:** 6888

Communication, Swallowing Disorders

Problem #1: Aphasia	**Date of Onset:** 8/11/00
Problem #2:	**Date of Onset:**
Problem #3:	**Date of Onset:**

Medical Information

Previous Medical History: Adult onset diabetes mellitus diagnosed 1991. Controlled by oral medications.
Hypertension diagnosed November 1993. Pt's wife mentioned brief episode of numbness in pt's RUE, March, '99. MD: "poss. TIA."

History of Present Illness: The patient apparently was in good health until the morning of August 11. He was dressing for work when he experienced sudden onset of right-sided weakness and slurred speech. He alerted his wife who called an ambulance which brought him to the emergency room at this medical center. On arrival he exhibited extreme weakness and exaggerated reflexes on his right side. His speech apparently was fluent with verbal paraphasias and some jargon, and his comprehension was grossly impaired. Since that time he apparently has been improving slowly, although he seems still to have a substantial aphasia. Nursing notes suggest that he is oriented and alert.

Laboratory Results: CT Scan: New area of decreased attenuation in the left temporo-parietal white matter, extending into cortex, c/w new occlusive infarct. No evidence of hemorrhage. Carotid u/s: Severe stenosis R ICA (60-79%), mild-moderate stenosis LICA (20-59%).

BP: 162/89.

Medications: tolbutamide, chlorothiazide

Other: Low fat low salt diet. Consult to SW: "Pls assist with d/c planning." Consult to Rehab: "RUE, RLE weakness, pls assess and make rec's."

Clinician: G. Becker, Ph.D, CCC-SLP	**Signature:** *G. Becker*	
SPEECH-LANGUAGE PATHOLOGIST	**Date:** 8/12/00	

Figure 3-7 ■ **Form used by the speech-language pathologist to record information from Mr. Shaw's medical record.**

Medical Record	Consultation Request/Referral	
To: Speech Pathology	**From**: Ward 2N Neurology	**Date**: 8/12/00 14:36

Provisional Diagnosis: LMCA CVA, global aphasia

Requested by: Ericsson, G. 4498	Place: Consultant's choice	Urgency: Routine

Reason for Request: 55 y/o R-H M 1 day s/p recent L MCA CVA. RUE, RLE weakn. Globally aphasic. Pls eval pt's sp & lang & make recs.

Consultation Report

Mr. Shaw's speech and language was evaluated in the Speech Pathology Clinic on 8/14/00.

Subjective Observations: Mr. Shaw is a 55-year-old man who experienced a left middle cerebral artery CVA on August 11, 2000. Mr. Shaw was brought to the speech pathology clinic in a wheelchair, although he later claimed that he can walk, although "I guess I'm a little unsteady on my feet." During the evaluation he was cooperative, attentive, alert, and task-oriented, although the presence of a severe auditory comprehension impairment markedly compromised his conversational and test-taking abilities.

Objective Measures: Several speech and language tests were administered. Mr. Shaw's performance suggested:
 - Severe impairment of listening comprehension. Mr. Shaw can correctly identify drawings of common objects named by the examiner on about 50% of trials. He can follow one-step commands ("Pick up the spoon") with about 50% accuracy, but cannot follow 2-step commands ("Point to the pencil and give me the key.")
 - Severe impairment of speech production. Mr. Shaw's speech, both in conversation and during testing, is vague, devoid of meaning, and littered with verbal paraphasias ("chair" for "table") and literal paraphasias ("spomb" for "comb"). Occasional neologisms (nonwords) are also observed. However, the mechanics of Mr. Shaw's speech production are relatively unaffected -- he speaks smoothly and effortlessly, with essentially normal rate, intonation, and stress patterns.
 - Severely compromised reading ability. Mr. Shaw can read a few simple concrete words ("man," "dog") but cannot read multisyllabic words or longer units. Failed attempts are characterized by paraphasias and neologisms.
 - Severely compromised writing ability. Mr. Shaw could copy his name, with effort, but could write nothing intelligible either spontaneously or to dictation.

Impressions and Conclusions: Mr. Shaw currently exhibits symptoms consistent with severe Wernicke's (receptive) aphasia. Because of the recent onset of Mr. Shaw's aphasia, the severity of his language impairments should diminish during the next several weeks, although he is likely to remain moderately aphasic even when full neurologic recovery has taken place. His return to employability appears, at this time, unlikely.

Recommendations:
 1. Additional assessment of Mr. Shaw's listening comprehension to determine the extent and nature of his comprehension impairments.
 2. A period of trial treatment to improve auditory comprehension and self-monitoring to determine Mr. Shaw's potential to benefit from treatment.
 3. Speech-language pathologist to meet with Mr. Shaw's wife and other concerned family members to answer questions and discuss Mr. Shaw's potential return home.

The patient was examined: [x] yes [ ] no
The patient's medical record was reviewed: [x] yes [ ] no

Signature and Title: *G Becker* G. Becker, Ph.D., CCC Speech-Language Pathologist		**Date:** 8/14/00
ID#: 133591	**Organization/Service:** Speech Pathology	**Reg #:** -	**Ward:** -
Patient Identification: Shaw, Arthur 5/17/45 503-42-9680 2K435-32-NEU		**SF 522 5/98 Consultation Request**

Figure 3-8 ■ **Speech-language pathologist's response to the consultation request by Mr. Shaw's physician.**

then describes the results of objective tests, interprets the test results, and offers an opinion regarding the nature of the patient's problems and their probable time course. The speech-language pathologist concludes with recommendations for dealing with the problems noted in the referral. The speech-language pathologist's response to the consultation request is brief and to the point (most physicians and other health care personnel are reluctant to take the time needed to read long and complex reports). Tests are described in everyday language, and examples of test items are provided. (The names of most tests of communication ability and scores on them have little meaning to most non-speech-language pathologists.) The format of the speech-language pathologist's report makes it easy for the person making the consultation request to get the information from the report quickly and effortlessly. This helps to ensure that the report will be read by the requestor (and others) and that those who read it will get the information they need to appreciate the effects of the patient's communication impairments on the plan of care. The impressions generated by the speech-language pathologist's review of the patient's medical record subsequently are put to the test when the speech-language pathologist interviews the patient.

INTERVIEWING THE PATIENT

The interview provides the speech-language pathologist's first direct look at the patient's communication abilities, physical condition, orientation and attention, visual and hearing acuity, behavioral inclinations, and other characteristics that might affect how (or if) the subsequent assessment is carried out. Getting the interpersonal relationship off to a good start usually is as important as the information-gathering function of the interview. There is no one best way to do this, and different clinicians may approach a given patient in different ways with equivalent results. The most successful, however, share two common attributes—they care about the patient and let it show, and they treat the patient

with respect. In addition to caring about and respecting the patient, good interviewers comply with the following general principles that govern how the interview takes place.

Do your homework before the interview. Before the interview, review the patient's medical record to get a sense of the patient's personal and medical history and medical problems. Talk with the patient's physician and nursing staff to get insights and observations that may not be in the patient's medical record. Your homework will help you ask the appropriate questions and make appropriate comments during the interview, and it will help you focus on the most relevant information for testing diagnostic questions. It also may help you avoid material that may elicit emotional responses from the patient or make them feel apprehensive or threatened.

Conduct the interview in a quiet place, free from distractions. Many first interviews are held at bedside, in the patient's room. This is fine if the room is quiet, without peripheral distractions, because the patient is likely to be more relaxed and comfortable in familiar surroundings. However, the advantage of familiar surroundings is lost if noisy or distracting activities are present. If the patient's room is not quiet and free of distractions, find another place nearby—a day room, a conference room, an empty patient room, or, if nothing is available on the patient's ward, move the interview to a quiet room off the ward.

Include family members or significant others in the interview. Family members and significant others should be invited to participate in the interview, especially if the patient's communication impairments are severe. If the patient's communication impairments are mild or moderate, family members and significant others can corroborate what the patient says and can help the patient remember, produce, or clarify information. If the patient's communication impairments are severe, family members and significant others may be the primary (or only) source of information, and the patient's role may be that of confirmation and corroboration. If a patient is able to communicate only rudimentary information, and that with great difficulty, the speech-language pathologist may schedule some time with family members and significant others to get the information that the patient cannot provide. The following suggestions relate to the patient interview, but they also apply to interviews with family members and significant others.

Tell the patient who you are. In teaching hospitals, patients are seen by a confusing mix of physicians, residents, medical students, interns, and others, many of whom pop in and out of the patient's room without introduction or explanation. Helping the patient sort out this mix usually makes for a more relaxed and less stressed patient. Regrettably, physicians sometimes neglect to tell patients that they are referring them to other specialists, so patients are surprised and concerned when the specialist arrives unannounced. Therefore it is important that you make certain that the patient knows right away who you are and why their physician asked you to see them.

> Boll (1994) recommends that the interviewer begin by asking the patient why the patient's physician has referred the patient to the specialist. According to Boll, the patient's response gives the interviewer a sense of the patient's comprehension of the circumstances, their level of interest and motivation, their comfort with the arrangements, and the adequacy with which the referral has been handled by the referring parties. According to Boll, it also gives the interviewer a sense of whether the patient has been informed about the nature of the interview, and whether the information has been understood, ignored, or forgotten.

Introduce yourself and tell the patient what your responsibilities are:

> I'm Ms. Smith. I'm from the speech clinic. Dr. Jones said that you might be having some problems speaking. I'll be working with you to find out if

you do, and we'll decide what we might be able to do about them.

Tell the patient how you fit into the treatment team:

> Your doctor will take care of your medical problems. The physical therapist will work on your walking and help you regain strength in your arm. I'll be working with you on talking, writing, and understanding.

Make the patient comfortable. Spend a few minutes in conversation to allow the patient to relax and talk about familiar topics. Ask the patient some general questions about themselves ("Where are you from?" "What kind of work do you, or did you, do?" "Are you married?" "Do you have children/grandchildren?") This usually helps put the patient at ease, especially if the interviewer can discover common ground—knowledge of the patient's home town, street address, mutual interests, and so forth.

> Some patients (in my experience, not many) react emotionally to questions about family and occupation because the questions make them despondent about compromised family and work relationships and responsibilities. The interviewer must be sensitive to the potential effect of such topics and should be prepared to move away from them if the patient shows signs of emotional upset.

Sit down during the interview. A standing interviewer conversing with a seated or recumbent patient can be intimidating, and, regardless of the length of the interview, standing during the interview may give the patient a feeling that you are on the way to somewhere more important and that the patient represents an unwelcome intrusion into your busy schedule. Try to give patients the sense that getting to know them and their concerns is important to you and that there is nothing that you would rather be doing than talking with them.

Get the patient's story. Begin with a general question ("How are you feeling today?"), following it with whatever additional questions or commentary seem appropriate. Then move on to the patient's communication problems ("Are you having difficulty talking? Tell me about it."). Find out how the patient feels about the problems. Some patients may be traumatized about communication abnormalities that most would consider minor annoyances, whereas others are unconcerned about impairments that seriously interfere with communication. Make mental notes of what the patient says and pursue any interesting leads. Note other significant aspects of the patient's condition and behavior—whether the patient is ambulatory and able to sit up and attend for the length of time needed for testing; the patient's mood, orientation, and mental status; the patient's visual and auditory acuity; and whether the patient wears eyeglasses or a hearing aid.

Be a patient, concerned, and understanding listener. Give the patient time to tell his or her story. Don't interrupt and don't lead, unless the patient gets bogged down in trivial details or goes off on tangents that clearly are unrelated to the purpose of the interview. Ask questions to follow up on potentially meaningful information, but do not steer the patient to provide the answers that you expect, based on your preconceptions. Don't be oversolicitous and overly sympathetic. Adult patients don't need and often resent overdone expressions of concern and sympathy. Receive what the patient says objectively and matter-of-factly and treat the interview as a problem-solving enterprise between the patient and the interviewer.

Talk to the patient at the patient's level. Use everyday language, and avoid jargon and technical terminology, which may confuse or intimidate the patient. Monitor the patient's alertness and understanding, and repeat and paraphrase if necessary. Pay careful attention to the patient's eye contact, facial expression, and body language as indicators of frustration, anxiety, or miscomprehension. Don't talk *at* the patient; talk

with the patient. Treat the patient as a partner in the interview. Accommodate the patient's interaction style, but avoid excessive familiarity. Be friendly, but objective. Use humor sparingly and judiciously, but do not avoid it. Judiciously used and properly timed humor can help to humanize the interview, dissipate tension, and reassure the patient without minimizing the seriousness of the patient's situation.

Treat the patient as an adult who merits respect. Never ask questions or convey an attitude that makes the patient feel inadequate, juvenile, or incompetent. Sometimes it helps to point out to the patient that their medical condition may make it difficult or impossible to do some of the things that the patient used to do easily, but that many other abilities remain unaffected. If a topic or line of questioning appears to embarrass the patient or make them anxious, it may be time to move on to a different topic. If the abandoned line of questioning appears important, you can come back to it later and lead into it more carefully.

An important, but subtle, indicator of respect is the way in which the clinician addresses the patient. It is never appropriate to address the patient by first name during the clinician's early contacts with the patient, but it may become appropriate later, when the clinician and the patient have gotten better acquainted, but even then the clinician should ask the patient how she or he would prefer to be addressed. Some older patients resent the use of their first names by those involved in their care, especially when the person providing care is appreciably younger than the patient.

Prepare the patient for what comes next. If you plan more testing, prepare the patient for it. Give the patient a general idea of the kinds of tests you plan to administer and why you are going to administer them. Tell the patient the day and time of testing if you know them. Answer the patient's questions and deal with concerns they express.

Reassure the patient. Be objective and straightforward about the patient's impairments, but emphasize the patient's retained abilities. If you believe that the patient will improve as time passes, say so, but do not give the patient false hope by offering an unduly optimistic prognosis. Discuss options for treatment with the patient and point out that all members of the patient-care team are there to help the patient regain physical, cognitive, and communicative abilities.

By the end of the interview the patient and the clinician should be comfortable with each other and the patient should be comfortable with the idea of being tested. The clinician should have a good idea of what tests to begin with and the approximate level of difficulty of the first few tests. Information from the referral, the patient's medical records, and the interview helps to determine which tests are selected. The clinician's experiences with the patient during the interview largely determine the level of difficulty at which testing begins.

TESTING THE PATIENT

Most testing is done in a private testing room, although screening tests may be administered in the patient's room. Before the testing begins, the clinician takes a few minutes to explain the purpose of the tests, answer the patient's questions, and obtain the patient's consent for testing. Lezak (1995) provides guidelines regarding what the patient should be told before any test is administered:

- Explain the purpose of testing. Tell the patient why testing is necessary and how the information from the tests will be used. (Some common purposes: to determine if the patient has a communication impairment, to understand the patient's communication problems, to decide about the need for treatment, to decide how to treat the patient's communication problems, and to measure the patient's progress.)
- Tell the patient what will be done to protect the patient's privacy and the confidentiality of test results. This usually means that only persons in the medical center who are involved in the patient's care will have access to the re-

sults of testing and that access will be given to others only with the written permission of the patient or the patient's legal representative.

- Tell the patient who will report test results to the patient and family and when they will report them. This usually is the speech-language pathologist, but occasionally may be the physician or another professional.
- Give the patient a brief explanation of test procedures (e.g., explain how long test sessions usually last; that the patient will be asked to do tasks involving speaking, listening, reading, and writing; that some tasks will be easy and others may be difficult; and that testing can be terminated if the patient becomes tired or wishes to terminate the test).
- Find out how the patient feels about taking the tests. Some patients may be uneasy or apprehensive about testing because they fear that poor performance will be seen as weakness, lack of intelligence, or childishness. Reiterating the purposes of testing may be sufficient to dispel the uneasy patient's concerns. However, the patient (or the patient's legal representative) always has the right to refuse any or all testing.

If audiotape or videotape recordings of the patient's test performance are made, the examiner must explain the purposes of the recording (e.g., to allow the patient and the speech-language pathologist to evaluate the patient's progress), who will have access to the recordings (e.g., the speech-language pathologist, the patient's physician, and student trainees), and what will be done with the recordings when the patient is no longer receiving speech-language pathology services (e.g., given to the patient or erased). Most facilities require that the patient, the patient's legal representative, or both read and sign a printed consent form giving permission for the recordings.

GENERAL CONCEPTS 3-1

- Skilled clinicians employ a structured approach when they evaluate adults who have neurogenic communication impairments. Most use some form of what is called *the clinical method.* The clinical method is a structured procedure for making clinical decisions about diagnosis, testing, prognosis, and treatment.

- The *referral* (consultation request) gives the speech-language pathologist an important first look at the patient. The referral usually provides personal information about the patient together with the physician's plans for the patient's care and indications of the patient's medical, physical, and behavioral condition; medical diagnoses; and probable length of stay.

- *Medical records* typically are divided into sections, with each section containing a different kind of information about a patient:
  —*Patient identification:* personal information about the patient, plus diagnostic or other codes
  —*Medical history:* information about previous medical conditions and a summary of the patient's current symptoms
  —*Physical and neurologic examination:* the physician's findings from examination of the patient
  —*Doctor's orders:* orders, instructions, special precautions, consultation referrals, requests for medications, requests for special tests
  —*Progress notes:* descriptions of the patient's physical, behavioral, and mental status and descriptions of significant events or incidents (e.g., falls, emotional outbursts)
  —*Laboratory reports:* results of tests such as x-ray studies, computerized tomography scans, analysis of blood

- The speech-language pathologist's initial interview with the patient provides a general sense of the patient's abilities and disabilities, personality, behavior, emotional state, attention and alertness, as well as information about the nature and severity of the patient's communicative impairments. During the interview the clinician may support, inform, counsel, and educate the patient and family members about the nature of the patient's communicative impairments; tell them how, when, and by whom decisions about treatment will be made; and provide them with a preliminary estimate of outcome.

- The speech-language pathologist's interview with the patient provides information that helps the speech-language pathologist decide what tests to give, the level of difficulty at which to begin testing, and what modifications of test procedures might be necessary. The interview may also permit the speech-language pathologist to make preliminary decisions regarding treatment.

- Testing brain-injured adults is a collaborative effort between the speech-language pathologist and the patient. The speech-language pathologist finds out what the patient's primary concerns are and gets the patient's opinions about what the directions of treatment might be.

- The speech-language pathologist explains the purpose of each test and how each test relates to the patient's problems and concerns. Helping the patient understand the nature of the impairments and pointing out areas of preserved abilities can be therapeutic.

- Before testing begins, the speech-language pathologist tells the patient why they are being tested, what kinds of tests will be given, who will have access to test results, and who will communicate the results to the patient and family members.

- The speech-language pathologist ascertains how the patient feels about being tested and asks the patient to consent to the testing.

- If audiotape or videotape recordings are made, the patient or the patient's legal representative must give consent to the recording.

BEHAVIORAL, COGNITIVE, AND EMOTIONAL EFFECTS OF BRAIN INJURY

Brain injury affects the way patients approach tasks, solve problems, and respond to stimuli. The effects of brain injury on a patient's behavior, cognition, and emotional tone reflect not only the brain injury itself, but the patient's premorbid personality, intellect, social skills, interests, and emotional predispositions, together with the coping strategies still available to the patient. The behavioral, cognitive, and emotional effects of brain injury may complicate interactions with the patient, affect the patient's performance in testing and treatment activities, and compromise the patient's daily life independence and self-sufficiency. Clinicians who work with brain-injured patients must not only be skilled in administering tests and conducting treatment, but also must be skillful in anticipating, recognizing, and managing the behavioral, cognitive, and emotional anomalies that many times accompany brain injury.

Altered Responsiveness

Slowed responding is one of the most common behavioral consequences of brain injury. Sometimes slowed responding is attributable to weakness or incoordination (the slowed speech of the dysarthric patient, the slow writing of the patient with rigidity), but more often is the visible result of slowed mental processing, which appears as slow reaction times, delays in responding to stimulation, or longer-than-normal times to complete tasks. Even patients with mild brain injury who seemingly have no residual impairments often complain of mental slowing.

> I'm still not as sharp as I used to be . . . I'm just generally slower on the uptake. Mentally, I mean.

Some brain-injured patients are passive and compliant, but tend not to initiate purposeful behavior. These patients typically respond appropriately to requests, especially in highly structured contexts. Some readily talk about plans and projects but fail to put their talk into action. Because these patients are capable of doing much more than they spontaneously do, caregivers, family members, and associates may regard them as lazy, unmotivated, uncooperative, or stubborn. Patients with severe initiation

problems produce almost no spontaneous purposeful behavior beyond that required for routine self-care and day-to-day household chores.

Some brain-injured patients are hyperresponsive and impulsive. Their responses to people, events, and situations are quick, indiscriminate, and often inappropriate. They seem to be caught up by their first impressions. They fail to appreciate subtle or abstract aspects of events or situations, which may lead them into misinterpretations. Patients' impulsiveness and concreteness may compromise their success in rehabilitation programs and may create problems in social, personal, and financial matters.

Some brain-injured patients behave as if they do not trust their perceptions and doubt their ability to handle challenges. Their self-doubts make them indecisive, hesitant, and slow to respond when they feel challenged or threatened, and when they do eventually respond, they revise, qualify, or elaborate on adequate and appropriate responses. Excessive cautiousness affects these patients' test-taking and their performance in treatment activities, wherein they often perform below their capabilities. Cautiousness often compromises these patients' social lives by leading them to withdraw from all but the most comfortable and predictable daily life relationships. Patients with mild brain injury are especially susceptible to excessive caution and timidity, perhaps because they are highly aware of minor lapses that would not be noticed by patients with more severe brain injury.

Perseveration

Perseveration denotes repetition of responses when they are no longer appropriate, as when a patient who has correctly named a pencil calls the next several objects pencils or when a patient who has correctly given her name in response to the examiner's request continues to give her name in response to the examiner's questions about her address and vocation. The frequency and persistence of perseverative responses are related to the severity of brain damage, although the relationship is not perfect.

Perseveration often appears in the first days and weeks following brain injury, but often diminishes (and sometimes disappears) as the patient recovers.

Diminished Response Flexibility

Many brain-injured patients have difficulty changing their responses when tasks or response requirements change. In test situations these patients show a pattern of performance in which the first few responses in a new task are less prompt, accurate, or complete than later responses in the task. The problem for some seems to be that they are slow at refocusing or reallocating attention when situational requirements change. The problem for others seems to be that they are slow at developing a strategy for dealing with the new task requirements.

Concreteness and Difficulty with Abstract Concepts

Concreteness, or what Goldstein (1948) referred to as "loss of the abstract attitude," is a common consequence of brain injury, especially diffuse brain injury. Goldstein was referring to brain-injured patients' failure to appreciate the abstract or implied meaning of events, situations, or spoken and written material. These patients frequently have difficulty appreciating figurative meanings such as idiom and metaphor ("a heavy heart," "the handwriting on the wall") and fail to grasp the implications of humor, sarcasm, proverbs, and other materials in which intended meaning cannot be represented by literal interpretations. Concreteness may contribute to some brain-injured patients' tendencies toward *egocentrism* (inability to appreciate another's point of view). Concreteness often has major effects on brain-injured patients' problem-solving because they see only the simplest and most obvious solutions. Sometimes apparent concreteness can be a result of impulsiveness, but more often it reflects an underlying cognitive impairment that prevents the patient from appreciating the implied meaning of abstract material.

Impaired Self-Monitoring

Many brain-injured adults do poorly at monitoring their performance, both in structured assessment and treatment activities and in unstructured social situations. Impaired self-monitoring can have wide-ranging effects, including obliviousness to errors during testing and treatment and inappropriate behavior in social situations. It is a common consequence of both focal and diffuse brain injuries. Many patients with impaired self-monitoring do better in highly structured situations where response choices are constrained than they do in situations in which they are left to their own behavioral devices.

Difficulty Focusing and Sustaining Attention

Many brain-injured adults are slow at focusing attention and cannot maintain attentional focus over time. Those who are slow at focusing attention have difficulty when tasks or response requirements change. When these patients are tested, they may miss the first items in a test or subtest but respond adequately to later items. Patients who have difficulty sustaining attention typically get worse as testing progresses, even when the difficulty of test items does not change. Some patients' attentional processes seem to fluctuate over time, so that intervals of poor performance alternate with intervals of adequate performance, with the changes in performance seemingly unrelated to changes in tasks, stimuli, or response requirements.

Disturbances of Personality and Emotion

Brain damage sometimes contributes to exaggerated swings in emotional expression, a condition called *emotional lability.* Emotionally labile patients' expressions of emotion are appropriate (they express sadness and happiness in appropriate contexts), but the magnitude of their emotional response is disproportionate to the eliciting stimulus. Emotional lability associated with brain damage frequently is expressed as uncontrollable crying in response to neutral or mildly emotional stimuli—for example, the patient who breaks into tears when asked if he has children. Neurologists and others sometimes call this phenomenon *pseudobulbar affect* because it can occur as a consequence of bilateral damage to corticospinal and corticobulbar tracts above the pons. (The pons is sometimes called the *bulb;* hence the term *pseudobulbar.*) For these patients, lability may represent loss of cortical inhibition of emotional responses originating in lower, phylogenetically more primitive structures. Emotional lability sometimes takes the form of inappropriate laughter in situations that are not humorous or excessive laughter in response to mildly amusing stimuli, especially when the patient feels stressed, challenged, or threatened.

> Emotional lability can occur in association with, or as a consequence of, conditions that have nothing to do with brain injury—for example, some psychiatric states, intoxication, or as a reaction to stress, confusion, or embarrassment.

Some brain-injured patients are prone to emotional outbursts, usually as a consequence of lowered frustration tolerance. These patients explode emotionally when stressed or pushed to their limits or beyond—a response that Schuell, Jenkins, and Jimenez-Pabon (1964) called *catastrophic reaction.* There are several differences between emotionally labile patients and patients with low frustration tolerance. Emotionally labile patients can be pushed into emotional breakdown by innocuous or mildly stressful events, but patients with low frustration tolerance typically lose control only when pushed too far. The emotional outbreaks of emotionally labile patients appear suddenly and without warning, but patients with low frustration tolerance often give visible signs of an impending explosion, becoming progressively agitated and showing other signs of autonomic arousal as they approach the threshold for an outburst. Those who live and work around patients with low frustration tolerance learn to recognize the precursors to emotional outbursts and may prevent the outbursts by changing the situation or by otherwise lowering the patient's level of arousal.

The foregoing effects of brain damage on cognitive, perceptual, and behavioral functions can influence brain-injured patients' responses to the interview and affect their test performance. The clinician who knows that brain damage can create cognitive, perceptual, and behavioral disturbances can plan for them and by planning for them can minimize their effects on clinician–patient interactions, on testing, and on treatment.

SOME GENERAL PRINCIPLES FOR TESTING ADULTS WITH BRAIN INJURIES

Testing adults who have brain injuries poses special challenges. Because brain-injured adults may exhibit a bewildering array of behavioral, cognitive, linguistic, and psychologic abnormalities, those who test them often are called on to exhibit unusual levels of patience, empathy, and understanding, in addition to being expert in test administration and skilled at interpreting patients' responses to test items. There is no substitute for experience in testing brain-injured adults, just as there is no substitute for experience in other complex activities such as making a soufflé or driving a taxicab in New York City. However, observation of the following set of general principles can help beginning clinicians compensate for lack of experience.

Do your homework. The conscientious clinician comes to the first test session with a plan for assessing the patient's communication, based largely on information from the patient's medical record and the interview. From the medical record the clinician has learned something about the patient's background, life situation, and current problems, and from the interview the clinician has gotten a sense of the patient's cognitive abilities, personality, social behavior, and communication impairments. The clinician may have formulated a tentative diagnosis and usually will have in mind a plan for where to begin and how to proceed with testing. Such a plan ensures that testing is systematic and efficient, so that each test builds on the one before, and ensures that all necessary tests, but no unnecessary ones, are administered.

Choose an appropriate place for testing. The test environment should be quiet, well-lit, and free from distractions. Furnishings should be comfortable but functional—a good-sized table and two comfortable chairs are a minimum requirement. The test materials should be accessible to the examiner but out of sight until they are needed. If audio or video recordings are made, microphones and cameras should be in unobtrusive locations.

Schedule testing to maximize the patient's performance. Most hospitalized patients have surprisingly busy schedules. Laboratory tests, appointments with counselors and social workers, physical and occupational therapy appointments, and other such activities fill the patient's day. To compound the problem, most brain-injured patients no longer have the stamina they had before their injury and by late morning or early afternoon are exhausted and need nothing so much as a nap. Consequently, the shrewd speech-language pathologist schedules testing sessions early in the day, while the patient is still fresh, and if testing sessions must be scheduled later in the day, ensures that the patient has had a chance to rest before the test session.

Make testing a collaborative effort. The examiner must never forget that the patient is an adult who may be anxious, apprehensive, bewildered, and perhaps frightened by their neurologic and behavioral symptoms. The clinician should point out that because the purpose of testing is to get a sense of the nature and severity of the patient's impairments, together with an accurate picture of what the patient can still do, both difficult and easy tests are necessary.

The clinician should prepare the patient for potential failure on tests that previously would have been easy for the patient by pointing out that failure is the result of what has happened to the patient and does not represent the patient's general competence or value as a person.

Testing should be approached matter-of-factly, but in an atmosphere of support and understanding. Pointing out to the patient that the assessment process is a collaborative effort by the patient and the clinician may help give the patient a sense that they are an active participant in the process. Schuell, Jenkins, and Jimenez-Pabon (1964) claim therapeutic benefits for testing when it is approached as a joint effort by the clinician and the patient:

> ...searching exploration of aphasic disabilities can be a therapeutic rather than a traumatic procedure. This is true because the process of testing establishes communication on a level that is highly meaningful to the patient. As a result, he feels less isolated and less anxious. By means of the tests, the examiner leads the patient toward objectivity by helping him understand the nature of his problems and their limits. The patient discovers things he is able to do, which tends to restore confidence and alleviate depression. Patients become less and less defensive as confidence in the clinician increases. (p. 168)

Select tests that are appropriate for the patient. Skilled clinicians usually have a general sense of the nature of the patient's probable impairments and the patient's likely level of impairment before testing begins. This knowledge helps the clinician focus testing on the patient's probable impairments and ensures that testing begins at a level appropriate to the patient.

The assessment process often begins with administration of a generic test battery (e.g., a standardized aphasia test battery). Generic test batteries provide a general description of a patient's performance in a variety of tasks and at various levels of difficulty within tasks. They are useful for identifying communicative or cognitive disabilities, estimating their severity, and describing their nature. Some can be used to assign patients to diagnostic categories. Some can be used to predict the eventual level of a patient's recovery. Generic test batteries provide broad coverage of a domain of linguistic, cognitive, or behavioral attributes in a reasonable amount of time (1 to 3 hours). Generic test batteries provide clinicians with a look at many aspects of a patient's communication performance (speaking, listening, writing, and reading), but the look does not always have great depth. Generic test batteries in some respects function as screening devices because they are good at detecting communication impairments, but not so good at specifying their exact nature or severity.

Weisenberg and McBride (1935), Schuell (1965), and Porch (1967) have each discussed characteristics that generic test batteries for brain-injured adults should have. The following list is a blend of recommendations made by Weisenberg and McBride, Schuell, and Porch:

- The test battery should sample a large number of performances at different levels of difficulty in several related tasks so that all potentially disturbed performances are evaluated.
- The test battery should allow the clinician to determine the level at which performance is error-free, the level at which performance completely breaks down, and several intervening levels within each test or subtest.
- The test battery should sample in a consistent way the input modalities through which test instructions are delivered, the mental processes needed to perform the tasks, and the output modalities necessary for carrying out the tasks.
- The test battery should be standardized so that results are reliable from test to test and examiner to examiner. It should provide for control of relevant variables such as method of stimulus presentation, nature of test stimuli, instructions to the patient, and response scoring.
- The test battery should record patient performance in such a way that the quality of responses, as well as their correctness, is recorded.
- Subtests in the test battery should include enough items to permit the user to reliably

determine a patient's average performance on each subtest and to control for the effects of sporadic fluctuations in the patient's performance.
- The test battery should suggest the reasons for a patient's deficient performance on test items.
- The test battery should permit predictions regarding a patient's eventual recovery.

Because no two brain-injured patients are likely to exhibit exactly the same pattern of deficits, clinicians rarely rely exclusively on a generic test battery for evaluating every patient within a diagnostic category. Most clinicians begin with a generic test battery to get a general impression of the patient's level of performance under well-controlled test conditions and to establish the general pattern and overall severity of the patient's deficits. Then they branch off with standardized or nonstandardized tests appropriate for the patient's pattern of impairments. The generic test battery permits them to get a look at the patient's performance under standardized test conditions, compare the patient's performance with that of norm groups, and establish reliable baseline levels of performance. The follow-up testing permits them to describe the patient's unique pattern of impairments and preserved abilities.

Let the patient's performance guide what and how you test. Skilled clinicians are alert to signals suggesting that they should branch off from their usual test routine. These signals come from many sources—the patient's history, the diagnosis, the clinician's previous experience with similar patients, the patient's current test performance, and sometimes from a clinical hunch. When skilled clinicians receive such signals, they diverge from their test routine to follow up on leads provided by the patient's performance. They modify standard tests or improvise new tests to specify the variables that affect the patient's performance. This sometimes requires that the focus of testing change throughout the examination until the nature and severity of the patient's impairments become clear.

An important part of this process is what Lezak (1995) calls *testing the limits*. Clinicians test the limits by going beyond the standard procedures for administering a given test to explore the reasons for a patient's compromised performance. For example, a clinician might allow a patient who fails a standard test of written spelling to spell the same words orally. Normal oral spelling performance would show that the deficient performance on the standard test was not because the patient could not spell, but perhaps because the patient could not write. If the patient were to fail the oral spelling test, the clinician might have the patient choose correctly spelled words from sets of printed words in which the correctly spelled word is shown with incorrectly spelled foils. According to Lezak (1995):

> The limits should be tested whenever there is suspicion that an impairment of some function other than the one under consideration is interfering with an adequate demonstration of that function. (p. 129)

An important benefit of personalizing tests and procedures to the patient is a substantial gain in efficiency. Patients and clinicians do not spend large amounts of time on tests in which the patient's performance is normal, nor do they spend time on too-difficult tests in which the patient experiences repeated failure. The results of tests in which the patient either makes no errors or makes only errors are of little diagnostic or therapeutic use, and administering them may be a waste of precious clinic time. Furthermore, administering tests that are outside the patient's range may have negative effects on the patient. Too-easy tests may bore or insult the patient and too-difficult tests may frustrate and anger them, interfering with performance on other tests that normally might be within the patient's capabilities.

Use standardized tests and test procedures judiciously and purposefully. Skilled clinicians do not avoid standardized tests and test batteries, although they rarely provide the detail needed to describe a particular patient's pattern of performance. There is no substitute for standardized tests when the clinician wishes to compare a patient's test performance with that of other patients or with that of non-brain-injured adults, compare a patient's performance across several test occasions, or communicate about the patient with other professionals. For any of these purposes, uniform test procedures are necessary, and standardized tests are more likely than nonstandardized tests to have them.

Standardized tests can contribute to efficiency in testing—most are structured to minimize redundancy; maximize precision; and minimize the complexities of test administration, scoring, and interpretation. However, standardized test batteries can contribute to inefficiency by forcing the patient to undergo more testing than necessary. Skilled clinicians often minimize this inefficiency by administering only selected subtests from standardized test batteries. The subtests are selected to target aspects of performance that the clinician finds most important for a particular patient. This method of targeting is most practical when norms are available for each subtest in the battery. The availability of subtest norms permits the clinician to compare the patient's performance with that of groups of individuals—usually a group of "normal" adults and one or more groups of adults representing various diagnostic categories (e.g., adults with aphasia)—subtest by subtest.

Consider the validity of standardized tests. Most standardized tests come with information about their *validity*—the degree to which they actually measure what they purport to measure. Various kinds of validity have been described in the literature, but the most often described kinds are *content validity* and *construct validity*. There is some overlap, but in general *content validity* relates to how well the content of a test (items, tasks, or questions) represents the domain of concern (e.g., intelligence), and *construct validity* relates to how well the content of a test represents an underlying theory, model, or concept of a process or structure. Consider, for example, a test for measuring comprehension of spoken discourse. To evaluate the test's *content validity* a test user would ask if the items in the test actually require comprehension of spoken discourse. To evaluate the test's *construct validity,* one would ask if the content of the test and the test procedures are compatible with one or more theories, models, or concepts of discourse comprehension. Clinicians tend to be concerned more with content validity than with construct validity. They want to know that a test of auditory comprehension actually tests comprehension, that a test of memory actually tests memory, and that a test of sustained attention actually tests a patient's ability to maintain attentiveness over time.

Consider the adequacy of norms for standardized tests. Scores on a test are, in themselves, of limited value unless there is a way of relating a given patient's performance to that of normal adults or to the performance of other adults in the same diagnostic category. For example, knowing that a traumatically brain-injured patient responded correctly to 15 of 25 items in a reading test is, in itself, not very informative. However, if one knows that non-brain-injured adults, on the average, correctly answer 23 of 25, one can say that the patient's performance is below the normal average. If one knows that only 10% of non-brain-injured adults get 15 or fewer items correct, one can say that the patient's reading performance would place the patient at the 10th percentile of a typical group of non-brain-injured adults. If one knows that the average fourth-grade student correctly answers 15 of 25 items, one can say that the patient's performance is equivalent to that of average fourth graders. And if one knows that only 10% of traumatically brain-injured adults correctly answer 15 or more of the 25, one can say that the patient's performance places him or her at the 90th percentile for traumatically brain-injured adults. Such comparisons of a patient with normal adults or with other patients having similar diagnoses are made by means of *norms.* Unfortunately, not all published tests provide norms, and some that do provide insufficient or inappropriate ones. It is not always easy to tell if the norms in a test manual

are adequate and appropriate. However, the following general indicators should help weed out the very deficient ones.

The *size of the norm group* must be large enough to ensure that the sample is representative of the population to which the norms apply and to ensure that statistics calculated on performance of the norm group are reliable and replicable. There is no simple answer to the question of how large a normative sample must be. It depends partly on how much variability in performance there is in the norm group and partly on how much error users are willing to tolerate in comparing individuals with the norm group. When there is little variability in performance among individuals in the norm group, a relatively small sample may suffice. This sometimes happens when a group of non-brain-injured adults is tested with a test designed for assessing adults with brain injuries—few of the non-brain-injured adults make any errors on the test, and those who do make very few. Because the performance of the non-brain-injured adults is extremely homogeneous, increasing the size of the norm group beyond that necessary to establish that non-brain-injured adults rarely make errors adds little if anything to the accuracy of the norms. In such cases, 10 or 20 individuals in the norm group may be sufficient.

Most statisticians and others concerned with making inferences from a sample to a population are uneasy about the validity of statistics calculated on samples smaller than 20. Consequently, one rarely sees norm groups smaller than 20, even when the performance of a group is extremely homogeneous. The issue of sample size in such situations may, in fact, be moot because statistics that assume normal distributions of scores cannot be calculated on extremely homogeneous data because such data are not distributed normally. Nevertheless, a sample size of 20 seems to represent the lower level of the "comfort zone" for most test designers and publishers.

The situation changes when there is appreciable variability in performance across members of the norm group. Then the principle becomes *more is better.* Because brain-injured adults are a heterogeneous group, their performance on any test sensitive to the effects of brain injury is likely to show substantial variability from patient to patient. For this reason, tests designed for brain-injured adults cannot get by with norm groups of 10 or 20. Norms based on brain-injured groups of less than 30 or 40 are likely to have marginal reliability, and test users should be careful about assuming that norms based on groups of less than 75 or 80 brain-injured adults will be highly accurate.

Evaluate the representativeness of the normative sample. The degree to which the characteristics of the individuals in the normative sample are representative of the population from which the sample is drawn is important. Which characteristics are important depends to some extent on the nature of the test and the population represented by the sample, but characteristics that may affect test performance are the most likely candidates. When the norm group represents an impaired population, the severity and nature of the impairments of those in the norm group should resemble the severity and nature of the impairments present in the population. When the norm group represents a "normal" population, the norm group should resemble the population on any variables that are likely to affect test performance (for tests of language and cognition, these variables almost always include age, education, and intellect).

Evaluate the appropriateness of normative statistics. The performance of individuals is compared with that of the norm group by means of *statistics.* The simplest statistics are the *mean* (the average score for the group) and the *range* of scores. With the mean, the user of a test can tell if a particular patient falls at, above, or below the average of the norm group, and with the range, the user can tell if anyone in the norm group scored higher or lower than the patient. However, neither of these statistics gives much precision in comparing a patient's performance with the norm group. More precise comparative statements can be made when the test

manual provides *standard deviations* or *percentiles* in addition to the mean for the norm group. Standard deviations are statistical abstractions based on the concept of the *normal curve.* Percentiles are calculated from means and standard deviations, and they permit test users to say exactly where in the norm group a given patient would fall—that is, what percentage of the norm group would fall above or below the patient's score. Most statistics books provide tables showing the percentage of observations that lie within various segments of the normal distribution. It is reasonably easy to use these tables to calculate percentiles from means and standard deviations.

Obtain a large enough sample of the patient's behavior to ensure test-retest stability. When brain-injured adults are tested with materials that challenge but do not overwhelm them, their performance often fluctuates from item to item within tests. For example, a patient asked to name a set of 10 line drawings on 3 successive presentations of the set may miss 3 items on the first presentation, 5 on the second, and 2 on the third. In general, increasing the number of items diminishes such test-to-test variability, at least up to a point, after which increasing the number of items has little effect on the stability of performance.

There is no answer to the question, "How many items are enough?" Most test designers and clinicians seem to agree that 10 items in a subtest are adequate for testing most brain-injured adults. Most also likely would agree that tests containing 5 or fewer items are too short to ensure adequate test-retest stability.

GENERAL CONCEPTS 3-2

- Brain injury often affects a patient's behavior, cognition, and emotional tone. The behavioral, cognitive, and emotional consequences of brain injury may affect the patient's performance in testing and treatment activities. These consequences may include:
  —Slowed responding, difficulty initiating purposeful behavior, hyperresponsiveness and impulsivity, or extreme cautiousness and self-doubt

—Perseveration (repetition of responses when they are no longer appropriate)

—Diminished response flexibility

—Concreteness, difficulty with abstract concepts

—Impaired self-monitoring

—Difficulty focusing and sustaining attention

—Disturbances of personality and emotion (emotional lability, lowered frustration tolerance)

- Experienced clinicians observe several principles when testing adults who have brain injuries:

  —They come to the first test session with a plan, based on previously acquired information about the patient.

  —They choose a quiet place for testing and schedule testing to minimize the effects of patient fatigue.

  —They make testing a cooperative effort between the clinician and the patient.

  —They select tests that are at an appropriate level of difficulty and that focus on the patient's likely areas of impairment.

  —They permit the patient's performance to guide them in the tests selected and in following leads revealed by the patient's performance as testing progresses.

  —They are prudent in their use of standardized tests so as not to subject a patient to more testing than is necessary and so as not to miss important aspects of the patient's performance.

  —They obtain a large enough sample of patient performance to ensure test-retest stability.

- Generic test batteries serve as general screening instruments, permitting the speech-language pathologist to sample patient performance in several domains and at several levels of difficulty. The results of a generic test battery provide the underpinning for in-depth testing in which the speech-language pathologist may test the patient's limits in key areas.

- Standardized tests are necessary if the clinician wishes to relate a patient's performance to that of other patients or to groups representing a population, including that of "normal" adults.

- A set of 10 test items at a given difficulty level in a performance domain, wherein the patient is challenged but not overwhelmed, ordinarily is sufficient to ensure adequate test-retest stability. A larger sample of performance may be necessary if a patient's performance varies greatly from item to item, and a smaller sample may be sufficient if a patient's item-to-item performance is homogeneous.

PURPOSES OF TESTING

The speech-language pathologist may test patients with neurogenic communication disorders for several reasons. The most common are to:

- Diagnose a patient's communication impairments.
- Arrive at a prognosis for a patient's recovery of communication abilities.
- Determine the nature and severity of a patient's communication impairments.
- Make decisions about the appropriateness and potential focus of treatment.
- Measure a patient's recovery of communication abilities.
- Measure the efficacy of treatment.

The initial evaluation of a patient's communication abilities typically is directed toward some combination of the first four reasons, and it may be impossible to separate them. Determining the severity and nature of a patient's communication disorder usually has implications for the diagnosis, the prognosis, and decisions about treatment. A diagnosis may have prognostic implications and may affect decisions regarding treatment, such as when the patient's communication disorder suggests a degenerative neurologic disease. Nevertheless, the speech-language pathologist may now and then have a more limited objective in testing a patient—for example, when a patient with a mild communication disorder is referred by a physician who needs help in determining if the patient has an underlying neurologic disease. In such a case the emphasis is on diagnosis, and prognosis and treatment are secondary or perhaps not considered at all.

Deciding on a Diagnosis

Diagnosing a patient's communication disorder means attaching a label to it. Diagnostic labels are "shorthand for characterizing the constellation of symptoms" (Albert, Goodglass, Helm, & associates, 1981, p. 19) and are an efficient way of communicating large amounts of information about a patient in a few words, provided, of course, that those reading the diagnostic labels understand their implications.

Diagnosis by speech-language pathologists takes several forms. Sometimes a speech-language pathologist wishes to differentiate a patient's communication disorder from other communication disorders that might resemble it (a process called *differential diagnosis*). For example, the speech-language pathologist may wish to determine if a patient's communication disorder represents aphasia, dysarthria, apraxia of speech, or some form of dementing illness. Sometimes a speech-language pathologist knows, based on a patient's history and medical record, that the patient's communication disorder represents a general class of communication disorders, but the speech-language pathologist wishes to arrive at a more specific diagnosis. For example, the speech-language pathologist may conclude that a patient is dysarthric based on information about the location of the patient's brain damage and the neurologist's description of the patient's speech, but may wish to determine which of several dysarthria syndromes best fit the patient's speech characteristics.

Labeling a patient's communication disorder often suggests the location of the nervous system abnormality responsible for the patient's symptoms. For example, the label *Wernicke's aphasia* suggests damage in the temporal lobe of the language-dominant hemisphere, and the label *hypokinetic dysarthria* suggests damage in the extrapyramidal system.

The speech-language pathologist's diagnostic label usually plays a minor role in specifying the location of the patient's neurologic damage because the neurologic examination and the results of imaging studies (CT, MRI) typically have localized the patient's nervous system pathology before the patient gets to the speech-language pathologist. Those involved in the patient's care (including the speech-language pathologist) often know the location and sometimes the nature of the patient's nervous system abnormality before the first test of communication abilities is administered.

Before they actually see the patient, speech-language pathologists sometimes make a provisional diagnosis of a patient's communication disorder based on information in the patient's medical record. For example, if a patient's medical record shows that the patient has had a brain stem stroke, it is likely that the patient will be dysarthric, but not aphasic and not demented (unless there is also a history of previous stroke or other neurologic disease affecting the brain). Davis (1993) was discussing aphasia when he wrote:

> In clinical practice, a test is seldom used to diagnose aphasia, in the sense that a clinician has no idea what the disorder is until the test is analyzed. . . . Having read a patient's chart, an experienced clinical aphasiologist need only talk to a patient before reaching an initial conclusion about not only the presence of aphasia but also the type of aphasia. (p. 211)

Davis's assertion is true not only for patients with aphasia, but also for patients with other communication disorders. By the time experienced speech-language pathologists have finished reviewing a patient's medical record and have completed the interview they usually have a diagnosis in mind. Testing the patient may serve only to confirm (and perhaps to elaborate on) the preliminary diagnosis.

For most speech-language pathologists the act of attaching a diagnostic label to a neurologically impaired patient's communication disorder is less important than determining the nature and severity of the patient's communication impairments and making decisions about the appropriateness and content of treatment. This does not mean, however, that diagnostic labeling has no place in the speech-language pathologist's professional repertoire. Those referring a patient to the speech-language pathologist may expect a diagnostic label, and using a diagnostic label in a report may substitute for lengthy description. For example, reporting that a patient exhibits behaviors consistent with *conduction aphasia* communicates extensive information about the nature of the patient's speech, their comprehension of language, and the probable location of the brain damage responsible for the patient's aphasia, all in two words. Likewise, reporting that a patient exhibits *flaccid dysarthria* says a lot about the probable nature of the patient's articulatory impairments as well as the probable location of the central nervous system damage responsible for the impairments. Some diagnostic labels also have implications for treatment planning. For example, reporting that a patient exhibits multi-infarct dementia (which typically increases in severity in stepwise fashion) suggests not only the general nature of a treatment program, but suggests that treatment may have to change as the severity of the patient's impairments increases over time.

Making a Prognosis

A prognosis is a prediction about the course (sometimes) and the eventual outcome (usually) of a disease or condition. A prognosis may represent no more than a clinician's best guess based on their clinical experience and intuition, or it may represent a somewhat more objective probability statement based on actuarial information from studies of groups of individuals who have the disease or condition. This actuarial information may come from prospective prognostic studies or retrospective prognostic studies.

In *prospective prognostic studies,* patients in the early stages of a disease or condition are identified and various characteristics of the patients (the prognostic variables) are assessed at the beginning of the study. The patients then are followed to determine outcome. At some predetermined future time, the outcomes are tallied and the relationships between the prognostic variables and the outcomes are evaluated to identify the prognostic variables that are most strongly related to outcome.

In *retrospective prognostic studies* the records of a group of patients who already have experienced outcomes are reviewed to evaluate the relationships between various prognostic variables (determined from the records) and outcome (also determined from the records). Retrospective studies are scientifically less robust than prospective studies because in retrospective studies the prognostic variables are not defined in advance of the study, the data are not collected using standardized procedures, and the definitions of outcome measures tend to be less precise than the definitions of outcome measures in prospective studies.

Most studies of prognostic variables related to recovery of communication and cognition by patients with nervous system abnormalities are retrospective. The records of groups of patients who have recovered various levels of communication ability are reviewed and the relationships between patients' recoveries (usually defined as scores on standardized tests of communication ability) and various prognostic variables are evaluated.

Numerous studies and opinion pieces have been published in the search for prognostic variables that might predict brain-injured adults' recovery of communication and cognition. These variables fall into three categories—*neurologic findings, associated conditions,* and *patient characteristics.*

Neurologic Findings In addition to their function as a shorthand for communicating information about the patient, many neurologic diagnoses have prognostic significance. Longstreth and associates (1992) link diagnosis, prognosis, and treatment when they assert:

> A diagnosis that has no prognostic implications does little more than describe a constellation of patient characteristics. Prognosis links diagnosis to outcomes and identifies the diseases that warrant treatment. Treatment becomes an intervention intended to modify prognosis. Thus . . . the concepts

of diagnosis, prognosis, and treatment are insepa-rable, with prognosis as the keystone. (p. 29)

This opinion might be regarded by some speech-language pathologists as extreme be-cause the prognostic implications of many diag-nostic labels for communication disorders are fuzzy at best. For example, diagnosing a patient's communication disorder as *Wernicke's aphasia* provides little in the way of prognosis, except that as a group, patients with Wernicke's aphasia recover slightly less well than those with Broca's aphasia (Benson, 1979; Goodglass, 1993; Kertesz, 1979). Many neurologic diagnoses carry consid-erably more prognostic weight because the de-velopment and outcome of many neurologic conditions are well documented.

The speech-language pathologist who wishes to predict a patient's recovery of communica-tion and cognition pays close attention to the neurologic diagnosis because changes in a pa-tient's communicative and cognitive abilities of-ten parallel changes in the patient's physical and medical condition. When the usual course of a patient's neurologic disease is well-known and highly predictable, the speech-language patholo-gist's prognosis for recovery of communication and cognition also is likely to be quite accurate (although perhaps redundant once the neuro-logic diagnosis has been made).

Notes or comments in a patient's medical record relating to the location and extent of a patient's nervous system pathology can affect the speech-language pathologist's prognosis. The location of the pathology is important be-cause such conditions affecting regions of the nervous system that are directly involved in lan-guage and related processes carry greater nega-tive implications than pathology affecting pe-ripheral regions. For example, damage in the central zone of the language-dominant hemi-sphere typically creates more severe and persis-tent aphasia than damage in peripheral regions. Likewise, unilateral damage in the brain stem that affects the motor and sensory systems serv-ing speech typically causes severe and persis-

tent dysarthria, whereas unilateral damage in fiber tracts above the brain stem usually pro-duces less dramatic consequences.

The extent of nervous system pathology also affects prognosis. Large lesions, multiple lesions, and damage disseminated throughout the ner-vous system or throughout parts of the nervous system important for communication are omi-nous. For example, a speech-language patholo-gist might revise downward the estimated com-municative recovery for a patient with a confirmed recent left-hemisphere stroke on learning that the patient's CT scan showed a previous stroke in the right hemisphere. Sometimes indicators of the extent of nervous system abnormalities are indirect. For example, the presence and duration of coma are consid-ered important prognostic indicators for patients with traumatic brain injuries (Jennett, Teasdale, Braakman, & associates, 1979) and, to a lesser ex-tent, for patients with aphasia caused by stroke (Caronna & Levy, 1983). Longer intervals of coma suggest greater destruction of brain tissue, greater impairment, and a poorer prognosis.

The neurologic diagnosis and the location and extent of the nervous system pathology re-sponsible for a patient's impairments provide the speech-language pathologist with two rea-sonably dependable prognostic indicators. Several other prognostic indicators, although less dependable, often play a part in determin-ing a patient's prognosis. These indicators may represent *associated conditions* or *patient characteristics.*

Associated Conditions Associated condi-tions are medical conditions or physical findings that do not directly affect communication, but which have indirect effects on the magnitude of the patient's impairments and may compromise the patient's recovery and response to treat-ment. Several associated conditions have been shown to affect recovery of communication and cognition following nervous system injury.

A patient's *general health* can have impor-tant effects on recovery of communication abil-ities following neurologic events. The presence of illnesses such as diabetes, heart disease, pulmonary disease, or other such chronic diseases is thought to impede physiologic and behavioral recovery from nervous system pathology (Candelise, Landi, Orazio, & associates, 1985; Eisenson, 1964; Marshall & Phillips, 1983).

Associated sensory and motor impairments also have some prognostic significance. The presence of hemiplegia, perceptual disturbances, seizures, and motor impairments all have been identified as indicating a poor prognosis (Keenan & Brassell, 1975; Van Buskirk, 1955), although some investigators have reported no relationship between the presence of hemiplegia or seizures and recovery from aphasia (Gloning, Trappl, Heiss, & associates, 1976; Smith, 1972).

Patient Characteristics Several patient characteristics (age, gender, education, occupation, premorbid intelligence, handedness, personality, emotional state) reputedly affect brain-injured adults' recovery of communication abilities. However, the relationships between specific patient characteristics and recovery of communication abilities tend to be weak, and most have been the subject of contradictory findings. (See Darley, 1982; Davis, 1993; and Rosenbek, LaPointe, and Wertz, 1989 for reviews of these findings.) The most that can be said in their favor is that they appear to have some weak effects on recovery, but the effects of any single patient variable are overshadowed easily by the more potent effects of variables such as the location and severity of nervous system pathology.

The nature of a patient's communication impairment often has prognostic significance. For example, there is evidence that patients with Broca's aphasia recover somewhat better than those with Wernicke's aphasia when aphasia severity is equivalent and that patients with traumatic brain injuries recover better than those with brain injuries caused by strokes. (That patients with traumatic brain injuries usually are younger than stroke patients no doubt makes an important contribution to this relationship.) The

overall severity of a patient's communication impairment at the time of testing is a reasonably dependable indicator of future recovery from neurogenic communication impairments. In general, patients with severe communication impairments recover less well than those with milder impairments, although there may be striking exceptions. However, making a prognosis based on the overall severity of a patient's communication impairment is in many respects a subjective process because the predictive validity of the standardized tests for measuring the severity of a patient's communication impairment has not been established (Tompkins, 1995).

> The relationship between severity of impairments and outcome is weaker in the first days (and sometimes weeks) following nervous system injury, but becomes stronger as the diffuse and transitory effects of nervous system injury resolve, leaving the permanent effects of destroyed nervous system tissue. Most clinicians hedge their prognostic bets in the early post-injury period and defer their ultimate prognosis until the patient's neurologic condition has stabilized.

A few tests provide systematic procedures for making prognostic statements based on a patient's test performance. Some make use of a *patient profile approach,* in which a test battery is administered and a profile of the patient's performance is developed. The clinician then matches the patient's profile with the profiles of previously studied groups of patients whose recovery is known, expecting that the patient's recovery should match that of previously studied patients with the same profile.

The *Minnesota Test for Differential Diagnosis of Aphasia* (MTDDA; Schuell, 1972) is an example of the patient profile approach to prediction. The MTDDA permits clinicians to assign aphasic patients to one of five major and two minor groups based on their test performance.

The MTDDA test manual gives a prognosis for each group based on the recovery of previously studied patients. For example, MTDDA Group 1 usually has "excellent recovery of all language skills" (Schuell, 1972, p. 9), whereas for MTDDA Group 5 "language does not become functional or voluntary in any modality" (Schuell, 1972, p. 14).

Other tests permit the use of a more sophisticated *statistical prediction approach* (Porch, Collins, Wertz, & associates, 1980). The statistical prediction approach, like the other approaches, makes predictions based on the characteristics of previously studied patients. Unlike the other approaches, the statistical prediction approach uses statistical analyses to determine the relative contribution of several variables, alone and in combination, to observed recovery. These procedures provide quantitative information about which variables are most strongly related to recovery and which combinations of variables provide the most accurate predictions. They also permit quite precise predictions regarding the actual level of recovery to be expected. However, the predictions are not perfect—there is always some error in prediction associated with even the strongest prognostic variables.

A good example of the *statistical prediction approach* is Porch's (1981a) *HOAP* (for high-overall prediction) procedure for predicting recovery from aphasia. In the HOAP procedure, the patient is tested at 1 month post-onset with the *Porch Index of Communicative Ability* (PICA; Porch, 1981a), which has 18 subtests. The clinician then calculates an average score for the 9 subtests with the highest scores. This average then is used to enter a table in the PICA manual, from which the patient's 6-month overall PICA performance can be predicted.

For patients tested at more than 1 month but less than 6 months post-onset, a variant on the HOAP method, called the *HOAP slope* method, can be used to predict recovery at 6 months. The patient is tested with the PICA and an average score for the 9 subtests with the highest scores is calculated. This score is used to place the patient on one of several recovery slopes (Figure 3-9), which permits the clinician to predict the patient's overall PICA performance at 6 months post-onset.

Even at its best, predicting brain-injured adults' recovery of communication can be an uncertain business. No prognostic variables have been unequivocally tied to recovery of communication, and many have been the subject of conflicting claims in the literature. Even the sophisticated *patient profile* and *statistical prediction* approaches (which are quite accurate when predicting the average recovery of groups of patients) often yield inaccurate predictions for individual patients (Aten & Lyon, 1978; Porch & Callaghan, 1981; Wertz, Dronkers, & Hume, 1993). For this reason, many clinicians opt for a short period of *prognostic treatment* (Rosenbek, LaPointe, & Wertz, 1989) to increase the precision of their predictions. In prognostic treatment the clinician and patient spend several sessions (usually three to five) in treatment procedures designed to determine if the patient can perform treatment tasks and can generalize from clinic sessions to daily life. Prognostic treatment is an intuitively reasonable way to predict whether a patient will benefit from treatment. It also seems to be a good way to predict a brain-injured patient's recovery, with or without treatment.

> Present-day restrictions on reimbursement may make it impractical for a clinician to spend many sessions in prognostic treatment because third-party payers may refuse to pay for it. However, it is true that many times the first few treatment sessions with a patient serve diagnostic and prognostic purposes, although diagnosis and prognosis are not listed as formal objectives.

Regardless of how it is done, predicting newly referred patients' recovery (or loss) of communicative or cognitive abilities is an important skill for speech-language pathologists.

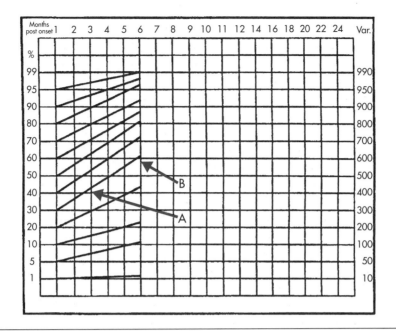

Figure 3-9 ■ High-overall prediction (HOAP) slopes. An aphasic patient's 6-month-post-onset Porch Index of Communicative Ability (PICA) overall percentile score is predicted by finding the patient's current PICA overall percentile score in the family of HOAP slopes and projecting the 6-month overall score based on the angle of the closest slope in the family. A patient who scored at the 40th percentile at 3 months post-onset *(A)* should improve to approximately the 58th percentile *(B)* at 6 months post-onset. (From Porch, B. E. [1967, 1981]. *Porch index of communicative ability.* Palo Alto, CA: Consulting Psychologists Press.)

Patients and their families, concerned about the potential effects of the patient's communication disabilities on familial, social, and financial conditions may press the speech-language pathologist for a prognostic opinion. Physicians and other health care workers may need the speech-language pathologist's prognosis to help them plan the patient's discharge and arrange for follow-up care. Social workers may need a prognostic opinion to make appropriate social and vocational arrangements for the patient and family. Attorneys may request a prognostic opinion to establish the patient's legal competence or lack thereof. Funding agencies may require that the speech-language pathologist provide evidence for a favorable prognosis before they will pay for the patient's treatment. Finally, the speech-language pathologist must decide on the patient's chances of recovery, with or without treatment, before deciding whether to treat the patient's impairments.

Measuring Recovery and Response to Treatment

Measuring patient performance across time is an important part of the clinical management of patients with neurogenic communication impairments. Such measurement permits clinicians to establish baselines against which the effects of treatment can be measured and to describe changes in a patient's performance during treatment. Well-defined baselines are the principal element in studies of the evolution of neurologic diseases or pathologic processes, and they often are the key to understanding the progression of a particular patient's impairments and predicting outcome for that patient.

Defining a baseline for a patient with a neurogenic communication disorder typically entails administering a test or set of tests at regular intervals to measure the patient's performance in the domain of interest. A patient with progressive dementia might be evaluated with a story-retelling test at 1-month intervals to evaluate the degree to which organization, recall, and production of story elements are affected by the patient's dementia. A semicomatose patient might be evaluated with daily tests of alertness and attention to determine when the patient might be a candidate for a more comprehensive evaluation. A patient with progressive muscle weakness might be evaluated with monthly tests of articulatory proficiency to monitor the course of the disease and to determine the effects of treatment on the patient's dysarthria.

Figure 3-10 shows how baseline measurements were used to help a neurologist decide on a diagnosis for a 63-year-old woman who was brought to the neurology clinic with vague complaints about difficulty concentrating and memory lapses. The patient's neurologic examination was unremarkable, and she scored within normal limits on a screening test of memory and cognition. The neurologist referred the patient to speech-language pathology with a request for help in determining if the patient had a progressive condition and, if so, whether the patient was in the early stages of progressive dementia or some other neurologic disease.

The speech-language pathologist chose three tests as baseline measures—a test of *proverb interpretation,* a *story-retelling* test, and a *picture-naming* test. The speech-language pathologist reasoned that performance on the proverb interpretation and story-retelling tests should be sensitive to dementing illness because they require analytic skills, abstract reasoning, and memory, which typically are affected early in the course of dementia. The picture-naming test was included because the speech-language pathologist knew

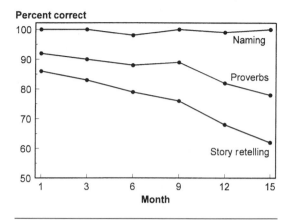

Figure 3-10 ■ Baseline measurements for a patient who eventually was diagnosed as having dementia. Naming performance remained stable throughout the period of baseline measurement, whereas performance on tests of proverb interpretation and story retelling gradually worsened.

that picture naming rarely is affected in the early stages of dementia. If the patient's performance on the proverb interpretation and story-retelling tests declined while her performance on the picture-naming test remained stable, a diagnosis of early dementia would become more plausible.

The speech-language pathologist tested the patient at 3-month intervals, concurrent with her appointments in the neurology clinic. The baselines in Figure 3-10 show the patient's performance across five test sessions. The patient's naming performance remained stable and within the normal range across all five tests, but her proverb interpretation and story-retelling performance gradually declined. The patient's neurologic examination remained unremarkable across the five test sessions, except for a questionable decline in performance on screening tests of cognition in the sixth session. The patient's baseline pattern of performance led the neurologist to conclude that the patient was in the early stages of progressive dementia, a diagnosis confirmed by subsequent evaluations during the following year.

GENERAL CONCEPTS 3-3

- Speech-language pathologists may test a patient with a neurogenic communication disorder to:
  —Diagnose the patient's communication impairments.
  —Arrive at a prognosis for the patient's recovery of communication.
  —Determine the nature and severity of the patient's communication impairments.
  —Make decisions about treatment.
  —Measure a patient's recovery of communication abilities or the efficacy of treatment.
- Diagnostic labels are convenient shorthand for summarizing several patient characteristics in a few words. Diagnostic labels, in themselves, do not lead directly to decisions about treatment, but they may convey information that suggests generic characteristics of treatment.
- Clinicians consider several categories of information when deciding on a prognosis:
  —The location and extent of a nervous system abnormality often has dramatic effects on a patient's recovery (neurologic findings).
  —A patient's general health and the presence of sensory and motor impairments also strongly influence the patient's recovery.
  —Patient characteristics such as age, education, and premorbid intelligence have relatively weak effects on recovery.
- The *patient profile approach* and the *statistical prediction approach* are two formalized procedures for generating prognoses. Both have greater accuracy for predicting the recovery of groups of patients than for predicting the recovery of individual patients.
- Establishing stable performance baselines followed by periodic testing of performance is an objective way to measure a patient's recovery of communicative abilities or their response to treatment.

Measuring the Effects of Treatment

Careful testing is crucial for establishing baseline performance, for measuring patients' responses to treatment, and for alerting the clinician to the need for changes in treatment procedures. Well-planned and well-executed testing helps clinicians determine the efficacy of their treatment for neurogenic communication disorders and for evaluating the extent to which changes in performance obtained in treatment generalize in a meaningful way to patients' daily life communication performance. These aspects of assessment will become more important as health care providers become increasingly preoccupied with balancing the costs of rehabilitation against its positive effects on patients' daily life independence. The concepts of efficacy, outcome, and *functional communication* are central to these considerations.

Efficacy and Outcome When the word *efficacy* is used in the rehabilitation literature, it refers to whether a treatment has a positive effect on a disease or condition. When the word *outcome* is used, it refers to whether treatment provides meaningful benefit to the patient in the patient's daily life environment. In speech-language pathology, efficacy usually is defined as a positive change on a standardized test of communication ability. That a treatment is *efficacious* does not necessarily mean that it has a *meaningful positive outcome.* Consider, for example, a treatment program that generates a significant increase in an aphasic patient's performance on the *Boston Naming Test* (Kaplan, Goodglass, & Weintraub, 2001). The Boston Naming Test requires the test-taker to provide the names of line drawings of common and uncommon objects. If one's measure of efficacy were improvement on the Boston Naming Test, the treatment could be called efficacious. However, the treatment might not have had a meaningful positive outcome because improved ability to name pictured objects may not provide meaningful benefit to the patient in the patient's daily life environment. To decide if a treatment is efficacious, one asks, "What happened to the patient's test performance?" To decide if a treatment has a positive outcome, one asks, "What happened to the patient's daily life performance?"

A treatment conceivably could have a meaningful positive outcome even though it had not been shown to be efficacious. This unusual situation could occur if, for example, one chose performance on the Boston Naming Test as the measure of efficacy for a treatment program that provided broad-based language stimulation and no naming training. One then might see no significant change in a patient's Boston Naming Test score (the measure of efficacy) but find a meaningful positive change in ratings of the patient's communicative success in daily life activities (a measure of outcome).

The issues of efficacy and outcome are exemplified by a study of the efficacy of aphasia therapy by Wertz, Weiss, Aten, and associates (1986). In this study, a *clinic* group of aphasic adults received 12 weeks of treatment by a speech-language pathologist followed by 12 weeks of no treatment. A *deferred* group received 12 weeks of no treatment followed by 12 weeks of treatment by a speech-language pathologist. (The design was more complex than this. These aspects of the study are chosen to illustrate the concepts of *efficacy* and *outcome*.) At the end of the first 12 weeks, the *clinic* group's overall percentile score on the PICA (Porch, 1981a) was 5.93 points higher than that of the *deferred* group—a statistically significant difference. This result led Wertz, Weiss, Aten, and associates to conclude that their treatment was *efficacious*—it yielded a statistically significant change in the chosen measure of treatment effect (PICA overall percentile). Whether the treatment had a meaningful positive *outcome* is not clear because no one knows if an improvement of 5.93 overall percentile points on the PICA yields a meaningful change in patients' daily life communicative functioning.

Most studies of treatment benefits for patients with neurogenic communication disorders are *efficacy* studies—the indicators of effectiveness are positive changes in performance on standardized tests of communication, per-haps because these tests are sensitive, reliable, and valid indicators of the communication performance of adults under carefully controlled test conditions. Few treatment studies of adults with neurogenic communication disorders have incorporated measures of *outcome* as indicators of daily life benefit, perhaps because few standardized outcome measures with proven sensitivity, reliability, and validity were available when the studies were carried out.

In contrast, many medical studies of treatment effects have incorporated measures that speak to both efficacy and outcome. Consider, for example, a study of the effects of treatment of hypertension (Veterans Administration, 1972). This study compared the effects of a combination of antihypertensive medications with the effects of a placebo administered to large groups of adults with hypertension. The measure of treatment effects was the frequency of occurrence of five adverse events—*sudden death, heart attack, congestive heart failure, increased hypertension,* and *ruptured aneurysm,* all known to be consequences of hypertension. At the end of the study 8.5 percent of the group given the antihypertensive medications had experienced adverse events, whereas 22.2 percent of the group given the placebo had experienced such events. Because the occurrence of these adverse events is likely to have profound negative effects on patients and their families, it is reasonable to conclude that the treatment regimen was both *efficacious* (the difference in the rate of adverse events between the groups was statistically significant) and that it had a *positive outcome* (the treatment improved patients' daily life well-being).

Although no direct measures of outcome were included in the foregoing study, few would argue that decreasing the occurrence of death, heart attack, heart failure, increased hypertension, and ruptured aneurysm would have no positive effects on the daily lives of the patients and their families.

The word *functional* is strongly associated with the concept of *outcome*—so much so that the combination *functional outcome* has become commonplace in the rehabilitation literature. When used in this context, *functional* means *affecting the patient's daily life competence or well-being,* making the combination *functional outcome* something of a redundancy. Hundreds of articles and dozens of measuring instruments with *functional* somewhere in their title have appeared in the literature in the past 15 or 20 years, and it is now true that in speech-language pathology an emphasis on functionality in writing clinical goals and outcomes is almost mandatory.

> It has become almost impossible to write a treatment plan or submit a claim to a third-party payor without using the word "functional." A speech-language pathologist must identify "functional" goals, using "functional" tasks, and show "functional" gains, or reimbursement for treatment is likely to be denied. (Elman & Bernstein-Ellis, 1995, p. 1)

Despite the frequency of the word *functional* in contemporary clinical writings and practice, no standard definition of *functional* exists, and its meaning varies, depending on who is using it and what their purposes are.

The label *functional communication* has been used by speech-language pathologists to describe an approach to assessment and treatment that focuses on patients' daily life communicative success or lack thereof. It emphasizes the means by which patients successfully get messages across, and it represents a movement away from a traditional emphasis on *language* to an emphasis on *communication*—the successful transfer of information from speaker or writer to listener or reader. This movement has been especially evident with regard to aphasia, but the emphasis on communication has spilled over to the other neurogenic communication disorders as well. The general idea is that successful communication does not depend on the linguistic or phonologic accuracy of messages, but that speakers (and writers) can communicate successfully in spite of errors in word choice, syntax, or the phonologic-graphemic form of messages. It is this sense of the term that underlies several "functional" approaches to treatment, such as *Promoting Aphasics' Communicative Effectiveness* (Davis & Wilcox, 1985). Functional treatment approaches typically rely on activities that are structured to resemble the patient's daily life communication environment and tend to focus on socially relevant aspects of communication, such as social conventions (greetings, farewells, and the like) and adherence to conversational rules.

When used by organizations that manage and pay for health care, *functional* often means *able to communicate basic needs and wants.* Because these organizations may be unwilling to pay for treatment to move patients beyond this level, defining the term in this way may save them money by eliminating their obligation to pay for treatment of patients with mild or moderate communication impairments (because the patients already can communicate basic wants and needs) and by ending payment for patients with more severe impairments as soon as they reach the minimal level of communicative competence represented by the provider's definition of *functional.*

Impairment, Disability, and Handicap
Much of current thinking about efficacy, outcome, and functional communication has been influenced by the concepts of *impairment, disability,* and *handicap* (World Health Organization, 1980). *Impairment,* according the World Health Organization, represents a structural or functional abnormality within a person. *Brain damage* and *hemiplegia* are examples of a structural abnormality and a functional abnormality that would be called impairments. *Disability* represents the effects of an impairment or collection of impairments on a specific skill or ability. *Aphasia* and *poor ambulation* are examples of disabilities that might be caused by brain damage and hemiplegia (their respective underlying impairments). *Handicap* represents the effects of one or more disabilities on the individual's ability to carry out daily

life roles. *Diminished ability to function as a spouse or parent* is an example of a handicap that might be caused by aphasia.

The World Health Organization is in the process of revising its classification system and has altered its terminology to reflect changes in attitudes toward the labels *impairment, disability,* and *handicap,* which are considered to carry negative connotations (World Health Organization, 2000). In the current version of the World Health Organization classification system the label *body function and structures* replaces *impairment, activity* replaces *disability,* and *participation* replaces *handicap.* Body functions are "the physiological or psychological functions of body systems" (p. 9). Body structures are "anatomic parts of the body such as organs, limbs, and their components" (p. 9). Activity is "the execution of a task or involvement in a life situation in a uniform environment" (p. 9). Participation is "the execution of a task or involvement in a life situation in an individual's current environment" (p. 9). The World Health Organization believes that the new labels have socially neutral connotations and allow for both positive and negative effects to be addressed.

The terms "uniform environment" and "current environment" are crucial distinctions. A "uniform environment" is one in which the full capabilities of the individual can be expressed. It provides neither hindrances nor enhancements that might affect the individual's performance. The individual's "current environment" is the context in which the individual currently lives, including society's response to the individual's performance in that environment. Performance in the "uniform environment" represents the individual's performance achieved under environmentally neutral conditions. Performance in the "current environment" represents the individual's performance in their current living environment, which may contain hindrances to performance or facilitators of performance.

The concepts of *impairment* (body function and structures), *disability* (activity), and *handicap* (participation) have had strong effects on contemporary thinking about the nature of health care services and how health care services should be paid for. The past decade has seen the development of numerous measuring instruments for assessing the level of handicap (effect on participation) created by diseases or conditions, for measuring the degree to which treatment serves to alleviate handicaps (increase participation), and for detemining a patient's level of handicap (participation) in a given domain. Most of these instruments are *rating scales* with which an observer subjectively estimates a patient's level of performance in selected domains. A few are *standardized tests* by which a patient's performance in a given domain can be scored objectively. The rating scales and standardized tests share a common attribute—that of focusing on what is called *functional outcome.*

Functional Outcome How functional outcome is measured greatly depends on the purpose of those doing the measuring. The two major reasons for functional outcome measures are *program evaluation* and *patient evaluation.* In *program evaluation* the primary objective is to identify the most efficient providers of health care service—"those who provide the greatest amount of functional improvement over the shortest period of time for the least cost" (Warren, 1992, p. 63). The concept underlying program evaluation is that in a competitive marketplace health care providers who reduce costs but maintain the quality of services and produce good outcomes will survive and prosper, whereas those who do not will vanish. The emphasis in program evaluation is on the financial health of the program rather than on treatment outcomes for individual patients.

The measures typically used for program evaluation are *rating scales.* Patients' functional abilities in the domain(s) of interest are rated when they enter the program and again when they leave the program. Judgments about the quality of the program are based on the amount of improvement in ratings of functionality between entry and exit and the average level of functionality of patients completing the program. The rating scales used in program evaluation are not specific to a given disease or condition such as stroke, and they are not specific to a given discipline such as speech-language pathology. They usually provide for global ratings of broadly defined categories of abilities likely to be important in daily life (for example, self-care). Most rating scales are insensitive to small changes in a patient's level of performance, and their global ratings do not typically capture changes in component skills that may underlie broadly defined categories of ability.

The best-known and most widely used measure of functional outcome in rehabilitation is a rating scale called the *Functional Independence Measure,* or FIM (State University of New York at Buffalo Research Foundation, 1993). The FIM was developed to measure outcome in rehabilitation medicine programs. It provides a 7-point scale to assess *self care, sphincter control, mobility, locomotion, communication,* and *social cognition* in 18 activities of daily life (Figure 3-11). The 7-point scale is divided into three levels. At the *independent* (no helper) level, patients do not need assistance to carry out an activity. Patients at the *dependent* (helper) level require help to carry out an activity. The *dependent* level itself is subdivided into two levels (*modified dependence* and *complete dependence*) based on the frequency with which assistance is needed by a patient.

The FIM has been criticized for poor reliability in rating levels of independence (Adamovich, 1990), and its use for rating functional independence in communication has been criticized because of its insensitivity to changes in communication abilities (Warren, 1992). Nevertheless, it remains the preeminent outcome measure for program evaluation in rehabilitation medicine.

The combination of increased emphasis on functional outcome by health care providers and dissatisfaction with the FIM as a measure of communicative adequacy led the American

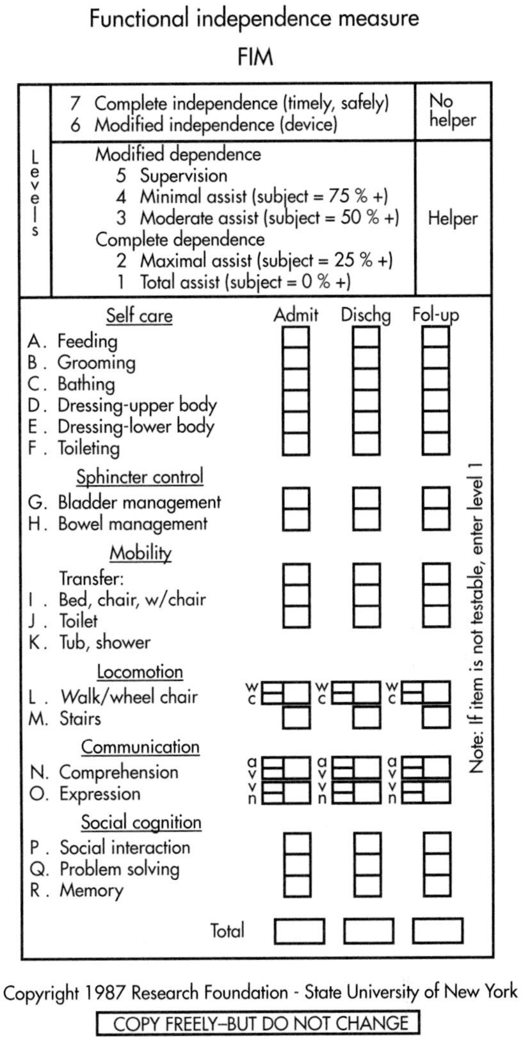
Functional independence measure
FIM
Levels
7 Complete independence (timely, safely)
6 Modified independence (device)
No helper
Modified dependence
5 Supervision
4 Minimal assist (subject = 75 % +)
3 Moderate assist (subject = 50 % +)
Complete dependence
2 Maximal assist (subject = 25 % +)
1 Total assist (subject = 0 % +)
Helper
Admit Dischg Fol-up
Self care
A. Feeding
B. Grooming
C. Bathing
D. Dressing-upper body
E. Dressing-lower body
F. Toileting
Sphincter control
G. Bladder management
H. Bowel management
Mobility
Transfer:
I. Bed, chair, w/chair
J. Toilet
K. Tub, shower
Locomotion
L. Walk/wheel chair
M. Stairs
w c
Communication
N. Comprehension
O. Expression
a v v n
Social cognition
P. Social interaction
Q. Problem solving
R. Memory
Total
Note: If item is not testable, enter level 1
Copyright 1987 Research Foundation - State University of New York
COPY FREELY–BUT DO NOT CHANGE

Figure 3-11 ■ Functional Independence Measure (FIM).

Speech-Language-Hearing Association (ASHA) to develop a measure of functional communication called *ASHA FACS,* for ASHA Functional Assessment of Communication Skills for Adults (Frattali, Thompson, Holland, & associates, 1995). ASHA FACS permits users to rate a patient's communicative adequacy in four domains: *social communication, communication of basic needs, daily planning,* and *reading/ writing/number concepts* (Table 3-1). The communicative adequacy of each behavior shown in Table 3-1 is estimated with a *7-point Scale of Communicative Independence* which, like the FIM, rates behaviors in terms of how much assistance is needed to perform them:

- Does with no assistance (7)
- Does with minimal assistance (6)
- Does with minimal to moderate assistance (5)
- Does with moderate assistance (4)
- Does with moderate to maximal assistance (3)
- Does with maximal assistance (2)

- Does not do, even with maximal assistance (1)
- No basis for rating

In addition to ratings of the individual communication behaviors shown in Table 3-1, ASHA FACS permits users to rate the *adequacy, appropriateness, promptness,* and *communicative sharing* aspects of a patient's overall performance in each of the four ASHA FACS domains.

The FIM and ASHA FACS, like most instruments designed for program evaluation, yield general estimates of a patient's functional ability in a small number of domains chosen because they are likely to be important in determining a patient's

---

T A B L E   3 - 1

Assessment domains for ASHA Functional Assessment of Communication Skills for Adults

Social communication	Communication of basic needs	Daily planning	Reading/writing/ number concepts
Uses names of familiar people	Recognizes familiar faces/voices	Tells time	Understands environmental signs
Expresses agreement/ disagreement	Makes strong likes/ dislikes known	Dials telephone numbers	Uses reference materials
Explains how to do something	Expresses feelings	Keeps scheduled appointments	Follows written directions
Requests information	Requests help	Uses a calendar	Understands printed material
Participates in telephone conversations	Makes needs/wants known	Follows a map	Prints/writes/types name
Answers yes-no questions	Responds in an emergency		Completes forms
Follows directions			Makes short lists
Understands facial expression/tone of voice			Writes messages
Understands nonliteral meaning and intent			Understands signs with numbers
Understands conversation in noisy surroundings			Makes money transactions
Understands TV/radio			Understands units of measurement
Participates in conversations			
Recognizes/corrects errors			

Data from Frattali, C. M., Thompson, C. K., Holland, A. L., & associates. (1995). *The Amercian Speech-Language-Hearing Association functional assessment of communication skills for adults (ASHA FACS).* Rockville, MD: American Speech-Language-Hearing Association.

independence in daily life. These instruments may provide reasonably accurate estimates of a patient's daily life independence and self-sufficiency in the domains addressed, but do not have sufficient sensitivity and do not provide enough detail to be very useful in planning treatment or in tracking a patient's response to treatment. Treatment planning and measuring a patient's response to treatment usually is better served by instruments designed for *patient evaluation,* rather than those designed for *program evaluation.*

The first measure of functional communication to be widely used for patient evaluation in speech-language pathology was the Functional Communication Profile (FCP; Sarno, 1969). According to Sarno, the FCP was designed to quantify the communication behaviors a patient actually uses when interacting with others, regardless of the severity of the patient's impairment. The clinician who wishes to rate a patient's functional communication with the FCP interviews the patient and then rates the patient on five categories of communication behavior considered common in everyday life (Table 3-2). The behaviors are rated on a 9-point scale in which the patient's current ability is rated as a proportion of their premorbid ability.

The Communicative Effectiveness Index (CETI; Lomas, Pickard, Bester, & associates, 1989) is a more recent rating scale for estimating aphasic adults' ability to communicate in several daily life situations. The situations selected by Lomas and associates were based on interviews with stroke survivors and spouses. In the interviews the stroke survivors and spouses were asked to identify situations in which a stroke survivor has to "get his meaning across and to understand what someone else means" (p. 115). The situations given by the stroke survivors and spouses then were partitioned into four categories, representing:

- *Basic needs* (such as toileting, eating, grooming, positioning)
- *Life skills* (such as shopping, home maintenance, using the telephone, understanding traffic signals)
- *Social needs* (such as dinner conversation, playing cards, writing to a friend)

- *Health threat* (such as calling for help, giving or receiving information about one's medical condition)

The list of situations generated by the stroke survivors and spouses then was refined to yield a list of 16 items (Table 3-3).

> Lomas and associates do not identify which items in the CETI represent each of these categories, and it is clear that the 16 items in the CETI are not distributed equally across the four categories. I counted 4 or 5 "basic need" items, 10 "social need" items, 1 "health threat" item, and 0 or 1 "life skills" items, using my own intuitions about which behaviors represented each category.

Results reported by Lomas and associates suggest that the CETI has acceptable internal reliability (CETI items test the same domain), adequate test-retest reliability (CETI results do not change unpredictably from test to test), and acceptable interrater reliability (different examiners rating the same patient agree). The procedures used to select items for the CETI support its face validity (it appears to measure what it was intended to measure), although strong evidence for its validity as a measure of daily life communication performance (such as correlations between ratings and actual daily life performance) is not provided in the published report.

> Lomas and associates reported strong and significant correlations between spouses' CETI ratings of their aphasic partner and spouses' ratings of their aphasic partner's overall communicative ability and considered those correlations evidence of CETI's construct validity. However, it seems that strong correlations would be expected because the same people did both ratings, apparently in the same rating session.

T A B L E   3 - 2

Abilities rated with the Functional Communication Profile

Category	Behavior	Category	Behavior
Movement	Ability to imitate oral movements	Understanding—cont'd	Understanding simple conversation with one person
	Attempt to communicate		Understanding television
	Ability to indicate "yes" and "no"		Understanding conversation with more than two people
	Indicating floor to elevator operator		
Use of gestures	Speaking		Understanding movies
	Saying greetings		Understanding complicated verbal directions
	Saying own name		Understanding rapid, complex conversation
	Saying nouns		
	Saying verbs		
	Saying noun-verb combinations	Reading	Reading single words
	Saying phrases (nonautomatic)		Reading rehabilitation program card
	Giving directions		Reading street signs
	Speaking on the telephone		Reading newspaper headlines
	Saying short, complete sentences (nonautomatic)		Reading letters
	Saying long sentences (nonautomatic)		Reading newspaper articles
Understanding	Awareness of gross environmental sounds		Reading magazines
	Awareness of emotional voice tone		Reading books
	Understanding of own name	Other	Writing name
	Awareness of speech		Time orientation
	Recognition of family names		Copying ability
	Recognition of names of familiar objects		Writing from dictation
	Understanding action verbs		Handling money
	Understanding gestured directions		Using writing in lieu of speech
	Understanding verbal directions		Calculation ability

Data from Sarno, M.T. (1969). *The functional communication profile.* New York: NYU Medical Center Monograph Department.

The FCP and CETI are subjective rating scales. Subjective rating scales are conducive to unreliability from test to test and from rater to rater. Most subjective rating scales also suffer from lack of sensitivity to small changes in patients' performances. *Communicative Abilities in Daily Living, Second Edition* (CADL-2; Holland, Frattali, & Fromm, 1999) differs from the FCP and CETI in that it scores a patient's actual performance in an interview and in various simulated

	TABLE 3 - 3

Situations rated by the Communicative Effectiveness Index

Item	Situation
1	Getting someone's attention
2	Getting involved in group conversations about him/her
3	Giving "yes" and "no" answers appropriately
4	Communicating his/her emotions
5	Indicating that he/she understands what is being said to him/her
6	Having coffee-time visits and conversations with friends and neighbors
7	Having a one-to-one conversation with you
8	Saying the name of someone whose face is in front of him/her
9	Communicating physical needs such as aches and pains
10	Having a spontaneous conversation
11	Responding to or communicating anything (including "yes" or "no") without words
12	Starting a conversation with people who are not close family
13	Understanding writing
14	Being a part of a conversation when it is fast and there are a number of people involved
15	Participating in a conversation with strangers
16	Describing or discussing something at length

From Lomas J., Pickard, L., Bester, S., & associates (1989). The Communicative Effectiveness Index: Development and psychometric evaluation of a functional communication measure for adult aphasia. *Journal of Speech and Hearing Disorders, 54,* 113-124.

daily life communication activities, rather than subjectively rating the patient's presumed ability.

The fact that the CADL is scored relative to getting a message across rather than to correctness or incorrectness per se is one of its major departures from traditional tests of language and communication. The CADL's other major departure is in its conceptualization of test items. Rather than being a series of acontextual attempts addressed to isolating a number of language modalities (e.g., speaking, reading, writing, comprehension), most CADL items are molecular communicative interactions not easily described by language modality. Additionally, many items are richly supplied with context and often require understanding of the context for appropriate communicating. Finally, a number of nonverbal communicative events are sampled. (Holland, 1980; p. 29)

CADL-2 testing begins with an interview, which begins with the examiner saying "Hello,

Mr./Mrs. ___" and waiting for a response from the patient. The interviewer then elicits personal information from the patient, occasionally making mistakes (for example, saying, "Your first name is [wrong name] isn't it?") and noting if the patient corrects the examiner. Following the interview the examiner asks the patient to respond to various test items relating to daily life activities by pointing to pictures ("Here's a bus schedule. What time in the afternoon does bus #3 leave Maintown?") or by speech or gesture ("How would you let someone know you are cold?").

Next the examiner gives the patient an appointment card for a pretend visit to a doctor's office and, by means of questions and pictorial props, tests the patient's understanding of the appointment card and the patient's ability to carry out the appointment. For example, the patient is shown a picture of the control panel of an elevator, while the examiner says, "Remember, Dr. Clark's office is on the third floor. Here's the elevator. What do you do after you step into the elevator?" (Pointing to the "3" button in the picture or an appropriate verbal response are acceptable.)

There follows a series of test items supported by pictorial or object props. The test items relate to traveling by car, grocery shopping, making change, and using a telephone and a telephone directory. (Examples: "Make a list of three things you might need from the grocery store." "Here's a map. How do you get from the bank to the post office?" "Please call time and temperature and let me know what time it is and what the temperature is.")

The patient's responses to CADL-2 items are scored on a 3-point scale. Failed communications are scored *0*, "in the ballpark" attempts are scored *1*, and fully successful attempts are scored *2*. The CADL-2 manual assigns individual CADL-2 test items to one or more of 10 categories (Table 3-4). Some of the 50 CADL-2 items represent a single category, and others represent

more than one. A table in the CADL-2 manual gives an item-by-item breakdown of which CADL-2 items represent each category.

The CADL-2 was standardized on a sample of 175 adults with neurogenic communication impairments. The test manual contains information about test-retest reliability, interexaminer reliability, and test validity. Information about the standardization of the original CADL (Holland, 1980) also is included.

GENERAL CONCEPTS 3-4

- In rehabilitation, the word *efficacy* refers to whether a treatment has a meaningful positive effect on a disease or condition. Efficacy often is defined as change in performance on a standardized test. The word *outcome* refers to whether a treatment has a meaningful positive effect on a patient's daily life competence.

- The word *functional* has no single established meaning in the rehabilitation literature, but usually means approximately "affecting the patient's daily life competence or well-being."

- The World Health Organization concepts of *impairment, disability,* and *handicap* have had strong effects on rehabilitation of brain-injured adults. *Impairment* denotes a structural or functional abnormality in a person. *Disability* denotes the effect of impairments on a skill or ability. *Handicap* denotes the effects of disability on a person's ability to carry out daily life activities. The World Health Organization recently has replaced the labels *impairment, disability,* and *handicap* with the labels *body function and structures, activity,* and *participation.*

- The *Functional Independence Measure* (FIM), a rating scale for measuring outcome, is widely used in rehabilitation medicine programs. It focuses on self-care activities such as bathing and personal care.

- The *Functional Communication Profile* and the *Communicative Effectiveness Index* are rating scales which provide an estimate of patients' daily life communicative abilities.

- The *ASHA Functional Assessment of Communication Skills for Adults* (ASHA FACS) and

---

T A B L E   3 - 4

Categories to which items were assigned in Communication Activities of Daily Living and the number of items assigned to each category

Category	# of Items
Reading, writing, or using numbers	21
Speech acts	21
Utilize context	17
Role playing	10
Sequential relationships	9
Social convention	8
Divergences	7
Nonverbal/symbolic	7
Deixis	6
Metaphor/humor/absurdity	4

Data from Holland, A. L., Frattali, C. M., & Fromm, D. (1998). *Communication activities in daily living* (2nd ed.). Austin, TX: Pro-Ed.

Communication Activities in Daily Living (CADL-2) are standardized measures of daily life communicative performance for adults who have communicative impairments. The *Functional Communication Profile* (FCP) and the *Communicative Effectiveness Index* (CETI) are rating scales designed for subjectively estimating daily life communicative performance.

- Increasing regulation and restrictions in health care financing make measurement of outcome increasingly important to practitioners who provide diagnostic and therapeutic services to brain-injured adults.

MANAGED CARE AND ASSESSMENT OF NEUROGENIC COMMUNICATION DISORDERS

The foregoing description of tests and procedures for assessment of brain-injured adults' language and communication is consistent with clinical practice during the past several decades. It may be a somewhat less accurate description of clinical practice in the next 10 years because changes in the way health care is paid for are having strong effects on how health care is provided and promise to affect the future delivery of health care services in important ways. Some of the most striking effects are likely to be on the scope and complexity of assessment and diagnostic procedures.

In *managed care,* organizations or institutions (such as Medicare) that pay for health care (*third-party payers*) pay a fixed price for services provided in caring for a patient or, more frequently, a group of patients. For example, a corporation with 1000 employees might contract with a health care provider (a group of physicians, allied health practitioners, and administrators) to provide 1 year of health care for its employees for, say, $850,000. In return for the $850,000, the provider agrees to provide comprehensive medical care (office visits, examinations, tests, medical and surgical procedures, rehabilitation services, and so on) for the corporation's 1000 employees and their dependents. Because most providers are in business to

make a profit, they expect their actual cost per employee to be less than $850. If the provider can care for the corporation's employees for an average cost of $600 per employee, they make $250,000 profit on the contract, but if their average cost is $950 per employee the provider loses $100,000. Thus, managed care has a built-in incentive for keeping down the cost of medical care (which is one of the primary purposes of managed care).

The positive side of managed care is that it rewards efficiency. Efficient providers make a profit, and inefficient ones go out of business. The negative side of managed care is that its emphasis on reducing costs can compromise the quality of care. Physicians may be encouraged to forego expensive tests that might provide potentially important information about the nature of a patient's medical problems, to substitute cheaper but less effective treatments for more expensive and more effective ones, to postpone elective procedures, or to change their traditional way of caring for patients to better fit the financial imperatives of the provider.

The effects of managed care are not confined to physicians. Psychologists, social workers, occupational and physical therapists, speech-language pathologists, and other allied health practitioners also are affected. Shortened in-hospital lengths of stay can make evaluation something of a race, with practitioners competing for the limited number of appointment times available during a patient's stay. Evaluations that at one time could be spread across several sessions now may have to be completed in a single test session. Comprehensive evaluation of a patient's impairments may be replaced by selective testing of a patient's most obvious deficits. Treatment options may be reduced. Some groups of patients who traditionally have received treatment may not receive it. Patients who do receive treatment may get it in fewer and shorter treatment sessions.

For the speech-language pathologist concerned with assessment and diagnosis of brain-injured adults' linguistic and communicative impairments, test administration time is likely to become increasingly important, given contemporary pressures from employers and health care funding agencies to increase efficiency and decrease costs. In a health care system that emphasizes economy and efficiency, tests requiring 2 to 6 hours to administer, score, and interpret will be at a significant disadvantage relative to shorter and quicker tests.

> One of the more often reported complaints from clinicians in recent months is the virtual elimination of standardized test batteries in patient assessments. Clinicians feel they no longer have the time to conduct the kind of comprehensive evaluations they were accustomed to and have been trained to do. (Golper & Cherney, 1999, p. 3)

There is no acceptable substitute for standardized tests that have documented reliability and validity, permit comparison of a patient with other patients in their diagnostic category, and permit comparison of a brain-injured patient's performance with the performance of persons without brain injury. Sensitive and reliable screening tests to detect communication impairments and give a general sense of the pattern of those impairments will become increasingly important. Comprehensive test batteries may have to be shortened and made more efficient, perhaps by providing norms for individual subtests or combinations of subtests. Some existing language test batteries provide subtest-by-subtest norms (e.g., the PICA, the Boston Diagnostic Aphasia Examination). Because they permit subtest-by-subtest comparisons of a patient with norms, language test batteries with subtest-by-subtest norms should prove particularly appealing to clinicians who wish to shorten a long standardized test.

Some test developers and publishers are creating shortened versions of standardized tests. The third edition of the Boston Diagnostic Aphasia Examination (Goodglass, Kaplan, & Barresi, 2001) includes a short version that shortens testing time to about 1 hour from the 3 to 5 hours required for the full BDAE. The

Discourse Comprehension Test (Brookshire & Nicholas, 1993) includes a short version that cuts test administration and interpretation time in half. Short forms of several standardized tests have been described in the literature, including the Boston Naming Test (Tombaugh & Hurley, 1997), the Western Aphasia Battery (Crary & Rothi, 1989), and the PICA (Disimoni, Keith, & Darley, 1980; Disimoni, Keith, Holt, & associates, 1975; Lincoln and Ellis, 1980). Most contemporary language test batteries could stand (and perhaps benefit from) some pruning. The danger is that the pruning may lop off too much, leaving clinicians with incomplete or inaccurate descriptions of their patients' impairments.

The days of comprehensive language testing may be numbered. If they are, speech-language pathologists and other practitioners must work to ensure that gains in economy and efficiency do not come at the expense of their understanding of their patients' impairments and do not compromise their ability to provide the most efficacious treatment for those impairments.

> Forming an accurate diagnosis and prognosis and confidently arriving at a plan for treatment that will benefit the patient require more information than can be gathered through cursory screening assessments, impressions gained from talking with family, or informal conversations with the patient. Further, the benefit of treatment is best determined through periodic testing. It is not appropriate to rely on cursory screening protocols to make a prognosis or design a treatment plan likely to benefit the patient, nor should cursory assessments be used to gauge treatment effects. (Golper & Cherney, 1999, p. 3)

Measures of functional communication are likely to become increasingly important in the future, as changes in the way health care is provided and paid for accentuate the need for reliable, sensitive, and valid indicators of daily life communication performance. Those who wish to be paid for services provided to patients with neurogenic communication disorders will be required to show that the services provide meaningful benefits to the patients served. Health care providers will require that treatment planning and treatment procedures explicitly address daily life communication performance. Consequently, development of efficient, sensitive, reliable, and valid measures that are indicators of daily life communication performance will be an important responsibility of those concerned with clinical management of neurogenic communication disorders during the next decade.

THOUGHT QUESTIONS

Question 3-1 You receive the following referral from a neurologist on a patient named Mrs. Olson: *63-year-old female, 1 day post-onset of suspected right-hemisphere stroke. Evaluation and recommendations please.*

You go to the patient's ward and find that Mrs. Olson's medical record is temporarily off the ward at a care-planning meeting. The nurse tells you that the patient is in her room so you decide to do a preliminary screening at bedside. When you enter the patient's room she is lying in bed with her eyes closed. You touch her on the shoulder and she opens her eyes and looks at you. You introduce yourself and ask her how she is feeling. She gestures weakly with her left hand and closes her eyes. You say, "Are you Mrs. Olson?" She shakes her head without opening her eyes. You touch her on the shoulder. She opens her eyes and looks at you. You say, "Are you Mrs. Olson?" She mumbles something incomprehensible and closes her eyes. You touch her on the shoulder. She does not respond. What would you do next? What are some potential reasons for Mrs. Olson's unresponsiveness?

Question 3-2 Describe some ways in which not having a sufficient number of items in a test might lead to inaccuracy in describing a patient's true performance. What are some ways in which a patient's performance might fluctuate over time? How might those fluctuations inter-

act with the number of test items to affect the accuracy with which a patient's true performance is specified?

Question 3-3 The following items constitute a screening test of oral reading for use with brain-injured adults. The test instructions are, "Now I'll show you some words on these cards. I want you to read each word aloud when I show it to you." What potential problems do you see in interpreting the results of the test?

1. cat
2. umbrella
3. dog
4. she
5. perambulator
6. the
7. yellow
8. seventy-two
9. its
10. slowly

Question 3-4 Consider the following interchange between a clinician and a brain-injured patient:

Clinician: *O.K. Mr. Chambers, now I'm going to say some words and sentences and I want you to ...*

Mr. Chambers: *O.K., fine, fine ...*

Clinician: *... and I want you to say them after me.*

Mr. Chambers: *Say them after you. O.K. O.K.*

Clinician: *Are you ready?*

Mr. Chambers: *Yes, yes, O.K. O.K.*

Clinician: *Here's the first one ...*

Mr. Chambers: *Fine, fine, O.K. O.K.*

Clinician: *The boy has ...*

Mr. Chambers: *The boy ...*

Clinician: *The boy has a dog.*

Mr. Chambers: *The boy has ... something or other.*

What do you think is happening here? What potential explanations do you see for Mr. Chambers's pattern of responses? What would you do next if you were the clinician?

Neuroanatomic Explanations of Aphasia and Related Disorders

THE LOCALIZATIONISTS

Neuroanatomic explanations of aphasia are based on models formulated during the nineteenth century by European physicians and neuroanatomists who, in addition to arguing fiercely among themselves about who was right, began the sometimes haphazard process of finding out which parts of the brain did what. The grist for the neuroanatomists' mill was provided by the brains of patients who had died following stroke or head trauma. Neuroranatomists laboriously accumulated information about brain-behavior relationships as they recorded their patients' symptoms, and when the patients eventually died, they dissected the deceased patients' brains to find out which parts had been damaged. When damage in a region of the brain produced a given pattern of impairment, it seemed reasonable to assign the impaired functions to the damaged region (*localization of function*).

The localizationist effort received its first major push from Franz Gall, a Viennese physician who in the early 1800s established what he called the science of craniology and published elaborate maps of the brain in which various human "faculties" such as *bravery, honesty,* and *love* were assigned to specific brain regions (Figure 4-1). Gall believed that brain regions responsible for unusually well-developed faculties were themselves unusually well developed and that manipulation of the skull could enhance mental faculties. He reasoned that hyperdeveloped brain regions pressed outward on the skull, creating bumps and ridges that a skilled practitioner could analyze, thereby determining the individual's unique pattern of talents and weaknesses.

Gall's methods were naturalistic and, by today's standards, naive. Gall obtained the evidence for his conclusions from observing friends, family members, and others, as well as his patients. Phrenology fell into scientific disrepute in the late 1830s but remained popular in England and the United States until the late 1800s. Today phrenologic maps are venerable curiosities, found primarily in treatises on the

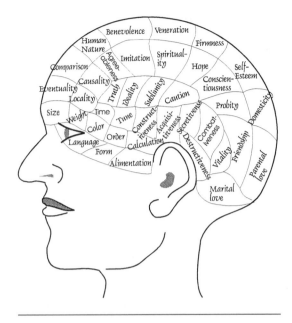

Figure 4-1 ■ Phrenologic diagram, showing the sites of various human "faculties" in the brain.

history of neurology and in advertisements for neurologic books and journals.

> Gall assigned responsibility for language to the frontal lobes because several of his acquaintances with well-developed verbal skills had protruding foreheads and bulging eyes.

Localizationist models specific to aphasia began with the work of Paul Broca, a French neurologist who in the 1860s published a series of papers in which he asserted that loss of "articulate speech" is caused by damage in the posterior inferior frontal lobe of the left hemisphere. Localizationist models of aphasia got another boost in 1874 when Karl Wernicke, a young German neuropsychiatrist, published a description of what he called "sensory aphasia," caused by lesions in the posterior temporal lobe. In subsequent publications Wernicke went on to construct an elaborate (for the time) account of the relationships between language functions and brain regions—an account that has survived in modified form until contemporary times.

The localizationists did not have the stage all to themselves. A vociferous group of antilocalizationists was active both in the clinics and in the medical literature of the time. The antilocalizationists asserted that the brain operates as an integrated whole, and they considered absurd the localizationists' obsession with fractionating mental activity and assigning it to various brain regions. The published work of Marie Jean-Pierre Flourens, a contemporary of Gall's, is considered by many to represent the beginning of the antilocalizationist movement. Flourens's beliefs subsequently were built on by others, including John Hughlings Jackson, a British neurologist, in the 1860s; Pierre Marie, a French neurologist, in the early 1900s; and Henry Head, another British neurologist, in the 1920s. The antilocalizationists had a point but had relatively little effect on the neurologic establishment, partly because the new localizationists were right somewhat more often than they were wrong and partly because localization provided neurologists with a reasonably reliable way of telling what part of a patient's brain had been damaged without having to take the brain out and look at it.

LANGUAGE AND CEREBRAL DOMINANCE

One of the earliest assertions of the localizationists was that the left hemisphere of right-handed adults is responsible for language. This assertion had its beginnings in Broca's case reports and was reinforced by repeated observations of language disturbances following left-hemisphere damage in right-handers. Based on a scattering of case reports (and, no doubt, on logic and a desire for symmetry) it became generally accepted that left-handers' brains were mirror images of right-handers' brains; namely, the right hemisphere of left-handers' brains carried the language load.

The mirror-image concept began to fall apart in the 1950s when published reports (Goodglass & Quadfasel, 1954; Penfield & Roberts, 1959) began suggesting that left-handers who became aphasic seemed not to have heard of the localizationists' assertions. At least half of these aphasic left-handers had damage only in the left hemisphere. Russell and Espir (1961) subsequently studied a group of 58 left-handed adults with traumatic brain injuries. According to the mirror-image theory, the left-handers with right-hemisphere damage should have language impairments and the left-handers with left-hemisphere damage should have intact language. Contrary to the mirror-image hypothesis, 36% of the left-handers with left-hemisphere damage had significant language impairments, whereas only 13% of the left-handers with right-hemisphere damage had language impairments.

The mirror-image belief was pushed further into disrepute by the results of a study by Milner (1975). Milner injected sodium amytal into the carotid arteries of a group of left-handed adults. Sodium amytal is an anesthetic, and injection of sodium amytal into a carotid artery anesthetizes the brain hemisphere on the side of the injection. The person undergoing amytal testing loses the ability to speak when the language-competent hemisphere is anesthetized. Only 18% of Milner's left-handers stopped talking when their right hemispheres were anesthetized, whereas 69% stopped talking when their left hemispheres were given the drug. Thirteen percent lost speech when either hemisphere was anesthetized, suggesting that their brain hemispheres shared language responsibilities. The results of a retrospective study by Naeser and Borod (1986) support Milner's findings. They reviewed the medical records of 31 left-handed aphasic adults. Only 4 (13%) had right-hemisphere brain damage.

It seems clear that most adults, regardless of handedness, depend on the left hemisphere for language. However, left-handers' brains may be more flexible than right-handers' brains about which hemisphere gets the language responsibilities. Left-handers who become aphasic seem to have less severe aphasia and seem to recover language better than their right-handed counterparts, regardless of which hemisphere is affected (Gloning, Gloning, Haub, & associates, 1969; Goodglass, 1993; Luria, 1970). Milner's (1975) finding that 13% of left-handed adults became aphasic when either hemisphere was anesthetized provides additional support for the notion that left-handers' brains are less constrained than those of right-handers when it comes to which hemisphere takes care of language.

The question of whether we are born with one hemisphere specialized for language has not been answered, although indirect evidence suggests that we are not. Studies of children and adolescents who acquire brain damage suggest that left hemisphere specialization for language develops as we mature, and that it is not complete before adulthood. A child born with a nonfunctional left hemisphere usually develops normal language, unless the child's right hemisphere also is damaged, and a child or adolescent who becomes aphasic almost always recovers far more language than an adult with comparable damage. The brain's ability to reassign functions served by damaged tissue diminishes with age. The older a patient is at the time of brain injury, the more severe the persisting consequences of the injury are likely to be (Lenneberg, 1967; Osgood & Miron, 1963).

> The brain's potential for reassigning to a different brain region functions that are lost when brain tissue is damaged is called *cerebral plasticity*. Children's brains are said to be more plastic than adults' brains because brain injuries that would cause lasting impairments in adults often leave children with little or no permanent impairment.

THE PERISYLVIAN REGION AND LANGUAGE

Connectionist explanations of language impairment following brain damage emphasize the importance of the region surrounding the Sylvian

fissure (called the *perisylvian* region) in the left hemisphere. The left hemisphere is dominant for speech and language in approximately 85% of adults. Permanent damage anywhere in the perisylvian region in the left hemisphere of adult brains almost always causes language impairment (except for the approximate 15% of left-handers whose right hemisphere is responsible for speech and language).

> In what follows I use "left hemisphere" instead of the technically more accurate, but tedious, "language-dominant hemisphere."

The perisylvian region in the left frontal lobe (sometimes called *the anterior language zone*) plays an important part in planning and performing expressive language actions (speech, writing, and perhaps gesture). The perisylvian region in the left temporal and parietal lobes (sometimes called the *posterior language zone*) is important for comprehending and recalling linguistic material and for formulating linguistic messages with appropriate syntactic structure and semantic content.

The heart of the anterior language zone is the posterior inferior frontal lobe, immediately in front of the primary motor cortex. This region of cortex is called *Broca's area* (Figure 4-2). It is named after Paul Broca, the French neurologist who first described its role in speech. Broca's area is next to the primary motor cortex that controls the muscles used to produce speech. Sometimes Broca's area is called the *motor speech area* because it plans and organizes speech movements to be executed by the primary motor cortex. *Broca's aphasia* is said to be a major consequence of damage in Broca's area.

The heart of the posterior language zone is *Wernicke's area* in the posterior superior left temporal lobe (see Figure 4-2). Wernicke's area is named after the German neuropsychiatrist who first described an aphasia syndrome caused by temporal lobe damage. Sometimes Wernicke's

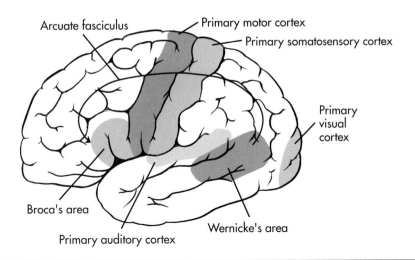

Figure 4-2 ■ **Important cortical regions and connecting pathways in connectionist explanations of how the brain produces language.**

area is called the *auditory association cortex.* It is thought to be important for storage and retrieval of the mental representations of words, for storage and retrieval of word meanings, and for knowledge and use of grammatic and linguistic rules. Damage in Wernicke's area may cause *Wernicke's aphasia.*

Wernicke's area receives a large part of its input from the *primary auditory cortex (Gyrus of Heschl),* on the top surface of each temporal lobe within the Sylvian fissure (see Figure 4-2). The two primary auditory cortices are responsible for perception and discrimination of auditory stimuli. Each auditory cortex receives information from both ears, although the contralateral ear has a slight advantage.

Wernicke's area communicates with Broca's area and other frontal regions of the brain by way of the *arcuate fasciculus,* a band of nerve fibers that runs between the mid temporal lobe and the lower regions of the frontal lobe via the parietal lobe (see Figure 4-2). The arcuate fasciculus is the primary route by which linguistic messages formulated in Wernicke's area reach Broca's area.

The region in and around the *angular gyrus,* at the junction of the temporal, parietal, and oc-

Destruction of the primary auditory cortex in one hemisphere does not cause lasting deafness; it causes only mild hearing loss (usually in the contralateral ear) and occasionally some difficulty localizing sounds. Destruction of the primary auditory cortex in both hemispheres causes cortical deafness, in which the patient initially loses all auditory sensitivity. For some patients with bilateral destruction of auditory cortex, some hearing sensitivity slowly returns and the patient's pure-tone audiogram may even reach normal. However, perception of speech and other complex auditory stimuli almost always remains profoundly impaired (Jerger, Weikers, Sharbrough, & associates, 1969).

cipital lobes, is important for processes involved in reading and writing. Damage to this region usually produces severe impairments in reading (called *alexia*) and severe writing impairments (called *agraphia*).

HOW THE BRAIN PERFORMS LANGUAGE

The connectionist model provides a metaphor for describing how the language-dominant hemisphere makes sense of incoming verbal messages and how it formulates, plans, and executes verbal and gestural responses. The connectionist model depicts the brain's processing of language as resembling a telephone system, in which various centers send messages here and there over a system of interconnected circuits.

> We know that the brain does not work like a telephone system, and we know that the connectionist model is simplistic and in some respects inaccurate. Nevertheless, it is a convenient metaphor for what actually happens, and it provides a practical way for students to get a general sense of how damage in the brain yields fairly predictable impairments of language and behavior.

Comprehension of Speech

To explore how the connectionist model works, consider a fictional normal adult. According to the connectionist model, when a normal adult (called Norman in this example) comprehends spoken messages, the message goes from Norman's ears via ascending fibers to the primary auditory cortices in each of his temporal lobes. The auditory cortices encode the acoustic information and send the encoded message off to Wernicke's area in Norman's left hemisphere. (The information from the auditory cortex in the right hemisphere gets to Wernicke's area by way of fibers passing through the posterior corpus callosum.)

When Wernicke's area recognizes the message as speech, it sorts through its store of semantic representations to find meanings for the words in the message. When Wernicke's area has located the word meanings, it consults its book of syntactic rules to determine the relationships among the words. Then it constructs a representation of the message's overall meaning. Norman's brain also evaluates the situation to determine if the literal meaning of the sentence actually represents the speaker's intent. (Some

sentences, such as "Can you open the window?" are implied requests and are not meant to be interpreted literally. A "yes" or "no" response usually wouldn't be appropriate.) When Wernicke's area has deduced the sentence's meaning and knows whether the message should be interpreted literally or figuratively, it sends instructions to other parts of Norman's brain regarding how he should respond—for example, talk, write, gesture, or open the window. (Norman's right brain hemisphere apparently plays an important part in identifying nonliteral statements.)

Comprehension of Printed Materials (Reading)

When Norman's brain has to get meaning from printed messages, the process resembles that for comprehension of speech, except that Norman's visual cortex is the first stop in the brain. Norman's visual cortex encodes the information coming from the eyes in a form that his Wernicke's area can understand and sends it to Wernicke's area. (The information from the visual cortex in Norman's right hemisphere gets to Wernicke's area via fibers passing through the posterior corpus callosum.) From Wernicke's area onward, the process resembles that for auditory comprehension. Wernicke's area constructs a representation of the message's meaning and sends the relevant information to the parts of Norman's brain that are to be involved in the response.

Spontaneous Speech

When Norman speaks a sentence spontaneously, Wernicke's area retrieves from the mental lexicon the words needed to express the message and constructs a sentence that complies with phonologic, syntactic, and semantic rules. Wernicke's area then sends the neurally coded sentence forward via the arcuate fasciculus to Broca's area. Broca's area translates the code into an action plan and sends the plan off to Norman's primary motor cortex. The primary motor cortex puts the finishing touches on the message and sends it down, via the pyramidal system, to Norman's cranial nerves, which set the speech muscles in motion. As the speech muscles produce the message, Wernicke's area monitors it to ensure that what it sent is what Norman actually says. If it is not, Wernicke's area shifts the system into repair mode.

Repetition

According to the connectionist model, repetition of words, phrases, and sentences tests the entire language circuit, from the primary auditory cortex through the motor cortex for speech. Suppose Norman is asked to repeat a phrase such as "Nelson Rockefeller drives a Lincoln Continental." The first stop in the brain is Norman's primary auditory cortex, where the incoming message is perceived and translated into a neural code that Wernicke's area will understand. Then the coded message is sent to Wernicke's area, where the meaning of the message (that Norman should say "Nelson Rockefeller drives a Lincoln Continental") is extracted. Wernicke's area then codes the sentence in a form that Broca's area can work with and sends it off via the arcuate fasciculus. When the message arrives at Broca's area, Broca's area recodes the phrase into an articulatory plan for the speech muscles and sends it off to the primary motor cortex. The primary motor cortex sends the message down pyramidal fibers to the cranial nerves, which move the speech muscles. Wernicke's area monitors the output and initiates corrective routines if necessary.

Oral Reading

If Norman is asked to read printed material aloud, processes similar to those involved in speech repetition take place once the message has reached Wernicke's area. However, Wernicke's area gets the message from the visual cortex rather than the auditory cortex.

Writing

When Norman writes a message, his Wernicke's area formulates a message containing the appropriate words in syntactically acceptable order,

gets the spelling right, and sends it via the arcuate fasciculus to the premotor cortex for Norman's hand and arm, which sets up the appropriate movement plans and sends them to his motor cortex. Norman's eyes and his Wernicke's area collaborate to monitor what he writes. If Wernicke's area is not satisfied, Norman may erase, revise, correct spelling errors, or make other repairs.

Gestural Responses to Spoken Commands

In this task, the neural processes are similar to those for speech, except that the information from Wernicke's area is sent to the premotor area for Norman's hand and arm located just above Broca's area in the premotor cortex, rather than to the premotor cortex for the speech muscles (Broca's area). If the gestural response is to be carried out by Norman's right hand and arm (contralateral to his left hemisphere), the message goes from Wernicke's area to the premotor cortex in Norman's left hemisphere and then to the motor cortex in the same hemisphere, which sends the message to Norman's right hand. If the response is to be carried out by Norman's left hand and arm (on the same side as his left hemisphere), the message goes from Wernicke's area to the premotor cortex in the left hemisphere, from whence it is sent, via the corpus callosum, to the motor cortex in the right hemisphere and then down the corticospinal tract to Norman's left hand. (The premotor cortex in Norman's left hemisphere plans volitional movements for both sides of his body.)

PATTERNS OF LANGUAGE IMPAIRMENT

Now we will consider how the connectionist model relates damage in certain brain regions to distinctive patterns of speech, language, and motor-planning disorders. Some of these patterns are caused by destruction of important centers such as Broca's area and Wernicke's area, and others are caused by damage in pathways connecting the centers such as the arcuate fasciculus. Those who classify aphasic patients into classic syndromes rely heavily on relationships among *speech fluency, paraphasia, repetition,* and *language comprehension.*

Speech fluency is an important concept for understanding the connectionist model because classic aphasia syndromes can be divided into two categories based on speech fluency. Patients with *nonfluent aphasia* typically have damage in the front half of the language-dominant hemisphere, anterior to the central sulcus (fissure of Rolando). Patients with fluent aphasia typically have damage posterior to the central sulcus in the language-dominant hemisphere.

When it is used to sort patients into connectionist aphasia syndromes, speech fluency refers to the prosodic or melodic characteristics of speech. Patients with fluent aphasia speak smoothly and effortlessly. They manipulate speech rate, intonation, and emphatic stress in much the same way as normal speakers do. Patients with *nonfluent aphasia* speak slowly, haltingly, and with great effort, pausing between syllables and words. The speech of patients with nonfluent aphasia has a measured, machine-like quality, owing to diminished or absent intonation and emphatic stress patterns.

Over the years, the terms *fluent* and *nonfluent* have acquired meaning that goes beyond the mechanics of speech to syntax, grammar, and semantic content:

> Fluent [aphasic] patients have normal or near normal speech rates, and use a variety of different grammatical constructions; function words and grammatical inflections are present, and usually syntactically appropriate. Intonation patterns are present and usually appropriate. Non-fluent [aphasic] patients have slow and labored speech. The variety of grammatical constructions is often restricted and intonation may be reduced or absent; function words and grammatical affixes may be omitted, and patients may rely a lot on nouns. (Howard & Hatfield, 1987, p. 147)

Paraphasia is another important concept in connectionistic models of aphasia. Paraphasia can be loosely defined as *speech errors produced by a person with aphasia.* (The circularity of this definition has not affected its durability in the literature.) Two kinds of paraphasia have been described, although there is some confusion about which speech errors qualify as paraphasia. *Literal paraphasias* (sometimes called *phonemic paraphasias*) are phonologic errors in which incorrect sounds replace correct sounds, as in *shooshbruss* for *toothbrush,* or in which sounds within words are transposed, as in *tevilision* for *television. Verbal paraphasias* (sometimes called *semantic paraphasias*) are errors in which an incorrect word (usually semantically related to the target) is unintentionally substituted for the target word, as in *door* for *window* or *knife* for *fork.*

Goodglass, Kaplan, and Barresi (2001) separate verbal paraphasia into three categories. *Semantic paraphasias* are substitutions of semantically related words for target words, as in *father* for *mother. Unrelated paraphasias* are substitutions in which the substituted words have no clear relationship to target words, as in *cigarette* for *motorcycle. Perseverative paraphasias* are substitutions in which a previously used word is unintentionally substituted for a target word in a new context, such as when an aphasic patient who has previously named a comb correctly subsequently calls a fork, toothbrush, and key a *comb.* Goodglass, Barresi, and Kaplan separate one-word circumlocution (deliberate use of a substitute word for a word that a patient cannot retrieve—for example, a patient who says *barn* for *cow*) from paraphasia because paraphasias are unintentional substitutions. (The reliability of this distinction seems suspect because it is not easy to tell when a patient's substitutions are deliberate or unintentional. However, the concept of the distinction has merit.)

According to Canter (1973), the term *literal paraphasia* denotes a *pattern* of articulatory errors, which means that the label should not be attached to individual articulatory errors, especially those made by patients who are dysarthric rather than aphasic. Consequently, the clinician must consider not only the nature of the speech errors, but the context in which they occur to tell if the errors are truly literal paraphasias. When an aphasic patient makes speech sound errors in a context of fluent, effortless speech they are likely to qualify as literal paraphasias. When they occur in a context of nonfluent, effortful articulatory posturing they are likely to represent the phonetic dissolution often associated with motor-planning impairments (apraxia of speech).

Aphasia Caused by Destruction of Cortical Centers for Language

Three of the most common aphasia syndromes (*Broca's aphasia, Wernicke's aphasia,* and *global aphasia*) are caused by damage in cortical regions considered important for comprehension, formulation, and production of language. These regions are located in the central region of the language-dominant hemisphere, which is served by the middle cerebral artery. Occlusion of the anterior branch of the middle cerebral artery causes Broca's aphasia, and occlusion of the posterior branch causes Wernicke's aphasia. Global aphasia is created by occlusion of the main trunk of the middle cerebral artery.

Broca's Aphasia As noted earlier, Broca's aphasia is caused by damage in Broca's area. Broca's area makes up the lower part of the *premotor cortex,* a strip of cortex just in front of the primary motor cortex. The premotor cortex seems to be responsible for planning skilled volitional movements for the primary motor cortices in both hemispheres. Because Broca's area is adjacent to the primary motor cortex for the speech muscles, it plays an important part in planning speech movements. Because Broca's area is close to the primary motor cortex for the face, hand, and arm, and because descending pyramidal tract fibers pass under Broca's area, patients with Broca's aphasia usually have right-sided hemiparesis or hemiplegia.

Broca's aphasia sometimes goes by other names, such as *expressive aphasia, motor aphasia,* and *anterior aphasia.* Patients with Broca's aphasia are nonfluent. They speak as if the motor plans for speech have gone awry. Their words come slowly, laboriously, and haltingly. They pause between words, and they often pause inappropriately between syllables. Their speech sounds monotonous because of diminished intonation and stress. Misarticulations are common, and some consonants and vowels are distorted (a phenomenon called *phonetic dissolution*). Patients with Broca's aphasia are laconic. Their utterances are short and consist mostly of content words (nouns, verbs, and an occasional adjective but rarely adverbs). Most function words (conjunctions, articles, and prepositions) are missing, leading some writers to describe their speech as *agrammatic* or *telegraphic.*

A patient with Broca's aphasia was asked to describe the "Cookie Theft" picture from the *Boston Diagnostic Aphasia Examination* (Goodglass & Kaplan, 1983; see Figure 5-22). Here is what she said:

> "uh . . . mother and dad . . . no . . . mother . . . dishes. . . uh . . . runnin over . . . water . . . and floor . . . and they . . . uh . . . wipin disses . . . and . . . uh . . . two kids . . . uh . . . stool . . . and cookie . . . cookie jar . . . uh . . . cabinet and stool . . . uh . . . tippin over . . . and . . . uh . . . bad . . . and somebody . . . gonna get hurt."

Patients with Broca's aphasia write as they speak—slowly and laboriously. Their written language typically consists of strings of isolated content words sprinkled with misspellings and distortions or omissions of letters. Letters are clumsily formed (perhaps in part because the presence of hemiplegia forces the patient to write with the nonpreferred hand). Patients with Broca's aphasia rarely write in cursive form. Their written sentences are produced with great effort and often slant downward across the page. Figure 4-3 shows a sample of writing from a patient with Broca's aphasia who is describing in writing what one does with the 10 test objects (*cigarette, comb, fork, key, knife, match, pen,*

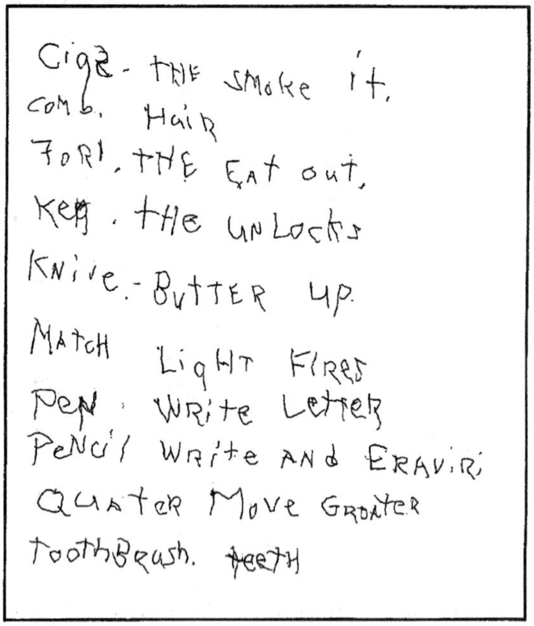

Cigr. the smoke it,
comb. Hair
Forl. the Eat out,
Keg. the unlocks
Knive.-Butter up.
Match Light Fires
Pen write Letter
Pencil write and Eravir,
Quater Move Grouter
toothBrush. teeth

Figure 4-3 ■ Sample of writing produced by a patient with Broca's aphasia.

pencil, quarter, and *toothbrush*) from the *Porch Index of Communicative Ability* (Porch, 1981a).

Patients with Broca's aphasia comprehend spoken and written language better than they speak or write, although they are slow readers, and careful testing almost always will reveal subtle impairment of both reading and listening comprehension. Their self-monitoring usually is well preserved. When patients with Broca's aphasia make errors in speech or writing or are unsuccessful in communicating, they typically repeat or attempt repairs. Patients with Broca's aphasia tend to be excruciatingly aware of their physical and communicative impairments and are easily upset by failed communication attempts, sometimes to the point of emotional outbursts. Patients with Broca's aphasia are cooperative and task-oriented in testing and treatment activities. They are good at remembering treatment procedures and goals from day to day and may spontaneously generalize the skills and strategies acquired in treatment to their daily life environment.

Wernicke's Aphasia Like Broca's aphasia, Wernicke's aphasia has several aliases, including *sensory aphasia, receptive aphasia,* and *posterior aphasia.* Wernicke's aphasia typically is caused by damage in the posterior superior temporal lobe of the language-dominant hemisphere. One of the most striking language characteristics of patients with Wernicke's aphasia is their impaired comprehension of spoken or printed verbal materials. Patients with severe Wernicke's aphasia fail to comprehend even simple spoken or written verbal materials, although some may get a smattering of what is said in conversations. Patients with mild or moderate Wernicke's aphasia usually get the overall point of conversations but miss the specifics.

Patients with Wernicke's aphasia often exhibit dissociations between the sound (or sight) of words and their meanings and in extreme cases may be unable to discriminate between phonologically valid nonwords (*spome*) and real words (*spoon*). Their language comprehension may be compromised by blurring of semantic distinctions among words, rendering them unable to appreciate differences between words with related meanings (*good* versus *wonderful*) and causing some patients with Wernicke's aphasia to lose their sense of semantic typicality (whether *carrot* is a more typical vegetable than *artichoke*).

Evidence of Wernicke's aphasic patients' confusion about semantic typicality comes from tests in which they must make typicality judgments about printed words. Their confusion does not extend to daily life. Patients with Wernicke's aphasia are unlikely to confuse real carrots and real artichokes when it comes time to peel, cook, or eat them.

The semantic impairments of patients with Wernicke's aphasia are exacerbated by impaired short-term retention and recall of verbal materials. Patients with Wernicke's aphasia perform poorly on tests of short-term memory in which they must repeat strings of numbers or recall word lists. When they are asked to perform sequences of manipulative or gestural responses to spoken or printed commands (e.g., "Put the pencil beside the spoon, and put the quarter beside the box.") their performance rapidly deteriorates as the commands become longer.

In contrast with the slow, laborious, and halting speech of patients with Broca's aphasia, patients with Wernicke's aphasia talk smoothly, effortlessly, and usually copiously. (Wernicke's aphasia is a *fluent* aphasia.) Patients with Wernicke's aphasia can produce long, syntactically well-formed sentences with normal intonation and stress patterns, although they may pause and muddle about when experiencing word retrieval difficulties, which are common. That the mechanics of speech are preserved in Wernicke's aphasia does not mean, however, that patients with Wernicke's aphasia have no difficulty communicating by talking. Their connected speech may be littered with verbal paraphasias (substitution of one word for another), occasional literal paraphasias (substitution or transposition of sounds within words), and *neologisms* (nonwords such as *carabis*). The speech pattern of patients with mild to moderate Wernicke's aphasia sometimes is called *paragrammatism.*

Clinician: "Tell me where you live."
Patient: "Well, it's a meender place and it has two ... two of them. For dreaming and pinding after supper. And up and down. Four of down and three of up ...."

Patients with severe Wernicke's aphasia may produce *jargon*—strings of neologisms with a sprinkling of connecting words.

Clinician: "What's the weather like today?"
Patient: "Fully under the jimjam and on the altigrabber."

Patients with severe Wernicke's aphasia often produce strings in which the major content words are replaced by neologisms, but in which the connectives (articles, conjunctions, prepositions) are real words (as in the preceding speech sample). The strings also seem syntactically well formed (Goodglass, 1993). Wernicke's aphasic patients with word-retrieval impairments may produce what is called *empty speech,* substituting general words such as *thing* or *stuff* or pronouns without referents for more specific words.

A patient with moderate Wernicke's aphasia was attempting to explain what he had done on a shopping trip the previous day. He concluded with, "I went down to the thing to do the other one and she was only the last one that ever did it, so I never did."

Some Wernicke's aphasic patients talk around missing words—a behavior called *circumlocution.*

A patient with moderate Wernicke's aphasia was attempting to tell the examiner what she had had for breakfast that morning. Unable to come up with the needed words, she circumlocuted to get her intended meaning across. "This morning for—that meal—the first thing this morning—what I ate—I dined on—chickens, but little—and pig—pork—hen fruit and some bacon, I guess."

The ease with which Wernicke's aphasic patients produce speech, their circumlocution, and their deficient self-monitoring may contribute to their well-known inclination to run on when they talk—a phenomenon called *press of speech* or *logorrhea.*

The handwriting of patients with Wernicke's aphasia usually resembles their speech. They write effortlessly and their letters are well-formed and legible. Most write in cursive form, rather than printing. Although their handwriting, like

> ### An Example of Press of Speech
>
> Clinician: "Tell me what you do with a comb."
> Patient: "What do I do with a comb . . . what I do with a comb. Well a comb is a utensil or some such thing that can be used for arranging and rearranging the hair on the head both by men and by women. One could also make music with it by putting a piece of paper behind it and blowing through it. Sometimes it could be used in art—in sculpture, for example, to make a series of lines in soft clay. It's usually made of plastic and usually black, although it comes in other colors. It is carried in the pocket until it's needed, when it is taken out and used, then put back in the pocket. Is that what you had in mind?"

their speech, may be mechanically normal, their handwriting, like their speech, is deficient in content. Patients who produce verbal paraphasias in speech produce them in writing. Patients who speak neologistically write neologistically. (The letters in neologistic words usually are grouped in clusters that are consistent with letter groupings for real words.) Patients with press of speech when they talk usually exhibit press of writing when they write. Figure 4-4 shows a writing sample generated by a Wernicke's aphasic patient with mild aphasia describing what one does with the 10 test items from the *Porch Index of Communicative Ability* (Porch, 1981a).

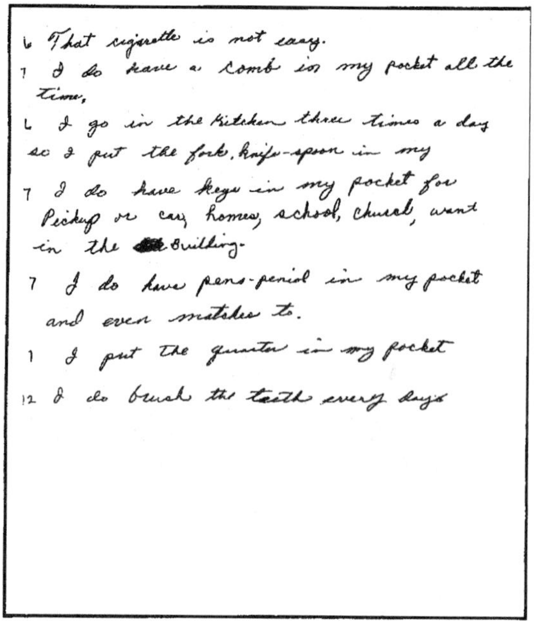
6 That cigarette is not easy.
7 I do have a comb in my pocket all the time,
6 I go in the Kitchen three times a day so I put the fork, knife-spoon in my
7 I do have keys in my pocket for Pickup or car, homes, school, church, want in the Building.
7 I do have pens-pencil in my pocket and even matches to.
1 I put the quarter in my pocket
12 I do brush the teeth every days

Figure 4-4 ■ **Sample of writing produced by a patient with Wernicke's aphasia.**

Most patients with Wernicke's aphasia are alert, attentive, and task-oriented. Those with mild Wernicke's aphasia are aware of their errors (at least most of them), the content of their speech is semantically appropriate, and they generally follow conversational rules such as those governing turn taking. Patients with moderate Wernicke's aphasia rarely notice errors or attempt repairs. They are attentive and cooperative in testing and treatment but may stray from the task unless the clinician intervenes to keep them on track. In conversations, patients with Wernicke's aphasia tend to wander off on verbal tangents and may talk at length about unrelated or trivial topics.

Most patients with severe Wernicke's aphasia are attentive, but their profound comprehension impairments greatly interfere with their performance of all but the simplest verbal tasks. Patients with severe Wernicke's aphasia are uniformly oblivious to errors and communication failure but appear sensitive at least to the basic rules governing conversational interactions. They acknowledge and attend to their conversational partner and respect turn-taking rules, although once they get the conversational floor they tend to talk excessively, tangentially, and sometimes neologistically.

Patients with Wernicke's aphasia usually show less outward concern about their communication impairments than do patients with Broca's aphasia. Part of their unconcern may relate to their lack of awareness, but many who do recognize errors and understand that they have communication impairments are remarkably complacent and unconcerned.

Because Wernicke's area is not close to the motor cortex, few patients with Wernicke's aphasia are hemiparetic or hemiplegic, unless the lesion responsible for the aphasia extends into the frontal lobe or affects descending pyramidal tracts (in which case the aphasia might be more appropriately labeled *global aphasia*). However, fibers in the optic tract pass under Wernicke's area on their way to the visual cortex. Lesions extending deep into the temporal lobe often destroy these fibers, causing contralateral visual field blindness (described in Chapter 2).

Global Aphasia As mentioned earlier, global aphasia most often follows occlusion of the trunk of the middle cerebral artery, which causes massive damage extending throughout the perisylvian region. However, cases of global aphasia have been reported in which either Wernicke's area or Broca's area is spared (Basso, Lecours, Moraschini, & associates, 1985; Vignolo, Frediani, Boccardi, & associates, 1986) and following subcortical damage in the thalamus and basal ganglia (Naeser, Alexander, Helm-Estabrooks, & associates, 1982).

Occlusion of the trunk of the middle cerebral artery has enormous effects on the patient. Globally aphasic patients invariably exhibit severe impairments in all language functions. Most cannot perform even the simplest tests of listening comprehension, and most cannot reliably answer simple yes-no questions, although some may respond to conversations in a way that suggests that they get at least a rudimentary sense of what is said.

Some globally aphasic patients who do not respond appropriately to any other spoken materials may respond appropriately to "whole body commands" such as "stand up," "turn around," "lie down," and so forth. The reason for this phenomenon is not clear, but Albert and associates (1981) suggest that it may be attributable to right-hemisphere participation in responses to such commands.

Few globally aphasic patients can read even simple words, and their reading of sentences or texts is invariably nonfunctional. The speech of globally aphasic patients is severely limited, usually consisting of a few single words, stereotypical utterances (such as *kakie-kakie-kakie*), overlearned phrases (such as *how-dee-do*), or expletives. Over time, some globally aphasic patients become proficient at communicating in a limited way with a combination of intoned stereotypic utterances, gesture, and facial expression, but verbal communication remains largely nonfunctional.

Most globally aphasic patients are attentive, alert, task-oriented, and socially appropriate (which helps to differentiate the globally aphasic patient from the confused or demented patient). They usually can perform nonverbal tasks (matching objects or pictures, matching pictures to objects) satisfactorily, and some may perform normally or nearly so on nonverbal (performance) tests of intellect.

Globally aphasic patients occasionally comprehend questions related to personally relevant information fairly well, compared with their universally poor comprehension of other spoken material. Some globally aphasic patients reliably answer spoken yes-no questions about family, personal information, and recent experiences but respond at chance levels to all other kinds of spoken materials (Goodglass, Kaplan, & Barresi, 2001).

Aphasia Caused by Damage to Association Fiber Tracts Important to Language

Several aphasia syndromes are caused by damage in association fiber tracts that connect Wernicke's area with Broca's area or by damage to tracts that connect Wernicke's area and Broca's area to the rest of the brain. In *conduction aphasia* the pathway connecting (language-competent) Wernicke's area to (speech-competent) Broca's area is affected. In the *transcortical aphasias,* pathways connecting the perisylvian region with other regions of the brain are affected. The brain damage producing these aphasia syndromes may involve the cortex but always extends beneath the cortex to affect association fiber tracts.

Conduction Aphasia Conduction aphasia typically is caused by lesions in the upper temporal lobe, lower parietal lobe, or insula that damage the arcuate fasciculus but spare Wernicke's area and Broca's area. The defining behavioral characteristics of conduction aphasia are *grossly impaired repetition* and *relatively preserved language comprehension.* Language comprehension is preserved in conduction aphasia because the primary auditory cortex and Wernicke's area are spared.

> That comprehension is *preserved* does not mean that conduction aphasic patients' comprehension is *intact.* They typically exhibit mild to moderate comprehension impairments. The point is that their ability to repeat phrases and sentences is strikingly worse than their ability to comprehend the same phrases and sentences.

Conduction aphasic patients have extraordinary difficulty repeating what they hear because of poor communication between Wernicke's area and Broca's area. When patients with conduction aphasia are asked to repeat words, multisyllabic words create more problems than monosyllabic words. Long and phonologically complex words tie most patients with conduction aphasia into verbal knots.

> Clinician: "Now I want you to say some words after me. Say 'boy.'"
> Patient: "Boy."
> Clinician: "Home."
> Patient: "Home."
> Clinician: "Seventy-nine."
> Patient: "Ninety-seven. No . . . sevinty-sine . . . siventy-nice . . ."
> Clinician: "Let's try another one. Say 'refrigerator.'"
> Patient: "Frigilator . . . no? How about . . . frerigilator . . . no . . . frigaliterlater . . . aahh! It's all mixed up!"

Conduction aphasic patients speak fluently (speech rate, intonation, and stress patterns are normal) but are prone to literal paraphasias and produce occasional verbal paraphasias. Their spontaneous speech is better than their repetition, although literal paraphasias and pauses generated by word-retrieval difficulties are common. Patients with conduction aphasia have difficulty reading aloud because oral reading, like repetition, depends on communication between Wernicke's area and Broca's area. Conduction aphasic patients' problems with oral reading do not extend to their reading comprehension, which, like their auditory comprehension, is relatively good.

Conduction aphasic patients' handwriting typically is well formed and legible, but self-formulated writing and writing to dictation usually contain spelling errors and transpositions of syllables and words. Just as they are better at saying what they think than repeating what they hear, they can write self-formulated material better than they can write what is said to them.

Conduction aphasic patients are alert, attentive, and task-oriented. They are aware of errors in speech and writing and attempt repairs. Conduction aphasic patients often seem surprised by paraphasias, and comments to that effect are not unusual. Patients with conduction aphasia typically produce conversational asides ("Why can't I say that?" "What's going on here?") normally and without conscious effort. Their first attempts at self-correcting a response often are unsuccessful, and long strings of unsuccessful repair attempts are common, with the patient often getting further and further from the target, until she or he throws in the towel or the examiner supplies the target word or words.

> A patient with conduction aphasia was trying to produce the word *circus.* "It's a kriskus. . . . No, that's not right, but it's near. . . . Sirsis . . . No. . . . This is very strange that I can't say this word. . . . How about kirsis? . . . No. . . . I'll have to by that. Kriskus? For some reason I can't say it right now. But I'm close. Kirsis? No . . ."

Transcortical Aphasia Transcortical aphasia (sometimes called *isolation syndrome*) is caused by dominant-hemisphere brain damage that spares the central region (Wernicke's area, Broca's area, and the arcuate fasciculus) but disconnects (*isolates*) all or parts of the central region from the rest of the brain. Because association fibers are compromised in the transcortical aphasias, Lichtheim (1885) called what we now know as transcortical aphasia *commissural dysphasia* or *white matter dysphasia.*

The disconnection causing transcortical aphasias usually is created by damage in the border zone (watershed region) surrounding the perisylvian region. Damage in the watershed region most often comes from severe narrowing of the middle cerebral artery, which produces hypoperfusion in the watershed region. Less frequently, watershed damage is caused by embolic strokes.

Preserved repetition is a defining characteristic of the transcortical aphasias. Because Wernicke's area, Broca's area, and the arcuate fasciculus are spared, repetition of spoken words, phrases, and sentences is preserved, although other language functions may be substantially compromised. Three kinds of transcortical aphasia have been described in the literature—*transcortical motor aphasia, transcortical sensory aphasia,* and *mixed transcortical aphasia.*

Transcortical Motor Aphasia The classic neurologic cause of transcortical motor aphasia is damage in the anterior superior frontal lobe of the language-dominant hemisphere. The defining characteristics of transcortical motor aphasia are *markedly reduced speech output, good repetition,* and *good auditory comprehension.* The reduced speech output of transcortical motor aphasic patients seems to be a consequence of their anterior frontal lobe involvement. The anterior frontal lobes are important for initiation and maintenance of purposeful activity. It follows, then, that patients with damage in the anterior frontal lobe of the language-dominant hemisphere are likely to have problems initiating and maintaining speech. Luria (1966) called what we know as transcortical motor aphasia *dynamic aphasia* and its behavioral manifesta-

tion *pathologic inertia.* Right hemiparesis (or less frequently, right hemiplegia) may accompany transcortical motor aphasia caused by large anterior frontal lobe lesions extending into the posterior frontal lobe. Wernicke's area is not affected in transcortical motor aphasia, so patients with transcortical motor aphasia comprehend language relatively well. The arcuate fasciculus is spared in transcortical motor aphasia, so patients with transcortical motor aphasia are good at repeating what they hear and good at oral reading.

Although they are attentive, task-oriented, and cooperative, patients with transcortical motor aphasia are poor conversationalists, content to sit silently while the conversational partner carries the communicative burden. When, after considerable urging, patients with transcortical motor aphasia eventually speak, they usually produce a perfunctory word or two and lapse into silence. However, if the interaction is highly structured and only a few highly predictable words are called for, these patients may respond fluently and without delay. The surprising thing about transcortical aphasic patients is how well they talk when asked to repeat phrases or sentences once they get started. Once started, these patients can repeat long and complex phrases and sentences fluently and without error.

> A patient with transcortical motor aphasia was asked, "What did you do for a living?" After a long delay he responded, "bakery," and lapsed into silence. Repeated requests by the examiner to "tell me more" elicited only the word *bakery.* When the examiner subsequently tested the patient's repetition, the patient repeated fluently and without delay, "Before I had my stroke I worked as a baker in a large wholesale bakery in Minneapolis, Minnesota."

Transcortical Sensory Aphasia Like transcortical motor aphasia, transcortical sensory aphasia (sometimes called *posterior isolation* *syndrome*) is caused by brain damage that spares Wernicke's area, the arcuate fasciculus, and Broca's area. The brain damage responsible for transcortical sensory aphasia is in the watershed region of the middle cerebral artery in the high parietal lobe of the language-dominant hemisphere. Like patients with transcortical motor aphasia, those with transcortical sensory aphasia do well when asked to repeat phrases or sentences after the examiner. Unlike patients with transcortical motor aphasia, those with transcortical sensory aphasia speak without having to be cajoled by their conversational partner. In fact, some patients with transcortical sensory aphasia seem compelled to repeat what is said to them, even when instructed not to do so (*echolalia*). In a test situation they often repeat what the examiner asks them to do before responding to the examiner's request, and in conversations they may incorporate what is said to them into their responses (Goodglass, 1993).

> In a test of sentence comprehension the clinician asked a patient with transcortical sensory aphasia, "Does the sun rise in the west?" The patient responded, "Does the sun rise in the west?—The sun rises in the west—in the west—the sun rises—Yes—I should think the sun does rise in the west—yes the sun rises in the west."

Because the brain damage that produces transcortical sensory aphasia isolates Wernicke's area from much of the parietal lobe and from the visual cortex, patients with transcortical sensory aphasia always have major impairments in listening comprehension and reading comprehension. In some ways patients with transcortical sensory aphasia resemble patients with Wernicke's aphasia—they speak fluently and their speech is empty and littered with verbal paraphasias. Most are unaware of their errors and do not attempt to self-correct. However, they usually do not exhibit *press of speech,* as many Wernicke's aphasic patients do, and their excellent repetition clearly differentiates them

from patients with Wernicke's aphasia. A striking characteristic of patients with transcortical sensory aphasia is their ability to repeat or read aloud long and complex sentences they are unable to comprehend. They may be at a loss when asked to perform even simple manipulations in response to spoken instructions but flawlessly repeat long and complex instructions.

> A patient with transcortical sensory aphasia was befuddled by simple commands such as "Pick up the pencil," but without hesitation repeated after the examiner, "Put the comb beside the matches, point to the quarter, and give me the spoon."

Because the brain damage that produces transcortical sensory aphasia involves the parieto-occipital-temporal junction and isolates Wernicke's area from the visual cortex, transcortical sensory aphasic patients invariably have severely impaired reading comprehension (although oral reading is preserved).

Mixed Transcortical Aphasia This rare syndrome sometimes is called *isolation of the speech area* (Geschwind, Quadfasel, & Segarra, 1968). Patients with mixed transcortical aphasia retain their ability to repeat what is said to them in the presence of profound impairment of all other communicative abilities. The prototypical patient with isolation of the speech area "is nonfluent (in fact does not speak at all unless spoken to), does not comprehend spoken language, cannot name, cannot read or write but can repeat what is said by the examiner" (Benson, 1979b, p. 46). These patients often have a striking tendency to repeat, in parrot-like fashion, what is said to them, and if the examiner says the first few words of familiar songs or rhymes, these patients often complete the phrase and may go on to provide one or more following lines.

Mixed transcortical aphasia is caused by damage that spares Broca's area, Wernicke's area, and the arcuate fasciculus but isolates those regions from the rest of the brain. Its most frequent cause is stenosis of the internal carotid artery, which compromises blood flow throughout the watershed area of the language-dominant hemisphere. Mixed transcortical aphasia also has been reported following cerebral hypoxia, severe cerebral swelling, and multiple embolic strokes affecting the peripheral branches of the left middle cerebral artery.

Clinician: "Hello, Mrs. Fenton."
Patient: "Mrs. Fenton. Yes."
Clinician: "How are you doing today?"
Patient: "How are you doing today?"
Clinician: "I'm very fine, thank you. How are you doing?"
Patient: "I'm very fine, thank you."
Clinician: "My name is Mary. I'll be working with you today."
Patient: "My name is Mary. I'm working today."

Anomic Aphasia: An Aphasia Syndrome Without a Clear Localization Whether *anomic aphasia* exists as a separate syndrome is not clear (Albert, Goodglass, Helm, & associates, 1981). Goodglass (1993) comments, "Of all the aphasia subtypes, anomic aphasia is the one that appears as a result of diverse causes and as a result of lesion sites that are remote from each other" (p. 214).

Clinician: "Do you have children?"
Patient: "I have a son and two daughters."
Clinician: "Tell me about them."
Patient: "My son ... Paul, he works in a ... he works at ... in the news ... but not TV. At the ... I don't know ... I know, but ... at the *Register* ... the *Register*. It's a paper ... a news ... newspaper. Paul is a ... he goes out and he talks to people. He does ... he does.... I guess you'd say he does interviews. People, you know. On the street and wherever ..."

The label *anomic aphasia* usually is applied to patients whose only obvious symptom is impaired word-retrieval in speech and writing. Anomic aphasic patients' spontaneous speech is fluent and grammatically correct but marred by frequent word-retrieval failures. These patients' word-retrieval failures generate unusual pauses, circumlocution (talking around missing words), and substitution of nonspecific words such as *thing* for missing words. Careful testing usually reveals that patients with anomic aphasia have subtle comprehension impairments and may have other mild language impairments.

Goodglass (1993) described four varieties of anomic aphasia, in which anomia appears in relative isolation. According to Goodglass, patients with *frontal anomia* represent mild versions of transcortical motor aphasia. The major characteristic of patients with frontal anomia is the remarkable degree to which their word retrieval improves if the examiner provides the first sound of the target word. Patients with *anomia of the angular gyrus region* speak fluently but with frequent word-retrieval failures. The phenomenon that sets this syndrome apart from the other anomic syndromes are intermittent occasions on which the patient who fails to retrieve a word fails to recognize it when it is supplied by the examiner. Patients with anomia of the angular gyrus often exhibit alienation of word meaning—repeating a word over and over without recognition. According to Goodglass (1993), anomia of the angular gyrus may be a mild form of transcortical sensory aphasia.

Clinician: "Tell me what the word *apple* means."
Patient: "Apple ... apple ... apple. Is that the word?"
Clinician: "Yes, apple."
Patient: "You mean apple? A-P-P-L-E?" (spells aloud)
Clinician: "Yes. Apple. A-P-P-L-E."
Patient: "I should know what it means, but I really don't ..."
Clinician: "Think about a fruit that you might put in a pie."
Patient: "Oh! Apple! It's round and red and it grows on trees and you put it in a pie!"

T A B L E 4 - 1

Characteristics of connectionist aphasia syndromes

Aphasia syndrome	Lesion location	Fluency	Speech	Word retrieval	Repetition	Comprehension
Broca's	Posterior inferior frontal lobe	Nonfluent, telegraphic	Phonetic dissolution*	Fair, but misarticulated	Labored, misarticulated, telegraphic	Fair to good
Wernicke's	Posterior superior temporal lobe	Fluent, empty	Verbal (semantic) paraphasia	Poor, with verbal paraphasias	Fluent, verbal paraphasias, grossly restricted retention span	Poor
Conduction	Parietal lobe	Fluent, sensical	Literal (phonemic) paraphasia	Fair, with literal paraphasias	Fluent, literal paraphasias, some restriction of retention span	Fair to good
Anomic	Temporal, parietal lobe	Fluent, sensical	Verbal (semantic) paraphasia	Fair, with verbal paraphasias	Good	Fair to good
Transcortical motor (anterior isolation syndrome)	Anterior superior frontal lobe	Fluent, sparse†	Variable	Variable, with delays in initiation	Good, but delays in initiation	Good
Transcortical sensory (posterior isolation syndrome)	Posterior superior parietal lobe	Fluent, empty	Variable	Poor	Good	Poor
Global	Large, perisylvian	Nonfluent	Literal, verbal paraphasia; verbal stereotypes	Poor	Poor; literal, verbal paraphasias; grossly restricted retention span	Poor

*Phonetic dissolution is *distortion* of consonants (and sometimes vowels) as a result of disrupted articulatory programming (apraxia of speech). In contrast, literal paraphasia involves *substitution* of a correctly articulated, but inappropriate, sound for another.
†But with unusual delays in initiation. Utterances tend to be one or two words long.

Patients with *anomia of the inferior temporal gyrus* have severe word-retrieval problems but speak fluently and grammatically and have near normal reading, writing, and presumably (although Goodglass does not mention it) near normal auditory comprehension. Patients with *anomia as an expression of residual aphasia* probably represent the most common anomic aphasia syndrome. These are patients who have passed through a more severe form of any of the other aphasia syndromes and have recovered nearly normal language function but continue to exhibit mild to moderate word-retrieval impairments. Goodglass, Kaplan, and Barresi (2001) recommend the label *residual aphasia* rather than *anomia* for these patients.

It is not clear if Goodglass's anomic aphasia syndromes are unique syndromes or if they simply represent milder versions of other aphasia syndromes, which seems likely. Anomia certainly is not a localizing phenomenon. As Goodglass notes, it can occur with damage in many different regions of the brain and in combination with a variety of other aphasic symptoms.

Table 4-1 summarizes the important characteristics of the connectionist aphasia syndromes. Figure 4-5 shows the proportions of patients exhibiting various aphasia syndromes in a group of 444 patients seen in the Aphasia Research Center at the Boston Veterans Administration Medical Center during a 10-year period (Benson, 1979a).

GENERAL CONCEPTS 4-1

- Localizationist models of aphasia began in the early 1800s. The observations of Paul Broca and Karl Wernicke laid the foundation for contemporary connectionist models of aphasia and related disorders.
- For most adults the left brain hemisphere has major responsibility for speech and language. This relationship is stronger for right-handers than for left-handers. Nearly 100% of right-handed adults are left-hemisphere dominant for speech and language, compared with about 85% of left-handed adults.

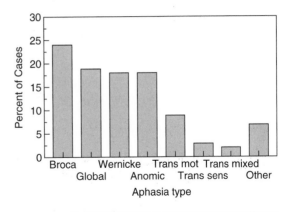

Figure 4-5 ■ **Percentages of patients exhibiting various aphasia syndromes in a group of 444 aphasic adults seen in the Aphasia Research Center, Boston Veterans Administration Medical Center.** (From Benson, D. F. [1979]. *Aphasia, alexia, and agraphia.* New York: Churchill-Livingstone.)

- The *perisylvian zone* in the central region of the language-dominant hemisphere serves many important speech and language functions.
- *Broca's area,* in the posterior inferior frontal lobe of the language-dominant hemisphere, plays an important part in organizing movement sequences for the speech muscles.
- *Wernicke's area,* in the mid temporal lobe of the language-dominant hemisphere, plays an important part in language comprehension and in rule-governed aspects of language.
- The *arcuate fasciculus,* a band of nerve fibers connecting Wernicke's area with Broca's area, is thought to provide a pathway by which Wernicke's area communicates with Broca's area.
- *Paraphasias* are errors in spoken (or written) word production. *Verbal* (semantic) *paraphasias* are substitutions of one word for another (e.g., "table" for "chair"). *Literal* (phonemic) *paraphasias* are substitutions or transpositions of sounds within a word (e.g., *naftersoon* for *afternoon*).
- *Broca's aphasia* is caused by damage in the posterior inferior frontal lobe of the language-

dominant hemisphere. Patients with Broca's aphasia speak slowly and with great effort, often leaving out function words (a combination called *agrammatism* or *telegraphic speech*). Patients with Broca's aphasia usually comprehend language better than they speak or write it.

- *Wernicke's aphasia* is caused by damage in the central or posterior regions of the temporal lobe in the language-dominant hemisphere. Patients with Wernicke's aphasia typically have problems comprehending spoken and written language. They speak effortlessly and with essentially normal rate. However, their speech may contain paraphasias and word-retrieval failures.

- *Global aphasia* is caused by massive damage in the perisylvian region of the language-dominant hemisphere. Patients with global aphasia have profound impairment of all speech, language, and comprehension, although some may get a rudimentary sense of simple conversations.

- *Conduction aphasia* is caused by damage in the parietal lobe of the language-dominant hemisphere, affecting transmission of information from Wernicke's area to Broca's area via the arcuate fasciculus. Patients with conduction aphasia typically have fairly good language comprehension but grossly impaired repetition. They speak fluently but with literal paraphasias.

- *Preserved repetition* is a defining characteristic of *transcortical aphasias* (sometimes called *isolation syndromes*).

- *Transcortical motor aphasia* is caused by damage in the watershed region of the anterior frontal lobe in the language-dominant hemisphere. Patients with transcortical motor aphasia have markedly reduced speech output, good repetition, and good listening comprehension.

- *Transcortical sensory aphasia* is caused by damage in the parietal watershed region of the language-dominant hemisphere. Patients with transcortical sensory aphasia speak effortlessly, but many are echolalic. They have

few problems repeating what is said to them but have significantly impaired language comprehension.

- It is not clear whether *anomic aphasia* represents a distinct aphasia syndrome or is simply a milder version of other aphasia syndromes. The primary characteristic of anomic aphasia is impaired word retrieval in speech and writing, with relative preservation of other speech and language functions.

RELATED DISORDERS

Nonlinguistic disorders sometimes occur in combination with the linguistic disorders characterizing the aphasia syndromes. *Disconnection syndromes* appear when the language-competent brain hemisphere is isolated from its nonlinguistic counterpart. *Visual field blindness* may accompany aphasia caused by temporal lobe or parietal lobe damage. *Apraxia* often occurs in combination with aphasia caused by frontal lobe damage. A variety of perceptual impairments, called *agnosias,* may follow cortical damage in association areas.

Disconnection Syndromes

Disconnection syndromes are created when nerve fiber tracts crossing between the hemispheres in the corpus callosum are damaged or destroyed. Most *complete disconnection syndromes* are created by neurosurgeons who cut the connections between the hemispheres (a procedure called *commissurotomy*) to keep epileptic seizures originating in one hemisphere from spreading across the corpus callosum to the other hemisphere. Most *partial disconnection syndromes* are caused by strokes or tumors. The most common causes of partial disconnection syndromes are occlusions of the anterior or posterior cerebral arteries, which provide most of the blood supply to the corpus callosum. Occlusion of the anterior cerebral artery produces *anterior disconnection syndrome* and occlusion of the posterior cerebral artery produces *posterior disconnection syndrome.*

Right-handed patients with *anterior disconnection syndrome* exhibit an unusual collection of symptoms caused by isolation of somatosensory and motor cortex in the right hemisphere from the language-competent left hemisphere. Patients with anterior disconnection syndrome cannot carry out verbal commands requiring responses by their left hand (a condition called *unilateral limb apraxia*) because the right hemisphere (which controls the left hand) cannot comprehend the command and the meaning of the command cannot be sent over from the left hemisphere. Patients with anterior disconnection syndrome cannot talk about or name objects held out of sight in the left hand because sensory information from the left hand cannot reach the language-competent left hemisphere. These patients easily name objects held out of sight in the right hand. Some patients with anterior disconnection syndrome who cannot name, describe, or talk about objects palpated with the left hand may provide a few bits of rudimentary description (e.g., "It's small." "It's long and thin.").

If a patient with anterior disconnection syndrome is blindfolded, given objects to palpate in one hand, and then is allowed to choose the palpated object from a group, they choose correctly when the palpated object and the choice objects are palpated with the same hand but not when the test object is palpated with one hand and the choice objects are palpated with the other. This differential performance happens because the brain cannot send the sensory information from the hand that palpated the object across the corpus callosum to tell the other hand what to search for. Patients with anterior disconnection syndrome also can draw, demonstrate the function of, or choose an unseen palpated object from a group, provided they use the hand with which they palpated the object.

Right-handers with anterior disconnection syndrome can name objects held out of sight in the right hand. (The tactile information goes to the language-competent left hemisphere.) If they are allowed to name the object they hold, they then can choose the correct match with either hand because both hemispheres have

heard the spoken name. Likewise if they can sneak a peek at the test object from under the blindfold, they can choose the correct object with either hand because the visual information gets to both hemispheres. If a brain injury causing anterior disconnection syndrome extends laterally into the left frontal lobe, a patient may exhibit signs of transcortical motor aphasia.

The most common impairments of patients with *posterior disconnection syndrome* are visual impairments attributable to isolation of the visual cortex from the language-competent left hemisphere, caused by destruction of visual fibers crossing in the posterior corpus callosum. These patients' visual impairments are measurable only by special testing in which printed words or pictures are flashed into the eyes in such a way that the image goes only to the right hemisphere. A patient with posterior disconnection syndrome can report seeing words or pictures flashed into the right hemisphere but cannot name them, talk about them, or write about them. If the patient is allowed to choose a picture that has been flashed into the right hemisphere from among several pictures, the patient can choose the correct picture with the left hand but not the right. If printed commands calling for arm or hand movements are flashed into the right hemisphere, the patient cannot carry out the commands. If the commands are flashed into the left hemisphere, the patient responds correctly with the right hand but not the left.

Patients with *complete disconnection syndrome* (sometimes called *split-brain syndrome*) exhibit a symptom complex that is a combination of anterior and posterior disconnection syndromes. Patients with complete disconnection syndrome, like patients with anterior disconnection syndrome, are unable to name objects held out of sight in the left hand because the sensory input from the hand goes into the mute right hemisphere, which cannot transfer the information to the verbal left hemisphere. They also exhibit visual impairments like those of patients with posterior disconnection syndrome, in which the patient cannot verbalize about visual stimuli restricted to the right hemisphere.

Commissurotomized patients do not ordinarily encounter situations outside the clinic or laboratory that restrict stimulus input to one hemisphere. Consequently, they usually get along normally in daily life.

> Commissurotomies are performed in only a few centers and are reserved for patients with intractable seizures that have resisted less dramatic intervention. Because their disconnected brain hemispheres provide neuropsychologists and neurophysiologists with such fascinating insights into hemispheric functions, commissurotimized individuals are in such great demand as study participants that some have retained agents to negotiate fees with interested investigators.

Patients with posterior disconnection syndrome sometimes have an unusual reading impairment called *alexia without agraphia* (also known as *occipital alexia* or *pure word blindness*). Patients who have alexia without agraphia have ". . . a serious inability to read contrasted with an almost uncanny preservation of writing ability" (Benson, 1979a, p. 110). These patients may write personal letters or, in a test, write long and grammatically accurate narrative paragraphs, but they cannot subsequently read aloud what they have written. Some may retain the ability to read and comprehend highly familiar words, such as their name and the city and state where they live. Patients who exhibit alexia without agraphia have great difficulty copying written material but can spell aloud and instantly recognize words spelled aloud by the examiner. Some patients who have alexia without agraphia can "read" slowly and laboriously by reading individual letter names aloud and identifying words by this oral spelling, which gets to the brain through the ears rather than through the eyes.

Alexia without agraphia is caused by a complex lesion (or combination of lesions) that destroys the left visual cortex and cuts the tracts in the posterior corpus callosum that connect the right visual cortex with the left hemisphere (Figure 4-6). The left hemisphere cannot see the material, and visual information from the language-incompetent right hemisphere (which can see the material) cannot reach the language-competent left hemisphere. The patient can write because the connections between Wernicke's area (which formulates verbal messages) and the anterior motor planning and control regions (which do the writing) are intact. Patients with posterior disconnection syndrome do not exhibit the tactile disconnection symptoms seen in anterior disconnection syndrome. They can name, describe, and talk or write about unseen objects pal-

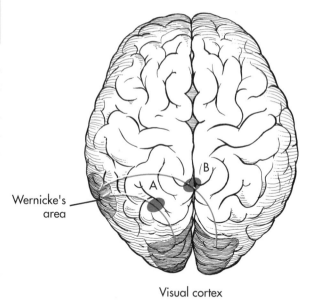

Wernicke's area

Visual cortex

Figure 4-6 ■ How brain damage produces alexia without agraphia. The visual cortex in the left and right hemispheres is isolated from Wernicke's area by one lesion that destroys the left visual cortex or disconnects the left visual cortex from Wernicke's area *(A)* and another lesion that interrupts the visual fibers crossing through the posterior corpus callosum from the right visual cortex *(B).*

pated with either hand. Because the left visual cortex is no longer functioning, patients with alexia without agraphia invariably exhibit right homonymous hemianopia. Strokes affecting the posterior cerebral artery are the most common cause of alexia without agraphia. Tumors and arteriovenous malformations are less common causes.

Another syndrome, *alexia with agraphia* (sometimes called *parieto-temporal alexia*), is caused by lesions in the region of the angular gyrus, at the posterior end of the Sylvian fissure. These lesions disconnect the visual cortex from Wernicke's area and disconnect Wernicke's area from anterior motor planning and execution areas. Consequently, visual information from printed materials cannot be communicated either to Wernicke's area or from Wernicke's area to the anterior motor planning and execution areas, leaving the patient unable either to read or to write. Oral reading is grossly impaired, and these patients cannot identify words spelled aloud by the examiner. Copying printed materials is much better than writing to dictation, but most patients with alexia and agraphia are unable to translate printed material to cursive or vice versa. Alexia with agraphia is a common component of many aphasic syndromes, and its isolated occurrence is extremely rare.

Visual Field Blindness

Patients with posterior temporal lobe damage or low parietal lobe damage often exhibit contralateral visual field blindness. (See Chapter 2 for more on how lesions in the visual system cause perceptual problems.) Because the visual fibers pass through the inferior parietal lobes and the superior temporal lobes on their way to the visual cortex, many patients with Wernicke's aphasia or conduction aphasia experience visual field blindness. Patients with anterior aphasias (Broca's aphasia, transcortical motor aphasia) rarely have visual field blindness, and such blindness is unusual for patients with transcortical sensory aphasia because lesions in the watershed regions of the brain usually do not affect vi-

sual fibers. When visual field blindness does occur in combination with transcortical sensory aphasia, it usually is an inferior quadrantanopsia (blindness in the lower quadrant of the visual field). Patients with global aphasia often experience visual field blindness because of temporal lobe and parietal lobe damage.

APRAXIA
Characteristics of Apraxia

Apraxia (from a Greek word meaning *unable to do*) is a label for several different syndromes characterized by difficulty carrying out volitional movement sequences in the absence of sensory loss or paralysis sufficient to explain the difficulty. Apraxia often accompanies aphasia, especially aphasia caused by damage in the frontal lobe or anterior parietal lobe.

Liepmann (1900) described two kinds of apraxia, which he called *ideational apraxia* and *ideomotor apraxia* (ideomotor apraxia is sometimes called *ideokinetic apraxia*). Liepmann characterized *ideational apraxia* as a disruption of the *ideas* needed to *understand* the use of objects. Individuals with ideational apraxia are unable to carry out movement sequences that lead to a given result. Liepmann attributed ideational apraxia to damage in the left parietal lobe, but many contemporary writers consider ideational apraxia a sign of diffuse or bilateral brain damage. Ideational apraxia always affects both sides of the body, and because ideational apraxia is a conceptual impairment, patients with ideational apraxia are unable to perform movement sequences on command even if they are given real objects to use in the movements.

> . . . a defect of purposeful movements, where the ideational project or plan appeared to be disordered, although engrams for individual movements were considered to be intact. Instead of accomplishing the desired object, a false one is realized. The patient puts the match into his mouth in trying to light a cigarette, tries to drink from a cup by leaning over or under it, etc. Here, the whole series of actions is impaired due to the conceptual disturbance. (Kertesz, 1979, p. 234)

In contemporary times the meaning of apraxia has drifted away from the concept of ideational apraxia. Most contemporary writers and practitioners consider apraxia a motor-planning impairment and would reject Liepmann's *ideational apraxia* as not a true apraxia. Readers who see the unadorned word *apraxia* in contemporary works safely can assume that the authors are referring to ideomotor apraxia and not to ideational apraxia.

Ideomotor apraxia represents disruption of the *plans* needed to *demonstrate* actions. Ideomotor apraxia usually is caused by frontal lobe damage in the language-dominant hemisphere, and the resulting apraxia may be either unilateral or bilateral, although it usually is bilateral. Patients with ideomotor apraxia can carry out movement sequences if they are given real objects to use in the movements. The patient with ideomotor apraxia may be unable to show the examiner how one would use a hammer when asked to pretend using it but performs the movements fluently and effortlessly when given a hammer, some nails, and a board. Patients with ideomotor apraxia also are better at carrying out movements when the movements are a spontaneous response to natural environmental conditions (e.g., waving goodbye as someone drives away in an automobile) than when the movements are elicited by command (e.g., waving goodbye in response to an examiner's request during a test situation).

Several varieties of ideomotor apraxia have been identified, including *buccofacial apraxia, limb apraxia,* and *apraxia of speech.* (A fourth, so-called *dressing apraxia* sometimes seen in patients with right hemisphere pathologic conditions, is not a true apraxia.)

Apraxia is one of the most consistently misused terms in medical literature. Most of the types of apraxia currently described by medical and paramedical workers (e.g., verbal, constructional, dressing) represent fixed motor or visual-spatial disturbances and should not be defined by the term apraxia any more than a hemiplegia should. Despite the widespread misuse of apraxia to de-

note many types of motor performance failure, the presence of motor [ideomotor] apraxia in individuals with aphasia is almost routinely overlooked. (Benson, 1979a, p. 172)

Patients with so-called *dressing apraxia* have difficulty getting into articles of clothing. They may put articles of clothing on backward or inside out and may attempt to put their arms through trousers legs or their legs through shirt or blouse sleeves. Dressing apraxia apparently represents a combination of disrupted body image and disturbed appreciation of the body's relationship to surrounding space and is not a problem with planning and executing movement sequences. Patients with so-called *constructional apraxia* have difficulty drawing complex figures. Constructional apraxia apparently represents disordered visual-spatial perception.

In *buccofacial apraxia* (sometimes called *oral nonverbal apraxia*) the patient is unable to demonstrate on command volitional sequences of movements such as whistling, blowing dust off a shelf, sucking up through a straw, and sniffing a flower. Buccofacial apraxia may be the most common form of ideomotor apraxia. DeRenzi, Pieczuro, and Vignolo (1968) reported the presence of buccofacial apraxia in 90% of patients with Broca's aphasia.

In *limb apraxia* the patient is unable to demonstrate on command volitional movements with the arm, wrist, and hand. Limb apraxia usually is bilateral, but the presence of hemiplegia usually masks the limb apraxia on one side. The presence of limb apraxia is revealed by asking the patient to demonstrate movement sequences such as flipping a coin, winding a watch, thumbing a ride, using a hammer, and waving goodbye.

Limb apraxia is more severe *distally* (away from the torso) than *proximally* (near the torso). Consequently, when patients with limb apraxia are asked to perform a movement sequence requiring shoulder, elbow, wrist, and finger movements, they perform shoulder and elbow movements better than wrist and finger movements. This means that tests requiring movements of the wrist and fingers (e.g., coin flipping, watch winding) are more sensitive to the presence of limb apraxia than tests that require movements of the shoulder and elbow (e.g., saluting, drinking from a glass).

For many years, the presence of apraxia was taken as evidence for damage in the premotor cortex, regarded as the center for motor planning. In recent years this view of the cause of apraxia has been somewhat modified. Buckingham (1979) and Geschwind (1975), for example, have postulated two kinds of apraxia, which I will call *center apraxia* and *disconnection apraxia. Center apraxia* is caused by damage to a cortical center for praxis. *Disconnection apraxia* is caused by disconnection of regions of the left hemisphere that comprehend spoken commands from regions that plan and execute responses to the commands.

According to Buckingham, the key difference between these syndromes is in patients' responses to nonverbal requests for movements of apractic body parts. Patients with center apraxia are unable to execute movements in response to the examiner's requests whether the movements are requested verbally by asking the patient to perform them or nonverbally by showing a picture depicting the requested movement. This is because the center for planning the movements is damaged. Patients with disconnection apraxia are unable to perform movements in response to verbal requests but can do them if the requests are made nonverbally because making the request nonverbally bypasses the pathways involved in comprehension of the request. (Patients with disconnection apraxia are likely to exhibit conduction aphasia because of the location of the brain damage. In 1966 DeRenzi and associates reported the presence of apraxia in one third of patients with conduction aphasia.)

Both sides of the body routinely are tested for limb apraxias, unless one side is paralyzed. The nondominant limb is tested first because limb apraxia can be unilateral, and if it is, the nondominant limb is the unilaterally apraxic one. If a patient is unilaterally apraxic and the examiner tests the (unaffected) dominant limb first, the patient may be able to perform the movement sequence with the apractic nondominant limb by watching the performance of the dominant limb and imitating it with the nondominant limb.

The relationship between dominance and unilateral apraxia is interpretable by a connectionistic model. According to the model, the left hemisphere pathways from the primary auditory cortex to Wernicke's area and from Wernicke's area to the premotor cortex and motor cortex (via the arcuate fasciculus) are crucial for performing motor movements in response to spoken commands. (To keep things simple, the patient is assumed to be right-handed.)

According to the model, the spoken request for the movement is first perceived at the primary auditory cortex (Figure 4-7). The message then is sent to Wernicke's area, where its meaning is deduced. A neurally coded response to the message then is sent via the arcuate fasciculus to the premotor cortex, where the plan for the movement sequence originates. If the patient is to carry out the movement sequence with the right (dominant) hand and arm, the plan is sent from the premotor cortex in the left hemisphere to the primary motor cortex in the same hemisphere. If the patient is to carry out the movement sequence with the left (nondominant) hand and arm, the plan is sent from the left hemisphere premotor cortex across the corpus callosum to the motor cortex in the right hemisphere. (The left premotor area for the hand and arm plans movement sequences for the limbs on both sides of the body, just as Broca's area in the left premotor cortex plans all speech movements.)

Destruction of Wernicke's area prevents the patient from comprehending the meaning of spoken requests for limb movements. The patient fails to execute the movement with either limb but not because the patient is apraxic. Damage in the arcuate fasciculus prevents the sense of the

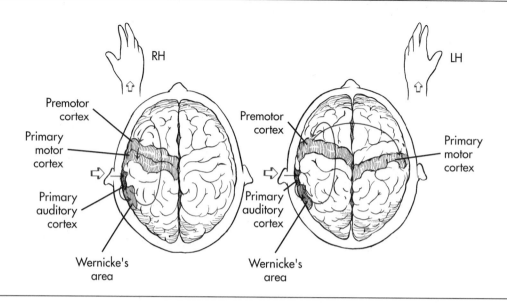

Figure 4-7 ■ **Connectionist explanation for limb apraxia. The spoken command requesting a limb movement is perceived by the primary auditory cortex, comprehended by Wernicke's area, and sent via the arcuate fasciculus to the premotor cortex for the hand, where a plan for the movement is formulated. The premotor cortex sends the plan to the motor cortex for execution. If the movement is to be carried out by the right hand, the plan is sent to the motor cortex in the left hemisphere. If the movement is to be carried out by the left hand, the plan is sent across the corpus callosum to the motor cortex in the right hemisphere.**

command from getting to the premotor cortex. The patient fails to execute the movement with either limb and exhibits disconnection apraxia. (These patients also cannot write with their left hand.) Destruction of the motor planning region in the premotor cortex causes center apraxia, and both right-side and left-side limbs are apraxic. If Wernicke's area, the arcuate fasciculus, and the left premotor cortex are intact but the crossing fibers that connect the premotor cortex in the left hemisphere with the motor cortex in the right hemisphere are interrupted, the patient exhibits unilateral apraxia of the left hand because the patient's left hand is isolated from the motor plans for the response. (Also, the patient may have other signs of anterior disconnection syndrome.)

Diagnosis of Ideomotor Apraxia

The examiner must be careful to exclude alternative explanations for an apparent apraxia be-

fore concluding that a patient is apraxic. *Paralysis, weakness,* or *incoordination* of muscles needed for volitional sequenced movements sometimes leads clinicians astray by making the movement sequences clumsy or distorted. Apraxic patients can perform familiar movement sequences fluently and effortlessly when the movements are a spontaneous response to natural occurrences in the environment or are part of automatic movement sequences, but patients with weak, paralyzed, or incoordinated muscles cannot.

Comprehension impairment sometimes may lead an unwary clinician toward a diagnosis of apraxia. The clinician who suspects comprehension impairment may estimate a patient's comprehension and test the patient's familiarity with movements requested in an apraxia test by demonstrating various movements and asking the patient a question such as, "Am I using a hammer?" If the patient responds appropriately, the clinician can assume that auditory comprehension and knowledge of the movements requested are good enough to eliminate them as explanations for the movement abnormalities observed. A patient's successful performance in screening tests of auditory comprehension also eliminates comprehension impairment as the culprit.

AGNOSIA

Agnosia is a generic label for a group of perceptual impairments in which patients fail to recognize stimuli in a sensory modality, although perception in the modality is unimpaired. Patients with *visual agnosia* do not recognize objects visually although they can see, which they can prove by matching identical objects or forms, and although they are familiar with the visually unrecognized objects, which they can prove by recognizing them when they feel them or hear the sounds they make. Visual agnosia characteristically is caused by damage (usually bilateral) in the occipital lobes, in the posterior parietal lobes, or in the fiber tracts connecting the visual cortex to other areas in the brain. Visual agnosias usually are incomplete, intermittent, and inconsistent, and patients with visual agnosias usually function reasonably well in daily life. Because they can see, they do not bump into things and grope their way about, and they usually recognize and respond appropriately to familiar visual cues in their daily life environment.

Patients with *auditory agnosia* do not appreciate the meaning of sounds, despite adequate hearing acuity. Patients with auditory agnosia respond to sound by turning toward its source, and they are startled by loud sounds. However, they cannot match an object with the sound it makes, although they recognize the object when it is shown to them or when they are permitted to feel it. Auditory agnosia, like visual agnosia, may be incomplete or intermittent. Auditory agnosia suggests damage (usually bilateral) in the auditory association areas. Patients with auditory agnosia may sporadically respond appropriately to sounds or may respond appropriately to certain sounds or categories of sounds.

Patients who have brain damage that isolates Wernicke's area from the auditory cortex in both hemispheres sometimes exhibit *auditory-verbal agnosia* (sometimes called *pure word deafness*). Pure word deafness is a rare phenomenon in which comprehension of speech is severely compromised but other language skills (reading, writing, speaking) are retained. Patients who have pure word deafness fail to appreciate the meaning of spoken words but respond appropriately to nonverbal sounds such as ringing telephones or sirens. They are aware of spoken words but do not understand their meaning, although they comprehend them in printed or written form. Patients with auditory-verbal agnosia often respond to speech as if their native language is unknown to them, but their speech usually is appropriate both in content and form.

Patients with *tactile agnosia* cannot recognize objects by touch and palpation, although their tactile perception is intact. They immediately recognize the objects if the objects are presented in other sensory modalities. Tactile agnosia usually is caused by parietal lobe damage that isolates the somatosensory cortex from other parts of the brain. Patients with tactile agnosia can report touch, pinprick, and other simple stimulation of the cutaneous receptors in the hands, but they cannot name, describe, talk about, or demonstrate the use of objects palpated with the hands. Patients with tactile agnosia can draw or demonstrate the shape and size of palpated objects, and they can choose matching objects from a group of objects when vision is blocked. The term *astereognosis* is a synonym for tactile agnosia, but sometimes it is (erroneously) used in a broader sense to denote loss of tactile recognition in the presence of sensory impairment.

Prevalence of Agnosia

True modality-specific agnosia is rare, despite its frequent mention in the literature. Some cases of agnosia reported in the literature may not be true agnosias but perceptual impairments or sensory discrimination impairments, comprehension impairments, cognitive impairments, or psychogenic symptoms. Therefore, in arriving at a diagnosis of agnosia, the clinician must exclude several alternative explanations:

- Sensory deficits that interfere with perception in the affected modality. A diagnosis of agnosia requires that sensory function in the affected modality be adequate for perception.
- Comprehension disorders that prevent the patient from understanding what is required in the test for agnosia.
- Expressive disturbances that prevent the patient from verbally identifying test stimuli.
- Unfamiliarity with test stimuli that prevents the patient from relating the stimuli to knowledge and previous experience. If the patient recognizes the stimuli in another modality, one can conclude that unfamiliarity does not explain the agnosia.

GENERAL CONCEPTS 4-2

- *Disconnection syndromes* are caused by damage in the corpus callosum. The damage prevents communication between the brain hemispheres.
- Right-handed patients with *anterior disconnection syndrome* cannot name, describe, write about, or talk about objects palpated out of sight with the left hand because sensory information from the left hand cannot reach the language-competent left hemisphere.
- Right-handed patients with *posterior disconnection syndrome* cannot verbally respond to visual information that is presented only to the right hemisphere. Some patients with posterior disconnection syndrome have *alexia without agraphia,* in which reading is grossly impaired but spontaneous writing and copying are preserved.
- Patients with *complete disconnection syndrome* (split-brain syndrome) exhibit impairments that combine the impairments caused by anterior and posterior disconnection syndromes.
- Patients with posterior temporal lobe or low parietal lobe damage often experience contralateral visual field blindness.

- *Apraxia* denotes difficulty in carrying out sequences of volitional movements in the absence of weakness, paralysis, sensory loss, or incoordination in the muscles used for the movements.
- *Ideational apraxia* denotes the loss of the ideas needed to understand and demonstrate the use of objects. Ideational apraxia is not considered a true apraxia by many contemporary writers.
- *Ideomotor apraxia* denotes disruption of the motor plans needed to demonstrate actions. Ideomotor apraxia is much more common than ideational apraxia.
- *Buccofacial apraxia, limb apraxia,* and *apraxia of speech* are forms of ideomotor apraxia.
- Diagnosis of ideomotor apraxia requires that alternative explanations for the movement disorder be eliminated. Alternative explanations include weakness or paralysis, sensory loss, incoordination, and comprehension impairment.
- *Agnosia* denotes a condition in which patients fail to recognize otherwise familiar stimuli in a sensory modality although basic perception in that modality is preserved. Visual agnosia, auditory agnosia, and tactile agnosia (astereognosis) are the three basic agnosia syndromes described in the literature.

LIMITATIONS OF CONNECTIONIST EXPLANATIONS OF APHASIA AND RELATED DISORDERS

With the advent of brain imaging technology—such as computerized tomography (CT), magnetic resonance imaging (MRI), and positron emission tomography (PET)—cerebral damage came to be localized with greater accuracy and in greater detail than ever before (except, of course, for postmortem examination of patients' brains). The use of brain imaging technology has created new insights into the relationships between brain damage and aphasia syndromes. Numerous reports on the relationships between aphasia and lesions located and measured with brain imaging technology have appeared in the literature during the last two decades (Cappa, Cavallotti, Guidotti, & associates, 1983; Cappa, Cavallotti, & Vignolo, 1981; Knopman, Selnes, Niccum, & associates, 1983; Knopman, Selnes, Niccum, & associates, 1984; Naeser, Hayward, Laughlin, & associates, 1981; and others). These reports have led to several modifications to the classic concepts of the relationships between brain damage and aphasia syndromes. Two of the most important are as follows:

- Damage confined to Broca's area or Wernicke's area usually does not produce chronic Broca's or Wernicke's aphasia.
- Aphasia can be caused by damage deep in the brain, below the perisylvian cortex and its association fibers.

Several reports have suggested that lesions confined to Broca's or Wernicke's area do not produce persisting Broca's or Wernicke's aphasia. Mohr and associates (1978) studied 22 cases of aphasia in which the site and extent of brain damage was documented, and reviewed 83 published reports in which the brains of aphasic patients came to autopsy. They concluded that lesions confined to Broca's area do not produce chronic Broca's aphasia; instead they produce transitory mutism progressing to rapidly resolving articulatory targeting and sequencing impairments (apraxia of speech), with no significant persisting impairments in language. According to Mohr and associates, lesions must extend beyond Broca's area to produce persisting Broca's aphasia. Knopman and associates (1983) reported findings consistent with those of Mohr and associates. They reported that patients with lesions confined to Broca's area exhibit transient nonfluent speech without persisting Broca's aphasia. According to Knopman and associates (1983), persisting Broca's aphasia requires a lesion extending from Broca's area into the primary motor cortex or parietal lobe.

Similar doubts have been raised concerning the relationship between damage confined to Wernicke's area and chronic Wernicke's aphasia. Selnes and associates (1983) measured recovery of language by 39 aphasic adults with single left hemisphere lesions. They tested the patients' language comprehension once a month for 5 months. Patients with damage confined to Wernicke's area recovered near-normal language comprehension. Patients with persisting severe language comprehension deficits characteristically had damage extending beyond Wernicke's area into the inferior parietal lobe.

Selnes and associates (1985) later reported that the most striking persisting consequence of damage confined to Wernicke's area is impaired repetition. They studied 10 patients who were judged to have Wernicke's aphasia at 1 month post-onset. Eight of the 10 subsequently were judged to have conduction aphasia at 6 months post-onset. They had poor speech repetition and relatively good (although not normal) comprehension.

Classical connectionist models attribute aphasia to damage in key regions of the cerebral cortex or in fibers connecting one key region with another and disregard the possibility of aphasia resulting from deep subcortical damage. However, it is now apparent that right-handed patients with damage in the left basal ganglia or left thalamus can develop aphasia (Alexander & Lo Verme, 1980; Cappa & Vignolo, 1979; Mohr, Walters, & Duncan, 1975; Naeser, Alexander, Helm-Estabrooks, & associates, 1982; Ojemann, 1975; and others).

Naeser and associates (1982) studied nine cases of aphasia caused by damage in and around the left basal ganglia and reported three subcortical aphasia syndromes based on the front-to-back location of damage. Patients with an *anterior syndrome* (caused by damage in the internal capsule, the lenticular nucleus, and extending into anterior white matter) exhibited hemiplegia; slow, dysarthric speech with good phrase length and prosody; good comprehension; good repetition; poor oral reading and writing; and poor confrontation naming.

Patients with a *posterior syndrome* (caused by damage in the putamen and internal capsule, extending into posterior white matter) exhibited hemiplegia, fluent speech without dysarthria, poor comprehension, good single-word repetition, poor sentence repetition, impaired reading and writing, and poor confrontation naming. Naeser and associates' posterior syndrome resembles Wernicke's aphasia except for the presence of hemiplegia in the subcortical syndrome.

An *anterior-posterior syndrome* (caused by capsular-putamenal damage with both anterior and posterior extension) is characterized by a mixture of symptoms consistent with both Broca's and Wernicke's aphasias, "although they did not completely resemble cases of Broca's, Wernicke's, global, or thalamic aphasia in CT scan lesion sites, or language behavior" (Naeser, Alexander, Helm-Estabrooks, & associates, 1982, p. 2).

Cappa and associates (1983) also described an anterior aphasia syndrome and a posterior aphasia syndrome caused by damage in the internal capsule and adjoining basal ganglia. Their patients had smaller lesions than those of Naeser and associates, and their patients' aphasias were milder but resembled those of the patients studied by Naeser and associates. The current evidence suggests that patients with aphasia caused by damage in the basal ganglia exhibit a variety of disruptions in speech and language (Robin & Scheinberg, 1990) and that the three syndromes described by Naeser and associates do not account for all the varieties of aphasia that may be caused by lesions in the basal ganglia.

Aphasia caused by lesions in the left thalamus also has been described, and the role of the thalamus in language has received considerable attention (Mohr, Walters, & Duncan, 1975; Ojemann, 1975; Cappa & Vignolo, 1979; and others). Patients with aphasia caused by thalamic lesions are almost always hemiplegic because of damage to pyramidal tract fibers in the internal capsule. They have difficulty initiating spontaneous speech, and their spontaneous speech is sparse, echolalic, and neologistic. Their vocal intensity tends to decrease progressively during utterances. Their auditory comprehension and reading usually are good. Their writing usually is impaired, and word-finding problems are com-

mon. Patients with left thalamic damage tend to be perserverative, and their performance tends to fluctuate from task to task and moment to moment.

Murdoch (1990) has commented that aphasia syndromes resulting from thalamic lesions resemble transcortical motor aphasia, in that repetition and comprehension tend to be preserved but self-initiated speech tends to be reduced. According to Murdoch, the language impairments of patients with left subcortical damage usually are mild, and patients with subcortical aphasia have a better prognosis for recovery than patients with aphasia caused by cortical damage.

Naeser and associates (1989) reported that two left hemisphere fiber tracts—the *medial subcallosal fasciculus* (deep in the anterior frontal lobe) and the *periventricular white matter* (beneath the sensory and motor cortex for the mouth)—are important determinants of aphasic adults' recovery of spontaneous speech. They studied the relationship between recovery of speech by 27 aphasic adults and the location of their brain damage as indicated by CT scans. They reported that destruction of the subcallosal fasciculus and periventricular white matter always caused permanent severe impairment of spontaneous speech.

Although aphasia syndromes follow subcortical damage, it is not clear that the damaged subcortical structures are directly involved in language. In many of the patients studied, damage was not confined to subcortical structures, but it extended to the cortex. Dewitt and associates (1985) asserted that MRI scans of patients with subcortical aphasias usually reveal involvement of cortical tissue not shown by CT scans. Metter and associates (1983) reported that PET studies of patients with subcortical aphasia almost always reveal decreased cortical metabolism in areas of the left hemisphere without observable structural damage. Alexander, Naeser, and Palumbo (1987) studied 18 patients with only subcortical damage and retrospectively reviewed the cases of 61 more. They reported that damage confined to the thalamus does not cause persisting aphasia but may cause mild word-retrieval impairments. They suggested that subcortical lesions causing aphasia must involve deep nerve fiber tracts connecting subcortical regions with one another or nerve fiber tracts connecting subcortical regions to cortical regions.

THE EXPLANATORY POWER OF CONNECTIONIST MODELS

Despite the seeming objectivity of connectionist explanations of aphasia, they do not and probably cannot provide a complete explanation of brain-behavior relationships. As Jackson (1873) pointed out, symptoms appearing after brain damage identify the brain location in which damage produces a *symptom* and do not necessarily identify the location in the brain of the underlying *function* or *process* to which the symptom relates. Kertesz (1979) extends Jackson's assertion, saying ". . . only lesions causing impairments are localizable, not the impairment itself" (p. 142).

When symptoms are produced not by destruction of functional regions of cortex but by destruction of association fibers, localizationist interpretations are likely to go astray. For example, damage in the left hemisphere at the parieto-occipital-temporal junction (the angular gyrus region) is known to cause reading impairments. From this evidence a strict localizationist might conclude that the parieto-occipital-junction in the left hemisphere is a center for reading. The conclusion would be naive because reading is a complex process that requires the participation of several brain regions. Reading impairments and damage in the region of the angular gyrus of the left hemisphere tend to co-occur because damage there disrupts communication between the visual cortex and Wernicke's area, not because the angular gyrus region is a center for reading. Few would argue that the lesions producing transcortical motor aphasia do so by destroying a center for initiation of speech, but most would agree that these patients' reticence is caused by isolation of regions responsible for speech from regions responsible for activation and arousal.

According to Goodglass (1993) connectionist syndromes represent "the result of modal tendencies for the functional organization of language in adult human brains" (p. 218). Goodglass believes that adult human brains are to some extent "hard-wired," but as an individual matures, the individual's brain develops its own most efficient neural organization for carrying out the processes involved in language. According to Goodglass, there are common (modal) patterns of brain organization toward which brains gravitate (presumably these common patterns are the result of the hard wiring). These modal patterns produce enough consistency in brain organization to suggest relationships between brain damage and language impairments that are sufficiently predictable to make connectionistic explanations of brain-behavior relationships useful. However, according to Goodglass, individual differences in how the brain has organized itself for language may be superimposed on these modal patterns, producing exceptions, contradictions, or incomplete representations of the classic connectionist aphasia syndromes in individual patients.

Because of these individual differences, connectionist explanations of aphasia work better for groups than for individuals. If a large group of right-handed adults with left temporal lobe damage was to be tested, the overall pattern of performance would almost certainly match the classic pattern for Wernicke's aphasia. The patient's comprehension would be impaired, they would produce paraphasic speech errors (especially verbal paraphasias), they would produce inordinate numbers of vague and indefinite words, and they would say more than necessary to communicate a given amount of information. However, there would undoubtedly be some in the group who produced few or no paraphasic errors, some who produced few vague and indefinite words, some who did not exhibit press of speech, and perhaps a few whose comprehension was relatively good.

The uncertainty of connectionist models increases not only as one moves from groups of aphasic patients to individuals, but as one moves from global characteristics (such as speech fluency) to more specific aspects of language (such as the behaviors seen as a consequence of word-retrieval failure). The fuzziness of connectionist models with regard to specifics is apparent when aphasia test batteries designed expressly to classify aphasic patients into connectionist syndromes prove unable to classify unambiguously from 15% (Poeck, 1983) to 40% (Benson, 1979) or up to 80% (Goodglass & Kaplan, 1983) of patients into classic connectionist syndromes based on their language behaviors.

Despite these shortcomings, connectionist aphasia syndromes and their terminology are useful to the clinician who wishes to communicate efficiently or to venture a guess about the location and severity of a patient's brain damage from a patient's observed symptoms. Goodglass (1993) has commented that classic patterns of Wernicke's or Broca's aphasia usually point unambiguously to damage in the temporal lobe (in the case of Wernicke's aphasia) or the posterior inferior frontal lobe (in the case of Broca's aphasia), but when the classic patterns are mixed or incomplete, predicting the location of the brain damage underlying the symptoms becomes uncertain. Often, those who use the connectionist model will be surprised by patients who do not fit the model, but their predictions will be supported by enough patients who do fit the model to make it a convenient tool.

The connectionist model is in many respects a fiction, but it remains a useful one for the speech-language pathologist who wishes to understand the basic relationships between symptoms of aphasia and their source in the nervous system. The speech-language pathologist who understands the relationships between connectionist aphasia syndromes and various patterns of language impairments can use the presence of a connectionist aphasia syndrome to help them plan assessment of the patient's communication impairments. In addition, knowledge of the connectionist model helps speech-language pathologists communicate with neurologists and other professionals who make referrals and talk in the language of the model.

GENERAL CONCEPTS 4-3

- Contemporary evidence suggests that brain injury must extend beyond Broca's area to cause persisting Broca's aphasia and must extend beyond Wernicke's area to cause persisting Wernicke's aphasia.
- Patients with brain injury deep in the subcortical regions of the language-dominant hemisphere may become aphasic. It is not clear whether their aphasia is caused by damage to deep-brain structures themselves, by disruption of neural communication between deep-brain structures and the cortex, or by extension of damage from deep-brain structures into the cortex.
- Connectionist models of aphasia are better at describing brain-behavior relationships for groups of patients than for predicting an individual patient's aphasic symptoms. Connnectionist models predict global symptoms such as speech fluency better than they predict specific impairments such as word-retrieval failure.

THOUGHT QUESTIONS

Question 4-1 A patient exhibits no paralysis of either hand or arm but exhibits unilateral limb apraxia of the right hand and arm. Is this what one would expect? Speculate as to the location of the neuropathology that might yield such a pattern of signs.

Question 4-2 A right-handed stroke patient with presumed alexia without agraphia and no other neurologic signs has intact visual fields. The patient has no previous history of neurologic problems. Is this possible?

Question 4-3 What non-language problems would you expect in the presence of transcortical motor aphasia? What non-language problems would you expect in the presence of transcortical sensory aphasia?

Question 4-4 Jack Johnson is a 72-year-old right-handed man who 3 days ago had a stroke in the posterior branch of his left middle cerebral artery. Joanna Redmond is a 56-year-old right-handed woman who 3 days ago had a stroke in the posterior watershed region of her left middle cerebral artery.

- Compare Mr. Johnson's and Ms. Redmond's probable speech and language impairments.
- Describe any associated nonlanguage impairments each is likely to exhibit.
- Describe any differences you might expect in their "spontaneous recovery."

Assessing Aphasia and Related Disorders

ASSESSING LANGUAGE AND COMMUNICATION

The assessment begins when the referral appears on the speech-language pathologist's desk. The assessment proceeds through several phases (medical record review, a patient and family interview, and perhaps bedside screening tests) before formal testing begins. Formal test-ing usually begins with a comprehensive language test battery to get a general sense of the patient's linguistic and communicative impairments, followed by one or more free-standing tests to analyze in more detail the patient's specific impairments. In this chapter, some widely used comprehensive language tests and some popular free-standing tests of specific abilities are described, and some ways in which comprehensive language tests and free-standing tests of specific abilities complement each other in assessment of brain-injured adults are discussed.

Language Test Batteries

Language test batteries permit clinicians to measure patients' communication performance in the two primary input modalities (vision and audition) and three output modalities (speech, writing, and gesture) at various levels of difficulty within modalities or combinations of modalities. Language test batteries permit clinicians to identify and describe communication impairments and to estimate their severity. Some permit prediction of a patient's recovery. Most help clinicians make a diagnosis.

Albert and associates (1981) described a model for designing language test batteries that provides for assessment of all stimulus input and response output modality combinations related to language (Table 5-1). Most language test batteries include subtests for assessing the combinations shown in the unshaded cells of Table 5-1, but none has subtests assessing verbal or gestural responses to tactile stimuli.

Although the subtests contained in most language test batteries can be partitioned according to Albert and associates' schema, clinicians (and patients) are more likely to divide communicative activities into traditional *speaking, listening, reading,* and *writing* categories. The following list of subtests likely to be found in many language test batteries is arranged according to those categories.

Speech
- Recite days of the week and months of the year and count aloud.
- Name objects or pictures indicated by the examiner.
- Complete incomplete phrases or sentences spoken by the examiner.
- Repeat words, phrases, and sentences spoken by the examiner.
- Formulate and produce single-sentence utterances.
- Formulate and produce multiple-sentence utterances.

Auditory Comprehension
- Answer spoken questions.
- Point to objects or pictures named by the examiner.
- Follow spoken directions.
- Answer questions about spoken discourse.

T A B L E   5 - 1

A schema for constructing comprehensive language tests

Stimulus	Response			
	Point	Say	Write	Do
See objects	Visual matching	Naming	Written naming	Pantomine
Hear words (sentences)	Word discrimination, sentence comprehension	Word repetition, sentence repetition, answering questions	Writing from dictation	Follow commands
See words (sentences)	Word-object matching	Oral reading	Copying	Follow written commands
Feel objects	Visual-tactile matching (stereognosis)	Tactile naming	Tactile-written naming	Pantomine

Data from Albert, M. L., Goodglass, H., Helm, N. A., Rubens, A. B., & Alexander, M. P. (1981). *Clinical aspects of dysphasia.* New York: Springer-Verlag.

Reading

- Match pictures, letters, or geometric forms.
- Match printed words to pictures.
- Read aloud printed numerals, letters, words, and phrases.
- Answer printed questions.
- Silently read and answer questions about printed sentences and paragraphs.

Writing

- Copy letters, geometric forms, and words.
- Write letters, words, and sentences spoken by the examiner.
- Formulate and produce written narratives.

Language test batteries for adults are designed for assessment of adults with aphasia, but most can be used to assess language performance of adults with other linguistic or communication impairments. In fact, several aphasia tests provide norms for other populations, such as adults with right-hemisphere damage or dementia. The major language test batteries are similar in content, but there are important differences in intent, scoring, and interpretation. The following descriptions illustrate some of these differences.

Minnesota Test for Differential Diagnosis of Aphasia The *Minnesota Test for Differential Diagnosis of Aphasia* (MTDDA; Schuell, 1965) was one of the pioneers in aphasia testing. It was one of the first tests for aphasia to emphasize the importance of qualitative scoring of responses, rather than simply counting errors. According to its authors, the MTDDA was designed to meet several criteria:

- Permits users to explore differences in the behavior of aphasic adults in all language modalities
- Includes tests of graduated difficulty within each language modality
- Includes a variety of nonlanguage tasks to measure processes underlying language behavior
- Is both comprehensive and detailed to differentiate among clinical syndromes caused by brain damage

The MTDDA serves three basic clinical purposes, according to its authors. It provides the following:

- An operational definition of aphasia
- An objective method for evaluating changes resulting from treatment
- An instrument for use in longitudinal studies

The MTDDA is one of the longest and most detailed of the standardized aphasia test batteries, with 47 subtests divided among five sections—*auditory disturbances* (9 subtests), *visual and reading disturbances* (9 subtests), *speech and language disturbances* (15 subtests), *visuomotor and writing disturbances* (10 subtests), and *disturbances of numerical relations and arithmetic processes* (4 subtests). The MTDDA is heterogeneous with regard to the number of items in subtests and the pattern of difficulty within subtests. The number of items within subtests ranges from 5 to 32. In some subtests, items increase in difficulty as the subtest progresses, and in others the items are of approximately equal difficulty. Because of its length and the time it takes to administer and score the entire MTDDA (3 to 6 hours), clinicians who are pushed for time (as most are) tend not to administer the complete test.

Schuell (1957) suggested a *baseline–ceiling* procedure for shortening an unpublished version of the MTDDA. First, the examiner estimates the patient's probable level of performance in each performance category (listening, speaking, reading, writing, and calculating). The examiner selects a performance category (e.g., *listening*) and begins testing with the most difficult subtest the examiner thinks the patient can complete with no more than one error. If the patient makes more than one error on a subtest, the examiner administers progressively easier subtest until the patient performs a subtest without error (this defines the patient's *baseline*). Then the examiner administers progressively more difficult subtests until the patient makes 90% errors, at which point testing ends (the *ceiling*) and the examiner moves on to another category.

The patient's performance on the MTDDA is recorded in a test booklet. Most responses are scored plus-minus (correct-incorrect) with some longhand notation, although errors made in two subtests (matching printed words to pictures, matching printed to spoken words) can be categorized as *semantic confusions, auditory confusions, visual confusions,* or *irrelevant responses.* As the MTDDA is administered, the examiner records the number of errors made by the patient adjacent to each subtest in the test booklet. After the test is completed, the user transfers the subtest scores to a *Summary of Test Scores* section on the face sheet of the test booklet, where they are entered as number correct.

> This change in record-keeping for the MTDDA can create transcription errors for the unwary. Many users ensure against transcription errors by writing the number correct next to the number of errors for each subtest, as in *12/15.*

The MTDDA provides few standardized procedures for interpreting patients' performance. The test manual provides mean scores, standard deviations, and subtest-by-subtest percentage of subjects making errors for a group of 50 nonaphasic adults and six groups of aphasic adults representing five major categories of aphasia and one minor syndrome. The norm group of aphasic adults ranges from 31 to 157 patients, depending on the subtest. Most subtests are normed on 75 aphasic adults. The MTDDA manual provides no procedures for profiling patterns of impairment and has no percentiles, either for individual subtests or the MTDDA as a whole, although some statistical information can be found in Schuell, Jenkins, and Jiminez-Pabon (1965). The test manual does provide a list of *signs* and *most discriminating tests,* which enables the user to assign patients to one of five major and two minor categories of aphasia:

- Simple aphasia
- Aphasia with visual involvement
- Aphasia with sensorimotor involvement
- Aphasia with scattered findings compatible with generalized brain damage
- Irreversible aphasic syndrome

- Minor syndrome A: aphasia with partial auditory imperception
- Minor syndrome B: aphasia with persisting dysarthria

The MTTDA manual provides no standardized prognostic procedures, although general descriptions of the patterns of expected recovery for the seven categories of aphasia are included. The subjective nature of procedures for assigning patients to diagnostic categories gives users of the MTDDA considerable latitude in making these decisions, which may contribute to unreliability. The MTDDA test manual provides no information about either interexaminer reliability or the reliability of its patient categorization procedures.

Porch Index of Communicative Ability
The *Porch Index of Communicative Ability* (PICA; Porch, 1981a) was designed, according to Porch because of:

> ...the pressing need for a tool which could sensitively and reliably quantify the patient's ability to communicate, for only if such a tool were available could an experimenter measure the effects of treatment, drugs, surgery, time, and the myriad of other variables of communication (Porch, 1981a).

The PICA differs from other language test batteries in several ways. With 180 test items in 18 subtests, it can be administered in about 1 hour for most aphasic adults. Unlike other language test batteries, the PICA uses the same 10 test stimuli (*pen, pencil, matches, cigarette, key, quarter, toothbrush, comb, fork, knife*) in all 18 subtests.* The order in which PICA subtests are given differs from other language test batteries, which usually administer subtests in groups representing different communicative abilities (e.g., listening, reading, speaking, writing). Subtests in

---

* A revised version of the *Porch Index of Communicative Ability* was recently announced (Porch, 2001). In the revised version the cigarette test item is replaced with scissors; administration procedures are updated; and constructs, models, and terminology related to the test are revamped. Information about the revised PICA may be obtained at www.picaprograms.com.

the PICA are arranged so that patients receive as little information as possible about the answers to succeeding subtests as they proceed through the PICA. (This ordering of subtests is mandated because the same objects are used throughout the test. For example, if Subtest 12, in which the patient repeats the names of test items after the examiner, were to precede Subtest 4, in which the patient names each test item, the patient has gotten a head start on Subtest 4 by previously having heard the names in Subtest 12.)

> Another result of this ordering of PICA subtests is that the subtests are arranged in general order of decreasing difficulty. Because of this arrangement the patient's initial experience is on tests in which failure is most likely, which may prove discouraging to some patients. Porch (1981a) comments, however, that "administering the tests in order of decreasing complexity, or increasing information, progressively increases the chance of the patient being motivated by a successful performance as he moves from test to test." (Porch, 1981a, p. 16)

The PICA also differs from other standardized aphasia test batteries in the constraints it places on administration procedures. The instructions to the patient are specified word by word for each subtest, and the circumstances under which the examiner can repeat a test instruction or offer a prompt or cue are stipulated. Every patient response is scored with a 16-category, binary-choice (yes or no) system (Table 5-2). A set of diacritic markings (circles, squares, and triangles around scores; marks through scores; superscript letters) can be used to augment the 16-category system, thereby increasing the descriptiveness of PICA scoring (e.g., drawing a square around a score shows that the response was produced with motoric distortion or awkwardness). The complexities of administration and scoring procedures for the PICA require that new users get 40 hours of training to become reliable in admin-

istering and scoring the PICA. The training, together with tightly controlled administration and scoring procedures, ensures high reliability across clinicians and clinics.

Each response to a PICA item is scored with the 16-category scoring system, and the score is written on a score sheet. A mean score for the entire test (the *Overall Score*) can be calculated, as can modality mean scores for *writing, copying, reading, pantomime, verbal, auditory,* and *visual* subtests. Profiles may be plotted on a *Rating of Communicative Ability* form (Figure 5-1), which groups subtests according to each of the modalities.

Profiles also may be plotted on a *Ranked Response Summary* graph (Figure 5-2), which plots subtest scores in order of decreasing subtest difficulty across the page.

Changes in a patient's performance over time can be recorded on an *Aphasia Recovery Curve* form (Figure 5-3), on which the overall percentile score and intrasubtest variability can be graphed.

The PICA is normed on 357 left-hemisphere-damaged adults, 96 right-hemisphere-damaged adults, and 100 bilaterally damaged adults. Duffy and associates (1976) have published norms for a group of 130 non-brain-injured adults. Volume I of the test manual contains information about the development of the PICA, interscorer and test-retest reliability, and internal consistency. Volume II contains percentiles for overall scores, subtest scores, and various combinations of subtests within modalities.

The PICA manual provides procedures for predicting the recovery of aphasic patients by plotting a recovery curve, which allows predictions about eventual recovery of communicative ability based on the patient's performance 1 month or more after onset of aphasia. Porch calls this method *HOAP,* for *high overall prediction.* It is described in Chapter 3.

Shortened versions of the PICA have been described in the literature (Disimoni, Keith, & Darley, 1980; Disimoni, Keith, Holt, & associates, 1975; Lincoln & Ellis, 1980). However, Holtzapple and associates (1989) reported sig-

T A B L E   5 - 2

The 16-category, binary-choice scoring system used in the *Porch Index of Communicative Ability*

Score	Level	Description
16	Complex	*Spontaneous, accurate, fluent elaboration* about the test item
15	Complete	*Complete, accurate, fluent* response to test item
14	Complete-distorted	*Complete, accurate* response to test item but with *reduced facility of production*
13	Complete-delayed	*Complete, accurate* response to test item but *significantly slowed or delayed*
12	Incomplete	Accurate response to test item but *lacking in completeness*
11	Incomplete-delayed	*Accurate, incomplete,* and *significantly slowed or delayed* response to test item
10	Corrected	Accurate response to test item *self-correcting a previous error* by request or after a prolonged delay
9	Repeated	An accurate response *after a repetition of instructions, by request,* or *after a prolonged delay*
8	Cued	*Accurate* response to test item *stimulated by a cue, additional information, or another test item*
7	Related	An *inaccurate* response to test item that is *closely related* to a correct response
6	Error	An *inaccurate* response to the test item
5	Intelligible	An *intelligible* response that is *not associated with the test item,* such as perseverative or automatic responses, or an expressed indication of inability to respond
4	Unintelligible	Different and *unintelligible* responses to the test item
3	Minimal	*Undifferentiated, unintelligible* responses
2	Attention	Patient *attends* to the test item *but gives no response*
1	No response	Patient exhibits *no awareness* of the test item

Data from Porch, B. E. (1967, 1981a). *Porch index of communicative ability.* Palo Alto, CA: Consulting Psychologists Press.

nificant differences between full PICA scores and scores on a shortened version (Disimoni, Keith, & Darley, 1980) for a group of 19 aphasic adults. They commented:

> We believe that as difficult as it is to obtain reliable retest results using the same measure, it is demonstrably more difficult when you eliminate a good portion of the test. . . . Our current recommendations are for caution. (p. 140)

Boston Diagnostic Aphasia Examination
The *Boston Diagnostic Aphasia Examination,*

Third Edition (BDAE; Goodglass, Kaplan, & Barresi, 2001) permits users to assign patients to classical aphasia syndromes (such as Broca's aphasia and Wernicke's aphasia). Goodglass, Kaplan, and Barresi believe that the nature of a patient's aphasia is jointly determined by the organization of language in the patient's brain and the location of the brain injury responsible for the patient's aphasia. According to Goodglass, Kaplan, and Barresi the BDAE permits clinicians to:

• Determine the presence of aphasia and the type of aphasia syndrome and make infer-

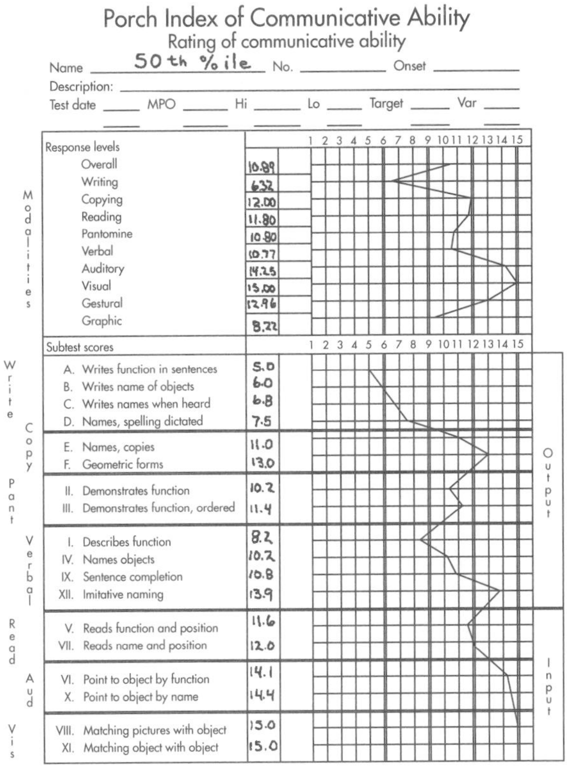

Porch Index of Communicative Ability
Rating of communicative ability

Name ___50th %ile___ No. _____ Onset _____

Description: _____

Test date _____ MPO _____ Hi _____ Lo _____ Target _____ Var _____

	Response levels		1 2 3 4 5 6 7 8 9 10 11 12 13 14 15
M o d a l i t i e s	Overall	10.89	
	Writing	6.32	
	Copying	12.00	
	Reading	11.80	
	Pantomine	10.80	
	Verbal	10.77	
	Auditory	14.25	
	Visual	15.00	
	Gestural	12.96	
	Graphic	8.22	

		Subtest scores		1 2 3 4 5 6 7 8 9 10 11 12 13 14 15
W r i t e	C o p y / P a n t / V e r b a l	A. Writes function in sentences	5.0	
		B. Writes name of objects	6.0	
		C. Writes names when heard	6.8	
		D. Names, spelling dictated	7.5	
		E. Names, copies	11.0	
		F. Geometric forms	13.0	
		II. Demonstrates function	10.2	
		III. Demonstrates function, ordered	11.4	
		I. Describes function	8.2	
		IV. Names objects	10.2	
		IX. Sentence completion	10.8	
		XII. Imitative naming	13.9	
R e a d		V. Reads function and position	11.6	
		VII. Reads name and position	12.0	
A u d		VI. Point to object by function	14.1	
		X. Point to object by name	14.4	
V i s		VIII. Matching pictures with object	15.0	
		XI. Matching object with object	15.0	

(Output / Input labels on right side)

Figure 5-1 ■ A *Porch Index of Communicative Ability (PICA) Rating of Communicative Ability* form for a patient with moderate aphasia. Mean scores (using the 16-category PICA scoring system) are written in the middle column and graphed in the cells on the right. (From Porch, B. E. [1981]. *Porch Index of Communicative Ability.* Palo Alto, CA: Consulting Psychologists Press.)

Figure 5-2 ■ A *Porch Index of Communicative Ability (PICA) Ranked Response Summary Form* for a patient with moderate aphasia. The diagonal line represents the hypothetical performance of a group of patients whose PICA performance places them at the 50th percentile of a large group of aphasic adults. The PICA subtests are arranged from left to right in order of decreasing difficulty. (From Porch, B. E. [1981]. *Porch Index of Communicative Ability.* Palo Alto, CA: Consulting Psychologists Press.)

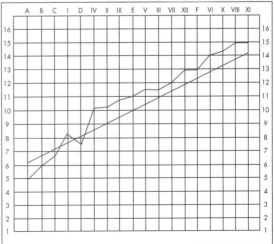

Porch Index of Communicative Ability
Ranked response summary

Name ___50th %ile___ Case No. _____

Description: _____ Onset _____

Test dates: Test 1 _____ Test 2 _____ Test 3 _____

	MPO	Target	OA	Writ	Copy	Read	Pant	Verb	Aud	Vis	Gest	Graph
1			10.89	6.32	12.00	11.90	10.80	10.77	14.25	15.00	12.96	8.22
2												
3												

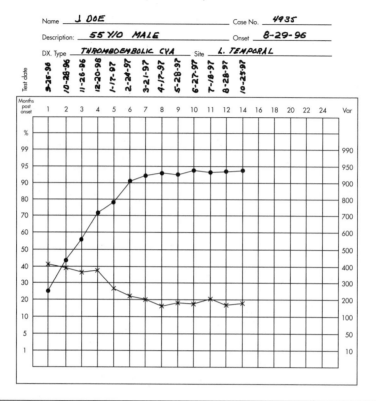

Porch Index of Communicative Ability
Aphasia recovery curve

Name __J DOE__   Case No. __4935__

Description: __55 Y/O MALE__   Onset __8-29-96__

DX. Type __THROMBOEMBOLIC CVA__   Site __L. TEMPORAL__

Figure 5-3 ■ *A Porch Index of Communicative Ability (PICA) Aphasia Recovery Curve* for a hypothetical aphasic patient with a left temporal lobe stroke. The *circles* denote the patient's overall mean percentile on the PICA and the *Xs* denote the patient's overall response variability on the PICA. The patient's overall PICA performance increases for the first 6 months and then plateaus. The patient's overall response variability gradually decreases during the first 8 months, after which it stabilizes. (From Porch, B. E. [1981]. *Porch Index of Communicative Ability.* Palo Alto, CA: Consulting Psychologists Press.)

ences concerning cerebral localization, linguistic processes that may have been damaged, and the strategies used to compensate for the damage.

• Measure a patient's level of performance across a wide range of tasks and several levels of difficulty within each task, both for initial evaluation and measurement of change over time.

• Assess a patient's assets and liabilities in all language skills as a guide to treatment.

The BDAE is a long test. The standard form consists of a structured interview, 27 subtests, a free-standing 60-item confrontation naming test called *The Boston Naming Test* (Kaplan, Goodglass, & Weintraub, 2001), and 9 rating scales. Administering the standard form of the BDAE takes from 1 to 5 hours. The average for aphasic adults is about 2 hours. A short form consists of selected items from 21 subtests of the standard form and takes from 40 to 60 minutes to administer. Individual subtests from a 28-subtest *Extended Testing* section can be added to the standard form of the BDAE for more detailed assessment of particular functions. (Examples of extended testing subtests include *story telling, comprehension of syntactically complex sentences, naming in categories,* and *oral spelling.*) A patient's BDAE subtest scores and an overall severity rating can be entered in a *Subtest Summary Profile* (Figure 5-4), from which percentile ranks for each subtest score can be read.

Norms for the BDAE are based on a sample of 85 aphasic adults and 15 elderly normal volunteers tested at a large number of clinical facilities across the United States. The results of several intercorrelation analyses and reliability coefficients among subtests are included in the test manual.

The BDAE is a comprehensive test of language and associated processes that permits clinicians to compare the performance of any aphasic patient with the performance of a large group of aphasic adults and to assign aphasic patients to neurodiagnostic aphasia syndromes based on their BDAE performance. However, users should be aware that many patients cannot be unambiguously classified on the basis of their BDAE performance.

Western Aphasia Battery The *Western Aphasia Battery* (WAB; Kertesz, 1982) is shorter and psychometrically more sophisticated than the BDAE, which it resembles in many respects, including an emphasis on classifying patients according to classic neurodiagnostic syndromes. The WAB uses what Kertesz calls a *taxonomic* approach to classification, in which patients are assigned to diagnostic categories (such as Broca's aphasia and Wernicke's aphasia) according to their scores on four language subtests—*spontaneous speech, auditory comprehension, repetition,* and *naming* (Figure 5-5). The WAB also includes subtests for evaluating reading and writing; one apraxia subtest; and several subtests

for assessing constructional, visuospatial, and calculation abilities.

No normative information is provided in the WAB test manual. The reader is referred to Kertesz (1979) and Shewan and Kertesz (1980) for information on standardization of the 1977 version of the WAB. Subtest mean scores and their standard deviations are reported in Kertesz (1979) for 365 aphasic and 162 nonaphasic adults from two standardizations of the WAB. The first, in 1974, included 150 aphasic patients and 59 control subjects. The second, in 1979, added 215 aphasic patients and 63 control subjects. Information on the reliability and validity of the WAB are provided in Kertesz (1979).

A patient's score on each WAB subtest is entered on a score sheet, which is the last page in the test booklet. A patient's scores on the auditory comprehension and speech subtests can be used to calculate an *Aphasia Quotient,* and both language and nonlanguage subtest scores are used to calculate a *Cortical Quotient.* The *Aphasia Quotient* is said by Kertesz to be a reliable measure of the severity of language impairment. The *Cortical Quotient* is said to be a measure of cognitive functions. Shewan and Kertesz (1984) described an additional summary score, called the *Language Quotient.* The *Language Quotient* is based on the WAB oral language subtest scores that contribute to the *Aphasia Quotient,* plus scores from the WAB reading and writing subtests.

Aphasia Quotient
- Spontaneous speech (rating of information content, fluency)
- Auditory comprehension

Language Quotient
- Spontaneous speech (rating of information content, fluency)
- Auditory comprehension
- Reading, writing

Cortical Quotient (entire test)
- Spontaneous speech (rating of information content, fluency)

SUMMARY PROFILE OF STANDARD SUBTESTS

NAME: _____ DATE OF EXAMINATION: _____

		Percentiles:	0	10	20	30	40	50	60	70	80	90	100
SEVERITY RATING			0	0	1	1	(1)	2	3	3	3	4	5
FLUENCY	Phrase Length (Rating Scale)		1	2 (4)		6	7	7	7	7	7	7	7
	Melodic Line (Rating Scale)		1	(2)	3	5	5	6	6	7	7	7	7
	Grammatical Form (Rating Scale)		1	2 (3)		4	5	5	6	6	7	7	7
CONVERSATION/	Simple Social Responses		0	3	5	6	6	6	7	7	7	7	(7)
EXPOSITORY SPEECH	Complexity Index		0	(0.1)	0.4	0.6	0.8	1.0	1.2	1.2	1.4	1.6	2.0
AUDITORY	Basic Word Discrimination		14	24	29	31	32	34	35 (36)		37	37	37
COMPREHENSION	Commands		0	6	10	(11)	12	13	14	15	15	15	15
	Complex Ideational Material		0	3	5	6	7	8	9	10	10 (12)		12
ARTICULATION	Nonverbal Agility		0	4	6	6	7	(7)	8	9	10	12	12
	Verbal Agility		0	3	6	7	(8)	9	10	11	12	14	14
	Articulatory Agility (Rating Scale)		1	2	3	3	4 (5)		6	6	7	7	7
RECITATION	Automatized Sequences		0	1	4 (6)		6	6	7	7	8	8	8
& MUSIC	Recitation		0	0	0	0	1	1	1	2	2	2	(2)
	Melody		0	0	1	(1)	2	2	2	2	2	2	2
	Rhythm		0	0	1	1	1	1	(1)	2	2	2	2
REPETITION	Words		0	3	6	7	8	9	9	(9)	10	10	10
	Sentences		0	0	1	(1)	3	4	7	8	9	10	10
NAMING	Responsive Naming		0	2	4	9	13	16	18	(18)	19	20	20
	Boston Naming Test		0	3	8	20	25	33	40 (43)	52	57	60	
	Special Categories		0	3	7	10	11	12	12	12	12	12	(12)
PARAPHASIA	Rating from Speech Profile		1	2	2	3	4	5	6	6	7	7	7
	Phonemic		27	15	9	6	4	3	2	1	(1)	0	0
	Verbal		19	12	9 (7)		6	4	3	2	1	0	0
	Neologistic		11	7	4	2	1	0	0	0	0	0	(0)
	Multi-word		15	7	2	0	0	0	0	0	0	0	(0)
READING	Matching Cases & Scripts		0	4	6	7	7	8	8	8	8	8	(8)
	Number Matching		1	8	10	11	11	12	12	12	12	12	(12)
	Picture-Word Matching		2	4	7	8	9	9	9	10	10	10	(10)
	Lexical Decision		0	2	3	4	5	5	5	5	5	5	(5)
	Homophone Matching		0	1	2	3	3	4	4	5	5	5	(5)
	Free Grammatical Morphemes		0	5	7	9	10	10	10	10	10	10	(10)
	Oral Word Reading		0	7	11	20	23	27	(27)	30	30	30	30
	Oral Sentence Reading		0	0	(1)	2	3	5	6	8	9	10	10
	Oral Sentence Comprehension		0	2	2	(3)	4	4	5	5	5	5	5
	Sent./Parag. Comprehension		0	3	5	6	7	8	(8)	9	9	10	10
WRITING	Form		7	(14)	15	16	16	18	18	18	18	18	18
	Letter Choice		7	(20)	22	23	24	24	25	26	26	27	27
	Motor Facility		6	(8)	9	11	15	17	18	18	18	18	18
	Primer Words		0	2	3	4	5	6	6	6	6	6	(6)
	Regular Phonics		0	0	0	1	2	3	4	(4)	5	5	5
	Common Irregular Words		0	0	0	1	1	(2)	3	4	5	5	5
	Written Picture Naming		0	0	1	3	5	(7)	8	9	10	11	12
	Narrative Writing		0	1	4	(5)	6	7	7	7	9	11	11

Figure 5-4 ■ A *Boston Diagnostic Aphasia Examination Summary Profile* for a patient with Broca's aphasia. (From Goodglass, H., Kaplan, E., & Barresi, B. [2001]. *The assessment of aphasia and related disorders* [3rd ed.]. Philadelphia: Lippincott Williams & Wilkins.)

Nonfluent			
Broca			
Global			
Isolation syndrome			
Transcortical motor			
Poor Comprehension		**Fair Comprehension**	
Global		Broca	
Isolation syndrome		Transcortical motor	
Poor Repetition	**Fair Repetition**	**Poor Repetition**	**Fair Repetition**
Global	Isolation syndrome	Broca	Transcortical motor

Fluent			
Wernicke			
Anomic			
Conduction			
Transcortical sensory			
Poor Comprehension		**Fair Comprehension**	
Wernicke		Conduction	
Transcortical sensory		Anomic	
Poor Repetition	**Fair Repetition**	**Poor Repetition**	**Fair Repetition**
Wernicke	Transcortical sensory	Conduction	Anomic

Figure 5-5 ■ How the *Western Aphasia Battery* assigns aphasic adults to classic neurodiagnostic categories. (From Kertesz, A. [1982]. *Western Aphasia Battery.* New York: Grune and Stratton.)

- Auditory comprehension
- Reading, writing
- Praxis (limb, buccofacial)
- Construction (drawing, block design, calculation, *Raven's Progressive Matrices*)

The accuracy and reliability of WAB procedures for classifying patients has been questioned. Swindell, Holland, and Fromm (1984) compared the WAB classifications of 69 aphasic patients with subjective classifications made by clinicians who had been trained to identify neurodiagnostic aphasia syndromes. They reported that the clinicians' judgments matched the WAB classification only 54% of the time. Wertz, Deal, and Robinson (1984) compared WAB and BDAE classifications for 45 aphasic patients. The two tests agreed on patients' classification only 27% of the time. Of the 45 patients, 28 were unclassi-

fiable with the BDAE, but only 5 were unclassifiable with the WAB. The WAB has been criticized for forcing patients into diagnostic categories. This may be one reason for the lack of agreement between WAB and BDAE classifications.

Other Language Test Batteries The BDAE, the MTDDA, the PICA, and the WAB are well known and widely used in the United States. Several other tests, although less widely used, are marketed in the United States and are the tests of choice for some clinicians. They include the *Neurosensory Center Comprehensive Examination for Aphasia* (NCCEA; Spreen & Benton, 1977), *Examining for Aphasia* (Eisenson, 1974), and *The Aphasia Language Performance Scales* (Keenan & Brassell, 1975).

Screening Tests of Language and Communication Assessment of brain-injured adults' language and communication does not always begin with a comprehensive language test. Many brain-injured adults are first seen at bedside, where the speech-language pathologist conducts a brief interview and may administer a screening test of speech, language, and communicative abilities. The interview gives the speech-language pathologist a general sense of the patient's background, problems, and concerns. The screening test gives the speech-language pathologist a general sense of the nature and severity of the patient's speech, language, and communicative impairments and sets the stage for more comprehensive testing that may follow.

Several screening tests for assessing adults' communication performance are on the market. Most are designed for adults with aphasia (Crary, Haak, & Malinsky, 1989; Fitch-West & Sands, 1987; Keenan & Brassell, 1975; Sklar, 1973), although a few are designed for adults in other diagnostic categories such as traumatic brain injury (Helm-Estabrooks & Hotz, 1991), right-hemisphere syndrome (Pimental & Kingsbury, 1989; Ross, 1996), or motor speech impairments (St. Louis & Ruscello, 1987). Davis (1993) suggests that published screening tests are not needed for screening communicative abilities at bedside:

> We do not need one of these tests to evaluate a patient's language abilities at bedside. All we need is a concept of what needs to be assessed, a few common objects, a pen, and some paper. We have the patient answer some yes/no questions, point to things, and name and describe some other things. If the patient cannot converse, we want to see if he or she can count or recite the days of the week. (p. 215)

However, Davis subsequently comments that published screening tests have advantages over informal tests because of their standardized administration, which contributes to consistency in measurement and interpretation. Although it is no doubt true that a skilled clinician can improvise a satisfactory bedside screening examination with a few common objects, something to write with, and something to write on, such

an unsystematic approach may lead the examiner to miss important signs and may invalidate comparisons of the patient's performance with that of other patients or with the performance of the same patient on subsequent tests.

Many experienced clinicians forego published screening tests in favor of locally designed tests, but few are content with informal, unstructured, and unsystematic screening routines. Most large speech and language clinics have formalized procedures for screening patients with impaired communication—usually with separate procedures for patients with aphasia, motor speech disorders, right-hemisphere syndrome, traumatic brain injury, or dementia. The use of standard screening procedures ensures that everyone in the clinic does the screening in the same way and that the results obtained by one clinician are equivalent to the results obtained by any other clinician in the clinic.

Figure 5-6 shows a protocol for screening patients with suspected language impairment (aphasia). It takes 10 to 20 minutes to administer and provides a general sense of the patient's orientation and memory, auditory and reading comprehension, production of automatized sequences, repetition, naming, oral reading, and writing, together with a rating of the patient's conversational connected speech.

Screening protocols such as the one in Figure 5-6 serve several purposes. Sometimes they help identify patients for whom no additional testing is appropriate (e.g., patients with no significant impairments; patients who have complicating conditions such as dementia, confusion, or illness that would make formal assessment impossible or meaningless; or patients with severe and irreversible impairments). More often screening protocols help the clinician plan which tests to administer and the level of difficulty at which formal testing will begin. Finally, screening protocols provide the clinician with enough information about the nature and severity of the patient's linguistic or communicative impairments to permit the clinician to respond to the consultation request and to write initial impressions,

Language screening assessment

Date:	Reason for referral, significant history

Orientation, memory

What year is it? _____ [__]   What day of the week is it? _____ [__]

What time is it right now? _____ [__]   What city are we in? _____ [__]

Three-word recall: _____ _____ _____ [__]   **Number Correct [__ /5]**

Auditory comprehension

Single-word ("Point to the. . .")

Chair[__]   Ring[__]   Shoe[__]   Key[__]   Pencil[__]   **Number correct[__ /5]**

Yes-no questions

Personal information: (1) Is your first name (correct name)?[__]   (2) Is your last name (incorrect name)?[__]

Immediate environment: (3) Are we in a bus station right now?[__]   (4) Is it nighttime right now?[__]

Factual information: (5) Is a dime worth ten cents?[__]   (6) Do carrots grow on trees?[__]

Number correct [__ /6]

Sentence comprehension ("Point to the one that best matches what I say.")

A shoe.[__](shoe)   A standard comb.[__](comb)   Children play with this one.[__](ball) It has rubber on one end and a point on the other.[__](pencil)   The flat surface of this one is ideal for doing a jigsaw puzzle.[__](table)   **Number correct [__ /5]**

Reading comprehension

Word to picture matching (foils are in parentheses)

Fox (box, coat)[__]   Frog (flag, fish)[__]   Cup (spoon, cap)[__]   Letter (city, ladder)[__] Television (thermometer, camera)[__]   **Number Correct[__ /5]**

Patient identification:

Speech Pathology: language screening assessment (Page 1 of 2)

Figure 5-6 ■ A language screening assessment form that may be placed in a patient's medical record.

Continued

Automatized sequences

Counting: 1[__] 2[__] 3[__] 4[__] 5[__] 6[__] 7[__] 8[__] 9[__]
10[__]

Days of week: Sunday[__] Monday[__] Tuesday[__] Wednesday[__]
Thursday[__] Friday[__] Saturday[__] **Number correct [__ /17]**

Repetition

Words: Boy[__] Dog[__] Cowboy[__] Gingerbread[__] Artillery[__]
Number correct [__ /5]

Sentences: It was raining.[__] Bill went to the store.[__] Please put the groceries in the
refrigerator.[__] Arthur was an oozy, oily sneak.[__]
Number correct [__ /4]

Confrontation Naming: Pictures

dog[__] broom[__] airplane[__] igloo[__] tambourine[__] **Number correct [__ /5]**

Oral Reading

Words Man[__] Book[__] Forever[__] Understanding[__] Conventional[__]
Number correct [__ /5]

Sentences: It was raining.[__] Mary baked a pie.[__] Under the table in the dining room. [__]
The little girl was happy to see the new puppy. [__] **Number correct [__ /4]**

Rating of connected speech

Fluency: Fluent[__] Nonfluent[__]

Average phrase length (words): 1-2[__] 3-4[__] 5-6[__] >6[__]

Literal paraphasia: Absent[__] Infrequent[__] Frequent[__]

Verbal paraphasia: Absent[__] Infrequent[__] Frequent[__]

Word-finding in connected speech: Normal[__] Moderate impairment[__]
Severe impairment[__]

Writing

Name[__]
Letters to dictation: F[__] M[__] D[__] X[__] Q[__] **Number correct [__ /5]**
Words to dictation: Man[__] Today[__] Carrot[__] Venture[__]
Number correct [__ /4]

Comments and impressions:

_____   _____
Speech-language pathologist   Date
Speech pathology: language screening assessment
(Page 2 of 2)

Figure 5-6, cont'd ■ A language screening assessment form that may be placed in a patient's medical record.

diagnoses, and recommendations in a progress note in the patient's medical record. (Some screening forms such as the one in Figure 5-6 are themselves progress notes that can be placed in the patient's medical record.)

Assessment of adults with neurogenic language impairments does not always begin with a screening test and end with a comprehensive language test. When a comprehensive language test confirms the presence of language impairments, the clinician may administer supplemental tests to obtain a more detailed picture of the impairments. The following material describes how brain-injured adults' speech, auditory comprehension, reading, and writing typically are assessed, beginning with subtests in language test batteries and progressing to free-standing supplemental tests of specific abilities.

ASSESSING AUDITORY COMPREHENSION

Impairments in auditory comprehension have for many years occupied a central place in models of aphasia. Schuell (1965) considered impaired auditory comprehension and shortened auditory retention span the essence of aphasia.

> *Auditory comprehension* includes both *comprehension* of spoken materials and their *retention* in memory.

Numerous other writers have, like Schuell, given auditory impairment special status in defining the nature of aphasia and have, like Schuell, given auditory impairment special attention in treatment programs. All language test batteries include auditory comprehension subtests, and several free-standing tests devoted exclusively to assessment of auditory comprehension have been published. Some assess comprehension of single words, either in isolation or at the end of short carrier phrases. Some assess comprehension of single-sentence questions or instructions. A few assess comprehension of spoken narratives.

Single-Word Comprehension

Single-Word Comprehension Subtests in Language Test Batteries The most common procedure for testing single-word comprehension is a *select-from-an-array* procedure, in which the examiner places an array of drawn or printed stimuli (usually line drawings of objects) or real objects before the patient and says the names of the items in the array one at a time. Then the patient points to or touches each item after the examiner names it. Figure 5-7 shows such an array.

> In most of these tests the examiner delivers the test word at the end of a short carrier phrase, such as "Point to the [blank]." Because the carrier phrase quickly becomes redundant, these tests qualify as tests of single-word comprehension rather than as tests of sentence comprehension.

Arrays of drawings are not always drawings of objects. Sometimes they include drawings representing actions, printed letters or numbers, geometric forms, or color swatches. Figure 5-8 shows an array of drawings that might be used to test comprehension of action names.

Sometimes single-word comprehension is tested by asking the patient to point to objects in the environment. Other times it is tested by asking the patient to identify body parts, either on their own body or the examiner's body.

The inclusion of tests for comprehension of color, form, number, and body-part names in some language test batteries may be a response to a study by Goodglass and associates (1966). They tested aphasic adults' comprehension of the names of objects, actions, numbers, colors, and letters. They reported that aphasic adults are best at comprehending the names of pictured objects and actions and worst at comprehending the names of numbers, colors, and letters.

The presence of color, letter, and geometric form subtests in some language test batteries also may reflect the influence of several pub-

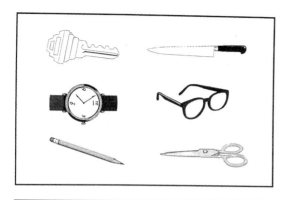

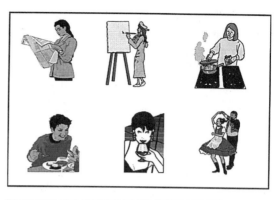

Figure 5-7 ■ A picture plate for testing single-word auditory comprehension. The examiner says the names of the items in random order and the patient points to a picture as the examiner names it.

Figure 5-8 ■ A response plate for testing verb comprehension. The examiner names in random order an action represented by a drawing and the patient points to the appropriate drawing.

lished case reports describing patients with unusual impairments in comprehending specific categories of words (e.g., color names). Although it may be clinically interesting and theoretically important to find a patient who comprehends color or letter names better (or worse) than the names of objects and actions, the relevance of such a finding to treatment planning or to estimation of the patient's daily life communicative competence seems enigmatic.

The single-word comprehension performance of most brain-injured adults who are tested using select-from-an-array procedures is not strongly affected by whether the items in the array are pictures or objects, although brain-injured adults with impairments in visual perception or visual discrimination tend to do better when arrays of real objects are used.

A study by Helm-Estabrooks (1981) suggests that aphasic adults may be affected by the nature of the array in which single-word comprehension stimuli are presented. Helm-Estabrooks tested aphasic adults' single-word comprehension in three conditions. In the *array* condition, 12 familiar objects (e.g., *book, spoon, cup*) were shown as individual line drawings on each of 12 cards arranged in three rows. In the *com-*

posite condition, smaller versions of the same 12 drawings were presented on a single card. In the *environment* condition, the 12 objects were distributed around the testing room. As a group the aphasic adults performed significantly better when pointing to pictured objects than when pointing to the real objects. Their performance was not significantly affected by whether the drawings were presented on individual cards or in a composite array. However, many subjects showed differences among conditions that were not consistent with group performance. Some were better in one of the picture conditions than the other, and some did better with real objects than they did with pictures.

Helm-Estabrooks commented that patients' difficulty *finding* objects distributed around the room, rather than difficulty *comprehending* their names, may have accounted for the differences between the pictured-object and real-object arrays. Helm-Estabrooks' report did not include the group's scores by conditions. Consequently, we cannot judge whether the statistically significant differences are also clinically significant. Nevertheless it seems important that clinicians keep in mind the potential effects of escalating demands on visual scanning and search as response arrays become larger and more widely distributed in the test environment.

> Statistically significant differences are not always clinically significant. The statistical significance of a difference depends on the magnitude of the difference, the number of observations contributing to the difference, and the variability among the observations. When variability among measures is small and many observations are made, a small difference may be statistically significant but clinically trivial. For example, a study of single-picture versus array conditions in a comprehension task might yield a mean score of 38/50 correct for the single-picture condition and a score of 36/50 correct for the array condition. If a large number of participants were studied and if their performances were relatively homogeneous, the 2-point difference might be statistically significant. However, most clinicians would consider the difference clinically trivial.

Free-Standing Tests of Single-Word Comprehension No free-standing tests of single-word auditory comprehension for brain-injured adults have been published, although picture vocabulary tests such as the *Peabody Picture Vocabulary Test-Revised* (PPVT-R; Dunn & Dunn, 1981) are, in a way, tests of single-word comprehension. However, picture vocabulary tests differ in content and purpose from single-word auditory comprehension tests for aphasic adults. Picture vocabulary tests include infrequent and unusual words (e.g., *lancinate, bumptiously*), some of which are known by few normal adults, whereas single-word comprehension tests for aphasic adults focus on common words that should be familiar to most normal adults (*fork, spoon, airplane*). The most common words represented in the early items of picture vocabulary tests may be equivalent to those in single-word comprehension tests for aphasic adults.

The norms for picture vocabulary tests are based on the entire test, and norms for performance on the more common items alone cannot be extracted, making partially completed picture vocabulary tests of limited use to clinicians who wish to compare an individual patient's performance with that of a norm group. A patient's performance on the common items in a picture vocabulary test could, however, serve as a baseline measure against which to measure the patient's response to the same items following treatment, and the patient's performance on the complete test may provide an estimate of the patient's available listening vocabulary, including a school grade level.

> Aphasic adults often make scattered errors throughout vocabulary test items that represent common words that most adults in the United States would know, followed by strings of consecutive errors when they reach less common items that many adults would not know. The early scattered errors probably represent something other than limited vocabulary—such as word retrieval failure, stimulus uncertainty, momentary inattention, and so on. Strings of consecutive errors when less common items are reached probably represent the limits of the individual's true listening vocabulary.

> Items in the last one third to one half of most vocabulary tests rarely occur in everyday communicative interactions. Consequently, impaired performance on those items may not suggest significant handicap in daily life interactions.

To carry the issue of how single-word comprehension may relate to daily life communicative competence a bit further, one might question the potential relevance of *any* test of single-word comprehension to daily life, given that in daily life one usually hears words in phrases or sentences and not in isolation. When one-word messages occur in daily life, they tend to be embedded in situational or linguistic context, and it is well known that brain-injured adults' comprehension of spoken material is enhanced by context. Consequently, it seems unlikely that brain-injured adults' performance on tests of single-word comprehension relates very strongly to daily life comprehension. Add to this the strangeness, in a daily life sense, of pointing to pictures or objects in response to their spoken names, and the potential relevance of tests of single-word comprehension to daily life comprehension becomes even more questionable.

Nevertheless most clinicians assess single-word comprehension as part of their testing routine for brain-injured adults. Tests of single-word comprehension are quick and easy to administer. The results of single-word comprehension tests may suggest unusual patterns of impaired performance, leading the clinician to revise a diagnosis or a treatment plan. For patients whose single-word comprehension is preserved, single-word comprehension tests may provide a comfortable lead-in to more challenging sentence-level and paragraph-level tests. For patients with severely impaired sentence comprehension, the results of testing at the single-word level may be the only indicator of the patient's spoken-language comprehension.

Variables That May Affect Brain-Injured Adults' Single-Word Comprehension

Frequency of Occurrence A word's frequency of occurrence in the language affects the ease with which aphasic listeners comprehend it (Figure 5-9). This effect can be seen in aphasic adults' performance on listening vocabulary tests such as the *Peabody Picture Vocabulary Test-Revised* (Dunn & Dunn, 1981), wherein most aphasic adults have inordinate difficulty with infrequently occurring words. However, see earlier comments on the potential implications of frequency of occurrence for comprehension in daily life. Because published norms for lexical frequency of occurrence are based on word frequency in printed materials, they may not accurately reflect frequency of oc-

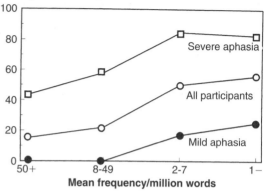

Figure 5-9 ■ The effects of word frequency on aphasic adults' single-word comprehension. As word frequency declines, error rates increase. (Data from Schuell, H. M., Jenkins, J. J., & Landis, L. [1961]. Relationship between auditory comprehension and word frequency in aphasia. *Journal of Speech and Hearing Research, 4,* 30-36.)

currence in daily life speech. Hayes (1989) has shown that printed materials contain a greater proportion of low-frequency (uncommon) words than do everyday spoken materials.

Semantic or Acoustic Similarity Between Target Words and Foils Semantic similarity between target words and foils usually has a much stronger effect on aphasic patients' accuracy in single-word comprehension tasks than does acoustic similarity. Schuell and Jenkins (1961), for example, reported that semantic confusions (such as *mother* for *father*) are far more frequent than either acoustic confusions (such as *dime* for *time*) or random errors (such as *motorcycle* for *cigarette*) when aphasic patients match spoken words to pictures (Figure 5-10).

Part of Speech Part of speech affects some aphasic adults' single-word comprehension, although the effect appears highly variable across individual aphasic adults. Miceli and associates (1988) studied aphasic adults' comprehension of nouns and verbs and found all possible patterns of noun versus verb comprehension in a group of

Percent of errors

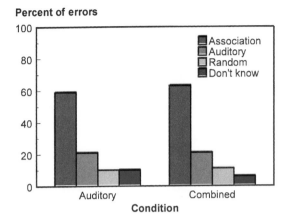

Figure 5-10 ■ **Performance on a test of single-word comprehension by a group of aphasic adults.** *Association errors* **are errors in which an individual chose a semantically related foil.** *Auditory errors* **are errors in which an individual chose a foil that sounded like the target word.** *Random errors* **are errors in which an individual chose a foil that had no semantic or acoustic similarity to the target. In** *auditory condition,* **the examiner said the target word and the aphasic individual chose one of two pictures. In** *combined condition,* **the examiner showed the aphasic individual a card on which the target word was printed and said the target word.**

75 brain-injured adults. Some did better on nouns than verbs, some did better on verbs than nouns, and some performed equally well (or poorly) on nouns and verbs. Consequently, clinicians can anticipate that part of speech may affect an aphasic adult's single-word comprehension, but the nature of the effect can be determined only by testing the patient.

Referent Ambiguity Referent ambiguity (ambiguity in pictured referents for spoken words) may affect aphasic patients' performance in matching spoken words to pictures. If pictorial referents are ambiguous or unclear, patients may respond inaccurately—not because they fail to comprehend the words, but because they are unable to deduce what the pictures represent.

Fidelity The fidelity of spoken messages (from words to discourse) can have important effects on aphasic listeners' comprehension (and, if the loss of fidelity is serious, on that of non-brain-injured listeners, too). Most aphasic adults' comprehension of spoken materials deteriorates in noisy listening environments or when speech is acoustically distorted. Answering the telephone can be a challenge for many aphasic adults because most telephones are low-fidelity instruments and many produce background noise.

Many audiotape recorders or players (especially inexpensive ones) have poor fidelity and create objectionable levels of background noise on playback. The distortion and interference created by these instruments can compromise aphasic adults' performance when they are used to play tapes in testing and treatment. Clinicians can minimize distortion and noise by using high-quality tape recorders and high-quality audiotape for materials used in testing and treatment.

Sentence Comprehension

Sentence Comprehension Subtests in Language Test Batteries All the major language test batteries include sentence comprehension subtests. Most require patients to perform gestural or manipulative responses to spoken commands. In some the patient points to one or more items in a set of pictures, objects, or body parts ("Point to the [pictured] dog, garage, and ladder. Point to the ceiling and then to the floor. Show me the one used for fixing hair. Point to your left ear and your right knee."). In others patients manipulate objects or body parts ("Ring the bell, close the box, and give me the key. Tap each shoulder twice with two fingers keeping your eyes closed.").

Most language test batteries also include subtests for assessing comprehension of spoken yes-no questions. The yes-no questions in these tests assess comprehension of different kinds of information. Some questions test personal information ("Is your last name Smith?"). Some test the patient's perception of the surrounding environment ("Are the lights on in this room?"). Some test knowledge learned in school ("Was Abraham Lincoln the first President of the United States?"). Some ask for opinions, inferences, or abstractions ("Should children disobey their parents?" "Is it possible for a good swimmer to be drowned?"). Some test general knowledge ("Do apples grow on trees?"). Questions that test general knowledge can be further divided into questions that test comprehension of temporal relationships ("Does March come before June?"), numerical relationships ("Are there seven days in a week?"), and comparative relationships ("Are towns larger than cities?").

Free-Standing Tests of Sentence Comprehension The *Token Test* (DeRenzi & Vignolo, 1962) and its variants are among the most widely used free-standing tests of sentence-level auditory comprehension. In the original DeRenzi and Vignolo version of the *Token Test,* 62 spoken commands direct the patient to touch or manipulate 20 tokens (5 large circles, 5 small circles, 5 large rectangles, and 5 small rectangles in each of 5 colors—red, yellow, green, white, and blue). There are 5 levels in the original *Token Test,* and the length and complexity of commands increases from level 1 to level 5.

- Level 1: Touch the red circle.
- Level 2: Touch the large blue rectangle.
- Level 3: Touch the red rectangle and the blue circle.
- Level 4: Touch the large white circle and the small green rectangle.
- Level 5: When I touch the green circle, you take the white rectangle.

Responses are scored correct or incorrect, and the maximum score is 62. No norms are provided in the DeRenzi and Vignolo version (1962), although norms for adults and children can be found elsewhere (Gaddes & Crockett, 1973; Noll & Lass, 1972; Spreen & Benton, 1977; Wertz, Keith, & Custer, 1971).

Several modified versions of the *Token Test* have been published. One is a subtest of the *Neurosensory Center Comprehensive Examination for Aphasia* (NCCEA; Spreen & Benton,

1977). It contains 39 test commands similar to those in the original *Token Test* divided among six levels of length and complexity. The easiest level in the Spreen and Benton version contains commands such as "Show me a square" and "Show me a red one," which permits testing patients at a lower level than provided for in the original *Token Test* and also permits identification of patients with specific impairments in comprehension of color or shape names. The Spreen and Benton version of the *Token Test* allows users to score patients' responses according to how accurately they represent the critical elements in test commands. For example, the command "Point to the small white circle" is worth three points—one each for *small, white,* and *circle.* A perfect score on the Spreen and Benton version of the *Token Test* is 163 points. Norms for aphasic adults, non-aphasic but brain-injured adults, and non-brain-injured adults are provided in the NCCEA manual.

> Spreen and Benton replaced rectangles with squares, which brings the Token Test shape names closer together in terms of their frequency of occurrence in English. *Rectangle* occurs approximately 10 times per million words; *circle* and *square* each occur approximately 140 times per million words. Most users of the original version of the *Token Test* also replace rectangles with squares.

The Spreen and Benton version of the *Token Test* appears to be as sensitive to the presence of impaired auditory comprehension as the original DeRenzi and Vignolo version (Orgass & Poeck, 1966); is quicker to administer, score, and interpret; and gives partial credit for responses that include some but not all of the critical elements in test commands. Consequently, the Spreen and Benton version is more widely used in the United States and Canada than the DeRenzi and Vignolo version.

The *Revised Token Test* (RTT; McNeil & Prescott, 1978) is a longer and more elaborate version of DeRenzi and Vignolo's test. The RTT has

10 subtests, each with 10 equally difficult test commands. The first 4 subtests in the RTT are similar to the first 4 parts of the original *Token Test*. Tests 5 through 8 each consist of 10 items that test comprehension of positional relationships (*in front of, behind, above, below, to the right of*). Tests 9 and 10 test comprehension of complex grammatic relationships (*instead of, unless, if, either*). Patients' responses to RTT items are scored with a multidimensional system similar to that for the *Porch Index of Communicative Ability* (Porch, 1981a). Profiles for five "auditory processing deficits" are provided in the test manual. Several procedures for scoring and analyzing patients' responses are provided.

The *Revised Token Test* takes longer to administer, score, and interpret than the other versions (usually more than an hour). Its comprehensiveness and its psychometric integrity make it a powerful research tool, but its length and complexity may preclude its use in routine clinical evaluation of brain-injured adults' sentence comprehension.

The *Token Test* and its variants are sensitive measures of sentence comprehension. Even patients with mild comprehension impairments are likely to have difficulty on higher-level token test commands. However, this sensitivity makes the token tests difficult or impossible for patients with severe comprehension impairments. A few patients have inordinate difficulty with token tests, compared with their performance on other tests of auditory comprehension. Some have specific difficulty with color, shape, and size descriptors. Others have temporal sequencing impairments that prevent them from maintaining the temporal order of the responses required by token test commands. (These patients typically point to the correct tokens but in the wrong order.) A few patients may have motor planning impairments (limb apraxias), which prevent them from making the required pointing responses, even though they understand the commands.

To rule out problems with comprehension of color, shape, and size descriptors, patients can be pretested by asking them to point to *a red one, a circle, a small one,* and so on (a procedure included as the first level in the Spreen and Benton version of the *Token Test* and as a pretest for the *Revised Token Test*). To rule out temporal sequencing impairments and limb apraxias as the cause of deficient performance, the examiner can ask the patient to imitate sequences of pointing responses modeled by the examiner. If the patient is successful, temporal sequencing impairments and limb apraxia become unlikely explanations for the deficient performance.

> In my experience, few patients have such severe limb apraxia that they cannot point sequentially to test tokens. However, it should be kept in mind as a potential cause of poor performance on token tests and other tests requiring sequential pointing, gestural, or manipulative responses.

Some patients with poor comprehension improve their performance on tests like the token tests by visually fixating on items in the array as they are named by the examiner, thereby using visual strategies to compensate for impaired auditory memory. These patients' performances deteriorate if the target items are covered while the commands are spoken. If the examiner suspects that a patient is relying on a visual strategy in a test of comprehension with an array of visual stimuli, covering the array while test commands are spoken will ensure that patients' performances reflect only auditory comprehension and retention.

For patients with subtle comprehension and retention impairments, examiners can increase the difficulty of sentence comprehension tests by imposing a delay interval between test sentences and the opportunity for the patient to respond. A 10-second or 20-second delay usually reveals even the most subtle auditory retention impairments. However, testing patients using nonstandard procedures may preclude comparison of their performance with norms based on the standard procedures.

The *Token Test* and its variants test comprehension of a limited range of syntactic structures and provide little information about a patient's listening vocabulary. Other free-standing tests of sentence comprehension permit testing a greater variety of syntactic structures and a greater vocabulary range.

Some sentence comprehension tests designed for children can be used to test adults with suspected comprehension impairments. Most do not provide norms for either normal or brain-injured adults, but they permit detailed analysis of the effects of various grammatic and syntactic variables on comprehension. For this reason they occasionally are used to evaluate how brain-injured adults are affected by those variables, although no comparisons of brain-injured patients with an adult norm group are possible. However, the content and form of these tests can be child-like, and some adults may consider them demeaning.

The *Northwestern Syntax Screening Test* (NSST; Lee, 1971) is a screening test of sentence comprehension for use with children. The NSST contains 20 sentences and 10 picture pages with 4 choices on each page. The 20 sentences evaluate comprehension of various grammatic and syntactic forms (such as locational prepositions, negation, subject-verb agreement, and tense).

The *Test for Auditory Comprehension of Language, Third Edition* (TACL-3; Carrow-Woodfolk, 1999) is a 142-item comprehension test designed for use with children, although it contains guidelines for use with adults. The test permits assessment of patients' comprehension of *word classes and relations* (nouns, verbs, adjectives, adverbs), *grammatic morphemes* (noun-verb agreement, number, tense, and case), and *elaborated phrases and sentences* (interrogative, negative, and embedded sentences; partially connected sentences).

Variables That May Affect Brain-Injured Listeners' Sentence Comprehension

Length and Syntactic Complexity Although several variables can affect brain-injured listeners' comprehension of spoken sentences, two of the strongest are *sentence length* and *syntactic complexity*. As spoken sentences become longer or syntactically more complex, they become more difficult for aphasic listeners to comprehend, provided other sentence characteristics do not change. Syntactic complexity seems to have stronger negative effects on comprehension than either sentence length or vocabulary difficulty (Shewan & Canter, 1971; Goodglass, Blumstein, Gleason, & associates, 1979; Nicholas & Brookshire, 1983).

For example, Goodglass and associates (1979) presented two sets of spoken sentences to aphasic listeners. The sentences in one set were syntactically complex ("The man greeted by his wife was smoking a pipe."), and the sentences in the other set were syntactically simpler forms of the same sentences ("The man was greeted by his wife and he was smoking a pipe."). Aphasic listeners comprehended the syntactically simpler sentences better than the syntactically complex ones, even though the simple sentences were longer than the complex ones.

> Increasing sentence length may facilitate aphasic adults' comprehension if the increased length also adds redundancy—something clinicians should keep in mind when designing treatment procedures.

Syntactically simple active sentences ("The dog bit the boy.") are easier for aphasic listeners to comprehend than passive sentences ("The boy was bitten by the dog."). Conditional sentences ("If the cup is blue, give it to me."), negative sentences ("The dog is not chasing the rabbit."), sentences with locational or directional statements ("Put the cup behind the box."), and comparative or relational sentences ("Is the boy taller than the girl?") are difficult for many aphasic listeners. Embedded clause sentences ("The letter the girl wrote is on the table.") are very difficult for almost all aphasic listeners (and for many non-aphasic listeners). The relative difficulty of sentences with various syntactic structures appears to be similar for aphasic adults exhibiting different levels of aphasia severity (Figure 5-11). Aphasic adults usually exhibit the same pattern of difficulty across syntax types as non-brain-injured adults do, although they take longer to comprehend the sentences and they make more errors.

Reversibility and Plausibility Reversible sentences, in which subjects and objects can be transposed without creating implausible sentences ("The man is hugging the woman" reverses to "The woman is hugging the man"), are more difficult than sentences for which transposition generates an implausible sentence ("The man is carrying the book" reverses to "The book is carrying the man"). Sentences that are improbable (but not implausible) when subject and object are transposed ("The dog is chasing the cat" reverses to "The cat is chasing the dog") are likely to be of intermediate difficulty.

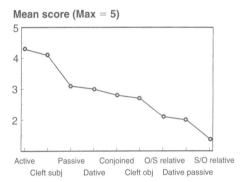

Mean score (Max = 5)

Active: The student hit the beggar.
Cleft subject: It was the student that hit the beggar.
Passive: The beggar was hit by the student.
Dative: The student gave the paper to the beggar.
Conjoined: The student hit the beggar and pushed the mailman.
Cleft Object: It was the beggar that the student hit.
Object/Subject Relative: The student that hit the beggar pushed the mailman.
Dative/Passive: The paper was given to the beggar by the student.
Subject/Object Relative: The beggar that the student hit pushed the mailman.

Figure 5-11 ■ Performance of a group of aphasic adults on a test of sentence comprehension in which the syntactic complexity of sentences was manipulated. As syntactic complexity increased, the performance of the aphasic adults declined. (Data from Caplan, D., Baker, C., & DeHaut, F. [1985]. Syntactic determinants of sentence comprehension in aphasia. *Cognition, 21,* 117-125.)

Caramazza and Zurif (1976) investigated the effects of reversibility on aphasic listeners' comprehension of embedded clause sentences ("The apple that the boy is eating is red."). They concluded that aphasic adults' sentence comprehension was poorer when sentences were reversible than when they were not, although their major finding was that their aphasic subjects relied heavily on plausibility to comprehend syntactically complex sentences.

Predictability Some sentences are predictable, in that they create expectations in the listener's mind, then violate the expectations. For this reason they are sometimes called *garden-path sentences*. Most garden-path sentences rely on the listener's (or reader's) more-or-less automatic syntactic processing to lead them astray, as in "The horse raced past the barn fell" (Caplan, 1987), in which the listener or reader first assumes that *raced* is the sentence's main verb, but later discovers that *fell* is actually the main verb, whereas *raced past the barn* is a phrase modifying *horse*. Normal listeners' comprehension of garden-path sentences has been intensively studied (Bever, Garrett, & Hurtig, 1973; Foss & Jenkins, 1973; Lackner & Garrett, 1972; Mackay, 1966; and others), primarily to construct or validate models of sentence processing. Not surprisingly, non-brain-injured adults take more time to comprehend garden-path sentences than straightforward ones, and they often miscomprehend them.

> To be led down the garden path is an idiomatic phrase meaning "to be led astray."

Personal Relevance The personal relevance of questions affects their difficulty for most aphasic listeners. Gray and associates (1977) and Busch and Brookshire (1982) evaluated aphasic adults' responses to three categories of spoken yes-no questions. Questions in one category referred to nonpersonal factual information ("Do apples grow on trees?"). Questions in another category referred to information about the immediate environment ("Are we in a hospital?"). Questions in a third category referred to personal information ("Is your name Smith?"). In both studies, aphasic adults' responses to personal information questions were more accurate than their responses to questions about the immediate environment, and their responses to questions about the immediate environment were more accurate than their responses to questions about nonpersonal factual information. Although similar studies have not been carried out with open-ended questions, it seems reasonable to expect that their difficulty would be affected similarly by personal relevance.

Semantic Variables Brain-injured adults often get into trouble when factual questions are falsified by substituting a semantically related word for a word that makes the sentence true. For instance, "Does the sun rise in the west?" from the MTDDA trips up many patients, whereas "Does the sun rise in the living room?" would mislead only those with severely impaired comprehension (or who have very large living rooms).

Reasoning and Inferences Questions that require reasoning or making inferences ("Is it possible for a good swimmer to be drowned?") are more difficult than questions in which reasoning or inference are not required if the length, vocabulary, and syntactic structure of the sentences are equivalent. Answering inferential questions adds to the processing load in comprehension by requiring that the patient (1) recognize that relevant information is not in memory in verbatim form, (2) construct the relevant information, using preexisting knowledge, (3) relate the relevant information to the question, and (4) produce the answer. Brain-injured adults may perform poorly on questions requiring inferences because they do not realize that an inference is called for, are unable to identify or retrieve from memory information relevant to the inference, are unable to construct the inference, or cannot produce the answer. Questions such

as "Why should children attend school?" also require longer and more complex responses, so that verbal formulation and production problems may compromise brain-injured adults' responses to such questions.

Rate Slowing the rate at which commands are spoken or placing pauses in test commands facilitates the performance of many aphasic patients (Parkhurst, 1970; Liles & Brookshire, 1975). Unfortunately, it is not clear which patients are most sensitive to rate or pause manipulations, and the effects are not always consistent from test to test, even for the same patient (Brookshire & Nicholas, 1984).

A study by Salvatore, Strait, and Brookshire (1978) showed that changes in the rate at which clinicians speak comprehension test sentences can have clinical consequences. Salvatore and associates had experienced and inexperienced examiners administer a token test to one group of patients who had mild comprehension impairments and another group of patients who had severe comprehension impairments. Salvatore and associates reported that the experienced examiners spoke test commands at a slower rate than the inexperienced examiners, that both experienced and inexperienced examiners spoke test commands at a slower rate when they tested severely impaired patients than when they tested mildly impaired patients, and that both experienced and inexperienced examiners spoke test commands at a slower rate following patient errors than following correct responses.

Because examiners' variability in delivering token test commands may affect patients' performance and because even experienced clinicians change their delivery of token test commands in response to patients' performance, clinicians who incorporate a token test into their testing routine may choose to record the test commands with uniform speech rate and consistent intonation, stress, and pauses and use the recording to test patients, rather reading the test commands aloud.

Redundancy The redundancy of spoken sentences also affects their comprehensibility for aphasic adults. West and Kaufman (1972) compared aphasic listeners' comprehension of token-test-like commands, in which some commands repeated key words (as in, "Show me the big **blue circle** and the little **blue circle.**"), with their comprehension of commands that did not repeat key words (as in, "Show me the big blue circle and the small red square."). The lexically redundant commands were easier for aphasic adults than were the lexically nonredundant commands.

Gardner, Albert, and Weintraub (1975) reported that *semantic* redundancy also affects aphasic listeners' sentence comprehension. Gardner and associates reported that aphasic listeners comprehended semantically redundant sentences ("You see a **cat** that is **furry.**") better than semantically neutral sentences ("You see a cat that is nice.") although the statistical analyses did not strongly support their conclusion.

Number, Similarity, and Nature of Response Choices The *number of choices* available for pointing or manipulation and *similarity among the choices* can affect the difficulty of tasks in which aphasic listeners point to or manipulate tokens, objects, or pictures in response to spoken directions. In general, increasing the number of choices increases the difficulty of the task. "Point to the red circle" is less difficult if there are three choices (red circle, blue square, yellow circle) than if there are six (red circle, blue circle, yellow circle, red square, blue square, yellow square). Increasing the similarity among choices also increases the difficulty of the task. "Point to the knife" is more difficult for aphasic listeners if the targets are semantically related (*fork, knife, spoon*) than when they are not (*knife, umbrella, hippopotamus*).

There is some evidence that brain-injured adults' performance on point-to tests of spoken-sentence comprehension is slightly better when the choice stimuli are real objects rather than tokens (Kreindler, Gheorghita, & Voinescu, 1971; Martino, Pizzamiglio, & Razzano, 1976; LaPointe, Holtzapple, & Graham, 1985). However, the differences between performance on token tests

and picture or object tests generally are small, and when results for individual subjects are reported, the performance of individual subjects often does not match that of the group. For most brain-injured adults it probably makes little difference whether tokens, pictures, or objects are used in point-to tests of sentence comprehension. On average, their scores on token tests are likely to be slightly worse than their performance on picture or object tests. This makes token tests slightly more sensitive to the presence of subtle comprehension impairments but also causes them to underestimate most patients' daily life comprehension.

> The chance probability of correct responses diminishes as the number of choices increases. When a patient has only two response choices, one of which is correct, one half of the patient's responses would, on the average, be correct if the patient were to respond randomly. Increasing the number of choices to four lowers the chance probability of correct responses to 1 in 4 (25%). The chance probability of a correct response in a 10-item array is 1 in 10 (10%), and so on.

Sentence Comprehension and Comprehension in Daily Life The items in most sentence comprehension tests are not very representative of what most adults are likely to encounter in daily life. In most sentence comprehension tests the patient hears a series of minimally redundant sentences, with no relationship among sentences in the series. The patient must remember the information from each sentence long enough to answer a question or point to tokens or a picture but then can forget it because each sentence is unrelated to the preceding sentences. In this respect sentence comprehension tests are similar to immediate-memory tests in which the examiner reads lists of numbers or words and the patient must recognize or reproduce them after a few seconds delay. In daily life adult listeners rarely hear strings of nonredundant sentences with no relationship to each other or to the listener's prior knowledge. They usually need only remember the gist of the sentences and not their verbatim form, and they usually have to remember the gist for more than a few seconds.

In daily life speakers relate new information to what they assume the listener already knows, and they relate the new information to preceding utterances and to a topic, thereby creating a semantic context for individual utterances. Single-sentence comprehension tests eliminate that context, no doubt to the detriment of the patient being tested, because brain-injured listeners, like non-brain-injured ones, use context to help them comprehend what they hear (Stachowiak, Huber, Poeck, & associates, 1977; Waller & Darley, 1978; Pierce, 1989; and others). Consequently, it seems unlikely that brain-injured patients' performance on sentence comprehension tests predicts a brain-injured patient's comprehension of what is said in typical daily life communicative interactions.

The results of several studies suggest that performance on sentence comprehension tests is not a dependable indicator of patients' comprehension of multiple-sentence spoken discourse (Stachowiak, Huber, Poeck, & associates, 1977; Brookshire & Nicholas, 1984; Wegner, Brookshire, & Nicholas, 1984; and others). These studies have shown that sentence comprehension test scores do reasonably well in predicting scores on other *sentence-level* tests of comprehension, but they are poor at predicting scores on tests of *discourse* comprehension. Consequently, clinicians should be cautious in making inferences about brain-injured listeners' daily-life comprehension competence based on their performance on single-sentence comprehension tests because brain-injured listeners are likely to perform better in daily life than their single-sentence comprehension test scores suggest that they should.

Comprehension of Spoken Discourse

Discourse Comprehension Subtests in Language Test Batteries Some language test batteries (e.g., the BDAE and the MTDDA) include subtests to assess comprehension of spoken discourse, albeit in a limited way. The items in these subtests are paragraphs read aloud by the examiner, followed by spoken questions about the paragraphs, as in the following example, which is part of a paragraph comprehension test item from the MTDDA.

Gold was first discovered in California by a millwright named James Marshall. Marshall was building a sawmill on the banks of the American River. One morning in January, 1848, as he was walking along the millrace, he saw some bright flakes at the bottom of a ditch. Marshall picked up a handful and took them back to the fort to show his partner, John Sutter. They turned out to be pure gold. Marshall and Sutter tried to keep the discovery a secret ...

In this story, did Marshall discover gold on the Rio Grande?

Did Marshall and Sutter try to spread the news of the discovery?

The BDAE discourse comprehension subtest includes four short paragraphs, two of which are factual narratives, similar to the one in the MTDDA, and two of which are humorous vignettes, such as the following.

A customer walked into a hotel carrying a coil of rope in one hand and a suitcase in the other. The hotel clerk asked, "Pardon me, sir, but would you tell me what the rope is for?" "Yes," responded the man, "that's my fire escape!" "I'm sorry, sir," said the clerk, "but all guests carrying their own fire escapes must pay in advance."

Was the customer carrying a suitcase in each hand?

Did the clerk trust this guest?

The BDAE and the MTDDA stories differ in several ways. The BDAE story seems more interesting, does not contain as much detailed information, and has an overall point (the punch line). It also resembles stories (or jokes) that are common in person-to-person interactions and on radio and television programs. Factual passages such as the MTDDA paragraph are more likely to be encountered in printed form in educational settings than in everyday spoken interactions.

A Free-Standing Test of Discourse Comprehension The *Discourse Comprehension Test* (DCT; Brookshire & Nicholas, 1993) is the only free-standing standardized test for assessment of brain-injured adults' spoken discourse comprehension. The DCT contains 10 tape-recorded narrative stories that are controlled for number of words and sentences, mean sentence length, speech rate, number of unfamiliar words, listening difficulty, and grammatic complexity.

Eight questions test the patient's comprehension and retention of information from each story in the DCT. Four questions for each story test main ideas and four questions test details. Two of the main idea questions and two of the detail questions for each story test information that is directly stated in the story. The remaining two main idea and two detail questions test information that is implied by information in the story, so that patients must make inferences to answer them correctly.

The DCT manual provides performance data for 40 non-brain-injured adults, 20 aphasic adults, 20 adults with right-hemisphere damage, and 20 adults with traumatic brain injuries. Cutoff scores for normal performance are provided for the full 10-story version of the DCT and for two 5-story short versions. Materials for administering the DCT as a silent-reading test are included, and performance data for 20 non-brain-injured adults for the reading version of the DCT are included in the test manual. Following is a story and questions from the DCT.

One day last Fall, several women on Willow Street decided to have a garage sale. They collected odds and ends from all over the neighborhood. Then they spent an entire day putting prices on the things that they had collected. On the first day of the sale, they put up signs at both ends of the block and another one at a nearby shopping center. Next they made a batch of iced tea and sat down in a shady spot beside the Anderson's garage to wait for their first customer. Soon a man drove up in an old truck. He looked around and finally stopped by a lumpy old mattress that was leaning against the wall. He gestured to it and asked how much they wanted for it. Mrs. Anderson told him that it wasn't for sale. Then she added that they were going to put it out for the trash collectors the next day. The man asked if he could have it. Mrs. Anderson said that he could. Then she asked, "Why do you want such a terrible mattress?" "Well," he said, "My no-good father-in-law is coming to visit next week and I don't want him to get too comfortable."

QUESTIONS
1. Did several women have a party? (No) [Stated main idea]
2. Were there a large number of things at the garage sale? (Yes) [Implied main idea]
3. Did the women put up a sign at a shopping center? (Yes) [Stated detail]
4. Was it cold the day of the garage sale? (No) [Implied detail]
5. Was the man driving a car? (No) [Stated detail]
6. Was the mattress in terrible condition? (Yes) [Stated main idea]
7. Was the man married? (Yes) [Implied detail]
8. Was the man fond of his father-in-law? (No) [Implied main idea]

Variables That May Affect Brain-Injured Adults' Comprehension of Spoken Discourse
Many of the variables mentioned earlier as affecting sentence comprehension also affect discourse comprehension, but not necessarily to the same degree as they affect comprehension

of isolated sentences. Because discourse permits listeners greater use of heuristic processes, variables such as word frequency and syntactic complexity, which can have strong effects on listeners' comprehension of sentences, do not have equally strong effects on their comprehension of discourse. However, several variables may have important effects on listeners' comprehension of discourse. Two of the most important are *salience* and *directness*.

Heuristic processes in comprehension denote processes in which the listener or reader uses world knowledge and previous experience to arrive at the meaning of spoken or printed materials. Heuristic processing is sometimes called top-down processing because the listener or reader begins with assumptions about the general meaning of spoken or printed materials and uses those assumptions to guide lexical and syntactic analyses.

Salience Speakers (and writers) make information salient by means of devices such as repetition, elaboration, and paraphrase and by establishing syntactic and semantic relationships among parts of the discourse. In this way speakers make important information stand out (the *main ideas*) and de-emphasize information that is less important to the overall sense of the discourse (the *details*). Both normal listeners and listeners with brain injury comprehend and remember main ideas in discourse better than details (Meyer, 1975; Meyer & McGonkie, 1973; Kintsch, 1974; Brookshire & Nicholas, 1984; Wegner, Brookshire, & Nicholas, 1984; Nicholas & Brookshire, 1995b; and others).

Directness Normal speakers do not always specify all the information needed for listeners to understand the speaker's meaning and intent (Clark & Haviland, 1977). Instead they may leave informational gaps and expect the listener to construct inferences and make assumptions to fill in the gaps. For example, a speaker might say,

"When I looked out the window, I saw the garage in flames. It took the firemen 20 minutes to get here, but by then it was too late."—expecting the listener to infer that the speaker called the fire department right away and that the garage was destroyed.

Several studies have assessed the effects of directness (whether information is directly stated or implied) on brain-injured adults' comprehension of information in spoken discourse (Nicholas & Brookshire, 1986; Nicholas & Brookshire, 1995; Katsuki-Nakamura, Brookshire, & Nicholas, 1988). In these studies brain-injured adults, like those without brain damage, had more difficulty with questions that tested implied information from discourse than they did with questions that tested stated information. The differences between questions about stated information and questions about implied information were greatest when the required inferences went beyond simple paraphrase of information in the discourse and required listeners to retrieve relevant information from memory and connect it with information provided by the speaker (Nicholas & Brookshire, 1986).

Redundancy Repetition, elaboration, and paraphrase increase the redundancy of discourse and highlight important information, making it easier for the listener to establish the overall theme or point of the discourse, organize it in memory, and recall it later. Repetition, elaboration, and paraphrase also contribute to the relatedness of information in discourse (its *cohesion*) and to the overall unity of the material (its *coherence*).

Cohesion and Coherence Cohesion denotes the degree to which the semantic units within discourse relate to each other. Cohesion is produced by linguistic devices called *cohesive ties*. Many kinds of cohesive ties have been described in the literature (Halliday & Hasan, 1976), but a few examples will suffice. *Pronominal* ties are created by pronouns that refer back to a previously mentioned referent ("The boy was lost. **He** stood in the center of the plaza, crying."). *Conjunctive* ties are created by conjunctions ("The horse was fast, **but** lost the race."). *Lexical repetition* ties are created by repeating words (or their synonyms) in nearby propositions ("The man and the woman got on the train. The **man** carried a large black suitcase. The **woman carried** flowers.").

Coherence denotes the overall unity of discourse. Multiple variables, which are not readily quantified, contribute to coherence. Cohesion and coherence contribute to heuristic, top-down comprehension processes. Consequently, cohesive and coherent discourse is much easier for both normal and brain-injured listeners to comprehend and retain in memory than noncohesive or noncoherent discourse.

Speech Rate and Emphatic Stress Speech rate and emphatic stress may affect aphasic listeners' comprehension of discourse. Pashek and Brookshire (1982) presented spoken paragraphs at slow speech rate (120 wpm) or normal speech rate (150 wpm), with either normal stress or exaggerated stress (extra prosodic emphasis on important words). They found (1) that both slow rate and exaggerated stress facilitated aphasic listeners' comprehension of the paragraphs, (2) that slow rate was slightly more effective than exaggerated stress in improving comprehension, and (3) that comprehension was best when slow rate and exaggerated stress were combined. Kimelman and McNeil (1987) replicated Pashek and Brookshire's study and reported similar results.

Nicholas and Brookshire (1986) reported that not all aphasic listeners' comprehension of discourse improves when speech rate is slowed and sometimes an aphasic listener benefits from slowed speech rate at one time and not at another. They presented narrative stories to aphasic listeners at slow (120 wpm) and fast (200 wpm) speech rates and tested their comprehension twice, with a week or more between tests. In the first session, slow speech rate improved comprehension of the aphasic listeners as a group. However, the facilitating effects of slow speech rate at the group level essentially disappeared by the second session, and there were many in-

stances in which individual subjects failed to demonstrate rate effects exhibited by their group.

GENERAL CONCEPTS 5-1

- Language test batteries provide a general sense of an individual's speech, auditory comprehension, reading, and writing. Most help clinicians identify communication impairments and plan treatment. Some help clinicians make a diagnosis and predict recovery.

- The *Minnesota Test for Differential Diagnosis of Aphasia* contains 47 subtests and takes 3 to 6 hours to administer. It permits users to assign patients to one of five major and two minor categories of aphasia.

- The *Porch Index of Communicative Ability* uses the same 10 test items in each of its 18 subtests. Users score responses with a 16-category, binary-choice scoring system. The PICA provides several procedures for charting patients' performance and predicting recovery.

- The *Boston Diagnostic Aphasia Examination* contains 27 subtests in its standard form, which takes from 1 to 5 hours to administer. A 21-subtest short form takes about 1 hour to administer. The BDAE permits users to assign patients to classic neurodiagnostic aphasia syndromes and to measure patients' performance across a large number of tasks.

- The *Western Aphasia Battery (WAB)* resembles the *Boston Diagnostic Aphasia Examination* but is shorter and psychometrically more sophisticated. Those who use the WAB may classify patients into classic aphasia syndromes with a taxonomic procedure.

- Although a commercially marketed screening test for aphasia may not be necessary, a standard procedure for screening aphasic patients is necessary to ensure uniformity across users within a facility.

- Screening tests help clinicians identify patients for whom treatment is not appropriate, plan subsequent testing, and respond to consultation requests.

- *Single-word comprehension* typically is tested by asking the patient to point to common objects or pictures of common objects named by the examiner. Most aphasic patients' performance is not greatly affected by whether the test stimuli are objects or pictures.

- Several variables may affect aphasic adults' single-word comprehension, including:
  - —*Frequency of occurrence* (low-frequency words are more difficult for most aphasic patients)
  - —*Semantic or acoustic similarity* between target words and foils (semantic similarity has stronger effects for most aphasic patients)
  - —*Part of speech* (nouns and verbs are perhaps easier than other parts of speech, but there is great variability across aphasic patients)
  - —*Referent ambiguity* (ambiguous pictured referents compromise patients' performance)
  - —*Fidelity* of spoken messages (low fidelity compromises performance)
- *Picture vocabulary tests* contain large portions of low-frequency words because they are designed to estimate an individual's receptive vocabulary rather than their daily life auditory comprehension.
- *Sentence comprehension* typically is tested by asking patients to perform gestural or manipulative responses to spoken instructions or to answer spoken yes-no questions.
- *Yes-no questions* may test *personal information, perception of surroundings, knowledge learned in school,* or *general knowledge.* General knowledge questions may test *temporal, numeric,* or *comparative* relationships. Some yes-no questions ask for *opinions* or *inferences,* which require extended speech, thereby compromising the performance of patients with speech-production problems.
- The *Token Test* is a widely used test of sentence comprehension for brain-injured adults. It requires manipulation of colored large and small circles and squares in response to the examiner's instructions. The Spreen and Benton version is shorter and permits scoring of critical elements within commands.

- Several variables affect the difficulty of sentence comprehension tests for aphasic adults:
  - —*Length and syntactic complexity.* Longer and syntactically more complex sentences are more difficult. Syntactic complexity usually has stronger effects.
  - —*Reversibility and plausibility.* Semantically reversible sentences are more difficult than nonreversible ones. Plausibility may allow patients to use general knowledge to enhance comprehension.
  - —*Predictability.* Syntactic or semantic constraints on sentence content contribute to ease of comprehension.
  - —*Personal relevance.* Sentences about personally relevant material are easier for most aphasic patients to comprehend than sentences about less personal material.
  - —*Semantic relationships.* Sentences that are falsified by substituting a semantically related word for a key word in the sentence are difficult for many aphasic patients to identify as false.
  - —*Rate.* Slow rate helps many aphasic patients comprehend spoken sentences, but the effects of slow rate may be variable across patients and within patients across time.
  - —*Redundancy. Lexical redundancy* (repeating key words) and *semantic redundancy* (providing semantically related words) enhance sentence comprehension for many aphasic patients.
  - —The need for *reasoning and inference.* Requiring reasoning and inference increases the difficulty of sentence comprehension for many aphasic patients.
  - —The nature of *response choices.* Adding foils and increasing the similarity of foils and targets makes sentence comprehension more difficult. Differences in the nature of response choices (tokens versus pictures versus objects) have minor effects on most aphasic patients' sentence comprehension.
- Performance on sentence-comprehension tests apparently does not predict the com-

prehension performance of aphasic adults in daily life.

- The *Minnesota Test for Differential Diagnosis of Aphasia* tests comprehension of spoken discourse with passages that resemble those found in school textbooks. The *Boston Diagnostic Aphasia Examination* assesses comprehension of spoken discourse with materials that seem more representative of daily life discourse.

- The *Discourse Comprehension Test* provides for comprehensive assessment of discourse comprehension, including comprehension of main ideas and details and comprehension of stated and implied material.

- Several variables affect aphasic adults' comprehension of spoken discourse:

  —*Salience.* Aphasic patients comprehend and remember important information (the *main ideas*) better than incidental information (the *details*) in discourse.

  —*Directness.* Aphasic patients comprehend and remember information that is *directly stated* in discourse better than information that is *implied.*

  —*Redundancy. Repetition, elaboration,* and *paraphrase* increase the redundancy of discourse and make it easier for aphasic patients to comprehend and remember.

  —*Cohesion and coherence.* Cohesive ties within discourse make it easier for aphasic patients to comprehend and remember. Cohesive ties contribute to the overall unity of discourse—its coherence.

  —*Speech rate and emphatic stress.* Slow speech rate and exaggerated emphatic stress usually enhance aphasic patients' comprehension, although the effects may vary across patients and across time within patients.

ASSESSING READING
Reading Subtests in Language Test Batteries

All language test batteries contain reading subtests. A few include *visual matching subtests,* in which the patient is shown a series of cards on each of which is printed a geometric form, a

letter of the alphabet, or a word. The patient then chooses the matching form, letter, or word from a card containing the test stimulus plus several foils. The test stimuli and target choices in these subtests are visually identical, permitting selection of the correct target based on visual form alone. When the test stimuli are letters or words, this means that patients can make correct choices by matching the visual form of stimuli and targets, without translating either into alphabet letters or words. Consequently, such letter-matching or word-matching subtests are best characterized as tests of visual perception and discrimination, rather than as reading tests. Figure 5-12 shows typical geometric-form-matching, letter-matching, and word-matching stimulus cards and response plates.

Most language test batteries assess *oral reading of printed words and sentences.* The patient is given a card on which a word or a sentence is printed and reads it aloud. These subtests provide an indication of a patient's ability to convert the graphemic forms of words into phonologic forms and to encode and produce the phonologic representations. They do not necessarily test reading comprehension because graphemes can be converted to phonemes without accessing the semantic representations of the words. Patients with speech production problems may make errors on oral reading tests because of their speech production problems rather than because of reading impairment.

Subtests in which patients *match printed words to pictures or objects* are the simplest tests of reading comprehension. These subtests come in several forms. In the most common form the examiner places a card containing several drawings in front of the patient and then shows the patient a card on which the name of one of the drawings is printed. The patient points to the drawing that matches the printed word *(word-to-picture matching).* Most often the drawings are of objects, but sometimes they portray verbs, colors, numbers, and geometric forms. In another less common form the patient is shown the printed name of an object and then

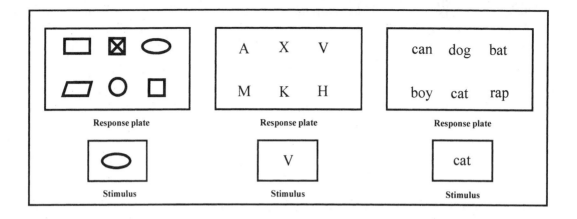

Figure 5-12 ■ Stimulus cards and response plates representing form-matching *(left),* letter-matching *(center),* and word-matching tasks *(right).* These tasks can be completed successfully without comprehending the linguistic value of the letters and words.

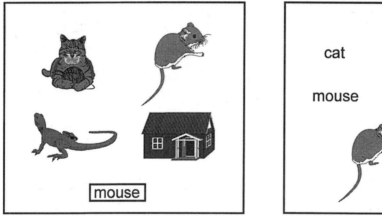
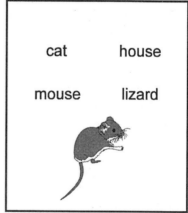

Figure 5-13 ■ An example of a word-to-picture matching task *(left)* and a picture-to-word matching task *(right).*

chooses the named object from a set of real objects *(word-to-object matching).*

Some comprehensive tests opt for a mirror-image version of the word-to-picture matching format by showing the patient a drawing of an object and asking them to choose the object's printed name from a card containing the name of the object plus the names of several other objects *(picture-to-word matching).* For most brain-injured adults it makes little difference which format is used. Word-to-picture and picture-to-word matching usually give equivalent results, and most patients perform similarly regardless of whether the printed words are matched to pictures or to real objects. (The exception is patients with impaired visual perception and discrimination.) Figure 5-13 gives an example of a word-to-picture test item and a picture-

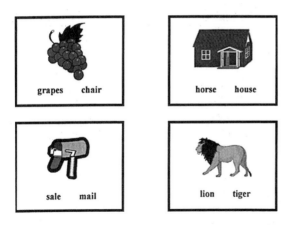

knees	lock
beans	peas
pens	eat

Figure 5-14 ■ An example of a two-choice picture-to-word matching task in which the relationship of foils to the target is manipulated to permit identification of random errors *(grapes/chair)*, visual confusions *(horse/house)*, auditory confusions *(sale/mail)*, and semantic confusions *(lion/tiger)*.

Figure 5-15 ■ A response plate from a single-word comprehension test in which the examiner says a word and the aphasic individual points to the word the examiner says. The target for this card is *peas*. Foils represent auditory confusion *(knees)*, semantic confusion *(beans, eat)*, and visual confusion *(pens)*. *(Beans* represents a semantic *category* error; *eat* represents a semantic *function* error.)

to-word test item in which foils represent semantically similar, visually similar, and unrelated choices.

Some language test batteries test single-word reading comprehension by showing the patient a series of cards. On each card is a drawing, beneath which are two printed words, one of which identifies the drawing. These tests sometimes are designed so that patients' errors can be identified as semantic confusions *(lion/tiger),* auditory confusions *(mail/sale),* visual confusions *(horse/house),* and irrelevant responses *(grapes/chair).* A less positive characteristic of this test format is that patients can get half of the items correct by chance because there are only two response choices for each item. Figure 5-14 gives an example of this test format.

Subtests in which patients *match printed words to spoken words* are somewhat more difficult than picture-to-word matching subtests for most brain-injured adults. Printed-word-to-spoken-word subtests come in different forms. The most common form is one in which a card on which several words are printed is placed be-

fore the patient, the examiner says the words in random order, and the patient points to each word as the examiner says it (Figure 5-15).

Tests for assessing *comprehension of printed sentences* also come in several forms. In one form the sentences are yes-no questions ("Do eggs come from chickens?"). Like the spoken yes-no questions previously described, printed yes-no questions may relate to personal information; general knowledge; knowledge acquired in school; or opinions, inferences, and abstractions. And, like the spoken yes-no questions previously described, the general-knowledge questions can be separated into questions that test comparative, temporal, and numeric relationships.

In another form of printed-sentence comprehension tests, patients choose from a list of words the one that best completes an unfinished sentence, as in:

A cowboy rides a . . . *cow horse house candlestick.*

(Foils often are selected to represent semantic, visual, or unrelated errors, as in this example.)

In yet another form of printed-sentence comprehension tests, the patient is given cards on which are printed instructions for manipulating test objects (or, less frequently, pictures). In the *Porch Index of Communicative Ability* (Porch, 1981a), for example, patients are given cards with instructions such as "Put this card to the left of the cigarette" or "Put this card under the one used for picking up food." Sometimes the printed instructions in language test batteries are similar to those in spoken-sentence comprehension tests ("Pick up the pencil, knock three times, and put it back.").

Several language test batteries provide subtests for assessing *comprehension of printed texts.* In the most common form, the patient is given several short printed passages to read. The final sentence in each passage is incomplete, and several phrases that might complete the passage are printed below it, as in the following item from the BDAE.

In the early days of this country, the functions of government were few in number. Most of the functions were carried out by local town and county officials, while centralized authority was distrusted. The growth of industry and of big cities has so changed the situation that the farmer of today is concerned with ...

Local affairs above all
The price of lumber
The actions of the government
The authority of town officials

A few language test batteries contain expository passages similar to those found in primary-school and secondary-school reading materials. The box in the next column contains a portion of the passage that makes up the MTDDA paragraph-reading subtest. The patient circles, underlines, or points to *yes* or *no* for each question.

The *Discourse Comprehension Test* (DCT; Nicholas & Brookshire, 1993) includes a reading comprehension subtest to assess brain-injured

adults' reading comprehension of 10 stories, together with normative information for 20 non-brain-injured adults who were tested with the reading version of the DCT.

Lawrence Griswold, a writer and scientist who lives in Minnesota, states that dragons really exist. In 1934, he and a classmate camped for eight months on Komodo, an island in Indonesia. Here they found dragons eighteen feet long, who walked on their hind feet like the ancient dinosaurs ...

Did Griswold go to Komodo in 1943? ...
Yes   No
Did he find dragons in Indonesia? ...
Yes   No

Free-Standing Tests of Reading Comprehension One free-standing test of brain-injured adults' reading comprehension is currently on the market. As the title suggests, the *Reading Comprehension Battery for Aphasia-Second Edition* (RCBA-2, LaPointe & Horner, 1998) is designed for evaluating aphasic adults' reading abilities. The *core section* of RCBA-2 contains 10 subtests with 10 items in each subtest. Subtests 1, 2, and 3 assess single-word reading from preschool to Grade 3 vocabulary levels. The foils in these subtests permit clinicians to identify visual confusions *(leaf/leap),* auditory confusions *(anchor/tanker),* and semantic confusions *(guitar/violin).* Subtest 4 tests functional reading of signs, labels, menus, calendars, recipes, and other such daily life material (Figure 5-16).

Subtest 5 is a reading vocabulary subtest in which the test-taker chooses synonyms for five common verbs and five common nouns, half of which are abstract and half of which are concrete. In Subtest 6 the test-taker reads each of 10 five-word sentences and chooses, from sets of three pictures, the one that best illustrates the meaning of each sentence (Figure 5-17). The sentences are controlled for vocabulary level, imageability, and concreteness.

Weather forecast
Turning much colder beginning today
Wednesday fair and cold
High today low 60s
Low tonight near 30
Chance of rain: 70%

Point to the part that tells how cold it will get tonight.

Figure 5-16 ▪ **A functional reading test item from the *Reading Comprehension Battery for Aphasia-Second Edition.*** (From LaPointe, L. L., & Horner, J. [1988]. *Reading Comprehension Battery for Aphasia* [2nd ed.]. Austin, TX: Pro-Ed.)

Figure 5-17 ▪ **A sentence comprehension test item from the *Reading Comprehension Battery for Aphasia-Second Edition.*** (From LaPointe, L. L., & Horner, J. [1988]. *Reading Comprehension Battery for Aphasia* [2nd ed.]. Austin, TX: Pro-Ed.)

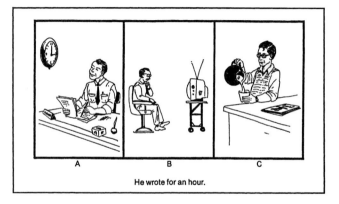

A   B   C

He wrote for an hour.

Subtest 7 contains 10 two-sentence, 25-word paragraphs in which the second sentence directs the test-taker to choose, from a set of three pictures, the one identified by the paragraph (Figure 5-18). The reading level of the paragraphs in Subtest 7 ranges from Grade 2.7 to Grade 4.8.

Subtests 8 and 9 present five 52-word paragraphs. The reading level of the paragraphs ranges from Grade 2.9 to Grade 6.7. The test-taker reads each paragraph and completes four statements about each paragraph by selecting a word or phrase from three choices for each statement (Figure 5-19). The first two questions for each paragraph assess comprehension of stated information and the last two assess com-

prehension of implied information. Scores on the 10 questions testing stated information are assigned to Subtest 8, and scores on the 10 questions testing implied information are assigned to Subtest 9.

> According to the RCBA-2 manual, correct answers are not obvious from the command sentence alone. However, in several items (including the ones in Figures 5-18 and 5-19) the correct answer seems obvious from the command sentences alone.

Subtest 10 is a sentence-to-picture matching task in which the subject chooses (from three

Figure 5-18 ■ **A two-sentence-paragraph comprehension item from the *Reading Comprehension Battery for Aphasia-Second Edition.*** (From LaPointe, L. L., & Horner, J. [1988]. *Reading Comprehension Battery for Aphasia* [2nd ed.]. Austin, TX: Pro-Ed.)

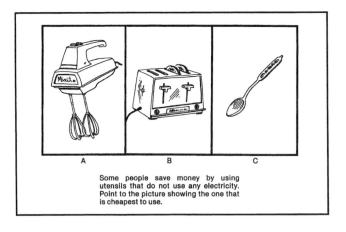

Some people save money by using utensils that do not use any electricity. Point to the picture showing the one that is cheapest to use.

Goose down
The soft and light feathers from the underside of a goose have so many uses. This material is called *down*, and it is used to fill some pillows. Goose down is used to fill sleeping bags and cold weather clothes, also. That is why you see so many naked geese walking around.

Soft goose feathers are called:
Down   Up   Pillows

This material is used to fill:
Weather   Sleeping bags   Time

A down-filled coat would be best in:
Summer   Winter   Cars

Goose down equipment can be used for:
Swimming   Music   Camping

Figure 5-19 ■ **A longer paragraph comprehension item from the *Reading Comprehension Battery for Aphasia-Second Edition.*** (From LaPointe, L. L., & Horner, J. [1988]. *Reading Comprehension Battery for Aphasia* [2nd ed.]. Austin, TX: Pro-Ed.)

sentences) the one that best describes a picture (Figure 5-20). The choice sentences differ in syntax, ranging from active declarative ("The player is hitting the ball.") to object embedded ("She threw the boy's dog the leash.")

The supplemental section of the RCBA-2 contains seven subtests: *single-letter visual discrimination, letter naming, letter recognition, lexical decision* (discriminating valid words from nonsense trigrams), *semantic categorization* (deciding if two words semantically go together), *oral reading of single words,* and *oral reading of sentences.*

Individual responses to RCBA-2 test items are scored correct or incorrect, and the time taken to complete each subtest is recorded. The number of correct responses for each RCBA-2 subtest can be plotted to create a graphic profile of a patient's RCBA-2 performance. The RCBA-2 test manual contains information about test construction, instructions for test administration and interpretation, and instructions for response scoring, together with a short list of references on reading impairments in aphasia. The test manual contains no normative information or documentation of the RCBA-2's reliability and validity, but some psychometric information is available elsewhere (VanDemark, Lemmer, & Drake, 1982; Pasternak & LaPointe, 1982).

Reading Tests for Non-Brain-Injured Adults and Children The reading tests in lan-

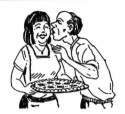

A. The man is kissing the woman who is holding the pizza.

B. The woman is kissing the man who is holding the pizza.

C. The man who is holding the woman is kissing the pizza.

Figure 5-20 ■ A sentence comprehension item from the *Reading Comprehension Battery for Aphasia-Second Edition.* (From LaPointe L. L., & Horner, J. [1988]. *Reading Comprehension Battery for Aphasia* [2nd ed.]. Austin, TX: Pro-Ed.)

guage test batteries and the RCBA-2, which were designed for brain-injured adults, are good screening tests to identify patients with moderate to severe reading impairments, but most do not provide enough detail to enable clinicians to detect subtle reading impairments or to describe the nature of a patient's reading impairments. For these purposes clinicians usually turn to standardized reading tests, which provide a comprehensive look at the severity and nature of a patient's reading impairments and permit the clinician to compare the patient with normal readers. Because brain-injured adults' reading abilities range from single-word reading to college level, clinicians who assess brain-injured adults' reading need tests that span a range from primary-grade to college level.

The *Gates-MacGinitie Reading Tests* (Gates, MacGinitie, Maria, & associates, 2000) span a range of reading skills from kindergarten through post high-school. The tests from Level 3 (third grade) through Level AR (adult reading) span a range that will permit testing most brain-injured adults. All have vocabulary and compre-

hension sections. The vocabulary section of each test takes 20 minutes to administer, and the comprehension section of each test takes 35 minutes to administer. Items in the vocabulary sections consist of short phrases with one word in the phrase underlined. The test-taker chooses one of four definitions that follow each phrase, as in this item from Level 3:

The others *peered* at it

looked closely
smiled
pecked
made loud noises

Items in the comprehension sections consist of reading passages taken from published books and periodicals representing fiction, nonfiction, science, and social studies and are written in a variety of styles. Passage content is selected to represent the interests and experiences of test-takers at a given grade level. Consequently, passages intended for testing lower grades tend to have juvenile themes, which some brain-injured adults may consider demeaning, as in the following excerpt from Level 3.

When I come home from school, my mother and father are still at work, so Gogo takes care of me. Gogo calls me her little tail because I follow her everywhere. She lets me carry her beautiful blue cloth bag in which she keeps her important things . . .
  Why does Gogo take care of the girl who is telling the story?

The girl has no parents.
Gogo gets lonely by herself.
Gogo is the girl's mother.
The girl's parents have jobs away from home.

Comprehension items at Level 7 and above have more adult-like content and probably would be suitable for testing most brain-injured adults who can read material at this level. The following excerpt is from Level 7.

> My earliest clear memory of my mother is her tall figure standing alone in the center of the lawn behind the house, looking down at the grass, turning in a slow circle, scanning the ground. I knew this to be a mild sign of trouble for my mother, trouble for the family . . .
> *What was the author doing?*
>
> Watching.
> Helping his mother.
> Copying his mother.
> Trying to stop his mother.

The reading comprehension subtest of the *Peabody Individual Achievement Test-Revised* (Markwardt, 1989) can be used to test the sentence-reading comprehension of brain-injured patients representing a range of reading impairments. The clinician shows a page containing a printed sentence to the patient, then covers it with another page that contains four pictures, one of which represents the meaning of the sentence. The patient responds by pointing to one of the pictures. Sentences increase in length (from 5 to 30 words) and difficulty of vocabulary as the test progresses. Norms (grade equivalents and percentiles) are provided for non-brain-injured children and adults up to 23 years old. Most brain-injured patients can complete this test in less than 30 minutes, making the test useful for moderately to severely impaired brain-injured adults who might not tolerate longer tests.

The *Nelson-Denny Reading Test* (NDRT; Brown, Fischco, & Hanna, 1993) may be useful for testing brain-injured adults with mild reading impairments. The NDRT uses reading materials selected from high school through college-level humanities, social science, and science textbooks. Like the Gates-MacGinitie tests, the NDRT has vocabulary and paragraph comprehension sections. The NDRT permits users to classify paragraph comprehension test items according to whether they test *literal* (stated) *information* or *interpretive* (implied) *information,* as in the following test item, in which the first item tests literal information and the second item tests interpretive information.

> One of Jung's best-known contributions is his personality typology of two basic attitudes, or orientations, toward life: extraversion and introversion. Both orientations are viewed as existing simultaneously in each person, with one usually dominant. The extravert's energy is directed toward external objects and events, while the introvert is more concerned with inner experiences . . .
> *The concept of extraversion and introversion was one of Jung's*
>
> Earliest contributions
> Most controversial contributions
> Most widely known contributions
>
> *You would infer that extraverts would most likely be*
>
> Speakers
> Listeners
> Readers

Assessing Reading Rate and Capacity In their standard administration, reading tests are given with a time limit, and norms for the test are based on scores obtained within the time limit. Clinicians who are interested in brain-injured patients' reading usually want to know how much a patient can accomplish within the time limit so that their performance can be compared with the performance of the norm group. They also wish to know how much a patient can do if permitted to work without time constraints. This way of testing provides estimates of a patient's *reading rate* and *reading capacity.* Reading rate tells the clinician how much the patient can read and understand under normal time constraints and allows comparison of the patient with norm groups, whereas reading capacity tells the clinician how much the patient can read under optimal conditions. Most brain-injured adults' reading rate is slower than their premorbid rate, even when their vocabulary, word recognition, and single-word comprehension seem intact. Estimates of reading rate and reading capacity are important in planning treatment programs and in counseling the patient and family about the patient's probable daily life reading competence.

Reading rate and capacity are measured in the following way. The patient begins the test and works for the amount of time prescribed by the test manual. At the end of that time the examiner marks the last item completed by the patient, and the patient continues until he or she completes the test or can go no farther. The examiner records the time at which the patient finishes the test and marks the last item completed.

Measuring Component Skills One weakness of most reading comprehension tests for adults is that they do not measure component skills that may be necessary for different aspects of reading comprehension (e.g., *sound-to-letter conversion, getting main ideas, using context*). After administering most adult reading tests the examiner has a test score, perhaps a percentile rank, and a reading grade level but no real sense of which component skills are compromised and which are preserved.

There is no universal list of component skills for reading, but the *Specific Skill Series* of remedial reading materials (Boning, 1990) provides materials suitable for getting a look at some of the more important ones: *symbol-to-sound correspondences, following directions, using context, locating answers, getting facts, getting main ideas, drawing conclusions, recognizing sequences,* and *identifying inferences.* The *Specific Skill Series* includes materials at 10 levels of graded difficulty within each skill. Table 5-3 gives examples of items from the *following directions, getting main ideas, drawing conclusions,* and *identifying inferences* series.

The reading materials in the *Specific Skill Series* cover a wide range of reading levels (preschool to Grade 8). A set of placement tests enables users to place readers at the appropriate level within each skill. Some of the reading selections have juvenile themes, but the incidents and situations portrayed are sufficiently interesting that most adult readers should not find them demeaning. With its compartmentalization of the reading process into component skills and its wide range of reading levels within each skill, the *Specific Skill Series* provides a useful collection of materials for assessing and treating brain-injured adults' reading impairments.

Reading Test Format Those who design standardized reading tests for normal adults and children assume that potential test-takers have essentially normal (for their age) memory, organizational skills, problem-solving skills, and visual perception and are able to attend to and follow spoken directions. These assumptions permit users of the tests to conclude that impaired test performance signifies reading impairment and not impairment of some underlying or related ability. Because reading tests for normal children and adults were designed with these assumptions in mind, their format may make some of them unsatisfactory for testing brain-injured adults who have memory impairments, impaired organizational or problem-solving skills, visual perceptual impairments, or difficulties in following instructions.

Most standardized reading tests for normal adults and children do not require written answers to test items but allow the test-taker to check off, circle, or underline their choice from a multiple-choice array of possible answers. Consequently, brain-injured adults with mild to moderate impairments are likely to have little difficulty with the responses required. Tests with answer sheets that are scored by machine—in which the person taking the test must read a stimulus item, choose the correct answer from a group of possible answers, remember the number of the test item and the number or letter of the correct choice, find the corresponding set of

T A B L E 5 - 3

Examples of reading items from the *Specific Skill Series*

Following Directions

DIRECTIONS

There are four words in the left-hand column. To the right of each word are two more words. Choose
the one that is opposite in meaning to the word at the left. Circle it.

listen	—speak, hear
below	—beside, above
everyone	—lately, nobody
many	—few, some

Getting the Main Idea

There is a plant in our country that doesn't have any green leaves. This plant grows about eight inches
tall. At the end of each stem is a white flower. The stem is also white. The plant looks like many clay
pipes. It is called the Indian Pipe.

The story tells mainly

    (A) why American Indians smoke pipes

    (B) why American Indians named plants

    (C) what the plant called the Indian Pipe looks like

Drawing Conclusions

Horses don't live as long as people. A horse that lives to the age of thirty is very old. One year of a
horse's life is equal to three years of a person's. A thirty-year-old horse is as old as a person who is
ninety.

A horse of ten is equal in age to a

    (A) ten-year-old child

    (B) thirty-year-old person

    (C) three-year-old baby

Identifying Inferences

"That's a pretty jewel you have in your ring," said Karen.

"Thank you," said Martha, "It was given to me as a present. I have other rings, but this is my favorite. My
mother always gives me things that I really like."

Martha has more than one ring.	True	False	Inferred*
The ring was given to Martha by her mother.	True	False	Inferred
Karen didn't like Martha's ring.	True	False	Inferred

Boning, R. A. (1990). Specific skill series (4th ed.). New York: Macmillan/McGraw-Hill.
*True items are facts that are directly stated in the story. False items are not true, based on information in the story. Inferred
items are items that are probably true, based on the story and the reader's experience.

response choices on the answer sheet, and
blacken the appropriate area on the answer
sheet—often cause transcription and bookkeep-
ing errors, even for adults with no brain injury.
Consequently, they should be not be used to
test brain-injured adults unless the response format can be changed to eliminate demands on
competencies other than reading.

*The Passage Dependency of Reading
Tests* Passage dependency is a term coined by

Tuiman (1974) to reflect the extent to which readers must rely on information from printed texts to correctly answer items that test comprehension of the texts. Items that are answerable without reading the texts to which the items refer are *passage independent* because they do not depend on the test-taker's comprehension of the text. When reading test items have low passage dependency, the test is more likely a test of single-sentence reading skills than a test of multiple-sentence reading comprehension. When you look at the following example, read and try to answer the questions before you read the passage. If you can answer a question correctly without reading the passage, the question is not passage dependent.

Obesity is:

not prevalent in the United States.

a major social and medical problem in the United States.

a condition that primarily affects older people.

Some consequences of obesity are:

increased resistance to communicable disease.

increased risk of strokes, heart attacks, and diabetes.

increased ability to tolerate cold weather.

Obesity is a major social and medical problem in the United States. More than one-half of the United States population is considered overweight and about thirty percent are considered obese (excessively fat). Obesity increases risk of strokes, heart attacks, diabetes, and several other medical problems. Billions are spent in the United States every year for diet books and over-the-counter diet drugs, but experts assert that eating less and exercising more is the best and surest way to lose weight.

Nicholas, MacLennan, and Brookshire (1986) reported that the validity of most multiple-sentence reading tests for testing brain-injured adults is compromised by low passage dependency. They evaluated the performance of non-

brain-injured adults and aphasic adults on reading-test items from the multiple-sentence reading subtests from BDAE (Goodglass, Kaplan, & Barresi, 2001), the MTDDA (Schuell, 1972), EFA (Eisenson, 1974), the WAB (Kertesz, 1982), and the *Reading Comprehension Battery for Aphasia* (RCBA; LaPointe & Horner, 1979). First they had participants respond to the test items without having previously read the passages to which the items referred. On the average, aphasic adults correctly answered beyond chance level 58% of the test items from these reading tests without having read the test passages, and non-brain-injured adults correctly answered 64%. Only the items from one of the two RCBA subtests had acceptable passage dependency. However, this subtest contained only two-sentence passages and would be unlikely to predict performance on longer passages.

Tuiman (1974) suggested that passages for which test-takers can answer not more than 40% to 50% of test items without reading the passages have acceptable passage dependency.

It seems inappropriate for clinicians to shun language test batteries' multiple-sentence reading comprehension subtests and the RCBA-2 multiple-sentence test items because they have questionable passage dependency. These tests are no doubt sufficiently sensitive and have sufficient validity to make them acceptable screening tests of multiple-sentence reading comprehension. They appear well suited for identifying patients with reading impairments, who then can be tested with a more comprehensive free-standing reading test, if appropriate.

GENERAL CONCEPTS 5-2

- Most language test batteries include subtests to assess *oral reading* and *reading comprehension*. Oral reading tests typically require the patient to read lists of words and sentences. Success in oral reading does not require comprehension of what is read.

- Most language test batteries assess reading *comprehension of single words.* Single-word reading comprehension typically is assessed by asking the patient to match printed words to pictures or to match printed words to spoken words.

- Most language test batteries assess reading *comprehension of sentences.* Comprehension of printed sentences typically is assessed by asking the patient to respond to printed yes-no questions, to complete unfinished sentences, or to follow printed instructions requiring gestural or manipulative responses.

- The *Reading Comprehension Battery for Aphasia* is a free-standing test of reading comprehension that provides for assessing aphasic adults' comprehension of single words, sentences, signs, labels, and short paragraphs, plus supplemental tests for assessing letter and word skills related to reading. It is a good screening test of reading for brain-injured patients but may be too easy for patients with mild reading impairments.

- Reading tests for non-brain-damaged children and adults provide for more comprehensive assessment of aphasic adults' reading than is possible with items from language test batteries or the *Reading Comprehension Battery for Aphasia.* Most permit assessment of reading vocabulary and paragraph comprehension and allow calculation of a reading grade level.

- The *Nelson-Denny Reading Test* may be appropriate for patients with mild reading impairment. It permits assessment of a patient's ability to answer questions related to *literal information* and questions related to *interpretive information.*

- Measuring brain-injured patients' *reading rate* (how much the patient reads and understands within normal time constraints) and *reading capacity* (how much the patient reads and understands if given unlimited time to finish) is important for understanding the adequacy of brain-injured patients' reading skills.

- Materials that permit measurement of component reading skills (e.g., *using context, getting the main ideas*) are a useful adjunct to standardized tests of reading and permit clinicians to tailor remedial programs to a patient's specific pattern of impairment.

- Straightforward and easy-to-understand test format is important when choosing a reading test for use with brain-injured adults, who may not be able to comprehend and follow complex instructions and test format.

- The passage dependency of reading test materials in language test batteries is relatively low, suggesting that these materials may test patients' general knowledge as much as their reading comprehension.

ASSESSING SPEECH PRODUCTION

Speech production subtests are prominent in all language test batteries, and several free-standing tests of speech production for brain-injured adults are available. Speech production tests cover a wide range of content, from repetition of syllables and words to self-generated connected speech. Patients with severely compromised communication usually can do the easiest tests reasonably well, whereas the most difficult tests will challenge even patients with mild speech impairments.

Simple Speech Production Tests

The simplest speech production subtests are useful for testing patients with moderate to severe speech production impairments. They call on patients to *produce rhymes, recitations, and automatized sequences; complete sentences;* and *repeat words, phrases, and sentences* after the examiner.

Recitations, Rhymes, and Automatized Sequences These tests are among the easiest speech production tests for most brain-injured adults. They require the patient to produce highly practiced material such as counting or reciting the days of the week, the months of the year, or the alphabet. Even severely aphasic patients who produce little or no volitional speech often can produce highly practiced material. Those who cannot produce such material in response to the examiner's request often can continue if the examiner helps them get started.

> Clinician: "Now, Mrs. Ryder, I'd like you to count from one to ten for me."
> Patient: "Ah . . . umm . . . lahti . . . lahti . . ."
> Clinician: "Can you count from one to ten?"
> Patient: "Lahti . . . lahti . . . lahti . . ."
> Clinician: 'Let's count from one to ten. Are you ready? One..."
> Patient: ". . . two . . . three . . . four . . . five . . . six . . . seventy . . . eighty . . . ninety . . . tenty."

Sentence Completion Sentence completion tests usually are more difficult than tests calling for recitation, rhymes, and automatized sequences, but they are still within the range of most brain-injured adults' abilities. The stimuli in these tests are short, syntactically simple sentences, minus the final word, which is highly predictable from the rest of the sentence ("I like bread and ——." "Roses are red, violets are ——.")

Speech Repetition Speech repetition tests span a range of difficulty, from repeating monosyllabic words (such as "boy") to repeating simple phrases (such as "up and down"), to repeating phonologically complex phrases and sentences (such as "Please put the groceries in the refrigerator."). The longer and more phonologically complex the phrase or sentence, the more difficult it is for the patient to produce.

> A patient with conduction aphasia is trying to repeat "Nelson Rockefeller drives a Lincoln Continental.":
> "Neller Fahkahfeller . . . Nelson Farkareller . . . no . . . Nelson Fahkahfiller . . . aah! Nelson Rockereller drives a Lincoln Contalental . . . no . . . a Kinkel Lontimental . . . aah! I give up!"

Patients with conduction aphasia or apraxia of speech often become tied in knots when asked to repeat phonologically complex materials. Patients with Wernicke's aphasia sometimes have difficulty with such materials, not because of the phonologic complexity of the materials but because of their short retention span.

> A patient with conduction aphasia, when asked to repeat "please put the groceries in the refrigerator," responded with:
> "Pease put the gripperies in the . . . pease put the gorsheries in the refligalator . . . no . . ."
> A patient with Wernicke's aphasia, when asked to repeat the same phrase, responded with:
> "Please put the . . . please put the bread, etcetera in the shopping cart."

Naming

Naming Subtests in Language Test Batteries Naming subtests are found in all the major language test batteries and provide information about patients across the aphasia severity continuum. Naming subtests take several forms. The most common is *picture naming or object naming* (sometimes called *confrontation naming*), in which the patient is shown a series of pictures or objects and is asked to say the name of each. The stimuli in most confrontation naming subtests are drawings or objects, but naming subtests in which the stimuli are geometric shapes, colors, numbers, or body parts are included in some comprehensive aphasia tests.

> Letter-naming tests also are found in some comprehensive aphasia tests. However, I would categorize these as low-level *oral reading* tests.

Two variants on confrontation naming subtests are seen in some language test batteries. In *responsive naming tests* the examiner asks a question that can be answered with one or two words ("What do you write with?" "What do you do with soap?" "What color is snow?"). In *generative naming* (sometimes called *category naming*) patients are given a specified time interval (usually 1 minute) to say as many words as they can think of that either begin with a certain letter (such as *F, A,* or *S*) or represent certain semantic categories (such as *animals* or *tools*).

Free-Standing Tests of Naming Several free-standing tests for assessing brain-injured adults' naming have been published or described in the literature. One of the oldest is a generative naming test called the *Word Fluency Measure* (Borkowski, Benton, & Spreen, 1967), which was originally published as a research report and subsequently was included as a subtest of the *Neurosensory Center Comprehensive Examination for Aphasia* (NCCEA; Spreen & Benton, 1977). In the *Word Fluency Measure* the patient is allowed 1 minute in which to say as many words that begin with a specified letter of the alphabet as the patient can think of. The letter (either *F, A,* or *S*) is specified by the examiner. The patient's score is the total of all appropriate words spoken in the 1-minute interval.

> The letters *F, A,* and *S* yield the largest numbers of correct responses from non-brain-injured adults (Borkowski, Benton, & Spreen, 1967). No equivalent information is available for semantic categories.

The *Word Fluency Measure* is a sensitive indicator of brain injury, but it does not discriminate among aphasia syndromes or between aphasia syndromes and other neurogenic impairments of communication or cognition. A patient's performance on the word fluency measure has marginal value for planning treatment because the task is an unusual one, with little relationship to daily life communication. Some clinicians make up informal generative naming

tests in which the patient is asked to produce words within functional categories (e.g., furniture, foods, or flowers). Although no norms are available for these informal tests, they can provide useful insights into a patient's word retrieval and speech production and the state of the patient's semantic system.

Most brain-injured adults perform well below normal on generative naming tasks. Aphasic adults almost always produce far fewer appropriate words than non-brain-injured adults (and fewer than adults with right-hemisphere brain injury). One potential problem for clinicians who wish to use generative naming tasks in treatment is that there is great variability in the number of names non-brain-injured adults produce in generative naming tasks. For example, one group of non-brain-injured adults produced, on the average, 23 animal names in a 1-minute interval, but the scores of individual subjects ranged from 9 to 41 words (Goodglass & Kaplan, 1983).

The *Boston Naming Test* (BNT; Kaplan, Goodglass, & Weintraub, 2001) is a picture-naming test in which the examiner shows the person being tested 60 line drawings (one by one) and asks them to name each drawing. Word familiarity (the frequency of occurrence of target names) decreases as the test progresses. Each response is scored for latency, correctness, and whether a cue was given. Norms (means, standard deviations, and range of scores) are provided for 356 children (age 5 years to 12 years, 5 months) and 178 normal adults (age 18 years to 79 years). (Norms for 75 aphasic adults are provided in *The Assessment of Aphasia and Related Disorders, Third Edition* [Goodglass, Kaplan, & Barresi, 2001].) The BNT manual provides brief instructions for administering the BNT and scoring responses, but neither administration nor scoring instructions are explicit enough to ensure interexaminer or test-retest reliability, and the manual does not report either. Nicholas and associates (1989) published more explicit procedures for administering and scoring the BNT, together with intrajudge and interjudge reliability for their more explicit procedures.

The *Test of Adolescent/Adult Word Finding* (TAWF; German, 1990) is a comprehensive test of word retrieval and has norms for non-brain-damaged persons from age 12 to age 80. The TAWF provides for assessment of word-retrieval in five tasks: *picture naming-nouns, picture naming-verbs, sentence completion* ("The farmer milked the . . ."), *naming of descriptions* ("Something you write with"), and *category naming* ("Bananas, oranges, and apples are . . ."). The TAWF can be administered in 20 to 30 minutes for normal adults and should take no more than 1 hour for most brain-injured adults. A short version of the test takes less than 20 minutes for normal adults and should take no more than 30 minutes for most brain-injured adults.

Variables That May Affect Naming Accuracy

Frequency of Occurrence A word's frequency in the language may affect the ease and accuracy with which aphasic adults name objects or pictures (Weigel-Crump & Koenigsknecht, 1973; Rochford & Williams, 1965; Tweedy & Schulman, 1982; and others). More frequent words are easier to name than less frequent words. However, in most studies of word-frequency effects, confounding variables—length, abstractness, age of acquisition, or phonologic complexity of words—and the ambiguity or uncertainty of pictures were not controlled, making conclusions about the effects of word frequency by itself somewhat ambiguous.

As noted earlier, published word-frequency counts are based on frequency of occurrence in printed materials, and Hayes (1989) has shown that published word-frequency counts do not accurately represent frequency of occurrence in everyday speech because printed materials contain greater proportions of low-frequency words than does everyday speech. Investigators also generally agree that word-frequency norms based on printed materials do not accurately represent the familiarity of words to normal adults. Brookshire and Nicholas (1995) had normal adults rate the familiarity of the words in the

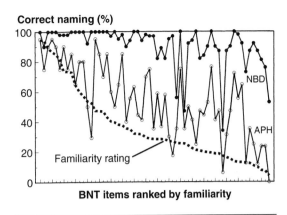

Figure 5-21 ■ **Non-brain-damaged adults' (NBD) and aphasic adults' (APH) performance on the *Boston Naming Test* (*BNT*), with test items arranged in order of diminishing familiarity. (Neither the frequency of occurrence nor the familiarity of BNT items diminish uniformly across the test.)**

Boston Naming Test. Then they tested a group of aphasic adults and a group of non-brain-injured adults with the test. The correlation between word frequency and aphasic adults' naming performance was $r = .37$, whereas the correlation between judged familiarity of words and aphasic adults' naming performance was $r = .71$. Figure 5-21 shows the performance of the aphasic adults and the non-brain-injured adults relative to word familiarity.

> Correlation coefficients range from 0 to 1.00. Larger correlation coefficients indicate stronger relationships. A correlation coefficient of .37 explains about 10 percent of the overall variability in scores. A correlation coefficient of .71 explains about 50 percent.

Length and Phonologic Complexity Length and phonologic complexity also affect aphasic adults' naming. Goodglass and associates (1976) found that aphasic adults' naming success decreased as the number of syllables in words increased. The true culprit may not be number of syllables but articulatory complexity because the number of syllables in a word is related to the ease with which it can be articulated. Word length and articulatory complexity affect the mechanical production of words, unlike variables such as word frequency or stimulus uncertainty, which are more likely to affect accessing words and retrieving them from memory. Patients with motor speech impairments (apraxia of speech) and phonologic selection and sequencing impairments (conduction aphasia) are most likely to be affected by word length and phonologic complexity.

Semantic Categories The semantic characteristics of items to be named may slightly affect how readily some aphasic adults name pictures and objects. Goodglass and associates (1966) evaluated aphasic adults' ability to name (and comprehend) words representing five semantic categories—*objects, actions, colors, numbers,* and *letters.* They reported that object names were hardest for aphasic adults to produce and that letters were easiest. (It is interesting that the spoken names of objects were easiest to comprehend and spoken letter names were hardest to comprehend.) However, the difference between object-naming and letter-naming was only 2 points of a possible 18, and it is almost certain that not every participant's performance pattern matched that of the group. Consequently, clinicians undoubtedly will choose to evaluate the strength of the effects of semantic categories on individual patients' naming before incorporating manipulations of semantic categories into their treatment procedures.

The Form of Visual Stimuli During the 1970s several investigators set out to determine if the *form* of visual stimuli (objects, pictures, photographs, or line drawings) affects the naming performance of brain-injured patients. Benton, Smith, and Lang (1972) asked aphasic adults to name real objects and line drawings of real objects and found a small but statistically significant difference in favor of real objects.

Bisiach (1966) asked aphasic adults to name either realistic colored pictures or line drawings of common objects. He reported a small but significant difference in favor of realistic colored pictures. Corlew and Nation (1975) reported contradictory results. They asked aphasic adults to name either real objects or line drawings representing the objects. They found no meaningful difference between participants' object naming and their naming of line drawings.

Most brain-injured adults are unlikely to perform much differently if they are asked to name objects, colored photographs, or line drawings. However, as in the case of comprehension tests, differences in the form of visual stimuli used in naming tests may be important for severely impaired patients or for patients with visual perceptual impairments. For these patients, real objects may elicit better naming performance than pictures or drawings and realistic photographs may elicit better performance than line drawings.

> The naming performance of some brain-injured patients improves in object-naming tasks if they are permitted to pick up the objects to be named. Apparently the tactile information supplied by handling adds information that enhances retrieval.

Context Context seems to have stronger effects on naming performance than the nature of the stimuli to be named. For many aphasic adults, naming of drawings, pictures, or objects improves when they are portrayed in a natural context. For example, an aphasic adult who cannot name a drawing of a horse portrayed in isolation may name it if the horse is shown harnessed to a cart. A patient who has difficulty naming cups, plates, knives, and forks presented in isolation or in an array of unrelated items may name them more easily if they are arranged in a place setting like those experienced in daily life.

Williams and Canter (1982) reported conflicting findings with regard to the effects of context on aphasic adults' naming. They asked aphasic adults to name line drawings of objects that were shown either in isolation or in a pictorial context. Adults with Broca's aphasia were better at naming the drawings of objects in isolation, and adults with Wernicke's aphasia were better at naming them in contexts. Other groups of aphasic adults exhibited no group preference for contextual or acontextual pictures, although Williams and Canter reported that individual aphasic adults in all groups showed marked differences in performance between the two conditions.

The presence of context can have negative effects on the naming performance of some patients with right-hemisphere brain injury, traumatic brain injury, or dementia. These patients may focus on trivial or tangential details of the context, with consequent negative effects on their naming performance. For these patients highly structured test procedures with minimally contextual stimuli may yield better performance than less structured procedures with contextually rich stimuli.

Sentence Production

Sentence Production Subtests in Language Test Batteries Sentence production subtests are included in all language test batteries. They take several forms. In *word definition* tests, the examiner provides a word and asks the patient to tell what the word means. ("Tell me what *onion* means.") In *make-a-sentence-from-a-word* tests, the examiner says a word and asks the patient to say a sentence containing the word. In *expressing ideas* tests, the examiner asks the patient to produce a sentence or two in response to the examiner's request. For example, in the MT-DDA *expressing ideas* subtest the examiner says to the patient, "Tell me three things you did today," and in the PICA *expressing ideas* subtest the examiner says to the patient, "As completely as possible, tell me what you do with each of these" ("these" being the PICA test objects).

Free-Standing Tests of Sentence Production The *Reporter's Test* (DeRenzi & Ferrari, 1978) is a reversal of the *Token Test* (DeRenzi &

Vignolo, 1962). In the *Token Test* the examiner asks the patient to manipulate large and small colored tokens. In the *Reporter's Test* the examiner manipulates the tokens and the patient describes the examiner's actions.

There are five levels in the *Reporter's Test,* similar to the five levels in the *Token Test.* In Level 1 (4 items) only large tokens are present and the examiner touches a single token ("You touched the green circle."). In Level 2 (4 items) large and small tokens are present and the examiner touches one of them ("You touched the small white circle."). In Level 3 (4 items) only large tokens are present, and the examiner touches two in succession ("You touched the red circle and the green square."). In level 4 (4 items) all tokens are present and the examiner touches two in succession ("You touched the large red circle and the small green square."). In Level 5 (10 items) only the large tokens are present and the examiner manipulates them in several ways ("You put the red circle on the green square. You touched all the circles except the green one. You put all the circles into the box.")

Responses to *Reporter's Test* items are scored either with a three-category system *(correct on first try, correct after a repeated demonstration, incorrect)* or with a weighted scoring system, which takes into account some of the qualitative characteristics of responses. Mean scores and standard deviations are included for normal (Italian) aphasic adults. DeRenzi and Ferrari assert that the *Reporter's Test* is a sensitive indicator of the presence of aphasia and that it is more sensitive to the presence of language impairment than confrontation naming, word fluency, picture description, or sentence repetition tests.

Wener and Duffy (1983) compared the *Reporter's Test* with other measures of speech production and language comprehension for English-speaking aphasic adults. Their results support DeRenzi and Ferrari's assertions about the test's sensitivity to language impairments. However, Wener and Duffy concluded that the *Reporter's Test* in combination with other tests is more sensitive to the presence of language impairments than the *Reporter's Test* alone.

Discourse Production

Discourse Production Subtests in Language Test Batteries The most common test format for eliciting discourse in language test batteries is *picture description,* in which the examiner shows the patient a drawing depicting several characters engaged in activities that should be familiar to most adults and asks the patient to describe the picture. The *Boston Diagnostic Aphasia Examination,* the *Minnesota Test for Differential Diagnosis of Aphasia,* and the *Western Aphasia Battery* include picture description subtests. Figure 5-22 shows the pictures that are used to elicit connected speech in those tests.

> The picture from the MTDDA is less story-like, more likely to elicit enumeration (naming of items in the picture), and less likely to elicit narrative than the WAB and BDAE pictures (Correia, Brookshire, & Nicholas, 1990).

Story retelling is sometimes used to elicit connected speech from aphasic adults. The patient reads (or, less frequently, hears) a narrative and then retells it to the examiner. The MTDDA is the only major comprehensive language test to provide a story-retelling subtest. The examiner reads aloud a 107-word paragraph about quicksand and the patient recounts as much of it as she or he can remember. The patient's narrative is scored with a seven-category system for number of ideas and amount of irrelevant material.

Story retelling makes heavy demands on comprehension and verbal memory. Consequently, poor performance on story-retelling tasks may not always be attributable to impaired speech formulation or production. Other connected-speech tasks that do not make such heavy demands on comprehension and memory usually are a better choice if the clinician's concern is with speech formulation and production and not with comprehension and memory.

Interviews and conversations are important parts of the *Boston Diagnostic Aphasia Examination* and the *Western Aphasia Battery.* The BDAE and the WAB base judgments regarding patients' aphasia type primarily on the characteristics of the speech they produce in an interview. In the interview the examiner asks the patient for personal information, such as the patient's name and address, and inquires into the patient's complaints or problems ("How are you today? Tell me a little about why you are here.") Then the examiner engages the patient in conversation about topics familiar to the patient ("What kind of work did you do before you became ill?"). The BDAE provides a *Rating Scale Profile of Speech Characteristics* (Figure 5-23) for rating melodic line, phrase length, articulatory agility, grammatic form, paraphasia, repetition, and word finding in the patient's connected speech (from the interview, conversation, and picture-description tasks). Voice loudness, voice quality, and speech rate also can be rated. The rating scale is subjective, but it can be used to construct a speech profile, which may be compared with profiles for major aphasia syndromes.

Examiners using the BDAE also consider connected speech when they rate the patients' overall aphasia severity.

0 No usable speech or auditory comprehension.

1 All communication is through fragmentary expression. There is great need for inference, questioning, and guessing by the listener. The range of information that can be exchanged is limited, and the listener carries the burden of communication.

2 Conversation about familiar subjects is possible with help from the listener. There are frequent failures to convey the idea, but the patient shares the burden of communication with the examiner.

3 The patient can discuss almost all everyday problems with little or no assistance. However,

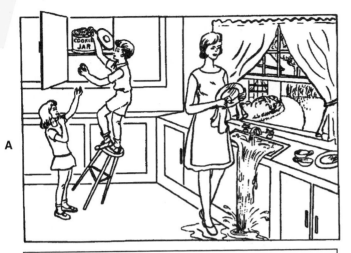

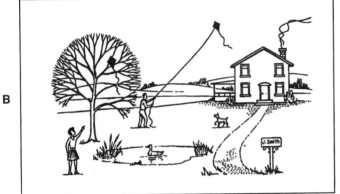

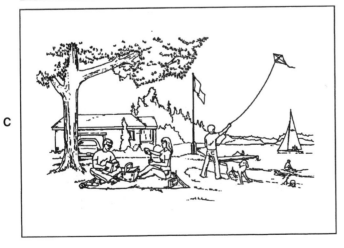

Figure 5-22 ■ The connected-speech elicitation pictures from **A,** the *Boston Diagnostic Aphasia Examination;* **B,** the *Minnesota Test for Differential Diagnosis of Aphasia;* and **C,** the *Western Aphasia Battery.* (**A** from Goodglass, H., Kaplan, E., & Barresi, B. [2001]. *The assessment of aphasia and related disorders* [3rd ed.]. Philadelphia: Lippincott Williams & Wilkins; **B** from Schuell, H. M. [1965]. *The Minnesota Test for Differential Diagnosis of Aphasia.* Minneapolis: University of Minnesota Press; **C** from Kertesz, A. [1982]. *Western Aphasia Battery.* New York: Grune and Stratton.)

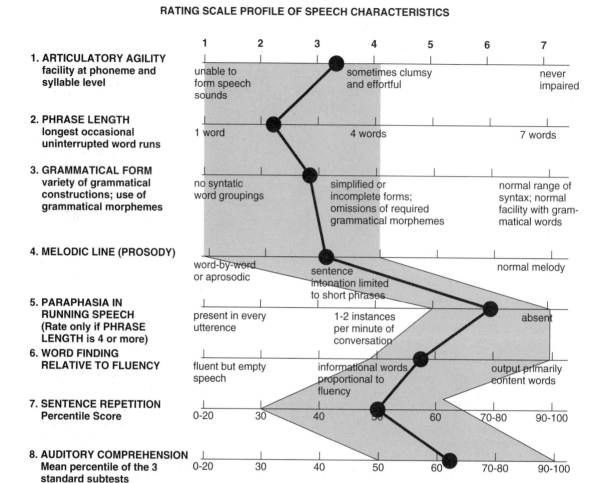

RATING SCALE PROFILE OF SPEECH CHARACTERISTICS

Figure 5-23 ■ A *Rating Scale Profile of Speech Characteristics* from the *Boston Diagnostic Aphasia Examination* for a patient with Broca's aphasia. (From Goodglass, H., Kaplan, E., & Barresi, B. [2001]. *The assessment of aphasia and related disorders* [3rd ed.]. Philadelphia: Lippincott Williams & Wilkins; p. 64.)

reduction of speech and/or comprehension make conversation about certain material difficult or impossible.

4 There is some obvious loss of fluency in speech or facility of comprehension, without significant limitation on ideas expressed or form of expression.

5 There are minimal discernible speech handicaps; the patient may have subjective difficulties that are not apparent to the listener.

The WAB provides two 11-point (0-10) scales for rating the speech elicited in the WAB connected-speech subtests. The examiner rates *information content* with one scale and *fluency, grammaticality,* and *paraphasias* with the other. Speech fluency is important in Kertesz's taxonomic approach, in which patients are assigned to diagnostic categories (e.g., Broca's or Wernicke's) according to their performance on the *Western Aphasia Battery.* Trupe (1984) questioned the reliability of the Western Aphasia Battery procedures for scoring spontaneous speech and the validity of assigning patients to diagnostic categories based on spontaneous speech scores.

Free-Standing Procedures for Assessing Discourse Production Several free-standing procedures for eliciting and scoring discourse produced by language-impaired adults have been described in the literature (Glosser & Deser, 1990; Glosser, Wiener, & Kaplan, 1988; Golper, Thorpe, Tompkins, & associates, 1980; Hier, Hagenlocker, & Shindler, 1985; Nicholas, Obler, Albert, & associates, 1985). These elicitation and scoring procedures are not actually *tests* of discourse. However, their materials and procedures may be useful for clinicians concerned with measuring (and treating) brain-injured adults' discourse impairments.

Yorkston and Beukelman (1980) published a system for measuring the amount of information conveyed by aphasic adults as they described the "Cookie Theft" picture from the *Boston Diagnostic Aphasia Examination* (see Figure 5-22). The central measure in their system is what Yorkston and Beukelman called *content units,* which they defined as elements of information that were mentioned by at least 1 of 78 non-brain-injured adults who described the BDAE picture.

> Yorkston and Beukelman's 1 of 78 criterion seems too permissive to me. It seems to me that including information mentioned by only 1 of 78 judges risks including tangential, irrelevant, or unimportant informational elements. Making the criterion more stringent (e.g., requiring mention by at least 10 of 78 judges) would, I think, provide a list of content units with greater validity when applied to a population of speakers.

Yorkston and Beukelman reported that *content units per minute* differentiated the speech of aphasic adults from that of non-brain-injured adults. (The aphasic adults produced fewer content units per minute.) Results reported by Yorkston and Beukelman for one aphasic adult suggested that both *number of content units* and *content units per minute* are sensitive measures of change in connected speech as a result of treatment.

Others have modified or expanded on Yorkston and Beukelman's content unit measures (Golper, Thorpe, P., Tompkins, & associates, 1980; Shewan, 1988). However, the content units measure and its variants are limited in application because they only can be used to analyze speech elicited with the BDAE "Cookie Theft" picture.

Nicholas and Brookshire (1993, 1995a) subsequently published a standard protocol for eliciting and scoring discourse from brain-injured adults, using several kinds of elicitation stimuli:

- The speech elicitation pictures from the *Boston Diagnostic Aphasia Examination* and the *Western Aphasia Battery* (see Figure 5-22)
- Two *single pictures* depicting story-like situations with a central focus and interactions among picture elements (Figure 5-24)
- Two *picture sequences,* each of which contain six pictures portraying a short story (Figure 5-25)
- Two *requests for personal information* ("Tell me what you usually do on Sundays" and "Tell me where you live and describe it to me.")
- Two *requests for procedural information* ("Tell me how you would go about doing dishes by hand" and "Tell me how you would go about writing and sending a letter.")

Nicholas and Brookshire (1993, 1995a) provided rules for scoring *words, correct information units,* and *main concepts* in speech samples elicited with the protocol. They defined *correct information units* as words that are accurate, relevant, and informative relative to the eliciting stimulus. They defined *main concepts* as statements that convey the most important information about a stimulus.

Nicholas and Brookshire (1993) reported that *words per minute, correct information units per minute,* and *percent of words that are correct information units* reliably discriminate aphasic adults from those without aphasia, but

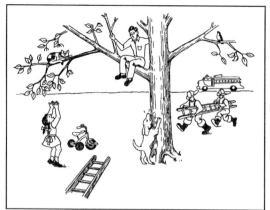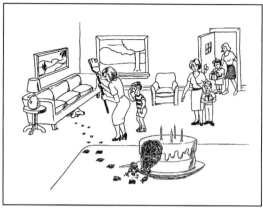

Figure 5-24 ▪ Connected-speech elicitation pictures. (From Brookshire, R. H., & Nicholas, L. E. [1993]. *The Discourse Comprehension Test.* Minneapolis: BRK Publishers.)

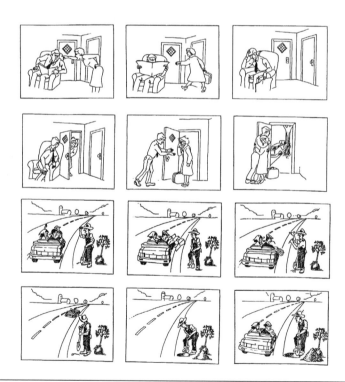

Figure 5-25 ▪ Prompted story-telling pictures. (From Brookshire, R. H., & Nicholas, L. E. [1993]. *The Discourse Comprehension Test.* Minneapolis: BRK Publishers.)

they suggested that combining a speech rate measure *(words per minute)* with an informativeness measure *(percent of words that are correct information units)* provides a better description of aphasic adults' connected speech than any single measure. They also reported that the number of main concepts mentioned did not reliably discriminate aphasic speakers' performance from that of non-brain-injured speakers. The *accuracy* and *completeness* of the main concepts aphasic speakers produced did, however, reliably discriminate them from non-brain-injured speakers (Nicholas & Brookshire, 1993). Nicholas and Brookshire's report contains normative information for non-brain-injured adults and aphasic adults.

Brookshire and Nicholas (1995a) described a rule-based system for scoring what they called *performance deviations* in the speech of adults with aphasia and reported the frequency of performance deviations in speech samples from 40 non-brain-injured adults, 10 adults with fluent aphasia, and 10 adults with nonfluent aphasia. They defined performance deviations as "features that make the connected speech of aphasic adults distinctive (e.g., inaccurate or vague words, revised utterances)..." (p. 118), and described nine categories of those features (Table 5-4).

Several categories of performance deviations distinguished non-brain-injured adults from those with aphasia. Non-brain-injured adults produced fewer inaccurate words, false starts, and

T A B L E   5 - 4

Performance deviation categories

Performance Deviations	Definition	Examples
Non-CIU Categories		
Inaccurate	Not accurate with regard to the stimulus and no attempt to correct	. . . on a ***chair*** (for stool)
False start	False start or abandoned utterance	. . . on ***a chair . . no.*** a stool
Unnecessary exact repetition	Exact repetition of words, unless used purposefully for emphasis or cohesion	. . . on a . . ***on a*** stool
Nonspecific or vague	Nonspecific or vague words or words lacking an unambiguous referent	. . . on a ***thing*** . . . on ***it*** (with no referent for "it")
Filler	Empty words that do not communicate information about the stimulus	. . . on a . . ***you know*** . . stool
The word "and"	All occurrences of the word "and"	. . . a boy ***and*** a stool
Off-task or irrelevant	Commentary on the test or the speaker's performance	***I've seen this one before. I can't say it.***
Nonword Categories		
Part word or unintelligible production	Word fragment or production that does not result in a word that is intelligible in context	. . . on a ***st . . sk . .*** stool . . . on a ***frampi***
Nonword filler	Utterance such as "uh" or "um"	. . . on a . . ***um*** . . stool . . ***uh.***

Data from Brookshire, R. H., & Nicholas, L. E. (1995). Performance deviations in the connected speech of adults with no brain damage and adults with aphasia. *American Journal of Speech-Language Pathology, 4,* 118-123.
CIU, correct information units.
*In the example, only nonwords and words printed in boldface italics are scored as performance deviations.

part-words or unintelligible productions than did the aphasic adults. The non-brain-injured adults also produced fewer instances of unnecessary exact repetition than did fluent aphasic adults and had fewer instances of the word *and* and less nonword filler than did nonfluent aphasic adults. There were no meaningful differences between a group of non-brain-injured adults and a group of adults with aphasia in the frequency with which they produced nonspecific words, filler words, or off-task words.

Brookshire and Nicholas (1995) suggested that measuring performance deviations in brain-injured adults' connected speech provides a useful supplement to measures of communicative informativeness and efficiency. Although Brookshire and Nicholas studied only aphasic adults, their categories of performance deviations and their scoring systems seem appropriate for quantifying the connected speech of brain-injured adults in other diagnostic categories.

Speech Fluency

Several methods for assessing brain-injured adults' speech fluency have been described in the literature. None has been standardized, and their reliability remains to be documented, but they do provide procedures with which speech fluency can be assessed in more or less systematic fashion.

Wagenaar, Snow, and Prins (1975) described 30 measures for quantifying various characteristics of aphasic adults' connected speech. Among their conclusions were the following:

- The most useful measure for classifying aphasia patients on the basis of their speech production is *fluency.*
- Patients can be classified as fluent or nonfluent on the basis of *speech tempo* (words per minute) and *mean length of utterance.*
- Telegraphic speech and empty speech are separate syndromes.
- Grammatic and articulatory errors are separate factors and not directly related to fluency.

Wagenaar and associates' procedures are too cumbersome for routine clinical use, but their list of measures and their findings may help clinicians develop systematic and practical procedures for analyzing aphasic patients' spontaneous speech.

Assessing Intelligibility

The speech of most patients with neurogenic language disorders caused by unilateral brain injury is intelligible, although its content may be anomalous. Consequently, assessment of intelligibility usually is not an important concern in evaluating these patients. When intelligibility is a concern, *Assessing Intelligibility of Dysarthric Speech* (Yorkston & Beukelman, 1981) permits its measurement. Yorkston and Beukelman's procedure is described in Chapter 11 of this book.

ASSESSING WRITTEN EXPRESSION
Writing Subtests of Language Test Batteries

All the major language test batteries include subtests for assessing written expression at several levels, but no standardized free-standing tests designed for assessment of brain-injured adults' writing are currently available. The writing subtests in language test batteries permit clinicians to assess written expression at four levels—*generating automatized sequences, copying, writing to dictation,* and *writing self-formulated material.* However, there are minor differences in test content within levels, and some language test batteries include writing subtests not seen in the others. For example, the MTDDA includes a subtest in which patients *orally* spell words dictated by the examiner in the *Visuomotor and Writing Disturbances* section, although no written output is required.

In *generating automatized sequences* subtests, the patient is asked to write overlearned sequences (usually the alphabet and numbers from 1 to 20 and sometimes the patient's name). Scoring of patients' responses differs across tests, but it usually involves counting misspellings, omissions, transpositions, and illegible productions. Producing automatized sequences usually is the easiest writing subtest for most brain-injured adults. Many can write strings of consecutive numbers and letters when they can produce little else in the way of written material. Signing one's name is a highly automatized activity for most adults, and many brain-injured adults who cannot generate strings of letters or numbers can write their name fluently and with little effort.

> Sometimes patients who cannot generate strings of letters or numbers or write their name in response to spoken requests can complete letter and number strings and complete their written name if given the first few letters or numbers in the series. Completing such automatized sequences often proves surprisingly easy for patients who seem completely at a loss when asked to generate them in response to the examiner's requests.

Copying subtests require patients to copy geometric forms, symbols, letters, printed words, or printed sentences. Adults with posterior brain injury often have unusual difficulty with copying subtests, perhaps because of impairments in visual perception and discrimination. Aphasic patients usually do well at copying simple stimuli such as forms, symbols, and letters, but their performance deteriorates when they copy words and sentences, wherein spelling errors, syntactic errors, and word substitutions may appear. Nonfluent aphasic patients who are weak or paralyzed in their preferred hand and arm usually produce distorted representations of stimuli in copying tests because of the mechanical difficulty of producing forms or letters with their nonpreferred hand and arm.

Writing to dictation subtests usually follow a letter-word-sentence progression. Patients are asked to write letters, then words, then sentences to dictation.

In *letter or number transcription* subtests the patient writes nonconsecutive strings of letters or numbers dictated by the examiner. The PICA includes a subtest in which the examiner

spells the names of the PICA test objects aloud, first at a moderate rate, pausing between syllables, and if the patient fails at that level, the examiner spells each word letter-by-letter, pausing while the patient writes each letter. The latter procedure is equivalent to the letter-transcription and number-transcription procedures in the other language test batteries. Tests in which patients must write words that are spelled aloud without pauses between letters make heavy demands on auditory memory and spelling ability, and for many brain-injured adults writing words dictated letter-by-letter is much more difficult than writing words to dictation.

All major language test batteries include subtests in which patients write words to dictation. The examiner may say a phrase containing the target word and then repeat it, as in the MTDDA ("I went to the dentist. Write went."), but most often the examiner simply explains the procedure to the patient then says the target words one at a time. ("Now I'll say some words, one at a time. I want you to write each word after I say it. Write banana.") Some language test batteries provide backup procedures when the patient cannot write a word. When a patient misses a word in the spelling subtest of the WAB the examiner orally spells the word while the patient writes it letter by letter, and if the patient still fails, the examiner provides anagram letters with which the patient can spell the word manually. Tests in which patients write words to dictation are primarily tests of spelling ability, although performance also may be affected by impaired auditory retention, compromised visual perception, or limb weakness or clumsiness.

The MTDDA and the WAB each provide a subtest in which patients write sentences to dictation. The MTDDA subtest includes seven sentences ranging in length from two words ("Come in.") to 13 words ("There is a church, a drugstore, and a filling station on the corner."). The WAB subtest contains a single unusual sentence ("Pack my box with five dozen jugs of liquid veneer."), which may prove challenging to some nonaphasic adults.

All major comprehensive aphasia tests include subtests in which patients write material for which the examiner provides no spoken model. For most brain-injured adults the easiest of these subtests are written confrontation naming subtests in which the patient is shown a drawing or an object and asked to write its name. (The WAB provides an object-based subtest as a backup for the writing words to dictation subtest. When a patient fails to write the name of an object in the writing-to-dictation subtest, they are shown the object and asked to write its name.)

The MTDDA and the PICA include subtests that require writing self-formulated sentences. In the MTDDA the patient is asked to create and write a sentence containing each of six printed words. In the PICA the patient is asked to write the functions of each of the 10 PICA test objects ("As completely as possible, write here what you do with each of these.")

> The difficulty of write-a-sentence-given-a-word tests depends greatly on the nature of the stimulus words provided. It is easier for brain-injured adults (and non-brain-injured adults) to write sentences when the stimuli are nouns or verbs than to write sentences when the stimuli are adjectives, adverbs, prepositions, or function words. Composing a sentence containing the word *man* requires much less mental effort than composing a sentence containing the word *slowly.*

The BDAE, the MTDDA, and the WAB each contain a written version of the *picture-description* subtest described earlier. In each, the patient is asked to write a paragraph about the picture they have previously described orally. (See Figure 5-22 for the pictures used in these subtests.) Writing words and sentences to dictation is easier for most aphasic patients than writing self-formulated sentences or paragraphs. However, a few patients may do better when their responses are not constrained to repro-

duce exactly what the examiner says. They may do better when they are free to choose their own words, construct their own sentences, and communicate their own thoughts and ideas.

Free-Standing Tests of Written Expression
Few free-standing writing tests are used commonly in evaluation of brain-injured adults' writing abilities, perhaps because the subtests in comprehensive aphasia tests are sufficient for most clinical purposes. However, written spelling tests, such as the spelling subtest of the *Wide Range Achievement Test* (Wilkinson, 1993), sometimes are used to evaluate brain-injured adults' written spelling. Using these tests permits the examiner to calculate a spelling grade level and sometimes a percentile rank for a patient's spelling performance.

GENERAL CONCEPTS 5-3
- *Recitations, rhymes, automatized sequences, sentence completion,* and *repeating short, simple phrases* are the easiest speech production subtests in language test batteries. Patients with moderate to severe speech production impairments often can perform acceptably (although not without error) in these subtests.
- Patients name pictures, drawings, or objects in tests of *confrontation naming.* Patients give one-word answers to questions such as "What color is snow?" in tests of *responsive naming.*
- The *Word Fluency Test* is a free-standing test of generative naming, in which the patient says all the words he or she can think of that begin with a certain letter (usually *F, A,* or *S*).
- The *Boston Naming Test (BNT)* is a free-standing, standardized test of confrontation naming. The words in the first part of the BNT are more common than the words in the last part.
- The *Test of Adolescent/Adult Word Finding* is a comprehensive test of naming. It permits assessment of naming in five tasks: *naming pictured nouns, naming pictured verbs, sen-*

tence completion, description naming, and *category naming.*

- Several variables affect the ease with which aphasic adults can produce words in tests of naming:

  —*Frequency of occurrence.* Frequently occurring words usually are easier for aphasic patients to retrieve and produce.

  —*Length and phonologic complexity.* Shorter and less complex words usually are easier for aphasic patients to retrieve and produce. Phonologic complexity is most likely to affect patients with speech motor control or phonologic selection and sequencing problems.

  —*Semantic characteristics.* Nouns may be slightly easier than verbs for aphasic patients to retrieve and produce.

- The *form* of stimuli to be named (drawings, photographs, real objects) has little effect on most aphasic adults' naming performance. Providing *context* for pictorial stimuli to be named has stronger effects, although there is considerable variability in the effects of context across aphasic patients.

- Language test batteries typically assess sentence production by requiring patients to define words, make sentences from words supplied by the examiner, or express simple ideas.

- The *Reporter's Test* is a free-standing test of sentence production in which the patient describes manipulations of tokens carried out by the examiner.

- *Picture description* is the primary means by which discourse is elicited from patients in language test battery subtests. Some test batteries also use *story telling* or *story retelling* tasks. However, brain-injured patients' performance in story retelling tasks may be compromised by their impaired comprehension and memory for the stories.

- Interviews and conversations are important speech production tasks in the *Boston Diagnostic Aphasia Examination* and the *Western Aphasia Battery.* Patients' performance in the interview and conversation is an important part of patient classification in those test batteries.

- Several free-standing procedures for assessing aphasic adults' *discourse production* have been reported in the literature. Measuring the *informativeness* (percentage of words that are informative) and the *rate* at which information is produced (content units per minute) provides a measure of communicative efficiency.

- Measuring *performance deviations* helps to capture the "aphasic" character of aphasic patients' spoken discourse.

- *Speech fluency* is important in the *Boston Diagnostic Aphasia Examination* and the *Western Aphasia Battery* procedures for classifying patients into neurodiagnostic syndromes. No standardized procedures for measuring fluency currently exist.

- *Speech intelligibility* usually is not a major problem for patients with unilateral brain injury.

- Language test batteries typically assess aphasic adults' ability to produce written language by asking them to *write automatized sequences, copy, write to dictation,* and *write self-formulated material.* Copying almost always is easier than writing to dictation for brain-injured patients. Most brain-injured patients are better at writing to dictation than they are at writing self-generated material.

THOUGHT QUESTIONS

Question 5-1 Andante Portofino, a right-handed patient with Broca's aphasia following a stroke, exhibits the following signs:

Right hemiparesis, arm greater than leg

Good auditory comprehension (85th percentile)

Poor oral reading (25th percentile)

Poor reading comprehension (30th percentile)

Is this pattern of performance what one would expect? Justify your answer.

Question 5-2 Corrina Aldeberan is a right-handed woman who has had a left-hemisphere stroke and has been diagnosed as aphasic. She is given a list of words to read aloud. Here is a sample of her performance.

Stimulus word	Patient reads
house	horse
cliff	stiff
tomorrow	tomorrow
store	stone
mother	mother
stand	stain
newspaper	newspaper

Speculate as to the reasons for Ms. Aldeberan's performance. What would you expect the nature of her aphasia to be?

Question 5-3 You administer the *Token Test* shown on the following pages to Jennie Smith, an aphasic patient. She receives the following scores:

Part A (7 points possible)	7	(100%)
Part B (8 points possible)	8	(100%)
Part C (12 points possible)	12	(100%)
Part D (16 points possible)	13	(81%)
Part E (24 points possible)	8	(33%)
Part F (96 points possible)	85	(89%)
Total	133	(82%)

(Words struck out denote parts of the commands that Ms. Smith missed. Underlined words are characteristics that are scored in Ms. Smith's response. Scoring is 1 point per characteristic correctly identified. The number of points possible in each part are in parentheses in the score boxes.)

There is something unusual about Ms. Smith's performance. Tell what it is and speculate about the reasons for the unusual performance.

Question 5-4 The following speech samples represent transcripts of two adults talking about the "birthday party" picture. They are typed without punctuation. The number of dots indicates the relative durations of pauses.

Mrs. Bloom produces the following speech sample. (She produces 105 words per minute.)

> and . . . um . . . what do you call it . . . but I guess the cat got into it and . . . uh he's hiding under the sitter and the mother is gonna . . . trying to get him out of there . . . and he cleaned up the rug and . . . uh the rest of the birthday cake . . . those ones there . . . children . . . boys and girls . . . are arriving and it's . . . um not too good a deal I'd say

Mr. Jones produces the following speech sample. (He produces 40 words per minute.)

> um . . . um . . . uh . . . cake . . . and . . . um . . . and . . . and dog . . . dog ate cake . . . and . . . and . . . trouble . . . mom is mad . . . and . . . and . . . um . . . um . . . kid is crying . . . and . . . and . . . neighbors . . . neighbors is coming

Is Mrs. Bloom aphasic? Is Mr. Jones aphasic? If so, what aphasia syndrome do they represent?

Question 5-5 The following writing sample was provided by a 56-year-old man who complained of sudden onset of reading and writing problems. He is describing the "Cookie Theft" picture from the *Boston Diagnostic Aphasia Examination*. Speculate as to the source of this patient's writing impairment.

> The woman iz at the senk drying dishez. The fauset iz on and woter is runing onto thi floor. Although her shoos are soaking, she seems knot to mind. Her young sun and daughter are steeling cockies from the cocky jar behind thi mother's bak. The sun is on a stul reaching for the cocky jar and thi daughter has her hand raised to git a cookie.

Patient Name: _____J. Smith_____

Date of Evaluation: _9/9/99_ Examiner: _____J. Doe___

Part A

#	Item	Score
1	Show me a <u>circle</u>.	1
2	Show me a <u>square</u>.	1
3	Show me a <u>yellow</u> one.	1
4	Show me a <u>red</u> one.	1
5	Show me a <u>blue</u> one.	1
6	Show me a <u>green</u> one.	1
7	Show me a <u>white</u> one.	1

Total: A (7)	7
Time (sec)	90

Part B

#	Item	Score
8	Show me the <u>yellow</u> <u>square</u>.	2
9	Show me the <u>blue</u> <u>circle</u>.	2
10	Show me the <u>green</u> <u>circle</u>.	2
11	Show me the <u>white</u> <u>square</u>.	2

Total: B (8)	8
Time (sec)	85

Part C

#	Item	Score
12	Show me the <u>small</u> <u>white</u> <u>circle</u>.	3
13	Show me the <u>large</u> <u>yellow</u> <u>square</u>.	3
14	Show me the <u>large</u> <u>green</u> <u>square</u>.	3
15	Show me the <u>small</u> <u>blue</u> <u>square</u>.	3

Total: C (12)	12
Time (sec)	95

Part D

#	Item	Score
16	Show me the <u>red</u> <u>circle</u> and the <u>green</u> <u>square</u>.	4
17	Show me the <u>yellow</u> <u>square</u> and the ~~<u>blue</u> square~~.	3
18	Show me the <u>white</u> <u>square</u> and the ~~<u>green circle</u>~~.	2
19	Show me the <u>white</u> <u>circle</u> and the <u>red</u> <u>circle</u>.	4

Total: D (16)	13
Time (sec)	125

Figure 5-26 ■ **Token Test score sheet.**   *Continued*

QUESTION 5-3: TOKEN TEST SCORE SHEET

Part E

#	Item	Score
20	Show me the ~~large white~~ circle and the ~~small green~~ square.	2
21	Show me the ~~small blue~~ circle and the ~~large yellow square~~.	1
22	Show me the large ~~green~~ square and the ~~large red~~ square.	3
23	Show me the ~~large white~~ square and the ~~small~~ green ~~circle~~.	2

Total: E (24)	8
Time (sec)	140

Part F

#	Item	Score
24	Put the red circle on the green square.	6
25	Put the white square behind the ~~yellow~~ circle.	5
26	Touch the blue circle with the red square.	6
27	Touch the blue circle and the red square.	6
28	Pick up the blue circle or the red square.	6
29	Move the green square away from the ~~yellow square~~.	4
30	Put the white circle in front of the blue square.	6
31	If there is a black circle, pick up the red square.	6
32	Pick up all the squares except the yellow one.	6
33	Put the green square beside the red circle.	6
34	Touch the squares slowly and the circles quickly.	6
35	Put the red circle ~~between~~ the ~~yellow square~~ and the ~~green square~~.	2
36	Touch all the circles except the ~~green~~ one.	5
37	Pick up the red circle --- no --- the white square.	6
38	Instead of the white square, pick up the yellow circle.	6
39	Together with the yellow circle, pick up the blue ~~circle~~.	5

Total: F (96)	85
Time (sec)	190

Total: A - F (163)	133
Time (min/sec)	725 / 12:05

Figure 5-26 cont'd ■ **Token Test score sheet.**

The Context for Treatment of Neurogenic Communication Disorders

THE TREATMENT TEAM

Contemporary medical care is oriented around the concept of the treatment team. Under the treatment team concept, the responsibility for a patient's overall care rests with a group, rather than with one person or with independently operating professionals, although one member of the team usually has primary responsibility for coordinating the team's activities. Which professions are represented on a patient's treatment team depends on the nature of the patient's physical and medical problems. For example, the treatment team for a patient with chronic obstructive pulmonary disease might include a pulmonary physician, a cardiologist, a respiratory therapist, an occupational therapist, a nurse, and a social worker. The treatment team for a stroke patient might include a neurologist, a nurse, a speech-language pathologist, a neuropsychologist, a physical therapist, an occupational therapist, a dietitian, and a social worker. Each member of a team has primary responsibility for a given aspect of the patient's care, but responsibilities often overlap, so planning, coordination, and communication among team members is crucial if the treatment program is to be efficient and effective.

Speech-language pathologists who participate in the care of brain-injured adults are likely to serve on teams with an assortment of other professionals, and, as noted above, the composition of the team for any given patient depends primarily on the patient's needs. Although one cannot always predict who will be on a given patient's treatment team, speech-language pathologists who work with brain-injured adults often serve on teams with representatives of the following professions.

Neurologists As described previously, neurologists have primary responsibility for the medical care of patients with brain damage or other nervous system pathology. Because their role in patient care has been described in detail earlier in this book, it will not be repeated here.

Physiatrists Physiatrists (or *rehabilitation medicine physicians*) have primary medical responsibility for patients admitted to rehabilitation wards. They help physically disabled patients regain the use of impaired muscles, and when restitution of function is not possible, they help the patient compensate for the muscular impairments. Physiatrists examine the patient; determine the patient's medical and rehabilitation needs; design comprehensive rehabilitation programs; and oversee the activities of physical, occupational, corrective, vocational, and recreational therapists.

Physical Therapists Physical therapists evaluate the patient's muscle strength and range of limb movement. Under the supervision of a physiatrist they also carry out programs to help patients retain or regain muscle strength and limb movement. When a patient is confined to bed, a physical therapist may see the patient at bedside and teach the patient how to turn over in bed, sit up, and transfer from the bed to a chair or wheelchair. Physical therapists carry out passive range-of-movement exercises in which bedbound patients' limbs are moved and muscles are stretched to prevent contractures (permanent shortening of muscles resulting from spasticity) and to preserve muscle strength and tone. Other physical therapy activities take place in the physical therapy clinic and include muscle strengthening and range-of-movement activities along with teaching patients how to transfer to and from a wheelchair; how to use braces, canes, and crutches; and how to get dressed. If a patient is about to be discharged home or to a nursing home, the physical therapist may help the family or nursing home staff prepare the living environment for the special needs of the patient and may provide the patient with exercise programs to do at home.

Occupational Therapists Occupational therapists help patients regain abilities necessary for activities of daily living, such as cooking, dressing, and grooming. Although both occupational and physical therapists work on muscle strengthening, occupational therapists usually work on muscles in activities that resemble those of daily living. A patient who needs to strengthen hand and arm muscles might sand boards, saw wood, or weave on a loom. A patient with visuospatial impairments might perform craft activities requiring eye-hand coordination. An important part of occupational therapists' responsibilities is to help the patient resume daily life activities such as cooking, cleaning, and making beds. Occupational therapists teach compensatory strategies, provide special tools and appliances, and modify standard tools and appliances to help patients compensate for their impairments. Occupational therapists also help patients develop leisure activities and hobbies, and they sometimes test and treat patients for sensorimotor and visuospatial disorders. Because occupational therapists often deal with visual perception and reading or writing, speech-language pathologists often collaborate with them on treating these aspects of the patient's needs.

Vocational Therapists Vocational therapists provide vocational testing and evaluation. They administer work aptitude tests and real or simulated on-the-job evaluations to determine if a patient can go back to work. Vocational therapists sometimes arrange work placements or modify a patient's work environment and responsibilities to enable them to perform work assignments successfully. In some medical facilities, occupational therapists provide vocational testing and evaluation.

Corrective Therapists Corrective therapists are primarily responsible for ambulation training. They collaborate with physical and occupational therapists to help the patient regain the strength, balance, and endurance needed for walking, and they may teach the patient how to use crutches and canes and how to climb and descend stairs.

Recreation Therapists Recreation therapists provide therapeutic recreational activities (usually arts and crafts) and may get the patient started in leisure activities that the patient may continue after discharge from the medical facility.

Neuropsychologists Neuropsychologists administer tests of cognitive functions (e.g., attention, memory, mental flexibility, intellect) that may help to discriminate between psychiatric and neurologic conditions, distinguish between different neurologic conditions, and predict the course of a patient's recovery. Neuropsychologists provide the treatment team with information about the patient's adjustment to disabilities and the patient's present and probable future cognitive and behavioral abilities and limitations. Neuropsychologists help to plan and carry out a plan of care for the patient and may have primary responsibility for assessing the effects of treatment on the patient's cognitive abilities. Neuropsychologists often collaborate closely with speech-language pathologists in a patient's care and may collaborate with speech-language pathologists in assessing brain-injured patients' cognitive and communicative status, with the neuropsychologist taking the lead in evaluating cognitive functions such as perception, attention, and memory, and the speech-language pathologist taking primary responsibility for evaluating communicative and linguistic abilities.

Clinical Psychologists Clinical psychologists administer and interpret tests of intelligence, cognition, and personality and provide the patient-care team with information about the patient's intellectual, cognitive, and emotional state. A clinical psychologist may help the patient and family deal with the emotional and psychologic effects of the patient's brain damage. When a patient is depressed or anxious, the clinical psychologist may help the patient and family understand and cope with the feelings.

Psychiatrists Some brain-injured patients develop symptoms of depression, psychosis, neurosis, or other personality aberrations. For these patients a psychiatrist may provide diagnosis, referral, and treatment (especially when medications to control a patient's psychiatric symptoms are appropriate).

Dietitians Dietitians evaluate patients' nutritional needs and recommend dietary adjustments to correct nutritional deficiencies. Dietitians work with the other members of the treatment team to ensure that the patient's food and liquid intake are sufficient to meet nutritional and hydration needs. Dietitians often collaborate with speech-language pathologists to set up special diets and feeding programs for patients with *dysphagia* (swallowing disorders) caused by neurologic or structural damage that disrupts the mechanics of chewing and swallowing.

Speech-Language Pathologists Speech-language pathologists provide assessment, treatment, and referral services for communication disorders and related impairments. Speech-language pathologists often play a prominent part on treatment teams for brain-injured patients with communication disorders because they are experienced in communicating with these patients. Because the speech-language pathologist's work with communicatively impaired patients often touches on the patient's personal concerns, they often learn a great deal about the needs and concerns of the patient and family. Consequently, the speech-language pathologist often plays an important part in communicating the needs and concerns of the patient and family members to the treatment team.

Social Workers Social workers coordinate and manage communication between medical facility staff and the patient and family. Social workers keep families informed about treatment and discharge plans. They suggest, initiate, and coordinate referrals to medical, financial, and social service agencies and programs, and they may provide patients and families with information about nursing homes, county and state medical and family services, and other social and community resources that help the patient and family adjust to altered financial, vocational, and social conditions. Social workers ensure that physicians' orders for wheelchairs and other prosthetic appliances are carried out, and the social worker may make arrangements for programs such as Meals on Wheels or public health nurse visits to the patient's home. Social workers coordinate evaluations of legal competence for patients whose competence is questionable and make referrals to psychologic and mental health services, chemical dependency programs, Social Security or Veterans Administration counselors, financial ad-

visors, vocational counselors, or family and marriage counselors. Social workers play a key role in coordinating interactions among the medical facility staff, the patient, the patient's family, and community and state agencies. Social workers help the patient and family adjust to changed lifestyles and ensure that the patient's post-hospital placement represents the needs, wishes, and current circumstances of the patient and the family.

The treatment team approach can improve significantly both the quality and the efficiency of patient care by ensuring that a comprehensive treatment plan addressing all important aspects of the patient's care is created and followed, by maximizing communication among members of the team, and by delegating important components of care to team members who are professionally qualified to assume responsibility for those components.

Candidacy for Treatment

The process of deciding which patients with neurogenic communication disorders should get treatment has received little attention in the literature, perhaps because of the number and complexity of variables that enter into the process and the subjective nature of the decisions. Although there are no immutable rules that permit clinicians to separate the good treatment candidates from the poor ones, there are several general principles that can be used to guide the decision-making process.

The amount and location of a patient's brain damage are important determinants of a patient's potential response to treatment. The greater the brain damage and the more it affects areas of the brain involved in communication, the less likely it is that a patient will recover communication abilities, with or without treatment. The size and location of a patient's brain damage can be estimated directly from laboratory measures, such as computerized tomography or magnetic resonance imaging scans, or indirectly from behavioral measures, such as tests of speech, language, memory, and cognition. However, the relationship between lesion size, lesion location, and behavioral deficits may be weak immediately following strokes or traumatic brain injuries, when temporary physiologic alterations such as bilateral reduction of cerebral blood flow, neurotransmitter release, cerebral edema, and diaschisis are present. For this reason clinicians may choose to wait several weeks before deciding not to treat a patient because of the severity of the patient's brain injury.

A patient's medical and physical conditions frequently affect decisions about treatment. Very ill, very depressed, or very weak patients often do not profit sufficiently from treatment to justify its cost. Patients who cannot sit up and attend to a task for 30 minutes may not be strong enough to tolerate intensive treatment, and the clinician may elect to forego treatment or at least to defer it until the patient recovers sufficient health and strength to participate gainfully in treatment activities.

A patient's enthusiasm and motivation to recover often have powerful effects on the outcome of treatment. Some highly motivated and resourceful patients benefit from treatment in spite of severe impairments. Some unmotivated or unconcerned patients fail to benefit from treatment although their impairments are not severe. A patient's life situation also may affect the outcome of treatment. A supportive, motivated, and caring family usually enhances the effects of treatment programs, whereas a nonsupportive, unmotivated, and uncaring family often compromises them.

Clinicians often resolve their doubts about the appropriateness of treatment for questionable treatment candidates by offering a short interval of trial treatment. If the patient responds well to the trial treatment, treatment continues, and if the patient responds poorly to the trial treatment, it is discontinued. If free to do so, most clinicians would offer trial treatment to all questionable treatment candidates to minimize the chances of missing patients who are good treatment candidates.

Given unlimited professional and financial resources, every patient with a neurogenic communication disorder might get at least a trial period of treatment. However, health care funding is increasingly limited, and health care providers face increasingly severe restrictions on who receives treatment and how much the treatment costs. This means that identifying the patients who are likely to benefit most from treatment, and doing so in a limited amount of time, will become an increasingly important part of the clinician's responsibilities. Limitations on resources will require that treatment be provided to those who are likely to receive the greatest benefit at the least cost and that decisions about who receives treatment must be made quickly. The issues of how benefit is defined and of what constitutes a reasonable cost-benefit ratio are complex, and, as in the tale of the blind men and the elephant, one's attitude depends greatly on the direction from which one looks at the problem. The issue is one that every clinician eventually must face, although few feel they have satisfactorily resolved it.

Patients have the right to refuse treatment, even though a clinician may feel that treatment is indicated. If a patient understands the nature of his or her communication impairments, the potential effects of the impairments on the patient and family, and the nature and potential benefits of treatment but refuses treatment, the patient's refusal must be accepted. If a patient is confused, intellectually impaired, or otherwise not competent to refuse potentially beneficial treatment, family members or others with the right to represent the patient may decide for the patient.

GENERAL CHARACTERISTICS OF TREATMENT SESSIONS
Frequency and Duration

Several variables affect the frequency and duration of brain-injured adults' treatment. One variable is the patient's medical and physical condition. Immediately after brain injury and for intervals that last anywhere from a few days to several weeks, many patients' physical and mental endurance are compromised by the physiologic effects of their brain injury. For patients in the early stages of recovery, short (15-minute to 30-minute) treatment sessions may be appropriate, with the length of sessions increasing as these patients recover their physical and mental stamina. Sometimes a patient may be scheduled for two or three short treatment sessions rather than one long one—for example, one 30-minute session in the morning and one in the afternoon.

> Many facilities bill for speech-language pathology services in 15-minute increments, making 15-minute treatment sessions a possibility. However, unless the patient is seen at bedside, the logistics of getting the patient to and from the speech pathology clinic usually make 15-minute sessions impractical.

The complexity of a treatment program also affects how long treatment sessions need be to accomplish treatment objectives. Some treatment programs may have only a single objective that can be accomplished by one or two treatment tasks (e.g., speech production drills to increase a dysarthric patient's speech intelligibility). For such programs 30-minute sessions may be sufficient. Complex treatment programs with several objectives typically need more time (e.g., treatment of a right-hemisphere-damaged patient to facilitate affective expression, improve abstract thinking, diminish tangentiality in spontaneous speech, and improve turn-taking behavior in conversations).

Logistics often play an important part in determining a patient's treatment schedule. Close by and accessible patients can reasonably be scheduled for shorter and more frequent appointments than those who are farther away or less accessible. Ambulatory hospitalized patients who can get themselves up, dressed, and to the clinic are logistically easier to schedule for multiple appointments than patients for whom a journey to the clinic requires that ward personnel get the patient up, dressed, and into a wheel-

chair, and that an escort must bring the patient to the clinic and return the patient to the ward. It usually is not practical for outpatients to come to the clinic more than once a day, and most have twice-a-week or three-times-a-week appointments. Outpatients who attend other clinics (e.g., physical therapy) on a regular schedule often can have their appointments scheduled so that they can have both appointments during one trip to the treatment facility.

> The policies of the agencies that pay for treatment are another important determinant of appointment schedules. For example, some agencies will pay for only a predetermined number of speech-pathology appointments for patients with a particular communication disorder. Speech-language pathologists frequently must work within such limits when setting up appointment schedules for their patients.

For patients who are approaching discharge, making treatment sessions shorter and increasing the time between sessions can provide a transition between intensive treatment and discharge. The emphasis becomes consolidation of the patient's current performance and extension of that performance to daily life. During this time the content of treatment sessions moves away from training new strategies and behaviors to enhancing generalization of already-learned strategies and behaviors to the patient's daily life. Shorter and more widely spaced sessions may contribute to the generalization process.

Format

Treatment sessions tend to have a consistent format. Most begin with a short interval of conversation (the *opening*), in which the clinician and the patient converse about what has happened since the last session. The patient recounts achievements, tells about significant happenings, and describes problems. The clinician applauds the achievements, discusses the happenings, and helps with the problems. The clinician also uses the opening to evaluate the patient's performance relative to previous sessions, to estimate the extent to which treated behaviors are generalizing to conversational interactions, and to appraise the patient's mood and energy level. The opening gives the patient time to settle in, get comfortable, and get problems and concerns out of the way and helps to establish and maintain personal rapport between the patient and the clinician.

The opening leads into a short interval of work on easy tasks in which the patient's performance is nearly error-free (*accommodation*). Accommodation tasks usually are tasks the patient has mastered in previous sessions. They get the patient into the sequence and timing of treatment procedures and provide the patient with a warm-up for the more difficult tasks that follow (*goal-directed work*).

Goal-directed work is the heart of the treatment session. Tasks become more challenging and are focused on specific treatment objectives. The clinician instructs, explains, delivers treatment stimuli, provides feedback, and records the patient's performance. The patient works at or near maximum capacity in each treatment task. The interaction between the clinician and the patient is governed by the treatment protocol—the clinician's contributions and the patient's responses are task directed. Except for transitions between tasks, there is little purely social interaction.

Many clinicians follow the work segment with some work on a few familiar tasks in which the patient is highly successful (*cool-down*). The patient's successful performance in cool-down tasks can contribute to a sense of accomplishment that generalizes to the session as a whole. Many clinicians end treatment sessions with a short interval of conversation about what happened in the session, what the patient plans to do before the next session, and what the clinician and patient plan to do in the next session (the *closing*).

The foregoing generic format describes how the focus of treatment activities changes as a typ-

ical treatment session unfolds. Not every clinician follows this format, and those who do may not follow it in every session. They may deviate from it or abandon it altogether, depending on what they perceive as the patient's needs.

GENERAL CONCEPTS 6-1

- Speech-language pathologists who work in medical facilities often serve on treatment teams with other professionals. The treatment team is responsible for planning, implementing, and evaluating a patient's care while the patient is in a medical facility.

- Several variables may affect the probability that a brain-injured and communicatively impaired patient will benefit from treatment, including *the nature and severity of the brain injury, the patient's medical and physical condition*, and *the patient's motivation and enthusiasm*. A few sessions of trial treatment often provide the most dependable indicator of a patient's response to treatment.

- The frequency and duration of treatment sessions are influenced by several variables, including *the patient's medical and physical condition, the complexity of the treatment program, logistics*, and *how close the patient is to completion of the treatment program*.

- Treatment sessions for communicatively impaired adults usually begin with general conversation (*the opening*), which leads into work on familiar tasks in which the patient has high success rates (*accommodation*). *Goal-directed work* follows with challenging tasks, focused on specific treatment objectives. A short *cool-down* segment with easy tasks and high patient success rates follows goal-directed work. A brief interval of conversation (*the closing*) ends the session.

ADJUSTING TREATMENT TASKS TO THE PATIENT

After more than a century of study, treatment of adults with neurogenic communication impairments remains as much art as science. Hundreds of databased studies of neurogenic communication impairments have been published, but only a small fraction are directly relevant to treatment. Many treatment procedures have been described in the literature, but most are little more than descriptions of the procedures, with anecdotes or the authors' opinions substituting for empirical evidence of the procedures' effectiveness. Consequently, most decisions about how to approach a given patient's communication impairments rely more on the clinician's experience and intuition than on empirical evidence.

Beginning clinicians are not, however, condemned to trial and error as their only guide while they accumulate the experiences and nurture the intuitions that lead to clinical expertise. The clinical and research literature reveals regularities in how adults with neurogenic communication impairments respond to manipulations of the clinical environment, and it shows that most patients with a particular pattern of communication impairments respond to the manipulations in predictable ways, although idiosyncratic responses often occur. For example, the performance of most brain-injured adults is affected adversely by noisy or distraction-loaded environments, but a few may perform as well in noisy and distracting conditions as they do in quiet ones.

The following section summarizes some regularities that permit clinicians to manipulate certain aspects of treatment to accomplish their clinical objectives. The section begins with a brief discussion of resource-allocation models of cognition and the application of these models to treatment of brain-injured adults.

Resource-Allocation Models and the Clinical Process

Many adults with brain damage have perceptual, attentional, cognitive, and performance impairments that compromise their ability to perceive and discriminate sensory input, diminish the flexibility and efficiency of their cognitive processes, and compromise the speed and accuracy of their responses to stimulation. Clinicians who work with brain-injured adults must deal with the effects of these impairments on the patient's performance throughout assessment and treatment.

Fortunately, there are many ways in which clinicians can manipulate procedures to lessen the effects of these impairments. However, knowing which characteristics of the procedures to manipulate requires that the clinician have an idea of why the patient is having trouble. If the clinician knows the *why*, the *how* becomes more apparent.

Resource-allocation models of cognitive processes provide a convenient metaphor for organizing the search for the causes of an impaired performance, which in turn contributes to an organized approach to improving the performance. Several resource-allocation models of cognitive processing have been described in the literature (Friedman & Polson, 1981; Kahneman, 1973; Norman & Bobrow, 1975). McNeil and associates (McNeil & Kimelman, 1986; McNeil, Odell, & Tseng, 1990) have described a resource-allocation model for adult aphasia. Although resource-allocation models differ in details, they share a common theme, which is that every human has a finite amount of cognitive resources available for carrying out mental operations such as perceiving incoming stimuli, comprehending messages, storing information in memory, and formulating responses. In resource-allocation models the mental operations are called *cognitive processes*, and the mental energy, which is contained in a *central pool*, is called *processing resources*.

Activation of any cognitive process depends on transfer of resources from the pool to the process. Processes of greater complexity require more resources than processes of lesser complexity. If several cognitive processes are simultaneously active, each draws resources from the pool. Consequently, the amount of processing resources drawn from the pool depends both on the number of active cognitive processes and their complexity. As more processes are activated and as the complexity of the active processes increases, more resources are drawn from the pool. If the demand for resources exceeds the amount available in the pool, some processes may be shut down or shortchanged, and the performance of the system suffers.

Because there is only one resource pool for all cognitive processes, and because the resources in the pool are limited, increasing the resources allocated to one cognitive process diminishes the amount available for others. When processing demands are low, this is not a problem because the pool contains enough resources to keep all the active cognitive processes in business. However, as processing demands reach the capacity of the pool, calls for more resources from individual processes may be ignored or resources may be diverted from other active processes to the one making the call. In either case, performance deteriorates.

> In some contemporary resource-allocation models, separate pools for different categories of cognitive processes are postulated. In these models, increasing the call for resources from one pool does not affect the resources available from the other pools, and the effects of shortages in a pool will be seen only on cognitive processes that depend on that pool. To keep it simple, this discussion will assume a single-pool model.

Some resource-allocation models propose that the availability of resources in the central pool is not constant; instead, it varies in quasirandom fashion across time. The reasons for this variability are not specified, but the individual's emotional state, the individual's level of fatigue, the metabolic activity of the individual's brain, and other such changeable conditions may contribute to it. By incorporating cyclical, quasirandom patterns of resource availability, resource-allocation models attempt to explain the variability in performance that customarily is seen when individuals are working at or near their processing capacity—for example, the university student whose comprehension of a lecture waxes and wanes across 20 or 30 minutes, although the complexity of the lecture does not change.

When resource-allocation models attempt to explain the performance of brain-injured adults, most assume that brain damage reduces the amount of processing resources in the pool.

Consequently, the pool runs out of resources at lower-than-normal levels of processing workload, causing brain-injured persons to perform poorly on many tasks that they could do easily before acquiring brain damage and causing them to perform poorly relative to adults without brain damage.

> Whether the brain damage reduces the amount of resources in the pool or compromises access to the resources in the pool without diminishing the volume of the pool is not known. In either case, the effects on performance would be similar, although not identical in all situations.

Resource-allocation models predict that when a brain-injured person is performing tasks in which the need for processing resources is well below the amount present in the person's resource pool, performance should be essentially normal. As the number or complexity of processing demands approach the capacity of the pool, the brain-injured person's performance begins to deteriorate, becoming progressively worse as the processing demands reach and exceed the available resources. If, however, some elements of the tasks are simplified, thereby diminishing demands for processing resources, the brain-injured person's performance improves. The following example shows how this works.

> A brain-injured aphasic patient who also has a visuoperceptual impairment is asked to point to black-and-white line drawings of objects when the clinician describes them by function ("Point to the one used for writing and erasing."). After 10 trials he has made 8 errors. When the clinician pauses after the tenth trial, the patient complains that he is having trouble making out what the drawings represent. The clinician trades the drawings for colored photographs and does 10 more trials. The patient makes only two errors in those trials.

This patient had trouble with two components of the task—auditory comprehension and visual perception of the line drawings. In resource-allocation terms, the patient's aphasia and visual perceptual problems combined to create a need for processing resources that exceeded the resources in the pool. By changing the stimuli from line drawings to more realistic colored photographs, the clinician reduced the complexity of the visual processing needed to perform the task, freeing resources that could be redirected to auditory comprehension, which then improved. If the treatment focus had been on perception and recognition of line drawings, the clinician could have facilitated the patient's identification of the line drawings by reducing the difficulty of the auditory comprehension aspects of the task, thereby freeing additional resources for visual processing.

This quid pro quo (one thing in return for another) characteristic of resource-allocation models has important implications for clinicians working with brain-injured adults. The general principle is that clinicians can focus treatment on a targeted process by controlling the processing load associated with incidental task variables that are not related to the treatment objectives. This is what happened in the preceding example, when the clinician facilitated the patient's comprehension (the targeted process) by lowering the processing load associated with perceiving the visual stimuli (an incidental task variable). Resource-allocation concepts help to sensitize clinicians to the unintended effects of incidental task variables when they design treatment tasks. Clinicians who are aware of these effects can control for them, so that treatment tasks focus on the intended processes and are not complicated by processing demands associated with incidental task variables.

Because cognitive processes are internal, they cannot be directly manipulated. However, clinicians can indirectly manipulate processing workload by manipulating the characteristics of task stimuli and by changing the specifications for the responses expected from the patient.

Stimulus manipulations permit clinicians to regulate the amount of resources the patient needs for perception, discrimination, and interpretation of task stimuli. Changing the specifications for the patient's responses permits clinicians to regulate the amount of resources needed for formulating and producing the responses. First we will consider how clinicians may regulate a patient's workload by manipulating stimulus input. Then we will see how clinicians may adjust the patient's workload by manipulating response specifications.

Stimulus Manipulations

Clinicians may manipulate the difficulty of treatment tasks by adjusting several characteristics of treatment task stimuli. These adjustments affect the workload associated with perception, discrimination, and comprehension of the task stimuli and move the task stimuli up or down a continuum of workload. These adjustments permit clinicians to design tasks that force the patient's processing system to operate at or near its maximum but do not overwhelm it. Clinicians may manipulate processing workload by adjusting the *intensity and salience,* the *clarity and intelligibility,* the *redundancy and contextual support,* or the *novelty and interest value* of task stimuli.

Intensity and Salience Increasing the intensity or salience of stimuli helps many brain-injured patients perceive, discriminate, and comprehend them. *Intensity,* as used here, refers to the perceived magnitude or strength of a stimulus. *Salience* refers to the perceived prominence or conspicuousness of a stimulus—how clearly it stands out from its surroundings. In some ways intensity and salience are related because making a stimulus more intense (louder, brighter, larger) usually makes it more salient. However, intensity and salience differ in that intensity is a property of the stimulus itself, whereas salience expresses a relationship between the stimulus and its surroundings. A loud auditory stimulus presented against a noisy background may be less salient than a soft auditory stimulus presented against a silent background, and a brightly colored visual stimulus presented against a brightly colored and cluttered background may be less salient than a stimulus with more subdued colors presented against a plain and colorless background.

> Stars in the night sky are easier to see when viewed in rural areas than in urban areas, where city lights raise the level of foreground illumination. The stars are more *salient* in darker night skies, although their *intensity* does not change.

Increasing the intensity or salience of treatment stimuli can help brain-injured patients whose impaired perceptual or attentional processes compromise their perception, recognition, or comprehension of the stimuli. For example, a patient with problems focusing and maintaining attention in the presence of distracting or competing stimuli may perform poorly in structured conversations when a radio is playing in the background. In resource-allocation terms, the mental effort required for the patient to attend to the conversation and ignore the radio draws processing resources from the pool. If resources are diverted from other processes (e.g., comprehension) to shore up attention, attention gets better and the processes from which the resources are diverted get worse (the patient attends but fails to comprehend). If the conversational partner increases the intensity of their contributions (by talking louder, moving in closer, adding gesture) or increases the salience of what they say (by turning down the radio or moving away from it), the patient's conversational performance improves because the resources no longer needed to overcome the distracting effects of the background noise can be redirected to comprehension and other conversational operations.

Clinicians sometimes increase the salience of treatment stimuli by presenting them in more than one stimulus modality (most commonly auditory plus visual, as when a clinician simultaneously says the name of an object and shows the patient a picture of it). Several studies have reported slight to moderate improvements in brain-injured adults' performance with multimodality stimulation (Gardiner & Brookshire, 1972; Halpern, 1965; Lambrecht & Marshall, 1983). However, in almost every study in which positive effects of multimodality stimulation have been reported for groups of brain-injured adults, the effects, although statistically significant, were not strong and not all of the participants in the groups exhibited the effects. This suggests that clinicians will know if multimodality stimulation will help a particular patient only by trying it and observing its effects on the patient's performance.

> Variability in the effects of a manipulation on the performance of individual participants is common in group studies involving manipulations of treatment stimuli. Although some manipulations seem to have relatively consistent effects across patients in the groups, exceptions almost always are encountered. Consequently, clinicians typically verify the effects of a manipulation by trying it with the patient.

Clarity and Intelligibility Indistinct or ambiguous stimuli are notoriously difficult for almost all brain-injured patients. Making stimuli clearer and more intelligible usually helps them—especially if a patient has impaired perception, recognition, or discrimination of sensory stimuli. The negative effects of indistinctness and ambiguity often are seen when treatment stimuli are line drawings representing common objects or situations. For patients with visual processing impairments, line drawings that seem unambiguous to the clinician may be ambiguous to the patient. For example, brain-injured adults have a tendency to misperceive the drawing of a harmonica in the *Boston*

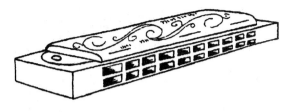

Figure 6-1 ■ **An example of a stimulus that sometimes proves ambiguous for brain-injured adults with visual perceptual impairments who often misidentify it as a building or factory.** (From Kaplan, E., Goodglass, H., & Weintraub, S. [2001]. *The Boston Naming Test.* Philadelphia: Lippincott Williams & Wilkins.)

Naming Test (Kaplan, Goodglass, & Weintraub, 2001) as a *building* or a *factory* (Figure 6-1).

Mills and associates (1979) studied the effects of what they called "stimulus uncertainty" on aphasic adults' naming of line drawings of common objects. Their measure of uncertainty for each drawing was the number of different names a group of 14 normal adults gave to the drawing. The more different names given to a drawing, the higher its uncertainty. When Mills and associates subsequently had a group of non-brain-injured adults and a group of aphasic adults name the drawings, they found that both groups took longer to name drawings with high uncertainty values and were more likely to misname them. The effects of uncertainty on response times and error rates were greater for the aphasic subjects than for the non-brain-injured subjects. Mills and associates recommended that item uncertainty be added to the list of variables that affect the speed and accuracy of aphasic adults' naming performance.

> The operational definition of uncertainty provided by Mills and associates provides an excellent way for clinicians or investigators to determine uncertainty values for stimuli used in their clinical activities or research.

Redundancy and Context The words *redundancy* and *context* denote similar and sometimes overlapping concepts. *Redundancy* refers to the presence of information in a stimulus beyond that needed to specify the target response under ideal conditions. For example, a clinician doing an auditory comprehension drill might increase the redundancy of a command such as "Show me the small red cup," by saying, "I want you to show me a *cup* that is *red* and *small*. Show me the *small red cup*." Stimulus redundancy usually improves the performance of brain-injured patients. For example, some patients perform poorly on point-to tasks in which they must point to objects named by the clinician ("Point to the cup."), but their performance improves if the clinician increases the redundancy of the commands by asking the patient to point to objects the clinician describes by function ("Point to the one you drink coffee from.") although the latter command is longer and syntactically more complex. Repetition, paraphrase, and multimodality stimulation are common ways of adding redundancy to task stimuli. (These manipulations no doubt also add salience to the stimuli.)

> Some brain-injured patients cannot handle the added information when task stimuli are made more redundant. The only way to find out who will profit from redundancy and who will not is to try adding redundancy on a few trials and see what happens.

Context refers to the presence of a background or a setting for a stimulus that provides information about the stimulus not found in the stimulus itself. For example, the clinician doing the auditory comprehension drill mentioned earlier might provide contextual support for the patient by changing the array of response choices from a group of randomly chosen objects to a group in which the cup is portrayed in its usual location in a place setting on a table.

The context in which responses are elicited often has potent effects on brain-injured patients' response accuracy. One of the most striking characteristics of the behavior of brain-injured adults is that responses that are difficult or impossible in one context can be astonishingly easy in another. Many brain-injured adults say more and say it better when they participate in natural communicative interactions than when they must talk in acontextual and unnatural situations. Similar effects of context on performance are seen in listening, reading, and writing. The major exceptions are distractible or impulsive right-hemisphere-damaged or traumatically brain-injured patients and some aphasic patients who cannot handle unstructured natural situations as well as they handle structured situations in which distractions are minimized and the focus of the interaction is carefully controlled.

Clinicians doing one-to-one treatment tasks with brain-injured adults typically keep treatment sessions orderly and predictable. The clinician's instructions and directions are concise but complete. Task stimuli are selected carefully and are consistent from trial to trial. The pace of stimulus delivery and responses is constant across treatment tasks. Background noise, distractions, and intrusions are minimized. Patients who perform flawlessly in such supportive contexts often break down when they leave the treatment room and have to deal with the less controlled and more chaotic situations of daily life. Clinicians sometimes help patients learn to deal with these less-than-ideal situations by making treatment tasks less orderly and predictable. For example, when a patient's auditory comprehension reaches normal levels in the clinician's quiet office environment, the clinician may add background noise or move the activity into a noisy common room to give the patient practice at comprehending in noisy environments like those the patient may face in daily life. In addition to building the patient's tolerance for noise, such replication of the elements of daily life environments helps to transfer skills learned in the clinic to daily life by letting the patient practice the skills in situations like those the patient is likely to encounter outside the sheltered clinic environment.

Novelty and Interest Value The novelty and interest value of treatment stimuli usually have less obvious effects on brain-injured patients' performance than other stimulus characteristics, and clinicians sometimes overlook novelty and interest value when they select stimuli for treatment tasks. This can be an important oversight because making treatment stimuli more novel and interesting often helps the patient toward better performance. Faber and Aten (1979) asked aphasic adults to "tell me what you see" in response to drawings that either depicted common objects in their normal state or in broken or altered states (e.g., a pair of eyeglasses with a broken lens as in Figure 6-2 or a shirt with a torn sleeve). The aphasic adults produced significantly more appropriate words and significantly longer utterances when they talked about the drawings of broken or altered objects than when they talked about the drawings of intact objects.

An item in the 1980 edition of *Communicative Abilities in Daily Living* (CADL; Holland, 1980) further illustrates the striking effects of novelty on

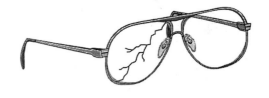

Figure 6-2 ■ **An example of how stimulus novelty may be increased by altering the appearance of familiar objects. An aphasic patient who was asked to "Tell me about this picture" when shown this drawing without a broken lens said, "That's glasses. A pair of glasses." Later, when asked to talk about the drawing shown here, he said, "That's a pair of glasses, but one side is broken. The glass there—the lens. It's broken. Somebody must have dropped 'em on the floor."**

brain-injured adults' attention and comprehension. The item is contained in a role-playing section of CADL, in which the clinician plays the role of a physician who is giving the patient instructions on lifestyle. The clinician says, "Okay, Mr./Ms.——, before our next visit I want you to smoke three packs of cigarettes and drink a bottle of gin a day. Okay?" Few brain-injured patients fail to do a double-take in response to this item, and most respond to it with more amusement, laughter, and commentary than is seen in their responses to more prosaic CADL items.

The experience of clinicians matches what Faber and Aten reported and replicates what occurs when patients respond to the lifestyle instructions in the CADL. Many brain-injured patients attend, comprehend, and respond more accurately and with less effort when treatment materials are novel or personally interesting than when the materials are mundane or have limited personal relevance to the patient. A patient whose speech output is limited to single-word utterances when obliged to talk about cups and spoons and keys and combs produces full sentences when asked to talk about family, hobbies, or profession. A patient who struggles to comprehend commands such as "Show me the white cup" easily gets the sense of longer and more complex utterances when they are personally relevant, as in "Tell me what the weather was like on the day you got married."

Cues Clinicians usually manipulate the stimulus characteristics described previously in a preplanned way. They specify the stimulus characteristics when they design the treatment task, and they keep the characteristics constant across trials within the task. However, when a patient has trouble the clinician often deviates from the routine. A clinician might intervene to facilitate a struggling patient's production of the word *pen* by saying, "It starts with *puh*," "It rhymes with *ten*," or "It has *ink* and you *write* with it." These clinician behaviors are called *cues* (Barton, Maruszewski, & Urrea, 1969; Li & Williams, 1990; Rochford & Williams, 1965; Stimley & Noll, 1991; and others).

Cues are hints a clinician gives when a patient is having difficulty getting a response out. Cues provide the patient with additional information that leads them in the direction of the target response without giving away the response itself. Strategic use of cues gives the clinician control over the pace of treatment tasks and permits the clinician to adjust the processing load associated with an individual treatment trial. More importantly, cues give the clinician a dependable way to intervene and get the patient back on track when the patient is momentarily defeated by a treatment trial. Cues give the clinician a tool for breaking up strings of error responses and keeping error rates at optimal levels. Cues are discussed in greater detail later, when treatment of specific communication impairments is addressed.

Response Manipulations

The second major way in which clinicians may control the processing demands of treatment tasks is by manipulating the characteristics of the responses required from their patients. By easing response requirements clinicians lower the need for resources associated with formulation and production of responses, and by requiring more complex and effortful responses clinicians escalate the processing workload associated with treatment tasks. The two most obvious contributors to response workload are the *length* and *complexity* of the responses required from the patient. Less obvious contributors are *familiarity and naturalness, response delay,* and *redundancy.*

Length and Complexity Length and complexity tend to interact, in that longer responses also tend to be more complex, although each can be manipulated separately. (Responses of the same length can differ in their level of complexity, and responses of different lengths can have the same overall level of complexity.) The length of responses usually is defined by measuring how many units (e.g., syllables or words) they contain, or, less often, how much time it takes the patient to perform the responses.

The complexity of responses can be defined in many ways, most of which are more subjective than counting units or measuring time. In treatment tasks for brain-injured adults, complexity may be defined *motorically* (i.e., the number of different articulatory movements per word or per unit of time), *linguistically* (i.e., the number of syntactic operations needed to determine the meaning of sentences), or *cognitively* (i.e., the presumed amount of abstraction or inference needed to produce appropriate responses to spoken messages). As a general rule, increasing the length or complexity of responses increases their appetite for processing resources, and if resources are in short supply, increasing response length or complexity leads to worsened performance. It is important to understand that the effects of increasing response complexity may not be limited to the adequacy of the responses themselves but may extend back to input processes such as perception, discrimination, and comprehension, depending on how the patient's system attempts to compensate for resource shortfall.

Familiarity and Meaningfulness The familiarity and meaningfulness of responses is related to the frequency with which a patient has performed the responses in the past. Highly practiced and socially meaningful responses (e.g., social greetings and farewells) usually are easier for brain-injured adults than infrequently practiced responses produced in unnatural contexts (e.g., naming objects or pictures), and many brain-injured patients who can say little else can get out highly practiced social verbalizations such as *hello* and *goodbye* in the appropriate settings. The effects of familiarity go beyond speech. Brain-injured patients with language comprehension impairments usually comprehend personally relevant material (e.g., questions about home and family) better than impersonal material (e.g., questions about the relative sizes of bicycles and locomotives). Brain-injured patients with impaired vocabulary typically are more successful at accessing frequently occurring words (e.g., *house* or *woman*) than infrequently occurring ones (e.g., *scholar* or *piccolo*).

Delay Many brain-injured adults have impairments in immediate memory that interfere with their ability to maintain information or action plans in memory for more than a few seconds. One consequence of these impairments is that the patient's performance deteriorates when the clinician imposes a timeout between the clinician's presentation of treatment stimuli and the opportunity for the patient to respond. A patient whose responses to spoken commands are quick and accurate when the patient is permitted to respond as soon as the clinician finishes saying each command may falter, equivocate, and fumble when the clinician requires a 5-second or 10-second wait before the patient can respond. A patient who flawlessly repeats phrases after the clinician under no-delay conditions may stumble, struggle, and grope about when forced to retain the clinician's model in memory for 10 or 20 seconds before producing it.

Sometimes imposing (or permitting) delays between stimuli and responses improves brain-injured patients' performance rather than detracting from it. Most brain-injured adults suffer from general slowing of cognitive processes. It takes them longer to retrieve the words they need to express their ideas. It takes them longer to combine words into meaningful strings. It takes them longer to recognize complex or unfamiliar stimuli and deduce the meaning of incoming messages. Their need for increased processing time causes them to respond slowly, creating delays between treatment stimuli and the patient's responses. Most brain-injured patients are excruciatingly aware of their slowness and feel obligated to get responses out as quickly as possible. Encouraging these patients to respond more quickly simply adds to their problems, whereas teaching them to resist the tyranny of the clock usually helps.

Some brain-injured patients try to compensate for their immediate memory problems by responding quickly, before the memory traces of the stimulus have time to decay. This strategy often leads them to "jump the gun"—respond before the clinician has finished delivering the stimulus.

This strategy rarely solves the patient's problems and often makes things worse because the patient almost invariably misses the material that comes in after they have begun to respond. Imposing short delays between stimuli and responses often improves the performance of these hyperresponsive patients (Yorkston, Marshall, & Butler, 1977).

Although it is not always obvious which patients will be hurt by response delay and which will be helped by it, the following general guidelines may help. When a patient's immediate memory is impaired and when a treatment task makes demands on immediate memory, imposing response delays adds to the patient's troubles. When a patient's internal processing is slow or inefficient and the treatment task calls on the slow or inefficient processes, permitting response delays may help the patient.

What does a skilled clinician do when a patient suffers both from immediate-memory impairments and slow or inefficient internal processes? If the clinician's purpose is to target immediate memory, then the clinician might take slow processing out of the picture by slowing the rate at which stimuli are presented, but he or she might enforce a delay between delivery of the stimulus and the time at which the patient is permitted to respond. If the clinician's purpose is to target the slow processing, the clinician might minimize memory demands by permitting the patient to respond immediately, and he or she might speed up the rate at which stimuli are presented to put the appropriate load on processing speed and efficiency.

Response Redundancy The redundancy of responses may affect the speed and accuracy of brain-injured patients' responses. Response redundancy comes in two forms. In one form elements are repeated within responses *(within-response redundancy)*. In another form responses are repeated across trials *(across-trials redundancy)*. Within-response redundancy is a prominent feature of many speech-articulation drills in which the patient is asked to produce strings of words in which the same articulatory positions are repeated within elements of each

string (as in *baby—bible—bobbin—beanbag*). Across-trials redundancy is common in tasks in which some characteristics of the patient's responses are the same from trial to trial (e.g., the pointing or gesturing responses called for on every trial of some auditory comprehension tasks). The ultimate in redundancy between task stimuli and the patient's responses happens when the clinician and patient produce responses in unison. One step down in redundancy are repetition tasks in which the patient's responses are direct copies of the clinician's productions, produced immediately after the clinician's productions.

GENERAL CONCEPTS 6-2

- Resource-allocation models of cognition assume that every human has a finite amount of cognitive resources available for carrying out cognitive processes. If the resources needed for active cognitive processes exceed the supply, performance deteriorates.

- Resource-allocation models of cognition assume that brain injury diminishes the available pool of processing resources. As a consequence, brain-injured adults are more sensitive to cognitive processing workload than are non-brain-injured adults.

- Clinicians may control the difficulty of treatment tasks by manipulating stimulus aspects such as *intensity and salience, clarity and intelligibility, redundancy and contextual support,* or the *novelty and interest value* of task stimuli or by manipulating response requirements such as *response length and complexity,* the *familiarity and naturalness of responses, response delay,* or the *redundancy of responses* required from patients.

- Clinicians often provide *cues* in impromptu, trial-by-trial fashion to help patients who are struggling with a specific item in a treatment task.

HOW CLINICIANS DECIDE WHAT TO TREAT

A clinician's decisions regarding what to treat come from the clinician's conclusions about the nature of the patient's communicative impairment, the clinician's attitudes about the nature and purpose of therapy, and the clinician's previous clinical successes and failures. There are no rules and few guiding principles, but a few general approaches to deciding what to treat have been described in the literature.

Perhaps the most commonly used approach to planning treatment is the *relative level of impairment approach,* in which the patient's performance on various tests is analyzed to identify "peaks" and "valleys" in the patient's performance profile. These peaks and valleys then are given special attention in treatment. Clinicians sometimes choose to treat in the valleys (areas of relative impairment) but are more likely to treat at the peaks (areas in which impairments are less pronounced). The relative-level-of-impairment approach has been most clearly explicated with reference to aphasia, but the principles apply equally well to treatment of patients with other neurogenic communication disorders.

Porch (1981b) described a relative-level-of-impairment approach based on variability in patients' performance within and across subtests of the *Porch Index of Communicative Ability* (PICA). Porch calls his measure of across-subtest variability the *high-low gap.* The high-low gap is calculated on the 18 subtests of the PICA. The average for the nine subtests with the highest scores and the average for the nine subtests with the lowest scores are calculated. The difference between the two averages is the *high-low gap.* The high-low gap, according to Porch, represents in part the amount of change that can be expected from treatment. Porch recommends that clinicians direct treatment toward processes represented by subtests in which patients exhibit slight to moderate impairments. Porch suggests that when the high-low gap is closed (a difference at or near zero) the patient has achieved maximum treatment benefits and may be ready for discharge.

Porch calls variability in performance within subtests *intrasubtest variability* (ISV). He defines intrasubtest variability as the number of different scores within a subtest. A 10-item PICA subtest in which a patient receives 8 scores of 13 (with the PICA 16-category scoring system) and 2 scores of 15 would have low ISV, whereas a subtest in which a patient's 10 responses included scores of 7, 9, 10, 13, and 15 would have high ISV. According to Porch, intrasubtest variability is related to a patient's potential for change in the task represented by the subtest, with greater potential for change on subtests with high ISV than on subtests with low ISV. According to Porch, intrasubtest variability decreases as the patient approaches the limits of his or her recovery potential.

In the *fundamental processes approach* to treatment, clinicians attempt to identify impairments in underlying processes that are thought to contribute to several related linguistic, cognitive, or communicative abilities. Treatment focuses on these processes, with the expectation that improving a process will improve the abilities that depend on the process. For example, Schuell, Jenkins, and Jimenez-Pabon (1965) have claimed that impaired auditory comprehension is a central problem in aphasia and that improving auditory comprehension leads to improvement in other language abilities. Clinicians who agree with Schuell and associates are likely to test auditory comprehension in detail and to make auditory comprehension disabilities the focus of treatment, expecting that as auditory comprehension improves, so will general linguistic and communicative abilities. Gardner and associates (1983) and Myers (1991) have suggested that impaired capacity to make inferences is a central problem for many right-hemisphere-damaged persons. Those who subscribe to this view might focus treatment on inference making, expecting that improvements there would generalize to other communicative abilities. Some practitioners believe that attentional impairments are a common problem for patients with traumatic brain injuries, and they focus treatment on rehabilitating attentional impairments, believing that improving attention will improve many skills that depend on attention.

Clinicians who use a *functional abilities approach* to treatment focus on skills that are likely to be important in patients' daily life communication. For example, a clinician might train a nonverbal patient to produce gestural *yes* and *no* responses because the patient's acquisition of dependable *yes* or *no* responses will enhance communication with others in the patient's natural environment. Clinicians using the functional abilities approach often invite patients and family members to help decide what is to be worked on in treatment. Because the focus of treatment is on communication in daily life, families and caregivers often participate directly in treatment procedures.

Most clinicians combine elements of the three approaches, and most consider functionality (the relevance of a skill, process, or ability to the patient's daily life) when deciding on a treatment approach. Clinicians rarely focus on fundamental abilities that have little relationship to a patient's daily life, and clinicians using the "relative level of impairment" approach usually consider how important a process or ability is in daily life when making decisions about what to treat.

TASK DIFFICULTY

Most clinicians structure treatment tasks so that patients are working at or just below their maximum performance level. In easy tasks (those that are well below a patient's maximum performance level), all (or nearly all) responses are prompt and accurate. As tasks become more difficult, responses become hesitant, tentative, or delayed, and false starts, revisions, self-corrected errors, and uncorrected errors appear. As task difficulty continues to increase, errors also increase, but cues or repetition of the stimulus by the clinician may elicit correct responses. When the difficulty of the task goes beyond the patient's maximum performance level, strings of uncorrected errors appear, and cues or repetition of stimuli have few beneficial effects.

Although there is considerable agreement that treatment tasks should target performance levels that challenge but do not overwhelm the patient, not everyone agrees on the precise level of difficulty at which treatment tasks should be constructed. Porch (1981b) asserts that treatment tasks should begin at levels where patients make no outright errors but produce combinations of immediate, correct responses and delayed but correct responses, self-corrected errors, distorted responses, or responses that are corrected after the clinician repeats the stimulus. He also declares that clinicians should not change tasks or response criteria until 100% of a patient's responses are immediate and correct because responses trained to less-than-perfect levels will deteriorate in real-life situations or in more difficult treatment tasks.

Porch's position, although logically reasonable, may not be appropriate for every brain-injured patient in every treatment task. Brain-injured patients differ in their tolerance for errors just as they differ in many other ways. Some fret and fuss over every misstep, whereas others remain serene in the face of repeated failure. Sensitive clinicians take such patient characteristics into account when deciding how hard to push a patient in treatment tasks. For the hypersensitive patient who is troubled by every mistake, the clinician may pitch treatment so that immediate, correct responses outnumber delayed, self-corrected, or prompted ones by a good margin. For the patient who is constructively challenged by failure, the clinician may permit greater proportions of delayed, self-corrected, and prompted responses and even some uncorrected errors.

For the "average" patient, a good general rule is to keep patient performance at 60% to 80% immediate and correct responses during the beginning of a given task and to increase the difficulty of the task when immediate and correct responses exceed 90% to 95% over two or three administrations of the task. Generally, if less than 10% of the average patient's responses are delayed and self-corrected across many trials, the clinician should consider making the task more difficult. One important exception is patients near discharge from treatment whose performance is plateauing. For these patients, clinicians may elect to stay with treatment tasks until all responses are immediate and correct to give patients extended experience in tasks calling for sustained effort at maximum performance levels, to give patients a strong sense of what successful performance at this level of effort feels like, and to build patients' confidence in their ability to handle situations that call for this level of performance.

Another reason for structuring treatment tasks to control the frequency of error responses is that error responses on one trial increase the probability of errors on subsequent trials. Brookshire (1972) found that when aphasic patients made an error in a picture-naming task, they had a strong tendency to misname following items, even when those items ordinarily were easy for them to name. Brookshire (1976) later found the same effect in a sentence comprehension task. Brookshire and associates (1979) found a similar effect in videotaped aphasia treatment sessions involving a variety of tasks. Regardless of the treatment task, when a patient made an error on one trial, the probability of errors on subsequent trials went up significantly. Strings of error responses proved to be especially disruptive to performance. When strings of error responses occurred, the probability of a correct response diminished with each error in the string, so that by the time three or four consecutive errors had occurred, the probability of a correct response on the next trial was near zero, unless the clinician changed the task or loosened response requirements.

As a general rule, it is a good idea to keep most brain-injured patients' percentage of uncorrected error responses at no more than 10% of all responses. However, clinicians (and patients) sometimes can tolerate higher error rates if the patient moves closer to the intended response with each attempt. Rosenbek and associates (1989) comment that a stimulus may be adequate even if it does not elicit a correct response provided that it leads to problem-solving or if a series of incorrect responses moves in the direc-

tion of adequacy. However, if there is no improvement across sequences of off-target responses (especially if the patient emits the *same* response on every trial), the patient is not learning much beyond what it feels like to fail, and the clinician should make the task easier.

INSTRUCTIONS AND FEEDBACK

Clinicians organize and regulate brain-injured patients' performance in treatment activities (and in assessment too) by *instructing* and providing *feedback. Instructions* tell the patient *what they are to do* in an upcoming activity. *Feedback* tells the patient *how they did* on a single treatment trial or a collection of trials. Although there is some functional overlap between instructions and feedback, each serves a different purpose. Clinicians who keep these purposes straight keep treatment activities focused and running smoothly. Clinicians who give feedback when they should be instructing or instruct when they should be giving feedback may confuse the patient and compromise the effectiveness of their treatment procedures.

Instructions

Instructions are the lead-in to treatment activities. They tell patients what they will be doing and (sometimes) why they will be doing it. Good instructions are clear and concise. They are delivered at a rate the patient can handle. They use language the patient can understand. They provide everything the patient needs to know (but no more). Many beginning clinicians (and some experienced ones) overdo instructions by providing more information than the patient needs or by unnecessarily repeating or paraphrasing until the patient is confused. Instructional excess can be avoided or at least minimized by monitoring the patient's apparent understanding and checking with the patient to see if they understand. Most brain-injured patients (including those with severe impairments) indicate their understanding or confusion by facial expression, gesture (especially head nods), and demeanor. Clinicians who attend to these sometimes subtle signs tend not to stray into instructional excess.

Experienced clinicians know that a little demonstration and a few practice trials can take the place of a lot of verbal instruction and are a good way to check a patient's understanding of instructions. The clinician begins with a concise explanation of the upcoming activity, followed by demonstration and a few practice trials to see if the patient has gotten the point. If the patient's performance on the practice trials shows that the patient knows what is expected, the clinician proceeds into the treatment activity. If the patient's performance shows that the patient does not know what is expected, the clinician provides more demonstration or explanation, guided by what the patient did during the practice trails.

A clinician is starting a new treatment activity with Mrs. Adair, an aphasic woman with a moderate language comprehension impairment and serious word-retrieval difficulties, both of which cause her great concern. Clinician: "Okay Mrs. Adair, now we'll be doing something different." (The clinician alerts Mrs. Adair to the upcoming change and gives her some time to make whatever mental adjustments are needed.) "I'm going to show you some pictures, one at a time. They're pictures of things you have in your kitchen at home, and they're the same ones you've been naming for me." (The materials are familiar to Mrs. Adair and relevant to her daily life. The clinician relates the new activity to one with which Mrs. Adair has had experience.) "I know that you can name them because you got all their names right last time and this time. Now let's see what else you can say about them." (The clinician tells Mrs. Adair the purpose of the new activity and provides her with time to process and make mental adjustments.) "Here's what I want you to do. I want you to tell me what you do with each one as I show it to you." (The clinician highlights the upcoming instruction with an alerting phrase.) "Are you ready?" (The clinician monitors Mrs. Adair's facial expression, eye movements, and other indicators of her understanding and readiness.) Mrs. Adair nods, and the clinician puts a picture of a broom on the table. Clinician: "See this one? Tell me what you do with it." (The clinician provides a lead-in question to highlight the request.) Mrs. Adair: "Broom." Clinician: "No, that's not what I had in mind. Tell me what you do with it." Mrs. Adair: "Sweep." Clinician: "Fine! Here's another one." (Puts down a picture of a food mixer.) Mrs. Adair: "Mixer." Clinician: "No, that's not what I'm looking for. Tell me what you do with it. I'll show you what I mean." (Turns over the next card, which is a picture of a knife.) Clinician: "This is something I'd use to cut things up. See what I mean? I didn't name it. I told you what I do with it. Now you try one. Remember, tell me what you do with it." (Turns over card to reveal a kettle.) Mrs. Adair: "Well, it's a kettle . . ., and I'd boil potatoes or make a stew in it." Clinician: "Great! Let's do another one . . ."

Several things about the clinician's behavior with Mrs. Adair are noteworthy. The clinician uses repetition, paraphrase, and lead-in phrases liberally to highlight important information and to give Mrs. Adair extra processing time. The clinician asks Mrs. Adair if she is ready before beginning the first trial. (For experienced clinicians this behavior is so routine as to be almost automatic. This is not so for beginners, who often move too fast and present stimuli before the patient is ready.) When Mrs. Adair responds to the first practice item with its name, the clinician gives her appropriate feedback, does not correct her, and repeats the instruction. When Mrs. Adair continues to name on the second practice trial, the clinician adds demonstration to repetition of the task instructions, at which point Mrs. Adair responds appropriately.

Feedback

Mrs. Adair's clinician combines instruction and explanation with response-contingent feedback to coach her into a new treatment activity with minimum fuss and confusion. When Mrs. Adair's responses to the first two practice items are not what the clinician intends, the clinician combines negative feedback ("no") with explanation ("that's not what I had in mind"), which elaborates on the feedback and also helps to soften its hard edges. Importantly, the clinician does not *correct* Mrs. Adair's unacceptable responses (as in "No. You sweep with a broom," or "No. You mix food with a mixer.") because the problem is not with the rightness of Mrs. Adair's responses but either with her understanding of the new activity or her ability to change her response set from naming to describing function. After two practice trials in which feedback and explanation fail to elicit the intended responses, the clinician moves on to demonstration combined with explanation. The switch in tactics succeeds and the clinician and patient continue into the new activity.

Knowing when to provide feedback and what kind to provide and knowing how to combine feedback, explanation, and demonstration are important clinical skills. Brookshire (1973) addressed the *what kind* question. He identified two major categories of response-contingent feedback in treatment activities—*incentive feedback* and *information feedback.*

Incentive Feedback   Incentive feedback can maintain (or eliminate) behaviors whose only purpose is to elicit (or avoid) the feedback. If the feedback stops, the behavior stops. Food pellets that drop into a hopper when a pigeon pecks a key are incentive feedback (sometimes called *positive reinforcement*) that keeps the pigeon pecking the key. Quarters that drop down the chute of a slot machine are incentive feedback that keeps the tourist from South Dakota putting in coins and pulling the lever. Disconnect the key from the pellet dispenser and the pigeon loses interest in the key. Program the slot machine to keep the tourist's coins and return none and the tourist (eventually) stops putting in coins and pulling the lever.

The power of incentive feedback over behavior depends strongly on the subject's real or apparent state of deprivation for the feedback stimulus. Feed the pigeon until it is no longer hungry and it loses interest in pecking the key. Give the tourist 40 million dollars, a new BMW, and a ticket to Bora Bora and the tourist loses interest in putting coins in the machine and pulling its lever.

Increasing the magnitude of incentive feedback or increasing the subject's level of deprivation often increases its effect on behavior, at least within certain ranges. Increase the payoff on the pecking key or the slot machine and their users respond faster and stay at it longer (unless the payoff is large enough to reduce the subjects' deprivation levels).

Incentive feedback is used in the clinic when the objective is a change in the frequency of behaviors that a patient can do but doesn't do often enough (such as making eye contact with listeners) or does too often (such as shouting at doctors and nurses). Many different stimuli can serve as incentive feedback, and what works as an incentive for one person may not work for another. Some stimuli, such as food (to hungry people), water (to thirsty people), electric shocks (to most), and loud noise (except for patrons of rock concerts) seem intrinsically rewarding or punishing—they serve as reward or punishment for most of the adult population. Other stimuli seem less intrinsically rewarding or punishing, and they work for smaller segments of the population. Verbal approval and reproof, for example, are not intrinsically rewarding or punishing, but they have rewarding and punishing properties for some individuals and not for others.

Information Feedback   Information feedback provides information about the appropriateness, correctness, or accuracy of the responses they follow. Information feedback comes in many forms, ranging from a tracing on an oscilloscope that tells a patient how close their vocal intensity is to a target, to the clinician's smile and spoken "good" that tells the patient that they have successfully communicated an intended message. Incentive feedback also can function as information feedback, as when the young traumatically brain-injured patient gets an M&M (his favorite candy) contingent on each successful detection of a target in a visual monitoring task. However, information feedback need not possess incentive characteristics to be effective in regulating the performance of brain-injured adults who are motivated to get better and for whom the payoff is not in the feedback but in the improved performance that comes with progress in treatment. For these patients it is the information about the appropriateness, correctness, or accuracy of the behaviors leading to the feedback that is important, and the incentive properties are an added attraction.

There are no specific rules for how and when feedback should be used in treatment of brain-injured adults because patients differ in their need for feedback and clinicians differ in their preferences with regard to what kind of feedback to deliver and when to deliver it. However, the following observations may help beginning clinicians get at least a general sense of how feedback functions in such treatment activities.

Incentive feedback does not play an important part in treatment of most brain-injured adults. Most brain-injured adults are motivated to get better and willingly do what is needed without external incentives. For these patients progress is its own reward. However, severely impaired, depressed, agitated, or confused patients who do not recognize progress in treatment activities or are not rewarded by progress may need incentive feedback. Incentive feedback often is needed in treatment of traumatically brain-injured patients in the early stages of recovery. These patients often are minimally responsive to their environment and have little tolerance for tasks that require mental or physical effort. Incentives for responding may be the only way to get these patients' cooperation in treatment tasks. Incentive feedback also may be needed when clinicians are working with patients in the late stages of dementia, when social rewards and penalties no longer function to maintain or change behavior.

General Encouragement

Most brain-injured adults appreciate general encouragement in treatment activities. General encouragement may be response-contingent positive feedback, or it may be occasional positive statements that are not contingent on any given response (e.g., "You're doing fine" or "You're doing much better today").

The effects of encouraging or discouraging comments by a clinician were demonstrated in a study by Stoicheff (1960). Stoicheff studied three groups of aphasic adults who performed picture-naming and word-reading tasks in three instructional conditions. One group received encouraging instructions ("...I'm very satisfied with what you have been able to do....I think that you will find the going much easier today....I expect that you will do just as well today if not better."). One group received discouraging instructions ("As I expected, you did even more poorly last time than the time before....I am disappointed in how much you have slipped behind....This seems to be harder for you each time instead of easier."). One group received neutral instructions ("I want you to do the same kinds of things as last time. We'll be working on different words/pictures.").

The clinician also made encouraging comments ("Good! You're doing fine!") to the encouragement group and discouraging comments ("You missed that one! That's wrong!") to the discouragement group during the tasks.

At the end of the study, Stoicheff explained to the subjects that they had participated in a study and reassured those in the discouragement and neutral groups to counteract any detrimental effects of their treatment on subsequent performance. It is unlikely that Stoicheff could have done this study today because of rules requiring that subjects be told, in advance, about the purposes and general conduct of any study in which they participate. It also seems unlikely that the discouragement group would welcome Stoicheff as their full-time clinician.

(The comments were not delivered contingent on acceptable or unacceptable responses.) After three sessions, the *discouragement* group performed significantly worse than the *encouragement* group. The performance of the *neutral* group fell between the other two groups but did not differ significantly from either. Stoicheff commented that subjects in the *discouragement* group were withdrawn, tense, and hostile by the end of the third session, whereas those in the *encouragement* group were spontaneous, friendly, and smiling.

How Clinicians Use Feedback

Many clinicians tend to avoid negative feedback, perhaps because they do not wish to discourage their patients. Brookshire and associates (1977) evaluated clinicians' use of feedback in 40 video-taped treatment sessions. They reported that clinicians provided positive feedback for more than 60% of acceptable responses but provided negative feedback for only about 10% of unacceptable patient responses. They were as likely to provide positive feedback as to provide negative feedback following *unacceptable* responses (Figure 6-3).

It is not clear why clinicians have this seeming aversion to negative feedback. Perhaps they wish to avoid discouraging their patients, as Stoicheff did with her negative instructions and comments. However, it is important to remember that Stoicheff's negative instructions and comments were not contingent on poor performance. It is not surprising that her subjects were tense and hostile following three sessions of negative instructions and criticism unrelated to their performance. Brain-injured adults, like the rest of us, are likely to be irritated by gratuitous negative commentary from another, but few are so sensitive that they cannot deal with negative feedback if it is delivered contingent on off-target responses and if the overall mood created by the clinician is supportive and reassuring.

It is true, however, that most clinicians (including this writer) deliver positive feedback at full strength but deliver negative feedback in di-

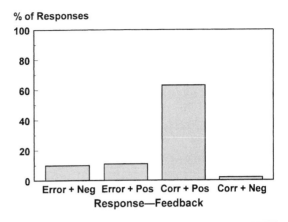

% of Responses

Figure 6-3 ■ **Percentage of aphasic adults' error responses receiving negative feedback (error + neg), percentage of aphasic adults' error responses receiving positive feedback (error + pos), percentage of aphasic adults' acceptable responses receiving positive feedback (corr + pos), and percentage of aphasic adults' acceptable responses receiving negative feedback (corr + neg).** (Data from Brookshire, R. H., Krueger, K., Nicholas, L., & associates. [1977]. Analysis of clinician-patient interactions in aphasia treatment. In R. H. Brookshire [Ed.], *Clinical Aphasiology Conference Proceedings* [pp. 181-187]. Minneapolis: BRK Publishers.)

luted form. One seldom hears clinicians say "Wrong!" or "No!" in response to inaccurate patient responses. They are more likely to say "Close!" or "Not quite!" and they sometimes sweeten the negative feedback even more by blending it with weak positive feedback, as in "Good try, but that's not quite it." Clinicians' positive feedback tends to be more emphatic. Exclamations such as "good," "great," "super," or "wonderful" commonly are heard in treatment sessions. By manipulating the strength of positive and negative feedback in this way, clinicians put more emphasis on the positive aspects of their patients' performance, contribute to their patient's self-confidence, and maintain an encouraging and supportive atmosphere in treatment activities.

As the patient and clinician become more familiar with each other and with treatment activities, feedback often becomes quite subtle. Once a treatment activity has achieved a consistent pace and rhythm in which the clinician's delivery of stimuli and the patient's responses have fallen into a regular temporal pattern, the clinician need only interrupt the pattern by withholding delivery of the next stimulus for a few seconds to signal to the patient that a response was off target. Similarly, clinicians who acknowledge on-target responses with a consistent head nod need only withhold it to signal that a response was not satisfactory. Most moderately impaired to mildly impaired brain-injured patients quickly become attuned to these subtle cues, but those with more severe impairments may need more conspicuous feedback, and they may need it after every response, rather than intermittently.

Patients often need feedback after each response when new treatment tasks are introduced and they are busy determining the point of the task and figuring out the criteria the clinician uses to decide what constitutes on-target responses. Consequently, feedback schedules tend to be more nearly continuous (feedback after every response) and feedback stimuli tend to be more overt and more intense at the beginning of new treatment tasks. As the patient gains experience with the task, feedback becomes intermittent and feedback stimuli often become more subtle.

Delivering overt feedback contingent on every response is rarely necessary once a treatment activity is a familiar routine with a consistent pace. Then intermittent positive feedback for on-target responses plus negative feedback for all, or nearly all, off-target responses usually is sufficient (unless the patient knows when responses are off-target, in which case negative feedback may be delivered on an intermittent schedule). Feedback schedules in which every patient response gets overt feedback soon become tiresome for clinicians and patients, and the effectiveness of the stimuli used as overt feedback often is diminished by overuse. However, as noted previously, most clinicians provide subtle indications of response acceptability even when they do not provide overt feedback, so in this sense it might be said that most clinicians provide some form of feedback for almost every patient response.

Keeping the purposes of *feedback* separate from the purposes of *instruction* is important. Feedback signals to the patient whether responses are acceptable. Instruction tells the patient what the patient is to do. Instructions usually come at the beginning of treatment tasks. If a patient's poor performance seems to be caused by incomplete understanding or misunderstanding of the task, the clinician gives more instruction on how to do the task. If a patient's poor performance represents an off-target response caused by system failure, the clinician provides information feedback regarding how or why the response was off-target. Providing negative feedback when deficient performance is caused by the patient's incomplete understanding or misunderstanding of task instructions is a procedural error on the part of the clinician, as is providing instruction when the patient already understands the task but makes off-target responses because of system failure.

GENERAL CONCEPTS 6-3

- Clinicians who use the *relative level of impairment* approach to treatment choose treatment activities based on a patient's test performance. Sometimes clinicians treat in areas of minimal impairment (the *peaks*). Less often clinicians choose to treat in areas of greatest impairment (the *valleys*).
- Clinicians who use the *fundamental processes* approach to treatment choose treatment activities to stimulate processes they believe underlie several related linguistic or communicative abilities.
- Clinicians who use the *functional abilities* approach to treatment choose treatment activities that target abilities they believe are important in patients' daily life communication.
- Clinicians usually adjust the difficulty of treatment activities for brain-injured adults so that

patients are challenged but not overwhelmed. This usually means that patients' responses include a mix of *immediate and correct* responses, *delayed* responses, and s*elf-corrected* responses, with *scattered errors.*

- Appropriate use of instructions and feedback is an important clinical skill. *Instructions* tell patients what will be expected of them in an upcoming activity. *Feedback* tells patients how they did on a particular trial or series of trials.
- *Incentive feedback* entails delivery of consequences that are intrinsically rewarding or punishing. *Information feedback* entails delivery of consequences that give the individual qualitative information about how a response (or series of responses) relates to the target responses.
- *General encouragement* (positive comments that may or may not be contingent on certain responses) helps clinicians keep treatment activities pleasant and rewarding for the patient.

RECORDING AND CHARTING PATIENTS' PERFORMANCE

Documenting what goes on in treatment by keeping organized and accurate records of patients' performance is an important clinical responsibility. Accurate records permit clinicians to establish stable baseline levels of performance to document the effects of treatment. Sensitive measures of changes in a patient's performance during the course of treatment permit clinicians to modify treatment procedures or introduce new ones to maximize treatment effectiveness. Good record-keeping contributes to the orderliness and efficiency of treatment because accurately and concisely recording a patient's performance in a treatment task requires that the task itself be orderly and easily described. Finally, those who pay for speech-language pathology services (insurance companies, governmental units) and health care accrediting agencies require that clinicians keep accurate and objective records of patients' performance and their response to treatment. Clinicians need

to be careful, however, that response scoring and record-keeping procedures do not become so elaborate, cumbersome, and intrusive that they disrupt the rhythm of treatment, compromise the naturalness of the interaction between the clinician and the patient, and divert the attention of the patient and the clinician from the primary objectives of treatment.

Record-keeping methods cover a range of complexity and sophistication, from simple paper-and-pencil routines devised by individual clinicians to elaborate standardized methods marketed commercially. Both personal and commercial record-keeping methods provide a way of labeling or describing the treatment activity, space for listing treatment stimuli (usually trial-by-trial), and space for entering the patient's responses to treatment stimuli. Figure 6-4 shows an example of a personalized record sheet for a treatment session, in which the clinician has recorded a patient's responses to 10 test stimuli across 3 trials in each of 6 treatment activities.

LaPointe's (1991) *Base-10 Programmed Stimulation* is an example of a commercially marketed system for task specification and response recording that formalizes the personalized record-keeping systems used by many clinicians. In Base-10 Programmed Stimulation, scores for patients' responses to treatment stimuli are entered in a *Base-10 Response Form* (Figure 6-5), on which the clinician also includes information about the treatment task, target performance criteria, the scoring system used, and the stimuli presented. The form also provides a graph on which a patient's performance can be charted over several treatment sessions. A different response form is used for each treatment task, so several response forms are needed to record what happens in treatment sessions with several tasks.

When doing treatment in Base-10 format, the clinician selects treatment tasks for the patient and writes a description of each task on a response form. A target behavior and a target level of performance are selected for each task and entered on the response form. Ten stimuli are se-

Patient: J. Smith   Date: 7/12/96   Clinician: M. Johnson

Task	Name			Point by name			Point by function			Imitation			Sentence completion			Point by two's		
Trial / Stimulus	1	2	3	1	2	3	1	2	3	1	2	3	1	2	3	1	2	3
Pencil	15	13	15	13	15	15	13	15	15	15	15	15	15	15	13	13	13	15
Bell	15	15	15	15	15	13	13	13	15	15	15	15	13	13	15	13	15	13
Comb	13	15	13	13	13	10	13	9	10	15	13	15	13	15	15	15	15	15
Knife	15	15	15	13	13	13	15	15	15	13	15	13	15	14	14	13	10	15
Flag	15	15	15	15	15	15	15	15	13	13	15	15	15	15	15	9	13	15
Book	15	15	15	5	15	15	13	15	15	15	10	15	14	14	14	13	15	13
Horn	13	15	15	10	15	15	10	15	15	15	15	15	15	15	15	13	13	15
Lamp	15	15	15	15	15	15	15	13	15	15	15	15	15	15	15	15	15	9
Brush	10	15	15	13	15	15	15	15	15	15	15	13	15	15	15	10	15	15
Candle	15	15	15	13	15	15	15	15	13	15	15	15	13	13	15	15	10	15
Mean score	14.6			13.7			13.9			14.5			14.4			13.4		

Figure 6-4 ■ A record sheet for recording patient performance in treatment tasks. Treatment stimuli are listed in the left-hand column, and treatment tasks are listed across the top. The clinician administered three consecutive trials, which elicited 30 patient responses within each treatment task.

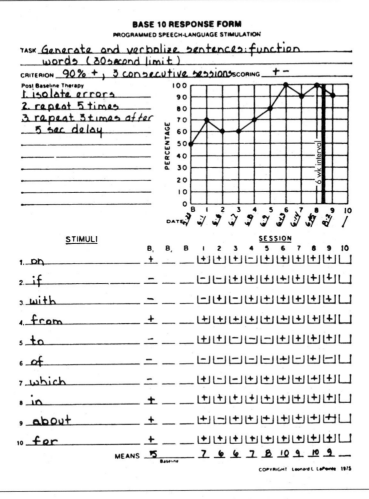

Figure 6-5 ■ The Base-10 task specification and response recording form. The task is described at the top left, the treatment stimuli are described at the bottom left, and the patient's responses are recorded on the bottom right. The columns labeled *B* are for entering the patient's scores in *baseline* conditions before treatment begins.

lected (hence the label *Base-10*) and described on the response form. As the treatment task is carried out, the patient's response to each stimulus is entered on the response form. After several sessions the clinician may graph the patient's performance to assess changes in performance over time.

In most didactic treatment tasks (e.g., pointing to pictures named by the clinician or writing words dictated by the clinician) the clinician controls the rate at which stimuli are delivered— the clinician does not deliver the stimulus for a new trial until the patient's response to the last trial has been scored. Consequently, it is relatively easy for the clinician to score every patient response as it occurs *(on-line scoring)*. The scoring situation is different in less structured treatment tasks such as conversations, in which target behaviors occur unpredictably and the clinician no longer controls the rate at which scorable responses occur. In such tasks, target responses may occur so rapidly that the clinician cannot score every response and get the score down on a record form without falling behind. In these situations the clinician has two options—*off-line scoring* and *sampling.*

In *off-line scoring* the clinician records the treatment activity on audiotape or videotape and does the scoring later, stopping and rewinding the tape as necessary to score every response. The advantage of off-line scoring is that every response can be scored without the need for the clinician to hurry transcription and scoring to keep up. There are some disadvantages to off-line scoring. It requires the use of videotape or audiotape recording equipment, which may not always be available. When recording equipment is available, its presence in the testing or treatment session may distract the patient or make the patient uneasy or tense. The time it takes to do off-line scoring may make it impractical for clinicians with busy schedules and pressing demands on their time.

Sampling provides an alternative to off-line scoring. Sampling permits clinicians to score a percentage of patient responses, rather than every response, and makes it possible for clinicians to score rapidly occurring responses on-line. (Sampling also can be used in conjunction with off-line scoring to decrease the amount of time expended in documenting the events in a treatment task.) Various formalized procedures for sampling have been described (Brookshire, Nicholas, & Krueger, 1978; Powell, Martindale, & Kulp, 1975; Repp, Dietz, Boles, & associates, 1976; Thomson, Holmberg, & Baer, 1974), but most clinicians opt for a less formalized approach in which they score as many responses as they comfortably can. They score the first occurrence of the target response, taking as much time as needed to decide on a score and enter it on a record form, ignoring any scorable responses that occur while they are doing this. When they get a score for that response on the record form, they look for the next scorable response, score it, and go on to the next one. The

proportion of a patient's responses that gets scored depends on the complexity of the scoring system and the rate at which scorable responses occur. Complex scoring systems and fast scorable response rates reduce the proportion of responses that gets scored.

There is no absolute proportion of responses that must be sampled to generate an accurate representation of patients' performance in a treatment task. Clinicians using the score-as-many-responses-as-you-can approach can expect to get half or more of scorable patient responses onto the record sheet in most treatment tasks. This proportion should yield accurate representations of patients' performance if the scored responses are fairly evenly distributed across the task. Brookshire, Nicholas, and Krueger (1978) reported that scoring only one response in five yielded records that deviated from patients' actual performance by less than 10%, provided that sampling was uniform across treatment activities. Consequently, it seems likely that scoring, on the average, every other response or every third response should almost always yield reliable indicators of patients' actual performance.

MEASURING THE EFFECTS OF TREATMENT

As mentioned in Chapter 3, measuring patient performance across time permits clinicians to establish baselines against which the effects of treatment can be measured and permits clinicians to describe changes in a patient's performance as treatment progresses. Establishing pretreatment baselines is particularly important for patients who may be experiencing spontaneous neurologic recovery because a patient's improvement on a communicative or cognitive task during (or following) treatment may reflect the effects of treatment, the effects of spontaneous recovery, or a combination of the two.

Clinicians providing treatment to patients who may be experiencing spontaneous neurologic recovery may choose from several procedures to ensure that treatment, and not some other variable, accounts for changes observed during a treatment program. Consider, for illus-

Although physiologic recovery is the most obvious and well-known source of spontaneous improvement in a brain-injured patient's communicative and cognitive abilities, these abilities may also improve as a patient learns to cope with and compensate for the effects of his or her neurologic condition. Many patients with central nervous system injury find ways to lessen the behavioral, cognitive, or communicative consequences of their injuries, either on their own or with help from family or friends. Like spontaneous physiologic recovery, these spontaneous behavioral compensations are most likely in the first weeks or months post-injury.

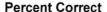

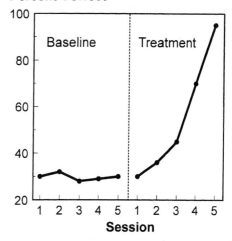

Figure 6-6 ■ **A baseline-treatment design. The behavior to be treated is measured several times in succession before treatment begins. Changes in the rate of behavior from baseline to treatment provide evidence regarding the effects of treatment.**

trative purposes, Mrs. Benchley, a fictional patient. She is 63 years old and is 1 month post-onset of aphasia caused by a thrombotic stroke. The results of testing suggest that Mrs. Benchley may benefit from treatment of auditory comprehension, so the clinician enrolls her in a treatment program designed to enhance Mrs. Benchley's auditory comprehension. Now let us examine the ways in which a clinician might measure the effects of the treatment program.

The simplest way to separate the effects of treatment from the effects of spontaneous recovery is called the *baseline-treatment design.* In a baseline-treatment design the patient's performance on tasks like those to be used in treatment is measured several times before treatment begins. Then the patient's performance is measured while treatment is provided, and the change (if any) in the patient's performance is evaluated. Figure 6-6 shows how this might work. Mrs. Benchley's performance in baseline is stable at approximately 30% correct responses across five baseline measurements. When treatment is provided, Mrs. Benchley's performance improves dramatically. After five treatment sessions her performance has improved to approximately 95% correct responses. That Mrs. Benchley's performance does not change until

treatment is provided suggests that treatment, and not some other variable, accounts for her improved performance.

The clinician may not be out of the proverbial woods yet, however, because the data in Figure 6-6 do not ensure that treatment is the only possible cause of Mrs. Benchley's improved performance. It is possible that a change in an incidental variable related to the onset of treatment—such as improved emotional state, the effects of general stimulation, increased sense of competence—could account for Mrs. Benchley's improvement during treatment.

Multiple-baseline designs were developed to deal with such issues. In multiple-baseline designs two or more behaviors are measured several times in baseline condition, then are measured periodically while treatment is applied to one of the behaviors. If the treated behavior changes and the nontreated behaviors do not, a treatment effect is assumed. Figure 6-7 shows

Percent Correct

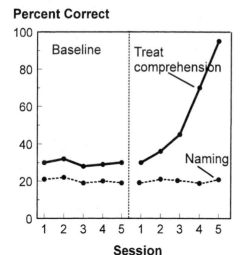

Figure 6-7 ■ **A multiple-baseline design. Two or more behaviors are measured under baseline conditions, then one of the behaviors is treated. If the treated behavior changes and the other behaviors do not change, an effect of treatment is assumed.**

how a clinician might specify the source of Mrs. Benchley's improved auditory comprehension by measuring a second, untreated, behavior (in this case, *naming*) during the baseline and treatment phases. Figure 6-7 shows that Mrs. Benchley's naming performance does not change during baseline or during auditory comprehension treatment, whereas auditory comprehension, stable during baseline, improves during treatment, making it unlikely that nonspecific changes in Mrs. Benchley's cognitive or communicative skills are responsible for her improved comprehension performance.

Now for a somewhat more complex but more powerful multiple-baseline design, called *crossover design*. In crossover design two or more behaviors are measured several times in baseline condition prior to treatment. Then one behavior is treated while the other behaviors remain in baseline condition. After the first behavior has been treated for a predetermined time (usually determined by a

criterion such as percent correct responses per block of *n* trials), treatment of that behavior ends and treatment moves on to one of the other behaviors. The first behavior now returns to baseline condition, in which it is periodically measured but not treated.

To illustrate how crossover designs work, consider a crossover treatment plan for Mrs. Benchley, in which a clinician evaluates the effects of treatment on three categories of language behavior—*auditory comprehension, naming,* and *spelling*. The clinician chooses these three behaviors because she does not expect much generalization of treatment effects from one behavior to another, permitting her to see treatment effects uncontaminated by generalization. The clinician establishes 90% correct responses per block of 20 trials as the criterion for ending one treatment phase and beginning another.

Figure 6-8 shows that all three behaviors are stable across five baseline sessions. The clinician begins by treating auditory comprehension, keeping naming and spelling in baseline condition. Mrs. Benchley reaches criterion in the auditory comprehension treatment phase within five sessions, and treatment shifts to naming. Auditory comprehension and spelling are now in baseline condition. Mrs. Benchley reaches criterion in naming treatment within five sessions, and her auditory comprehension performance remains at end-of-treatment levels. Treatment now shifts to spelling, with auditory comprehension and naming in baseline condition. Mrs. Benchley's spelling performance improves with treatment, but does not reach criterion within five sessions, so continued spelling treatment is indicated. Auditory comprehension and naming remain at end-of-treatment levels during treatment of spelling.

The data in Figure 6-8 provide compelling evidence for the effects of three different treatments on three categories of Mrs. Benchley's language behavior. All behaviors were stable in baseline conditions both before and after they were treated and each improved when it was

Percent Correct

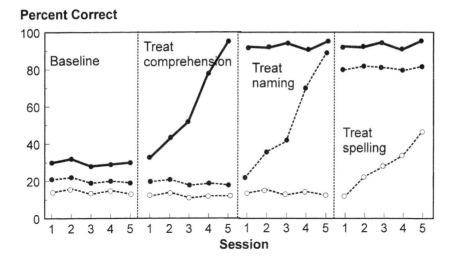

Figure 6-8 ■ **A crossover design. Two or more behaviors are measured under baseline conditions, then the behaviors are treated sequentially. If treated behaviors change when treatment is applied but untreated behaviors do not, an effect of treatment is assumed.**

treated. Neither spontaneous recovery nor any other general effect can explain the results in Figure 6-8. Mrs. Benchley's performance can be explained only by the discrete effects of the three treatments administered.

One more design and we can let poor Mrs. Benchley rest. The design is called *changing-criterion design*. Changing-criterion design is useful for tracking a patient's performance when stimuli or response requirements change during treatment. In changing-criterion design a target behavior is observed under baseline conditions to ensure that it is stable when not treated. A treatment program is designed in which criterion performance levels are specified and treatment stimuli or response requirements are systematically changed as the treated behavior reaches the criterion level. We return to Mrs. Benchley's auditory comprehension treatment program to illustrate how changing-criterion designs work (Figure 6-9).

Mrs. Benchley's ability to carry out gestural responses to one-step, two-step, and three-step spoken instructions is measured in baseline con-

dition *(Phase 1)* for three sessions. Her performance is stable, and her performance on one-step commands is better than her performance on two-step and three-step commands (see Figure 6-9). In *Phase 2* Mrs. Benchley participates in drills with one-step spoken instructions (e.g., "Give me the small pencil."). Her performance on two-step and three-step instructions is measured periodically while one-step instructions are treated. Her performance on one-step instructions improves and she reaches criterion in five sessions, ending Phase 2. In *Phase 3*, two-step instructions (e.g., "Touch the blue comb and pick up the red cup.") are the treatment focus, and Mrs. Benchley's performance on three-step instructions is measured periodically. Mrs. Benchley reaches criterion in Phase 3 in five sessions. Treatment with three-step spoken instructions (e.g., "Touch the small pencil, point to the white cup, and give me the large key.") follows *(Phase 4)*. Mrs. Benchley's performance improves and she reaches criterion in five sessions. The pattern of change in Mrs. Benchley's performance supports the effectiveness of the treat-

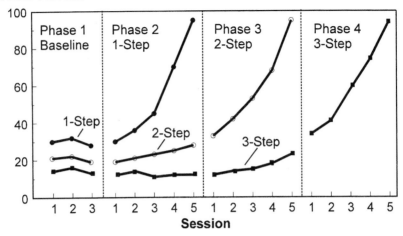

Figure 6-9 ■ A changing-criterion design. A patient's performance at several levels of task difficulty are measured under baseline conditions, then the behaviors are treated, beginning with the easiest level and progressing to the most difficult level. If behaviors representing the treated level change but behaviors representing other levels do not, an effect of treatment is assumed. (Generalization of improved performance from a treated level to an untreated higher level often occurs, as is seen in Phase 2 and Phase 3 of Figure 6-9.)

ment program in improving her ability to follow instructions of increasing length.

> Mrs. Benchley's performance on the baseline measures in Phase 2 and Phase 3 suggests that giving her practice with instructions of one length improved her comprehension of longer instructions. Mrs. Benchley's performance on two-step commands improved slightly when one-step commands were treated, and her performance on three-step commands improved slightly when two-step commands were treated (Figure 6-9). Such generalization across levels is common in treatment with a changing-criterion design and helps prepare a patient for the move from one level of complexity to the next.

Several other single-case design procedures are available to clinicians who provide treatment for neurogenic communicative disorders.

Most are elaborations on those described here. The interested reader may wish to consult a general source for single-case design such as Barlow and Herson (1984), Kazdin (1982), and Kratchowill (1978).

GENERAL CONCEPTS 6-4

- Structured procedures for specifying treatment tasks and recording patients' responses to task stimuli are an important part of treatment regimens for communicatively impaired adults. *Base-10 Programmed Stimulation* is a formalized record-keeping system.
- *On-line scoring* of responses is practical when response rate and complexity permit responses to be easily scored and recorded. If response rate or complexity makes on-line scoring impractical, clinicians may choose to do *off-line scoring* or *sampling*.
- In *baseline-treatment designs* a patient's performance in areas targeted for treatment is measured on several occasions before treat-

ment begins. Changes in performance from baseline to treatment are considered treatment effects.

- In *multiple-baseline designs* two or more behaviors are measured in baseline sessions, then are measured periodically while one of the behaviors is treated. If the treated behavior changes and the nontreated behaviors do not, a treatment effect is assumed.
- In *crossover designs* two or more behaviors are measured in baseline sessions. Then the behaviors are treated one after another. Changes in a behavior coinciding with treatment are considered treatment effects.
- In *changing-criterion designs* a target behavior is measured in baseline sessions, then it undergoes treatment in which stimuli or response requirements change as the patient reaches predetermined performance criteria.

ENHANCING GENERALIZATION FROM THE CLINIC TO DAILY LIFE

Treatment of communication disorders is not successful if the changes achieved in the clinic do not extend to the patient's daily life. Although most clinicians recognize that extension of treatment gains to daily life is important, until the 1970s most aphasia clinicians seemed to operate largely on the *train and hope* principle (Stokes & Baer, 1977), in which generalization of treatment effects from the clinic to outside contexts is hoped for but is neither actively pursued nor objectively measured. It is probably true that most aphasia clinicians (at least the better ones) either target communicative behaviors that are relevant to the patient's daily life environment or target underlying processes that are assumed to enhance daily life communicative behavior, but many do not pursue generalization in a systematic way, nor measure it carefully.

In the 1970s psychologists and behavior analysts began to address the problem of extending changes obtained in the clinic or training facility to outside environments. Literature on generalization developed, and procedures for enhancing generalization gradually made their way into clinical aphasiology. These procedures generally re-

semble those articulated by Stokes and Baer (1977), the first of which was *train and hope*. The others consist of the following eight procedures.

Using Natural Maintaining Contingencies

Stokes and Baer see this as "the most dependable of all generalization programming mechanisms" (p. 353). The easiest way to make use of natural contingencies is to target behaviors that naturally will elicit favorable consequences in the patient's daily life environment. For example, Thompson and Byrne (1984) trained patients with Broca's aphasia to produce various social conventions such as greetings, expecting that the patients' use of such social conventions would be naturally reinforced by others in daily life.

Sometimes natural contingencies are not present in the patient's daily life environment or are not consistent enough. Then one might redesign or restructure the patient's daily life environment so that the targeted behaviors receive enough pay-off to maintain them. An example of such restructuring is provided by an aphasic patient who learned to produce one-word and two-word requests in the clinic but continued to communicate at home with grunts and gestures, by which he usually succeeded in getting family members to do what he wanted. The clinician taught family members to respond to spoken requests and to ignore or delay responses to grunts and gestures unaccompanied by speech. This soon brought the patient's clinic-learned spoken requests into his home environment, after which natural contingencies maintained them both in the home and in the patient's interactions with other listeners.

Training Sufficient Exemplars

One way of training sufficient exemplars is to train a behavior in enough different settings that the behavior generalizes to all settings in which the behavior is desired. (*Exemplar* is technical jargon with various meanings. As used here it means, roughly, *stimulus-response-reinforcement triad.*) Once the behavior is established dependably in one context, the training systematically is extended to other contexts one or two at a time, with the expectation that at some point the behavior will generalize to all contexts of interest. Using social conventions as an example, one might first train social conventions in the clinic, then extend the training to other rooms, to other interactants, and to the patient's home or other community settings, expecting that at some point the patient's use of social conventions will generalize to all relevant communicative contexts.

Another way of training sufficient exemplars is to train enough different representatives of a class of responses to ensure that a class of responses, rather than a specific response (or subset of responses), generalizes. Using social conventions as an example, one might successively train several social conventions of a given kind (e.g., several different greetings) with the expectation that increasing the frequency of greetings might naturally lead to increases in the frequency of other conventions, such as questions ("How are you?") and self-disclosures ("I am fine.").

Loose Training

In loose training stimulus conditions, response requirements, and reinforcement contingencies are permitted to vary (within limits), to increase generalization across responses within a response class, and to increase generalization from the training environment to other environments. Loose training attempts to prevent a patient's responses from being tightly bound to specific contexts, which can often happen when treatment conditions are carefully controlled (as in many clinic treatment activities). In loose training a variety of stimuli are used to elicit targeted responses, sometimes in different situational contexts; a range of responses within a predefined response class is considered acceptable; and response contingencies vary both in kind and in schedule.

Loose training is *not* unsystematic treatment. Specific response classes are targeted, eliciting stimuli and situational contexts are planned in advance, and response contingencies and their schedule are predefined. Well-done loose train-

ing is as carefully thought out and as carefully controlled as more traditional structured treatment procedures.

Thompson and Byrne (1984) used loose training to train aphasic adults' use of social conventions. The social conventions first were established by asking the aphasic adults to imitate the clinician's production of the social conventions. Then the eliciting stimuli were systematically broadened to requests by the clinician (e.g., "Tell me hello."), naturalistic prompts given by the clinician (e.g., the clinician said "hello" and waited for a response from the patient), and role-playing situations structured to resemble natural conversations. Verbal feedback (e.g., "nice job") was provided contingent on responses, and the schedule of feedback gradually was loosened, from feedback for every response in the early stages of training to a variable schedule (feedback for an average of one response in four) in the later stages. Thompson and Byrne reported that loose training increased their patients' production of social conventions and that the increased production of social conventions generalized to novel social interactions. Although Thompson and Byrne's procedures departed somewhat from prototypical loose training (they targeted specific responses for intervention), their study is a good example of how loose training may be incorporated into treatment procedures for brain-injured adults.

Sequential Modification

In sequential modification (Stokes & Baer, 1977) generalization across contexts is obtained by carrying out training in every context to which generalization is desired. For brain-injured adults sequential modification may be practical when a communicative behavior is appropriate (or important) in only a few contexts or when there are only a few contexts in which the brain-injured person will be communicating and it is practical to carry out training in each context. It usually is difficult, however, to identify all potential communicative contexts for a given brain-injured person, and it is almost always impractical in terms of time and resources to carry out training in every context. Consequently, sequential modification usually has limited usefulness in treating neurogenic communication impairments (except, perhaps, for some patients with restricted communicative environments, such as those confined at home or in a nursing home who have contact with only a few others, and for patients with communication limited to a small range of topics).

Using Indiscriminable Contingencies

Stokes and Baer suggest that generalization to settings outside the treatment setting is enhanced if the response contingencies in treatment are altered gradually to make them more like those that can be expected in natural settings. These alterations may include (1) changing the schedule of contingencies from continuous (for every response) to intermittent (for every nth response) to intermittent and variable (for every nth response on the average, but varying around the average); (2) interposing delay between responses and their contingencies; and (3) choosing contingencies that resemble those expected in natural settings. Many clinicians routinely include such alterations in contingencies in their treatment procedures to increase the likelihood of generalization to natural contexts. Making contingencies indiscriminable also is an important part of other techniques such as loose training.

Programming Common Stimuli

Programming common stimuli means that the context in which behavior is trained is purposely made to resemble the context(s) to which the behavior is to generalize (the target context). Programming common stimuli manipulates *stimulus control* to enhance generalization across contexts. *Stimulus control* refers to how stimuli or stimulus complexes govern the occurrence of behavior. A pigeon reinforced with food pellets for pecking a key when a green light is on but not when a red light is on soon pecks the key only when the green light is on. The pigeon has learned to *discriminate* the reinforcement condition

from the nonreinforcement condition. To extend stimulus control to a patient's daily life environment, a clinician might incorporate stimuli from the patient's daily life environment into training, expecting that when the patient encounters the stimuli in daily life, she or he will be more likely to perform the trained behavior. The greater the similarity between the training environment and daily life, the more likely it is that the trained behavior(s) will generalize to daily life. The extent to which the training environment and the target environment resemble each other usually is decided subjectively. In most cases certain key elements (such as eliciting stimuli, surroundings, and sometimes people) are selected to resemble elements in the target environment. As is true for alterations in contingencies, programming common stimuli can be incorporated into any treatment approach to increase the likelihood of generalization to natural contexts.

Mediating Generalization

Mediation refers to the elicitation of one response by another response. Mnemonic devices are one example of mediation. One attaches easily remembered verbal labels (the mnemonic devices) to difficult-to-remember material and uses the mnemonic devices to retrieve the difficult-to-remember material (as in the rhyme for remembering the names of the cranial nerves). In mediated generalization easier responses are used to elicit more difficult responses. For example, an aphasic person might be taught to retrieve words by imagining their visual images. Most of the literature on mediated generalization has studied verbal mediation (Stokes & Baer, 1977), and verbal mediation may be inappropriate for many brain-injured adults with language impairments. However, verbal mediation sometimes is useful in treatment programs for persons with right-hemisphere syndrome or traumatic brain injuries.

Training Generalization

Sometimes patients "spontaneously" generalize during treatment activities. For example, a patient who is working on improving syntax in written work may begin using better syntax in spoken utterances. These spontaneous generalizations might themselves be targeted for reinforcement, and reinforcement contingencies might be modified gradually so that such responses receive a greater proportion of reinforcement than rote responses to training stimuli.

SOCIAL VALIDATION

Social validation is a procedure for evaluating the functional significance of changes created by a treatment program. Social validation attempts to determine whether a patient is better in a real-world sense than he or she was before treatment. It can be accomplished in two ways (Kazdin, 1982). One way is to compare the (socially relevant) behavior of the person receiving treatment with the behavior of a normal group of peers. The greater the progression toward normalcy, the more "clinically significant" the change in behavior. The other way is to obtain subjective evaluations of the behaviors of interest from persons in the patient's natural environment.

Although clinicians have for years carried out informal social validation by soliciting family members' opinions about how the patient is communicating at home, structured procedures for socially validating the effects of treatment on neurogenically impaired patients' communication only recently have been described (Doyle, Goldstein, & Bourgeois, 1987; Thompson & Byrne, 1984).

Doyle and associates, for example, trained four adults with Broca's aphasia to produce sentences with various syntactic forms in response to pictures. All improved on measures of accuracy, grammaticality, and utterance length. Doyle and associates then evaluated the social validity of the improvements by playing audiotape recordings of the aphasic adults' picture descriptions to five adults who did not know the aphasic people and who knew nothing about the study. Some of the recordings were made before treatment began and others were made after treatment had ended, and they were arranged so

that pre-treatment and post-treatment samples occurred in random order. The judges were asked to tell whether each sample was "adequate" or "inadequate." Despite subjects' improvements on measures of accuracy, grammaticality, and utterance length during treatment, the social validation procedure revealed no general increase in judgments of adequacy by the judges, although there were significant increases in judgments of adequacy for some syntactic forms. Doyle and associates concluded that social validation measures are crucial for evaluating the effectiveness of treatment programs and that they may be useful as pre-treatment measures for selecting behaviors to treat.

Thompson and Byrne (1984) used a peer-group-comparison method to assess the social validity of changes in the use of social conventions (such as *greetings, farewells,* and *introductions*) by their aphasic participants. They had each aphasic participant engage in a conversational interaction with a normal adult whom the aphasic participant had not met before. Then they compared the aphasic participants' use of social conventions with that of the normal adults. Before treatment the aphasic participants' use of social conventions was well below the range of the normal subjects, but at the end of treatment it approximated normality.

Social validation in clinical management of adults with neurogenic communication disorders is in its infancy, but it promises to become an increasingly important aspect of management as structured, reliable procedures for assessing and quantifying social validity are created, improved, and validated and as assessment of clinical results focuses more and more on changes in patients' daily life communicative competence.

GENERAL CONCEPTS 6-5

- Clinicians may promote *generalization* of treatment effects to a patient's daily life environment by:
  —Targeting behaviors that will be naturally rewarded in the daily life environment

—Training in several settings to which generalization is desired

—Training in all settings to which generalization is desired

—Allowing training conditions to vary within limits

—Altering the training environment, task stimuli, or response contingencies to make them increasingly similar to daily life

—Using easy responses to elicit difficult responses

—Rewarding patients' "spontaneous" generalization of clinic-acquired skills or behaviors to daily life

- *Social validation* is a way of evaluating the real-world significance of changes created by treatment. One approach to social validation is to measure how much closer to normal a patient is after treatment than before the treatment. Another approach is to have observers make subjective comparisons of samples of pre-treatment and post-treatment behaviors, without knowing which samples are from pre-treatment and which are from post-treatment.

THOUGHT QUESTIONS

Question 6-1 What weaknesses do you see in strict *treat the peaks* or *treat the valleys* approaches to selecting treatment activities?

Question 6-2 An administrative directive declares: "To ensure functional outcomes of speech and language treatment for brain-injured adults, henceforth all treatment activities must mimic daily life communicative interactions." You are asked to respond. What would you say?

Question 6-3 Consider the following interaction between a clinician and an aphasic patient.

Clinician: "Now I'll say a word and I want you to give me a word that means the opposite. Here's the first word. 'Up.'"

Patient: "Up. Up the road."

Clinician: "No. Give me a word that means the opposite. So if I say 'up,' you say 'down.' O.K., try this one. White.'"

Patient: "White. White as snow."

Clinician: "No. I want you to give me the opposite. For 'white' that would be 'black.' Do you understand?"

Patient: "Black. Black as coal."

Clinician: "No, when I say a word, you say its opposite—its antonym. If I say 'white,' you say 'black.' Let's try another one. What's the opposite of 'in'?"

What problems do you see represented in this interaction? What would you do to improve it?

Question 6-4 Consider the following interaction between a clinician and a patient.

Clinician: "Tell me the name of this one." (Shows a drawing of a book.)

Patient: "Writer."

Clinician: "No. That's not it. It's a book. Say 'book.'"

Patient: "Book."

Clinician: "Good! Now here's another one." (Shows a drawing of a chair.)

Patient: "Sitter."

Clinician: "No. It's a chair. Say 'chair.'"

Patient: "Chair."

Clinician: "Fine! How about this one?" (Shows a picture of a spoon.)

Patient: "Coffee."

Clinician: "No, it's not coffee. It's a spoon. Say 'spoon.'"

Patient: "Spoon."

What do you think of this interaction? Would you do anything differently?

Treatment of Aphasia and Related Disorders

This chapter describes in a general way how clinicians go about treating adults with aphasia and related communication impairments. The concepts and procedures described in this chapter also may apply to treatment of communication impairments other than aphasia. They appear in this chapter because they relate directly to the treatment of aphasia; they are more peripheral to treatment of adults with other neurogenic communication impairments. The chapter begins with a discussion of some general issues. The first reflects an overarching concern: is what speech-language pathologists do in treatment of aphasic adults worth doing?

EFFECTIVENESS OF TREATMENT FOR APHASIA

The value of treatment for aphasic adults' communication impairments has been a source of controversy for many years. The skeptics (mostly neurologists and others in the medical profession) were skeptical that treatment for aphasia provided benefits beyond those created by aphasic patients' spontaneous neurologic recovery. The believers (mostly speech-language pathologists, aphasic patients, and their families) were convinced that treatment provided benefits that could not be explained away by neurologic recovery.

Evidence

A retrospective study by Butfield and Zangwill (1946) was one of the first to address the efficacy of treatment for aphasia. Butfield and Zangwill's primary purpose was to describe the course of recovery from aphasia; evaluating the effects of "re-education" was a secondary concern. Butfield and Zangwill reviewed the records of 70 aphasic patients, all of whom had received treatment for their aphasia. The number of treatment sessions received was not controlled and ranged from 5 to 290. Butfield and Zangwill concluded that treatment was beneficial because three to six times as many patients were "improved" or "much improved" than were "unchanged" at the end of treatment. (Butfield and Zangwill's outcome measure

was a 3-category rating scale: *much improved, improved,* or *unchanged.*) Although good news to speech-language pathologists, the quality of the evidence provided by Butfield and Zangwill's study is not impressive. Their participants included stroke patients, tumor patients, patients with traumatic brain injuries, and patients with several other conditions. They described the nature of their "re-education" procedures only in general terms. Their outcome measure was subjective, insensitive, and of dubious reliability. It was a reasonable effort for its time but falls far short of contemporary standards of scientific precision and control.

Vignolo (1964) followed with a retrospective study of the records of 69 aphasic patients, each of whom had been tested at least twice with at least 40 days between the two tests. Vignolo's outcome measure, like Butfield and Zangwill's, was a three-category subjective rating: *unchanged, improved,* or *recovered.* Approximately 70% of participants who received treatment improved or recovered versus 56% of participants who were not treated. The effects of treatment were stronger for participants who began treatment at least 6 months post-onset. Vignolo reported that the differences between treated and untreated participants were smaller for participants who were less than 6 months post-onset than for particpants who were 6 months or more post-onset. He attributed the apparent smaller treatment effects for short-time post-onset participants to the effects of spontaneous neurologic recovery. Vignolo suggested that treatment for patients who are more than 6 months post-onset is most effective if it is continued for at least 6 months. Vignolo's study, like that of Butfield and Zangwill, was a reasonable effort for its time, but it does not meet contemporary standards for precision and control.

A study by Sarno, Silverman, and Sands (1970) provided grist for the skeptics' mill by placing severely aphasic patients into one of three groups: *traditional treatment, programmed instruction treatment,* or *no treatment.* The participants received from 7 to 46 hours of treatment (the average was 28 hours). There were no significant differences among the groups at the end of treatment, leading Sarno and her associates to conclude, ". . . severe aphasic stroke patients do not benefit from therapy" (p. 621). However, they also commented, "The fact that speech therapy of either type did not affect language recovery in this study is no doubt related to the severity of their aphasia" (p. 621).

Despite its popularity with the skeptics, Sarno and her associates' study provided no convincing evidence for or against the value of treatment for aphasia. They studied only patients who were severely aphasic, and severely aphasic patients are known to be notoriously unresponsive to treatment. Programmed instruction treatment, although in vogue at the time, essentially was abandoned in favor of other approaches to treatment within a few years, presumably because those who used it were disappointed in its results. Several outcome measures (e.g., *writing* and *connected speech*) used by Sarno and her associates may have been inappropriate for severely aphasic patients. Sarno and her associates' study was a well-intentioned attempt at getting at an important question in aphasiology, but its results said nothing about aphasia treatment in general and said little about treatment of severely aphasic adults.

Basso, Capitani, and Vignolo (1979) provided fresh ammunition for the proponents of aphasia treatment. Basso and her associates retrospectively compared the effect of "stimulation" treatment for a group of 162 aphasic patients with the effect of no treatment for another group of 119 aphasic patients. Their outcome measure consisted of the number of patients who improved or did not improve according to predetermined criteria for changes in performance on tests of auditory comprehension, reading, speech, and writing. A significantly greater percentage of patients who received treatment improved, compared with patients who received no treatment. The effects of treatment were somewhat greater for patients with severe aphasia than for patients with moderate aphasia.

Basso and her associates concluded that treatment had a highly significant positive effect on recovery from aphasia and that early treatment was better than later treatment. Basso and her associates' study was comparatively well designed and well executed. Its major weakness is that the no-treatment group was made up of aphasic persons who did not receive treatment because they lived too far from the clinic, had no transportation, were unwilling to participate, or had similar reasons for not participating, rather than being randomly assigned to the no-treatment group.

Wertz and associates (1981) prospectively studied the effects of individual treatment and group treatment on aphasic adults' recovery from aphasia. Aphasic participants were selected carefully, reliable outcome measures were chosen, and the nature of treatment was well controlled. Each participant was tested with a comprehensive battery of tests at intake and at 15, 26, 37, and 48 weeks after intake. Both groups improved significantly between intake and each subsequent test, with few significant differences between the groups at any test point. Wertz and associates asserted that both treatments were efficacious because both groups continued to improve beyond 24 weeks post-onset—when spontaneous neurologic recovery is assumed to be complete. Because no untreated control group was included, Wertz and his associates could make no claims regarding the benefits of treatment versus no treatment.

Lincoln and associates (1984) weighed in on the side of the skeptics with a prospective study of the effects of aphasia treatment on a group of 87 patients. A group of 74 patients who received no treatment served as a control group. Patients were tested with standardized tests at 4 weeks post-onset, 10 weeks post-onset (when treated patients entered treatment), 22 weeks post-onset, and 44 weeks post-onset. There were no significant differences between groups at any test point, leading the authors to conclude, "speech therapy does not improve language abilities any more than was achieved by spontaneous recovery" (p. 1199). Unfortunately for the authors' conclusions, serious flaws in design and execution make their study essentially worthless. Participants were not screened to exclude those with multiple lesions or with cognitive, emotional, or physical impairments that would compromise their response to treatment. Few treated patients received the prescribed number of treatment sessions. Of the treated patients, 48% received less than half of the prescribed 48 treatment sessions, and about three quarters of the treated patients would be considered dropouts in a well-designed study. Wertz, Deal, and associates (1986) subsequently commented, "The results indicated that when one does not treat patients who may or may not be aphasic, those patients do not improve" (p. 31).

Shewan and Kertesz (1984) added to the confidence of those who believe in treatment for aphasia when they reported the results of a prospective study in which they assigned aphasic adults to *language-oriented treatment, stimulation-facilitation treatment, unstructured treatment,* or *no treatment.* Each patient was tested with the *Western Aphasia Battery* (WAB) at 2 to 4 weeks post-onset and at 3, 6, and 12 months after the first test. There were no significant differences in the amount of improvement on the WAB among the groups at the 6-month test point, which Shewan and Kertesz attributed to the strong effects of spontaneous recovery. When the change in WAB performance from the first test to the 12-month test was measured, each of the three treated groups had improved significantly more than the untreated group. Shewan and Kertesz concluded that treatment administered by trained speech-language pathologists is efficacious.

Wertz, Weiss, and associates (1986) provided more good news for proponents of aphasia treatment. They compared the effects of clinic treatment, home treatment, and deferred treatment on aphasic adults' recovery from aphasia. The *clinic treatment* group received 8 to 10 hours of treatment provided by a speech-language pathologist each week for 12 weeks, followed by 12 weeks of

no treatment, with periodic testing. The *home treatment* group received 8 to 10 hours of treatment provided by a family member or friend in the patient's home, supervised by a speech-language pathologist, each week for 12 weeks, followed by 12 weeks of no treatment, with periodic testing. The *deferred treatment* group received no treatment for 12 weeks, followed by 8 to 10 hours of treatment provided by a speech-language pathologist each week for 12 weeks. At 12 weeks the clinic treatment group had made significantly greater improvement on the criterion measure (the overall percentile score on the *Porch Index of Communicative Ability*) than either of the other two groups. At 24 weeks the deferred treatment group had caught up with the other two groups; there were no significant differences among the groups at the 24-week test (Figure 7-1).

Poeck, Huber, and Willmes (1989) also concluded that aphasia treatment is efficacious

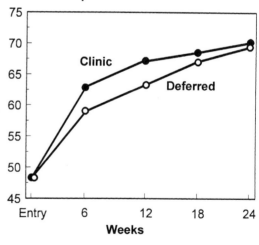

PICA overall percentile

Figure 7-1 ■ Change in PICA overall percentile for participants in the Clinic Treatment group and the Deferred Treatment group from entry in the study to 6, 12, 18, and 24 weeks after entry. (From Wertz, R.T., Weiss, D.G., Aten, J.L., & associates [1986]. A comparison of clinic, home, and deferred language tratment for aphasia: A VA cooperative study. *Archives of Neurology, 43,* 653-658.)

based on the results of a well-designed study in which they provided 6 to 8 weeks of intensive treatment to 68 aphasic adults. A control group of 92 aphasic adults received no treatment but were tested on the same schedule as the treated subjects. (Poeck and his associates used an ingenious statistical procedure to control for the effects of spontaneous recovery.) Both the treated group and the untreated group improved significantly on measures of speech and language, but subjects who received treatment improved significantly more than those who did not, even when the effects of spontaneous recovery were controlled for.

In addition to group studies of the effects of aphasia treatment, a number of well-designed single-case design studies (e.g., Kearns & Salmon, 1984; Thompson & Byrne, 1984) show that individualized treatment programs produce meaningful changes in targeted aspects of aphasic patients' performance and that generalization of the changes to patients' daily life environments can be obtained. Thompson and Byrne, for example, trained two adults with Broca's aphasia to use social conventions *(greetings, self-disclosures, questions)* in conversations. Training progressed from traditional clinician–patient treatment in a therapy room to role-playing situations. Generalization of participants' use of social conventions to conversations with unfamiliar partners was assessed. Training resulted in increased use of social conventions by both aphasic participants, and both participants generalized their use of greetings and self-disclosures (but not questions) to conversations with unfamiliar partners.

Robey and associates (1998, 1999) have reported results from two meta-analyses of treatment literature in aphasia. Meta-analysis is a statistical procedure for finding converging evidence within a group of independent studies—in this case, evidence related to treatment efficacy in studies of aphasia treatment. Robey and associates' results suggest that recovery of communication by treated aphasic adults is approximately twice that of untreated aphasic adults when treatment begins in the first month post-onset of aphasia, with a smaller, but statistically significant, benefit for aphasic adults whose treatment begins after the first month post-onset.

The Outcome

The evidence from group and single-case studies clearly supports the efficacy of treatment for aphasia, provided that several conditions are met:
- The treatment is delivered by qualified professionals.
- Patients with irreversible aphasia are excluded.
- The content, intensity, duration, and timing of treatment are appropriate for those receiving treatment.
- Sensitive and reliable measures are used to track changes in performance.

This does not mean, however, that speech-language pathologists are off the effectiveness hook because the emphasis has shifted from *efficacy* (whether treatment yields a significant change on one or more tests) to *effectiveness* (whether treatment causes meaningful changes in daily life communication performance). When the concepts of efficacy and effectiveness are separated, it becomes clear that most existing studies of aphasia treatment are efficacy studies—their measures of the effects of treatment are changes on one or more tests of communication ability. Consequently, the evidence supports the *efficacy* of aphasia treatment but not necessarily its *effectiveness*. The issue of effectiveness now has taken center stage, and investigators are at work developing measures of treatment effectiveness and planning studies to determine if aphasia treatment is *effective* as well as *efficacious*.

THE TIMING OF INTERVENTION

Another question that has bedeviled clinical aphasiology relates to the timing of intervention—namely, is treatment begun a month or more post-onset of aphasia as efficacious (or effective) as treatment begun soon after a patient becomes aphasic? Scientific studies of early versus late intervention have yielded equivocal results. Several

Holland (1996) asserted that changes on standardized language tests do, in fact, reflect changes in functional communication because the standardized measures are significantly correlated with functional performance. The validity of Holland's assertion depends on the strength of the correlation. A significant correlation does not necessarily mean that the correlated phenomena are strongly related—it simply means that the coefficient of correlation is significantly greater than zero. Holland presumably based her assertion on correlations of 0.84 and 0.93 between aphasic patient's performance on *Communicative Abilities in Daily Living* (CADL; Holland, 1980), a measure of functional communication, and performance on two standardized language assessment batteries. Correlations of this magnitude suggest that performance on the standardized language assessment batteries is a relatively strong indicator of functional communication.

investigators have reported that delaying treatment by 2 months or more after the onset of aphasia has significant negative effects on patients' eventual recovery (Butfield & Zangwill, 1946; Sands, Sarno, & Shankweiler, 1969; Vignolo, 1964; Wepman, 1951). Vignolo, for example, studied the recovery of 69 aphasic patients. Some received treatment and some did not. Vignolo concluded that it is important that treatment begin while physiologic recovery is most rapid. "Only the period which extends from 2 to 6 months after the onset of aphasia seems to provide a ground where intrinsic capacity for recovery can be highly enhanced by the intervention of planned training" (p. 366).

Poeck and associates (1989) reported that neither age nor time post-onset of aphasia significantly affected aphasic adults' *recovery of language*. However, time post-onset appeared to affect the magnitude of patients' *response to treatment*. Of those who began treatment within the first 4 months post-onset of aphasia, 78% improved significantly on a standardized

aphasia test, whereas 46% of those who began treatment from 4 to 12 months post-onset improved significantly on the same test, even when subjects' test scores were corrected for the effects of spontaneous neurologic recovery. The results of Robey's (1998) meta-analysis of 21 aphasia treatment studies also suggested that treatment begun in the first few weeks post-onset of aphasia produces greater improvement than treatment begun after that time.

Others have concluded that delaying treatment has no major effects on outcome. Wertz and associates (1986) concluded that delaying treatment for 12 weeks had no irreversible effects on aphasic patients' eventual *Porch Index of Communicative Ability* overall scores because the performance of patients who received treatment after a 12-week delay approximated the scores of patients who received treatment on entry into the study. As this is written, we do not know if delaying treatment has important or irreversible effects on aphasic adults' recovery of communicative abilities. Group studies have reached conflicting conclusions, and single-case studies have not addressed the question.

If delaying treatment were to have few or no significant effects on patient's scores on standardized tests of language and communication (the criterion used in published studies), it may not be legitimate to conclude that delaying treatment has no negative effects on the patient or the patient's family. Clinicians do more than treat specific speech and language behaviors in the first weeks following the onset of a patient's aphasia. They educate patients and families about the causes of the patient's aphasia and provide them with strategies for dealing with communication breakdown. They make referrals to other disciplines and help the patient and family make use of community resources. They provide reassurance, advice, and support to patients and families.

Education, counseling, and support may not affect an aphasic patient's scores on standardized tests, yet they are important to patients and families immediately after onset of aphasia. Consequently, it cannot be said that clinicians have little to contribute to aphasic patients during the first 10 or 12 weeks post-onset that cannot just as well be done later. It may be that delaying treatment is not fatal to aphasic adults' recovery of communicative abilities as measured with standardized tests, but it seems highly likely that delaying or eliminating counseling, education, and support during the first weeks after the patient becomes aphasic may have important and irreversible negative effects on the patient and the patient's family.

CANDIDACY FOR TREATMENT

Not all adults with aphasia receive treatment for their aphasia, and not all should. Some have such mild impairments that spontaneous neurologic recovery leaves them with no significant linguistic or communicative impairments. Some are too ill or too weak to tolerate treatment. Some are so severely impaired that existing treatment procedures offer no hope of recovery sufficient to justify the cost of treatment. Some who would otherwise be candidates for treatment refuse it. And, regrettably, some who are treatment candidates do not have the money or the insurance coverage to pay for it. Patient refusal and financial coverage are not under the clinician's control, so the clinician's decision about offering treatment usually depends on the clinician's best guess as to whether treatment will produce improvements in the patient's communication performance sufficient to justify its cost.

Schuell (1965) described the test performance of a group of aphasic adults who exhibited what she called *irreversible aphasic syndrome,* which she characterized as "almost complete loss of functional language skills in all modalities" (p. 14). According to Schuell, patients with irreversible aphasic syndrome cannot reliably point to common objects named by the examiner, cannot follow simple spoken directions, cannot read aloud nor comprehend simple printed sentences, cannot name objects or give simple biographic information, and cannot write simple words either spontaneously or to dictation. A few can match some simple words to pictures, some produce a

few automatic and overlearned speech responses such as counting or profanity, and some can copy simple drawings. Schuell commented that a few patients with irreversible aphasic syndrome make limited gains in auditory comprehension, but she asserted that none recover functional language in any modality.

Presumably Schuell was referring to verbal language (auditory comprehension, reading, speaking, writing) and not gestural communication, body language, or other nonverbal means of communication, which often are retained by patients with severe aphasia.

What Schuell calls *irreversible aphasic syndrome* others call *global aphasia.* Collins (1991) characterizes global aphasia as follows:

Global aphasia is a severe, acquired impairment of communicative ability across all language modalities, and often no single communicative modality is strikingly better than another. Visual nonverbal problem-solving abilities are often severely depressed as well and are usually compatible with language performance. It [global aphasia] usually results from extensive damage to the language zones of the left hemisphere but may result from smaller, subcortical lesions. (p. 6)

Goodglass and Kaplan (1983) likewise characterized aphasia as loss of almost all verbal communication.

In global aphasia, all aspects of language are so severely impaired that there is no longer a distinctive pattern of preserved versus impaired components. It is only articulation that is sometimes well preserved in the few words or stereotyped utterances that are preserved. Global aphasics sometimes produce stereotyped utterances that may consist of real or nonsense words. Some patients produce a continuous output of syllables that employ a limited set of vowel-consonant combinations that make no sense, even though they are uttered with expressive intonation . . . Auditory comprehension of conversation concerning material of immediate personal relevance may appear fairly good in comparison to the patient's poor performance on all the formal auditory comprehension subtests. (p. 97)

The foregoing descriptions are remarkably consistent. They portray the globally aphasic adult as one who has limited comprehension of personally relevant spoken language but little usable expressive language beyond a few stereotyped utterances.

The healing effects of time apparently have little effect on the language abilities of most patients who remain globally aphasic beyond the first month or so post-onset. Studies by Brust and associates (1976); Kertesz and McCabe (1977); and Prins, Snow, and Wagenaar (1978) suggest a grim prognosis for most patients who remain globally aphasic at 1 month or more post-onset.

Brust and associates reviewed the medical records of 177 aphasic stroke patients. Of those who were diagnosed as globally aphasic at onset, 75% remained globally aphasic 1 month to 3 months later. Kertesz and McCabe reported that 83% of patients who were globally aphasic at 1 month post-onset remained globally aphasic at 1 year post-onset. Prins, Snow, and Wagenaar found that 80% of patients who were globally aphasic at 3 months post-onset remained globally aphasic at 1 year post-onset.

Collins (1991) reminds us, however, that global aphasia can be acute, evolving, or chronic. According to Collins, many aphasic patients are globally aphasic at onset and immediately thereafter. Those with acute global aphasia evolve to less severe forms within the first week or so post-onset. Those with evolving global aphasia are globally aphasic at onset, but over a period of months or years they slowly evolve to less severe forms of aphasia (usually Broca's aphasia with coexisting agrammatism). Those with chronic global aphasia experience profound communicative impairments for the rest of their lives.

There seems little doubt that the presence of global aphasia in a neurologically recovered pa-

tient is an ominous prognostic sign. Only about one in five achieve some functional use of language, and most who do regain some functional language remain markedly aphasic with functional verbal communication limited to communication of basic needs and comprehension limited to bits and pieces of simple conversational interactions on highly familiar topics.

> I will use the appellation "neurologically recovered" to denote patients for whom "spontaneous" physiologic recovery is mostly complete. For most patients with occlusive strokes, physiologic recovery is essentially complete within 4 to 6 weeks, although slow improvement beyond that time is common. For patients with hemorrhagic strokes and for those with traumatic brain injuries, physiologic recovery may last longer, but usually is essentially complete within 3 to 6 months.

Not surprisingly, globally aphasic patients perform poorly on language test batteries. Their overall test performance places them well below the 25th percentile for aphasic adults (usually around the 10th to 15th percentile) and their performance across subtests is consistently poor, with no subtest or group of subtests yielding strikingly better performance than other subtests. Figure 7-2 summarizes the performance of a globally aphasic patient on the *Porch Index of Communicative Ability* (Porch, 1981a). The patient makes no intelligible, accurate, stimulus-related responses on any subtest except Subtest X (pointing to objects by name), Subtest VIII (matching pictures to objects), and Subtest XI (matching objects to objects).

Universally poor performance across all subtests in language test batteries is one sign of global aphasia. In addition to their poor performance on all tests of speaking, listening comprehension, reading, and writing, globally aphasic patients typically exhibit other signs of severe impairment that may become evident before formal testing begins, when the clinician in-

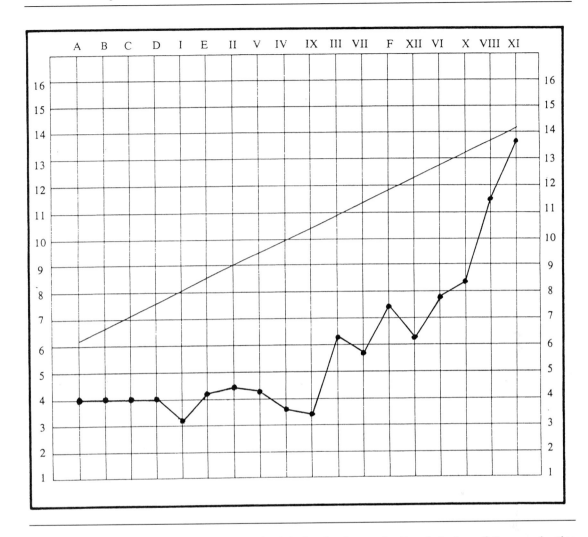

Figure 7-2 ■ Performance of an adult with global aphasia on the *Porch Index of Communicative Ability* (PICA; Porch, 1981a). The subtests are arranged from left to right in approximate order of difficulty. The patient makes no intelligible responses (represented by PICA scores of 5 or below) in the 10 most difficult subtests. The patient makes intelligible but inaccurate responses (represented by PICA scores of 6 or 7) on the next five less difficult subtests. The patient makes accurate but prompted or delayed responses on the three easiest subtests—pointing to test objects by name (X), matching pictures to objects (VIII), and matching identical objects (XI).

terviews the patient, or during screening tests of communication, memory, and cognition.

They may utter *verbal stereotypies.* Repetitive, stereotypical utterances (e.g., *me-me-me-me, oh boy-oh boy-oh boy-oh boy*) are common in the speech of patients with global aphasia, and verbal stereotypies often are the only spontaneous speech produced by globally aphasic patients. Some patients with severe Wernicke's aphasia also produce verbal stereotypies, but the stereotypies alternate with, or occur within, words, phrases, or sentences that convey meaning, although the meaning may not be appropriate to the context.

They may be *unable to match identical objects or pictures and objects.* Many globally aphasic patients cannot match identical common objects (e.g., forks, pencils, keys) or cannot match common objects to pictures—tasks that patients with less severe aphasia easily accomplish. Failure to match objects to objects or objects to pictures is considered a sign of bilateral brain damage by some practitioners.

Aphasic patients with posterior brain injury and visual impairments caused by damage in the visual cortex or visual association regions may fail visual matching tests. These patients have great difficulty in tasks that depend on visual input, but their performance improves in tasks in which visual input is not crucial.

They may give *unreliable* yes *or* no *responses.* Many globally aphasic patients cannot reliably indicate (or learn to indicate) *yes* and *no* by speech, by gesture or head nod, or by pointing to cards showing words or symbols representing *yes* and *no.* Most aphasic patients who are not globally aphasic can acquire reliable *yes* or *no* responses to simple *nonverbal* stimuli with an hour or two of training, but many globally aphasic patients seem unable to grasp the concepts of *yes* and *no* or are unable to match the concepts with the appropriate gesture or with the words *yes* and *no.*

They may produce *jargon and meaningless speech without self-correction.* Some globally aphasic patients' spontaneous speech consists primarily of jargon (nonwords such as *kalimfropper*) or meaningless strings of true words (such as *that's Sheila's aunt in a full subscription*) uttered uncritically whenever the patient is moved to speak. Patients with severe Wernicke's aphasia or severe transcortical sensory aphasia also produce jargon and meaningless word

strings, but as mentioned previously, these patients also produce some words, phrases, or sentences that convey meaning, although the meaning may not be appropriate to the context.

Treatment options for patients with chronic global aphasia are limited. Globally aphasic patients do not become competent speakers, listeners, readers, or writers, no matter how tenaciously the clinician tries. Some globally aphasic patients' daily life communicative adequacy may be enhanced by a few sessions of intensive training dedicated to modest goals with a reasonable probability of success, such as those recommended by Collins (1991), who comments that they should be minimal goals for all globally aphasic patients. I have arranged Collins's goals in what I consider to be descending order of importance:

1. Improve speech production to make the patient's *yes* and *no* consistent, reliable responses in structured situations.
2. Improve the patient's production of simple, unequivocal gestures, which may include gestures to express *yes* and *no.*
3. Ensure that the patient can convey a small, basic set of communicative intentions in one or a combination of modalities.
4. Improve the patient's auditory comprehension to permit comprehension of one-step commands (e.g., *hand me the pencil*) in controlled situations with contextual cues.
5. Improve the patient's writing of a few simple important daily life words.
6. Improve the patient's drawing to permit simple unequivocal messages.

Not every globally aphasic patient will accomplish all of the foregoing goals. Some may have to rely on gestures, rather than speech, to express basic needs. Some with artistic talent may find it feasible to communicate by drawing. Some may be able to write a few important words they cannot say. Which goals are attainable depend on each patient's abilities, needs, motivation, and life situation. The clinician, the patient, and caregivers collaborate to choose appropriate goals and to devise treatment procedures that address the goals.

THE FOCUS AND PROGRESSION OF TREATMENT

Aphasia test batteries typically partition communication among traditional verbal processes (listening, speaking, reading, and writing) and provide tasks that test various input and output modalities (auditory, visual, and sometimes tactile input; oral, gestural, and graphic output). Such partitioning of communication can prove attractive to novice clinicians who are searching for a rationale to guide treatment and may lead them to adopt a *treat-to-the-test* approach to treatment, in which the clinician identifies tests in which a patient's performance is deficient and constructs treatment tasks that mimic the content and structure of the tests.

The clinician who uses a treat-to-the-test approach may distribute treatment tasks across processes or modalities to increase the generality of treatment and may select tasks in which the patient's performance is somewhat deficient but not completely erroneous to ensure that the treatment tasks are at an appropriate level of difficulty. If a simple *treat-to-the-test* approach is to be effective (which means that it has positive effects on the patient's daily life communication), the tasks in the test serving as the model for treatment must represent processes or skills that operate in the patient's daily life. If they do not, the treatment may improve a patient's test scores but have little effect on their daily life communication. (The treatment is *efficacious* but not *effective*.)

A more sophisticated version of the *treat-to-the-test approach* is the *selective treat-to-the-test approach*. Clinicians using this approach consider deficient performance in some tests more important than deficient performance in other tests. For example, those who believe that impaired auditory comprehension is a central problem in aphasia pay particular attention to patients' performance on tests of auditory comprehension, and they design treatment to mimic the auditory comprehension tests on which a patient's performance is deficient. The *selective treat-to-the-test approach* assigns greater impor-

tance to some tests than others based on some underlying rationale, but the tasks included in treatment closely resemble the tests that led to their inclusion in the treatment program.

Clinicians who believe that impaired auditory comprehension is a central problem in aphasia often enroll their aphasic patients in auditory comprehension drills in which the patient must carry out gestural responses to the clinician's spoken commands. Some mimic the *Token Test* by asking the patient to point to or manipulate colored geometric forms (a tedious business for patient and clinician). Others ask the patient to point to or manipulate picture cards or pictures of objects in response to spoken commands ("Point to the spotted dog, the red book, and the fat man.").

The major problem with *treat-to-the-test* approaches is that the tasks in aphasia test batteries may have little to do with patients' daily life communication needs. Consequently, *treat-to-the-test* approaches run the risk of wasting the clinician's and the patient's time, energy, and resources in treatment tasks that have little or no positive effect on the patient's life beyond escalation of the patient's test scores (an escalation that often proves temporary—when treatment stops, the patient's test scores decline).

The *treat underlying processes approach* orients clinicians toward underlying cognitive processes assumed to be responsible for a patient's impaired test performance. Most clinicians and investigators agree that aphasia is not a loss of vocabulary or linguistic rules—instead it is the result of impairments in processes necessary for comprehending, formulating, and producing spoken and written language. For example, comprehension impairments in aphasia may be caused by reduced speed and efficiency in attaching meaning to words, rather than loss of word meanings; impaired naming may be caused by reduced speed, efficiency, or accuracy of retrieval of words from memory, rather than by loss of vocabulary; and speech production problems may be caused by disruptions of word retrieval or phonologic selection and sequencing, rather than loss of words or syntactic rules.

Clinicians who believe that aphasia represents a reduction in the speed and efficiency of processes underlying language, rather than loss of language, focus treatment on *reactivating* or *restimulating* language processes, rather than on *teaching* specific responses (Schuell, Jenkins, & Jimenez-Pabon, 1964). For example, if an aphasic patient has impaired reading, the clinician might attempt to determine whether the problem is related to:

- Eye movements and visual search
- Single-word comprehension
- Use of syntactic rules
- Ability to deduce main ideas, make inferences, or draw conclusions
- Storage and recall of information gained from printed materials

After a deficient process is identified, treatment focuses on the process. One of the major advantages of a process-directed approach to treatment is that stimulating a general process may affect several specific communicative abilities that depend on the process. For example, improving a patient's auditory retention span by means of *point-to* drills may improve a patient's comprehension of spoken sentences and discourse and also may enhance reading comprehension because both auditory comprehension and reading comprehension depend on retention of verbal information in immediate memory.

Schuell, Jenkins, and Jimenez-Pabon (1964) offered the following principles for stimulating disrupted processes in aphasia:

- Provide repetitive sensory stimulation.
- Provide intensive auditory stimulation, but combine auditory and visual stimulation to maximize patients' responses.
- Ensure that treatment stimuli are strong enough to get into the patient's brain via compromised sensory systems.
- Ensure that treatment stimuli are strong enough to get and hold the patient's attention.

- Ensure that every stimulus elicits a response.
- Elicit responses. Do not force them. (If stimulation is adequate, responses follow.)
- Stimulate, rather than correct. (Error responses do not appear if stimulation is adequate.)

Schuell, Jenkins, and Jimenez-Pabon comment that the clinician's role is not to teach but to communicate with the patient and to stimulate disrupted processes to function maximally.

THE GOALS OF TREATMENT

> The primary objective in treatment of aphasia is to increase communication. What the aphasic patient wants is to recover enough language to get on with his life. (Schuell, Jenkins, & Jimenez-Pabon, 1964, p. 333)

As Schuell suggests, complete recovery of language and communicative abilities is not an option for most aphasic adults. Most will be left with persisting language and communicative impairments. Treatment may enhance aphasic adults' recovery of language and communicative abilities, and when recovery stops, treatment may help aphasic adults compensate for their residual impairments. The objective of most aphasia treatment is to help aphasic adults to be effective communicators despite their residual impairments.

How this is accomplished differs across clinicians and treatment venues. From the 1940s to the late 1970s aphasia treatment customarily relied on didactic methods in which aphasic patients participated in drills designed to reactivate language processes. The general objective of such didactic treatment was to help aphasic adults become better communicators by improving the linguistic and grammatic quality of their communication.

In the late 1970s and the 1980s many clinicians began to move away from traditional linguistically oriented, didactic treatment toward treatment that emphasized functional communication in natural contexts—a trend that has continued to the present. Holland (1977) observed that traditional didactic treatment approaches tend to focus on linguistic correctness and propositional accuracy ...

. . . by means of activities such as matching, naming, and helping aphasics to comprehend utterances defined by their linguistic structure, instead of their likelihood of being heard in everyday communication . . . Most therapy is disproportionately centered on the propositionality of an utterance, not on its communicative value. (p. 171)

Holland went on to recommend that treatment focus on *communicative competence*—a person's use of language in naturalistic contexts.

Functional communication treatment programs downplay traditional didactic drills and emphasize communication in natural contexts to encourage generalization from the clinic to the patient's daily life. Clinicians and patients might act out daily life situations such as making a purchase in a department store, calling for information about airline schedules, and the like. Patients are encouraged (or taught) to communicate nonverbally (e.g., with gestures and facial expression) and to enhance their comprehension by using the information provided by others' gestures and facial expressions and by situational contexts. Functional approaches to treatment recognize that aphasic persons need not be perfect speakers or perfect listeners to communicate adequately.

Despite their intuitive appeal, there is no strong empirical evidence that functional approaches to treatment are more successful than traditional approaches in improving daily life communication. It seems intuitively reasonable that functional approaches would improve patients' daily life communicative adequacy. However, it also seems intuitively reasonable that traditional didactic process-directed approaches might lead to comparable improvements in daily life communication if the skills targeted for treatment are important in daily life communicative interactions. That the *procedures* used in treatment resemble natural communicative interactions may be less important than that the *skills* (or processes) targeted for treatment are relevant to daily life communication. For example, it seems reasonable that providing activities in which an aphasic person must quickly adjust to changes in stimuli or changing response requirements might enhance comprehension in daily life interchanges in which topics and speakers change without warning, even though the activities themselves do not mimic daily life interactions.

The important issue here is that of *generalization,* or the transfer of what is accomplished in the clinic to the aphasic person's daily life. Regardless of how one approaches treatment, generalization to daily life often does not occur unless procedures for enhancing generalization to daily life are part of the treatment program. Because improvements in communicative ability that do not extend outside the clinic are of little value, it behooves the clinician to plan for, to work for, and to test for generalization of skills, strategies, and behaviors acquired in the clinic to the patient's daily life.

Treatment procedures that mimic daily life may have an advantage when it comes to generalization because of what behaviorists call *stimulus control*—the tendency for behaviors learned in the presence of certain stimuli to recur when the individual next encounters the stimuli. The aphasic patient who acquires communicative skills in a clinic setting that resembles the patient's daily life environment may have a leg up on generalization, compared with an aphasic patient who acquires similar skills in a less naturalistic setting. (Chapter 6 provides more information on generalization and how to obtain it.)

GENERAL CONCEPTS 7-1

- Early group studies of the effectiveness of treatment for aphasia yielded conflicting results. Recent and better-designed studies suggest that treatment of aphasia in adults is efficacious provided that the following criteria are met:
  —The treatment is delivered by qualified personnel.
  —Patients with irreversible aphasia are excluded.
  —The intensity, content, duration, and timing are appropriate for the recipients.
  —Sensitive and reliable measures are used to document the effects of treatment.

- Single-case design studies show that specific treatment procedures provide meaningful changes in targeted skills and that generalization of changes to patients' daily lives may be obtained.
- Early intervention (within a few weeks of the onset of aphasia) appears to be somewhat more efficacious than late intervention.
- The primary objective of aphasia treatment is to improve aphasic adults' daily life communication, not simply to change their test scores.
- Some aphasic adults may not be candidates for treatment, including those who are too ill or too weak, those who are too severely aphasic, and those who elect not to participate in treatment.
- Globally aphasic adults have severely impaired comprehension and little expressive language beyond stereotypic utterances. Individuals who are globally aphasic at 1 month or more post-onset are likely to remain globally aphasic for the rest of their lives.
- The two most common generic approaches to treatment are the following:
  —The *treat to the test* approach (or the *selective treat to the test* approach) in which treatment tasks resemble the tests used to measure the aphasic patient's impairments
  —The *treat underlying processes* approach in which treatment tasks focus on cognitive processes that underlie several communicative skills
- Clinicians who believe that aphasia represents reduced speed and efficiency of underlying language processes focus treatment on *reactivating* or *restimulating* the processes.
- Contemporary aphasia treatment philosophies consider *functionality* (the daily life utility of skills) and *generalization* of skills learned in the clinic to a patient's daily life.

TREATMENT OF AUDITORY COMPREHENSION
Listening Comprehension and Memory

Listening comprehension and memory cannot be separated. Listeners cannot comprehend spoken language unless they can retain it in memory long enough to carry out the processes needed to de-duce its meaning, and they must retain the mental representation of its meaning long enough to respond. That listening comprehension and memory are related is clear. However, the relationships between memory and listening comprehension have not yet been well described.

During the 1960s several so-called *stages* models of memory were proposed. These models conceptualized memory as the transfer of information among several storage components, or stages. The models were called *stages* models because they portrayed information as passing through three stages, beginning with perception and culminating in long-term storage. These stages were given different labels in different models, and different models assigned slightly different responsibilities to stages, but the differences among models were mainly in the details and not in their general form. The first stage in most of these models is the *sensory register* (sometimes called *sensory memory*) in which traces of incoming stimuli are briefly stored in modality-specific form (auditory, visual, or tactile after-images). The sensory register has limited capacity and its contents decay within 1 or 2 seconds, after which the information is lost unless it is transferred to another stage. Information in the sensory register cannot be maintained by rehearsal.

The second stage in these models of memory is *short-term memory* (or *primary memory*). Short-term memory also has limited capacity, and information within it decays but at a slower rate than information in the sensory register (within several seconds to several minutes). Information can be maintained in short-term memory by rehearsal. Short-term memory capacity may be quantified as *retention span,* or the number of items of discrete information (numerals, letters, words) that can be held in memory at one time. Digit-span tasks and sentence-repetition tasks depend on short-term memory. Short-term memory is considered a passive storage space through which information passes on its way to *long-term memory* (or *secondary memory*)—the third stage. Long-term memory has very large (perhaps infinite) capacity, and information in long-term memory decays slowly, if at all. Long-term memory is conceptualized as a static repository for memories of our experiences and for our knowledge. The meanings of sentences are integrated into permanent memory at this stage.

> Semantic information, but not syntactic structure, is retained in long-term memory. An individual who is shown the sentence, "The white rabbit was chased by the brown dog," and after 30 minutes or so is shown the sentence, "The brown dog chased the white rabbit," may claim to have previously seen the latter sentence, although the syntactic structure differs. The individual remembers the meaning of the sentence and not its syntactic structure.

In the late 1960s and early 1970s some investigators (Baddeley, 1986; Shallice & Warrington, 1970; Warrington & Shallice, 1969) formulated the concept of *working memory* to denote a mental space wherein active processing of information coming from the sensory register or retrieved from long-term memory takes place. Working memory was conceptualized as a limited-capacity processing space in which cognitive processes (e.g., sentence comprehension) can be carried out. Working memory has many of the characteristics of what others call short-term memory, except that short-term memory is conceptualized as a static repository for information on its way to long-term storage, whereas working memory is a place where active mental processing goes on.

Some models of memory (such as that of Craik & Lockhart, 1972) reject the *stages* concept of memory in favor of a continuous *depth-of-processing* explanation. The general theme of depth-of-processing models is that the durability of information stored in memory is a function of the amount of active mental processing it received prior to storage. However, the general sense of how comprehension proceeds in depth-of-processing models is similar to that for stages models.

The exact role of memory in aphasic adults' comprehension impairments is not well understood. Most aphasic adults have impairments in short-term verbal memory that interfere with comprehension and recall of spoken or printed language. In fact, Schuell, Jenkins, and Jimenez-Pabon (1964) identified impaired short-term retention and recall as a defining characteristic of adult aphasia. There is little doubt that short-term verbal memory impairments affect comprehension of single-sentence messages such as those in the *Token Test* (DeRenzi & Vignolo, 1962) and other tests of single-sentence comprehension in which test takers must comprehend and retain unrelated sentences (e.g., "Touch the large yellow square and the small green circle" or "The thin girl with a bow in her hair chases the small black dog with no collar"). Aphasic adults' performance on such tests has been shown to correlate strongly with their performance on tests of short-term memory (Lesser, 1976; Martin & Feher, 1990).

Short-term memory impairment apparently does not account for aphasic adults' problems in comprehending syntactically complex sentences (e.g., "The dog the cat chased was white."). Nonaphasic adults with impaired short-term memory usually have little difficulty with comprehension of such sentences (Vallar & Baddeley, 1984), and aphasic adults' performance on tests of short-term memory is not meaningfully related to their performance on tests that assess comprehension of syntactically complex sentences (Martin & Feher, 1990). That aphasic adults comprehend longer sentences, such as "The man was greeted by his wife and he was smoking a pipe," better than shorter but syntactically more complex sentences, such as "The man greeted by his wife was smoking a pipe" (Goodglass & associates, 1979), also suggests that short-term memory does not fully explain aphasic adults' difficulties with syntactically complex sentences.

Models of Auditory Comprehension

Schuell, Jenkins, and Jimenez-Pabon (1964) considered impaired auditory comprehension and constricted auditory retention span central problems in aphasia. Since that time treating auditory comprehension impairments has had special status for many clinicians who believe that improving auditory comprehension is the most efficient way to improve aphasic adults' general language competence. The validity of this belief has not been confirmed by experimental evidence, but treatment of auditory comprehension impairments continues to occupy a prominent place in many approaches to aphasia treatment.

For many years auditory comprehension was thought to proceed through a series of stages, in which listeners analyzed the phonemic content of utterances, combined the phonemes into representations of words, retrieved the meanings of the words, determined the relationships among words, and constructed a mental representation for the meaning of the utterances. Such models of comprehension eventually became known as *bottom-up* models because listeners start with the physical characteristics of the message and work their way up through a series of levels until the meaning of the utterance becomes apparent.

During the 1960s and 1970s other models of comprehension were proposed, in which listeners' general knowledge and expectations played an important part in their comprehension of spoken and printed material. These models made it clear that comprehension is not simply the result of a series of computations by which listeners deduce the meaning of what they hear. For listeners in naturalistic situations, the words seem only to provide a starting point from which listeners go on to guess the speaker's intent, construct presuppositions, develop expectations, decide what is important and what is not, and relate what they hear to what they already know. These models became known as *top-down* models because listeners begin with general expectations about what a speaker is likely to say, use their general knowledge to prove or disprove their expectations, and resort to lower-level linguistic analyses only when higher-level processes leave the speaker's meaning in doubt.

Listeners seem to use lexical and syntactic processes primarily to establish what the speaker is talking about and to identify how the speaker's message relates to what the speaker has said previously. These lexical and syntactic processes sometimes are called *text-based processes* because they depend strongly on the words and syntax of what is said, in contrast with *knowledge-based* or *heuristic processes* in which the listener invokes general knowledge, intuition, and guessing to deduce the meaning of spoken material.

Text-based processes require more mental effort than knowledge-based (heuristic) processes. Heuristic processes lighten a listener's workload by allowing the listener to deduce a speaker's general meaning and intent without resorting to continuous word-by-word lexical and syntactic analysis. Normal listeners usually emphasize heuristic processes over text-based processes and resort to text-based processes only when forced to so do by the absence of extralinguistic sources of information, by unusual vocabulary, or by complex syntax.

Scripts often make an important contribution to heuristic processes. Scripts are mental representations of familiar daily life situations in which certain events typically occur and in which the events occur in a typical order. Consider, for example, a speaker who says to a friend, "Let me tell you about the party I went to last night." The listener with party-going experience can call on knowledge of what typically happens at parties to construct a set of expectations about what took place at the party. Once the listener has mentally activated a party script, expectations about what the speaker is likely to convey come into play:

- A number of people were there.
- Food and drink were served.
- There was a host or hostess.
- The party was at the host or hostess's home.
- Social conversations took place.

Normal listeners use such mental representations to organize information from discourse and to form expectations about what is likely to be conveyed in a sample of discourse (Adams & Collins, 1979; Bower, Black, & Turner, 1979; and others). Armus, Brookshire, and Nicholas (1989) have shown that aphasic adults' knowledge of scripts for common situations is preserved, and they have suggested that preserved script knowledge may at least partially account for some aphasic adults' good comprehension of spoken discourse in the face of substantially impaired performance on tests of single-sentence comprehension.

Script knowledge apparently does not help aphasic adults with poor single-word comprehension who also have poor comprehension of spoken sentences and spoken discourse. For them, treatment focused on single-word comprehension is a logical starting place.

Treatment of Single-Word Comprehension

The prototypical treatment for impaired single-word comprehension is pointing drill in which the clinician places an array of pictures or (less frequently) objects before the patient and asks the patient to point to each item as it is named. The clinician manipulates the difficulty of the task by manipulating the familiarity or abstractness of the stimulus words.

> Most clinicians put the stimulus word at the end of a short carrier phrase, such as "Point to the _____" or "Show me the _____." Although the clinician's utterances technically are sentences, the redundancy of the carrier phrase makes it irrelevant to successful performance.

Single-word comprehension drills are appropriate for patients with severe comprehension impairments who cannot comprehend phrase-length or sentence-length materials. Single-word comprehension drills usually serve as a starting point for drills in which the length, information density, and complexity of the treatment stimuli increase as the patient's comprehension improves.

Single-word comprehension drills are not appropriate for patients who can comprehend short phrases or sentences but have mild to moderate single-word comprehension impairments. These patients' single-word comprehension impairments usually relate to low-frequency words, and low-frequency words are not common in daily life conversations. Consequently, comprehension of most daily life spoken material seems unlikely to depend much on comprehension of low-frequency words. The context in which words occur often gives strong hints about their meanings, and the aphasic listener who can make use of context to deduce the meaning of uncomprehended words is unlikely to have much difficulty comprehending most daily life spoken material, even when it contains some low-frequency words.

A small number of patients with mild or moderate aphasia experience remarkable difficulties in attaching meanings to words they hear or read. They behave (usually intermittently) as if they do not know the meanings of spoken or printed words, even when the words are common in the language. Their performance is not word-specific. Sometimes they comprehend a word and at other times they do not. Sometimes they behave as if they are hearing words from a foreign language. They may repeat an unrecognized word over and over and may even spell the word while attempting to associate it with a meaning. When given a clue to the meaning of an unrecognized word (such as a synonym or an antonym), they often recognize the word.

> *Pure word deafness* is a rare syndrome in which comprehension of spoken language is severely impaired with preservation of speech, reading, and writing. Patients with pure word deafness have normal hearing for tones and environmental sounds but exhibit profound impairments in comprehension of speech. Pure word deafness is thought to be caused by isolation of an intact Wernicke's area from auditory input from the right and left auditory cortices.

Treatment for patients with impaired single-word comprehension usually consists of drills in which they match spoken words to pictures or give definitions, synonyms, or antonyms for spoken words. If such drills do not lead to improved single-word comprehension, these patients' single-word comprehension may be treated indirectly by working on short-term auditory memory and sentence comprehension and by teaching the patients to use context to arrive at the meaning of unrecognized words.

Understanding Spoken Sentences

Impaired sentence comprehension commonly is targeted in treatment programs for aphasic adults, not only because it seems to be important in daily life but because of the central role played by auditory comprehension in some models of aphasia. Treatment to improve comprehension of spoken sentences typically is accomplished by means of drills in which patients answer questions, follow directions, or verify the meaning of sentences.

Answering Questions The questions in question-answering drills can be either yes-no questions, to which patients can respond with spoken or gestural indicators of *yes* or *no,* or open-ended questions, which call for longer and more complex responses.

Yes-no questions may call on general knowledge ("Is Mason City the capital of Iowa?"), verbal retention span ("Are monkeys, horses, cows, and pigs animals?"), semantic discriminations ("Do you brush teeth with a comb?"), phonemic discriminations ("Do you wear a shirt and pie?"), syntactic analysis ("Do you wear feet on your shoes?"), or semantic relationships ("Is a banana a vegetable?").

Yes-no questions commonly are used for treating severely impaired patients who cannot produce enough speech to answer open-ended questions. Most of these patients can indicate *yes* and *no* verbally, by head movements, or by pointing to words or symbols signifying *yes* and *no,* which makes yes-no questions a reasonable treatment procedure.

Open-ended questions (e.g., "Why do people put locks on their doors?") permit clinicians to sample a greater variety of information and permit greater flexibility in the structure of the questions, but their validity as comprehension training items is compromised by the need for patients to formulate and produce longer verbal responses. Because of this, clinicians often use open-ended questions as vehicles for work on word retrieval and speech formulation, rather than as items in comprehension drills.

Following Spoken Directions Treatment tasks in which patients follow spoken directions are an important component of many clinicians' clinical repertoire. Following-spoken-directions tasks require patients to perform sequential pointing or manipulative responses in response to directions spoken by the clinician, as in "Put the spoon beside the pencil, put the quarter beside the comb, and give me the key." In following-spoken-directions drills, the length and complexity of the spoken directions are controlled so that the patient continuously is working at a level that taxes, but does not exceed, the patient's processing capacity. As the patient's comprehension improves, treatment progresses along a hierarchy of increasingly longer or syntactically complex sentences, such as the hierarchy described by Kearns and Hubbard (1977), who measured the average difficulty of 13 levels of spoken directions for a group of 10 aphasic adults. (The group's average scores on a 16-point scale are given in parentheses.)

1. Point to one common object by name. (14.30)
2. Point to one common object by function. (14.02)
3. Point in sequence to two common objects by function. (12.90)
4. Point in sequence to two common objects by name. (12.67)
5. Point to one object spelled by the examiner. (12.51)
6. Point to one object described by the examiner with three descriptors ("Which one is white, plastic, and has bristles?"). (12.23)
7. Follow one-verb instructions ("Pick up the pen."). (12.05)
8. Point in sequence to three common objects by name. (10.74)

9. Point in sequence to three common objects by function. (10.72)
10. Carry out two-object location instructions ("Put the pen in front of the knife.") (10.20)
11. Carry out, in sequence, two-verb instructions ("Point to the knife and turn over the fork."). (9.77)
12. Carry out, in sequence, two-verb instructions with time constraint ("Before you pick up the knife, hand me the fork."). (8.60)
13. Carry out three-verb instructions ("Point to the knife, turn over the fork, and hand me the pencil."). (7.53)

Kearns and Hubbard's 13-level hierarchy may be useful for setting up a hierarchy of task difficulty for individual patients, although the hierarchy for a given patient may not exactly match Kearns and Hubbard's, which was based on group average performance. Consequently, clinicians may elect to personalize a hierarchy for individual patients by assessing their performance with items representing levels in the hierarchy and selecting the level at which the patient's performance has the appropriate proportions of correct, nearly correct, and incorrect responses.

Following-spoken-directions drills primarily target patients' verbal retention span. Many clinicians believe that if an aphasic patient's verbal retention span improves, the patient's general language comprehension also will improve. No empiric evidence supports this assumption, and evidence from studies of normal language comprehension suggests that comprehending language in natural situations does not depend strongly on verbal retention span. Given that most utterances in daily life conversations are less than eight words long (Goldman-Eisler, 1968) and given that most utterances in daily life are not as informationally dense as the sentences in verbal retention span drills, it seems likely that improving aphasic patients' verbal retention span beyond six-word to eight-word moderately redundant utterances may have weaker effects on daily life comprehension than many clinicians believe.

This does not mean, however, that following-spoken-directions drills may not *indirectly* improve daily life comprehension by improving the operation of other processes that support comprehension. One likely candidate for such a supporting role is *attention.* Successful performance on following-spoken-directions drills requires that the patient quickly focus and maintain attention for the duration of the spoken directions. Patients who cannot quickly focus attention tend to miss information at the beginning of the directions, and those who cannot maintain attention miss information at the end of the directions. It seems reasonable that following-spoken-directions drills might enhance auditory comprehension by enhancing attentional skills that support comprehension.

Sentence Verification In sentence verification drills, the patient listens to spoken sentences and makes judgments about the relationship of each sentence to one or more pictures. In one form of verification (called *yes-no*), the clinician shows the patient a picture and says a sentence that may or may not match the picture. The patient then indicates whether the picture accurately portrays the meaning of the sentence. Usually each sentence is presented several times (not consecutively), sometimes with a picture that matches the sentence's meaning and sometimes with a foil. The foil pictures usually are chosen to contrast with the stimulus sentence in specified ways (e.g., differing from the stimulus sentence in subject, verb, or object, as in Figure 7-3).

In a second form of sentence verification (called *multiple choice*) each time the clinician says a sentence the clinician shows the patient a page containing several (usually four) pictures, one of which portrays the meaning of the sentence (Figure 7-4). The foil pictures usually contrast with the stimulus sentence in specified ways, as described previously. The patient points to the picture that represents the meaning of the sentence.

In most sentence-comprehension drills, foil pictures have systematic relationships to target

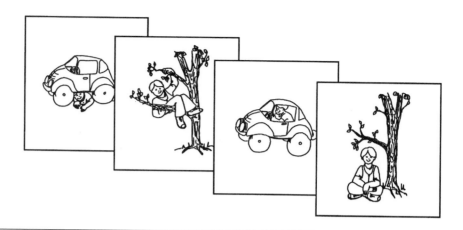

Figure 7-3 ■ Response cards that might be used in a sentence verification drill for the sentence, "The boy is in the tree." These four cards would be mixed with other cards, and the clinician would say the sentence whenever one of these cards came up.

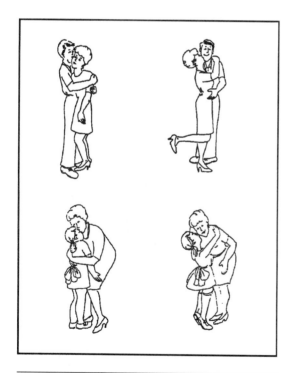

Figure 7-4 ■ A sentence-to-picture match-to-sample response card that might be shown as the clinician says, "The man is hugging the woman."

pictures. Figure 7-4 shows a set of four pictures that might accompany the sentence "The man is hugging the woman." To respond correctly, listeners have to perceive subject, object, or verb mismatches between foil pictures and the stimulus sentence. The difficulty of such an item for aphasic listeners depends primarily on the semantic closeness of foils to the target. ("The man is chasing the dog" as a foil for Figure 7-4 would be identified easily as a foil by most aphasic adults, whereas "The girl is hugging the man" would mislead many.)

Task Switching Activities Many aphasic adults are tripped up when they get into conversational interactions wherein they must maintain a sense of the overall purpose or theme of a conversation while simultaneously dealing with changes in topics, speakers, or conversational roles. Task-switching drills can help these patients. Task-switching drills are sentence-comprehension drills in which the form of the stimulus sentences and the nature of the responses expected from the patient change unpredictably from trial to trial, as in the following sequence:

Pick up the spoon.
Point to the black one.

Which one do you drink from?
Does Thursday come after Wednesday?
Make a fist and blink three times.
Put the key in the cup.
Is your name Fred?
    Drill continues in this way.

TREATMENT OF DISCOURSE COMPREHENSION

When planning treatment for patients with impaired discourse comprehension it is important to remember that the traditional concept of comprehension skills as progressing from words to sentences to texts (bottom-up processing) is inappropriate (Pierce, 1989). Words and sentences in discourse are easier to comprehend than words and sentences in isolation. When sentences occur in discourse, comprehension depends more on their relationship to the overall theme of the discourse and the degree to which the discourse relates to a given patient's knowledge and experience than on the length or syntactic complexity of the sentences.

The difficulty of a discourse comprehension task is determined not only by the content and structure of the discourse, but by what the patient is asked to comprehend and remember from the discourse. If patients are asked to comprehend and remember only the main ideas and the overall point of the discourse, they do better than if asked to remember details. If patients are asked to comprehend and remember only directly stated information, they do better than if asked to comprehend and remember implied information.

Most adults with mild to moderate aphasia are likely to have retained at least some of their discourse comprehension abilities. Most should get the main ideas, if the discourse is well-structured and unambiguous. Most should be able to construct the major inferences suggested by discourse, especially inferences that relate to main ideas or the overall theme of the discourse. However, the comprehension of patients with mild to moderate aphasia suffers when discourse is not well structured with clearly identified main ideas and an obvious topic or theme or if the information is outside their experience.

The Format of Discourse Comprehension Treatment

The typical format for discourse comprehension treatment is for the clinician to read aloud or play a recording of a sample of discourse, after which the patient answers questions about information in the discourse. The questions typically are yes-no questions, such as those in the *Discourse Comprehension Test* (Brookshire & Nicholas, 1993). Yes-no questions (e.g., "Did the women put up a sign at a shopping center?") typically are used because they minimize the effects of patients' memory impairments, speech formulation, and production problems on their discourse comprehension performance.

Yes-no questions test patients' *recognition* rather than their *recall* of information from discourse. To move patients toward recall yet keep memory, speech formulation, and speech production demands under control, yes-no questions can be replaced by *sentence completion* items, in which patients complete sentence fragments provided by the clinician, as in, "The women put up a sign at a _____." For patients who can handle the limited formulation and speech production demands, sentence completion places more demands on recall of information from discourse than yes-no questions do.

Open-ended questions ("What did the women do to advertise their garage sale?") provide fewer clues about the answer but require greater patient competence in speech formulation and production than yes-no questions or sentence-completion items. For patients who can handle the speech-production demands, open-ended questions are more flexible and more challenging than yes-no questions or sentence completion.

Retelling, in which patients recount as much as they can remember from a sample of discourse, requires patients to retrieve and produce information from memory without help from the content of the clinician's questions. Retelling provides the strongest indicator of patients' ability to comprehend, store, and retrieve information from discourse. Speech formulation and production impairments may, however, masquerade as comprehension impairments, making retelling inappropriate for treating comprehension in patients with limited speech.

Stimulus Manipulations in Treating Discourse Comprehension

Clinicians may regulate the difficulty of discourse comprehension tasks by manipulating several variables: *familiarity, length, redundancy, cohesion, coherence, salience, directness,* and *speech rate.*

Familiarity Treatment typically begins with material familiar to the patient. Familiar material permits patients to use preexisting knowledge to help them comprehend discourse. As a patient's comprehension of familiar material improves, the clinician may gradually introduce less familiar material, forcing the patient to depend less on preexisting knowledge and more on the content of the discourse itself.

Many familiar situations and routines (such as going to a restaurant, buying groceries, or taking a plane trip) can be represented by *scripts.* As previously described, scripts are mental devices by which individuals organize knowledge of common situations. They permit individuals to formulate expectations about what events are likely to occur in a situation and the order in which they are likely to occur. Armus and associates (1989) suggested that aphasic adults' knowledge of scripts be exploited to facilitate their comprehension of discourse by:

- Teaching patients and their families that some daily life spoken discourse is predictable based on what the listener already knows about the topic or situation being talked about
- Having patients practice identifying scripts that underlie samples of discourse
- Asking patients to predict what is likely to happen next in samples of discourse representing scripts

Length Treatment usually begins with short samples of discourse and progresses to longer ones. The samples should be long enough, however, to permit the patient to develop a sense of their overall theme and to identify the main ideas (100 to 200 words). As the patient's comprehension improves, the length of the materials in the treatment program increases.

Redundancy, Cohesion, and Coherence Treatment typically begins with samples of discourse in which repetition, paraphrase, and elaboration create substantial redundancy and high levels of cohesion and coherence. Redundancy, cohesion, and coherence establish relationships among ideas and help the listener determine the topic and identify the main ideas. Redundancy, cohesion, and coherence permit patients to substitute less effortful heuristic processes for more effortful lexical and syntactic processes as they strive to comprehend discourse. As the patient's comprehension improves, materials with less redundancy, cohesion, and coherence gradually may be introduced to increase the patient's ability to deal with less redundant and less coherent discourse.

Salience Treatment begins with material in which main ideas are easily identified and the focus of treatment is on identification of main ideas. As the patient's comprehension improves, the treatment focus gradually progresses to comprehension of details.

Directness Treatment begins with materials in which the important information is stated, rather than implied, and questions relate to information that is present in verbatim form in the discourse. As the patient's comprehension improves, questions that require simple inferences are introduced, followed by questions that require more complex inferences.

Speech Rate For those whose comprehension declines when materials are spoken at normal or fast rates, the rate at which discourse is presented may be slowed by placing pauses at strategic locations. As the patient's comprehension of slowly spoken material improves, the rate at which discourse is presented gradually may be increased, until the patient is working with materials spoken at a normal rate.

> Pauses after main ideas may help to highlight the main ideas and provide the listener with extra processing time for comprehending the main ideas and storing them in memory.

Nicholas and Brookshire suggested that increasing the salience (or redundancy) of information in discourse and stating information more directly are more dependable ways to improve aphasic listeners' comprehension of discourse than slowing the rate at which it is spoken because not all aphasic adults are helped by slow speech rate. However, they recommended that clinicians still advise those who communicate with aphasic patients to speak slowly because negative effects of slow speech rate are rare and because some aphasic listeners do benefit from slow speech rate. Nicholas and Brookshire also recommended that if a clinician intends to manipulate speech rate in treatment of aphasic adults' comprehension impairments, the clinician should pretest the patient to determine how that patient is affected by the manipulation.

GENERAL CONCEPTS 7-2

- *Stages* models and *depth-of-processing* models are two ways in which writers have conceptualized processes involved in memory.
- The role of memory in aphasic adults' comprehension impairments is not well understood, but most aphasic adults have short-term memory impairments that compromise their comprehension of noncontextual single-sentence utterances.
- Normal listeners rely on *top-down* (*knowledge-based* or *heuristic*) processes to comprehend language and resort to *text-based* processes (*lexical* and *syntactic analyses*) only when top-down processes fail to produce unambiguous meanings.

- *Scripts* are mental representations of familiar situations that may contribute to top-down comprehension processes.
- *Single-word comprehension drills* are most appropriate for patients with severe comprehension impairments who do not comprehend phrases or sentences.
- *Sentence comprehension drills* are a common treatment tool for clinicians who consider auditory comprehension an important language process. Sentence comprehension drills may require patients to *answer spoken questions, follow spoken directions,* or *verify the truth of spoken sentences.*
- *Discourse comprehension drills* may require patients to *answer questions* about samples of discourse or to *retell* what they remember from discourse. Clinicians may regulate the difficulty of discourse comprehension tasks by manipulating the *familiarity, length, redundancy, cohesion, coherence, salience, directness,* and *rate* of discourse materials.

TREATMENT OF READING COMPREHENSION

Aphasic adults almost always have impaired reading comprehension, and their reading comprehension usually is more impaired than their auditory comprehension. Aphasic adults may face an assortment of problems when confronted by printed texts. Most aphasic readers read slowly, misperceive letters and words, and rely on laborious word-by-word analysis to decode complex syntactic structures. Aphasic readers' impaired semantic and syntactic processes may cause them to misinterpret individual text elements and may prevent them from appreciating the overall meaning of printed materials. Aphasic readers' impaired short-term retention prevents them from establishing the overall topic or gist of printed materials or, having established the topic, causes them to lose it part-way through. Given the multiplicity of obstacles, it should not be surprising that reading comprehension is a major problem for most aphasic adults and that only those with very mild aphasia become recreational readers.

Processes in Reading

Word Recognition Recognizing and attaching meanings to words is a prerequisite for comprehending printed texts. Word recognition quickly becomes automatic as normal readers develop skill in reading, and only unskilled readers depend heavily on word-by-word reading. Skilled readers usually do not read sentences or texts word by word unless the material is complex or contains unfamiliar words.

Readers deduce the meaning of individual printed words in any of three ways:

1. In *whole-word reading* words are recognized as units and the reader does not analyze letters or letter strings within words. Whole-word reading requires that words be in the reader's reading vocabulary.

2. In *phonemic analysis* the reader segments words into letters or letter combinations, translates the letters or letter combinations into the sounds they represent, blends the sound representations together, and identifies the word represented by the sequence of sounds. Word recognition by phonemic analysis requires that the unfamiliar word be in the reader's listening vocabulary but not necessarily in the reader's reading vocabulary.

3. In *word recognition by context* the reader uses the meaning of the context in which a word appears to guess a word's meaning. Recognition by context does not require that the unfamiliar word be in the reader's reading or listening vocabulary.

Skilled readers read most words as whole words and use phonemic analysis and recognition by context only when they encounter unfamiliar words. When these methods fail, the reader may look up unfamiliar words in a dictionary.

Syntactic Analysis Syntactic analysis is the primary way in which readers deduce relationships among words. Syntactic analysis presupposes knowledge of syntactic rules and recognition of syntactic structures. Syntactic knowledge allows readers to combine word strings into units of meaning that can be stored in long-term memory. Failure to perform syntactic analysis overloads the reader's short-term memory, and errors in syntactic analysis lead to miscomprehension of sentence meanings. An important difference between failure to recognize a word and failure to recognize a syntactic structure is that readers usually know when they fail to recognize a word, but they may be unaware when they fail to recognize a syntactic structure.

There was once general acceptance of the idea that if readers could translate letters into their corresponding words, they could comprehend printed texts. This assumption is no longer considered valid because it neglects the role of syntactic analysis in reading. Reading depends on syntactic analysis more than listening does. In listening, syntactic information can be conveyed by pauses, intonation, and emphatic stress and by word order and syntactic markers. In reading, the reader depends completely on word order and syntactic markers to deduce syntactic structure. Most printed texts are more formal in style than spoken discourse, making them more difficult to comprehend than spoken discourse.

Semantic Mapping Semantic mapping is a process by which readers relate the writer's intended meanings to their own knowledge and experience. Semantic mapping is the stage at which a text can be said to make sense to the reader. In semantic mapping the ideas conveyed by a text are organized into a coherent and sensical whole, and the overall meaning of the text is integrated into memory. A reader's failure to organize the information in a text leads to confusion about which elements of the text are important and which are unimportant and may contribute to difficulty in getting the information into memory and retrieving it from memory. A reader's failure to relate meanings from texts to the reader's knowledge leads to problems in appreciating the true meanings of metaphor, idioms, and figurative language.

Most of the top-down processes that contribute to comprehension of spoken discourse also contribute to comprehension of printed texts. Readers, like listeners, use the lexical content and syntactic structure of printed texts to deduce relationships among units of information. From there they go on to use general knowledge and intuition to determine a text's overall meaning. Readers, like listeners, use heuristic processes to bypass continuous word-by-word lexical and syntactic analysis when permitted to do so by the structure and content of printed texts. Readers, like listeners, often emphasize heuristic processes over text-based processes and may rely on text-based processes only when pushed to do so by unfamiliar subject matter, complex syntax, ambiguity, or uncertainty.

Surface Dyslexia and Deep Dyslexia

Two patterns of word-reading impairment— *surface dyslexia* and *deep dyslexia*—sometimes accompany aphasia (Marshall & Newcombe, 1973). The concepts of surface dyslexia and deep dyslexia are based on a model of reading that postulates two routes from the visual form of words to word meanings. Readers who use the *direct* (lexical) route access the mental representations of words and their meanings directly based on the visual form of the words *(whole-word read-*

ing). Readers who use the *indirect* (phonologic) route access the mental representations of words indirectly by converting printed letters into their phonologic equivalents *(phonemic analysis)* and accessing meaning via these internal phonologic representations (Figure 7-5).

Individuals with *surface dyslexia* have lost (or are impaired in) the direct (lexical) route and depend on the indirect (phonologic) route, which requires letter-by-letter decoding to deduce the meaning of printed words. These individuals read regularly spelled words (such as *keep* and *banana*) accurately, but they misread irregularly spelled words by regularizing their pronunciation *(neighbor* may be read as *neg-bor).* Individuals with surface dyslexia can read aloud phonologically legitimate nonwords (such as *tobada*) accurately. Because analysis is letter-by-letter, long words take readers with surface dyslexia longer to identify than short words.

Individuals with *deep dyslexia* have lost (or are impaired in) the indirect (phonologic) route and depend on the direct (whole-word) route to deduce the meaning of printed words. These pa-

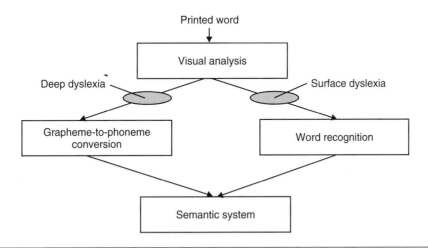

Figure 7-5 ■ A schematic diagram showing impaired processes responsible for surface dyslexia and deep dyslexia. In surface dyslexia the direct route from the printed stimulus to semantic representations is unavailable and the patient must depend on the indirect route (grapheme-to-phoneme conversion). In deep dyslexia the grapheme-to-phoneme conversion route is unavailable and the patient must depend on whole-word reading.

tients misread phonologically legitimate non-words *(tobada)*, and their misreadings of real words lead to semantic errors rather than phonemic errors (e.g., reading *chair* as *table*). Individuals with deep dyslexia may substitute morphologically related or visually similar words for target words (e.g., *steal* for *stealth, wise* for *wisdom*). Individuals with deep dyslexia have more difficulty reading *closed-class* (function) words (articles, conjunctions, prepositions) than *open class* (content) words (nouns, verbs, adjectives, adverbs). Semantically supportive context often helps these individuals recognize words they otherwise would fail to recognize.

The various forms of acquired dyslexia have received much attention from investigators who are interested in how the brain recognizes printed words and connects the visual images of words to their semantic representations. The models of the reading process constructed by these investigators provide a systematic approach to differential diagnosis of acquired reading impairments. Nevertheless, it is important to keep in mind that descriptions of acquired dyslexia focus on single-word recognition, whereas reading comprehension (at least for normal readers) is largely a top-down process. Consequently, the effects of word-recognition impairments, as typified in the various forms of acquired dyslexia, may not be as striking when the individual is reading texts as when reading single words. It seems likely that mild to moderate word-recognition impairment would not dramatically affect a reader's comprehension of printed texts if semantic and syntactic contexts give clues to the identity of words that are not recognized in isolation.

Treating Neurogenic Reading Impairments

Treating a brain-injured adult's reading impairment often begins with what Webb (1990) calls a *literacy history.* The literacy history comes from the patient, family members, caregivers, associates, or a combination of sources. The literacy history tells the clinician how much reading the patient did before becoming aphasic, identi-

fies reading topics of special interest to the patient, and gives the clinician a sense of the patient's level of reading competence before the onset of aphasia.

The clinician combines information from the literacy history, information about the patient's current reading skills, and the clinician's estimate of the patient's potential recovery to decide how (or whether) to make reading a focus of treatment. Patients for whom reading was a significant part of daily life, who have the requisite visual perceptual and language abilities, and who are motivated to regain reading are the best candidates for treatment of reading. Patients who were nonfunctional readers before they became aphasic will not become functional readers with treatment, and there is little point in attempting to make recreational readers of patients who were not interested in reading before they became aphasic.

Treatment of aphasic adults' reading impairments usually is most successful for patients with mild to moderate aphasia who were functional readers before the onset of aphasia. Patients with severe aphasia usually are more concerned with improving their speech production and enhancing their listening comprehension than with becoming recreational readers. Few patients with chronic severe aphasia regain functional reading of newspapers, books, magazines, or other printed texts. However, severely aphasic patients, and less severely aphasic patients who were not recreational readers before they became aphasic, may benefit from acquiring what have been called *survival reading skills* (Rosenbek, LaPointe, & Wertz, 1989; Webb, 1990).

Survival Reading Skills Survival reading skills are the skills needed to read materials commonly encountered in daily life, such as signs, labels, bills, checkbook registers, addresses, telephone listings, and menus. The first step in teaching (or reactivating) survival reading skills is to determine which daily life reading activities are most important to the patient. Rosenbek, LaPointe, and Wertz (1989) suggest that clini-

T A B L E   7 - 1

Lists of materials that an aphasic adult most wanted to read and wanted to read but could do without

Most want to read	Want to read but could do without
Mail	Messages
Checkbook	Signs
Medicine labels	Newspapers
Maps	Magazines
Phone book	TV guide
Elevator	Menus
Calendar	Bible
Product labels	Playing cards

From Rosenbek, J. C., LaPointe, L. L., & Wertz, R.T. (1989). *Aphasia: A clinical approach.* Boston: Little-Brown.

T A B L E   7 - 2

Reading activities ranked by importance by a group of non-brain-damaged British adults

Activity	Index of importance
Personal letters	188
Bills	171
Forms	168
Official letters	162
Advertisements	144
Phone numbers	140
Newspaper	136
Television listings	131
Books	130
Bank statement	130
Address book	125
Dosage instructions for medications	130
Recipes	118
Menus	107

Data from Parr, S. (1992). Everyday reading and writing practices of normal adults: Implications for aphasia assessment. *Aphasiology, 6,* 273-283.

cians ask aphasic patients and family members to make two lists. One list specifies the materials the patient most wants to be able to read, and the other identifies materials the patient wishes to be able to read but can do without. A list produced by one of Rosenbek and associates' patients is shown in Table 7-1. Rosenbek and associates focused treatment on the materials in the two lists, beginning with the items in the *most important* list, and when the patient could sight-read those items, treatment progressed to the second list.

Parr (1992) compiled a similar, but more generic, list by asking 50 non-brain-damaged British adults to make a list of daily life reading activities and to rate how important each activity was. Parr then calculated an index of importance for the group by multiplying the number of individuals who listed an activity by its average rating of importance. Table 7-2 shows Parr's ranked list.

Lists such as these provide a useful beginning point for the clinician who wishes to help an aphasic patient regain basic functional reading abilities. The clinician cannot assume, however, that an individual's needs will match those of groups of individuals who contributed to such lists. A patient with no bank account is unlikely to consider reading bank statements or checkbook registers important, and a patient who has no television is unlikely to be very concerned with reading television program listings. Consequently, the clinician must devise an individualized list of important daily life reading activities for each patient by asking the patient and family members to generate a list and to rank the items on the list. Treatment then can begin with the activities with the highest ranks and progress down the list as functional reading is achieved for each activity.

Functional reading for categories of everyday materials such as those in the lists in Tables 7-1 and 7-2 depends on the patient's acquisition of a sight-reading vocabulary of commonly occurring words for each category. A core sight-reading vocabulary for the instructions on medicine labels might contain only 15 or 20 words, whereas a core sight-reading vocabulary for advertisements in newspapers and magazines might contain several hundred words. When a sight-reading vocabulary has been selected, the clinician may test the patient to determine which words the patient cannot presently sight-read. The problem words then may be incorporated into treatment activities.

Drills in which the patient reads aloud core vocabulary words from flash cards are a popular way to train sight-reading of core vocabulary words. Flash-card drills give patients intensive sight-reading practice, but they may not be the most efficient way to promote sight-reading of vocabulary in daily life because training sight-reading of free-standing vocabulary words deprives the patient of contextual cues that may enhance word recognition. For example, the meaning of *tablet* is more readily apparent in "Take one tablet by mouth twice a day" than when printed by itself on a flash card. Furthermore, generalization to daily life is more likely if a patient acquires sight-reading vocabulary with natural materials.

Several computer-based programs to enhance sight-reading for vocabulary considered important in daily life activities have been designed. Such programs may prove useful in providing patients with intensive sight-reading drill without requiring the clinician's full-time participation (Katz & Nagy, 1983; Major & Wilson, 1985; Weiner, 1983; and others). However, their effectiveness has not been empirically demonstrated beyond a few case reports.

Treating Patients with Mild to Moderate Reading Impairments Treatment of patients with mild to moderate reading impairment begins with a literacy history followed by standardized tests to measure the patient's reading vocabulary, sentence comprehension, and paragraph comprehension. Clinicians typically measure both the patient's *reading capacity* (the level of vocabulary and complexity that the patient can comprehend) and the patient's *reading rate* (how quickly the patient can progress through a text with acceptable comprehension). Reading test scores often are defined by *grade level.* Grade level quantifies the difficulty of the reading materials in terms of the school grade at which average students can comprehend them. Most newspapers, popular books, and magazines are at grade 5 or grade 6 in reading difficulty. Consequently, those reading at 5th-grade to 6th-grade level or above are likely to comprehend most daily life reading materials (Chall, 1983).

Comprehension of Printed Words As noted earlier, many patients with acquired reading impairments have difficulty recognizing and assigning meaning to printed words. Problems in comprehending printed words can arise from several sources.

Many aphasic adults exhibit *deep dyslexia.* They struggle with phonemic analysis of printed words because they cannot convert the printed letters into their phonologic equivalents and cannot blend the individual sounds into sound patterns for words. These patients' printed-word recognition may be improved by exercises in which they:

- Orally sound out words and nonwords that have one-to-one grapheme-to-phoneme correspondence.
- Discriminate between words with similar phonologic structure (e.g., *cabbage/cottage*).
- Supply missing letters to complete regularly spelled partial words (e.g., *ban_na, an-niver__ry*).

Some aphasic adults have visual impairments that interfere with their perception of printed letters and words. They confuse words that look alike, and they may confuse letters with similar appearance (such as *b/c/d, m/w/n, e/f/k*). These patients may be helped by exercises in which they discriminate between visually similar words (e.g., *taxes/taxies, hear/clear*) or identify transposed or reversed letters within words (e.g., *birhtday, gadren*). Such single-word discrimination drills may not be needed if a patient can read and comprehend printed sentences because the context provided by the sentences may negate the effects of the patient's misperceptions on their comprehension of the sentences.

Although annoying to patients, scattered visual misperceptions may not seriously interfere with patients' comprehension of printed texts because the semantic and syntactic context provided by the texts may diminish the frequency of misperceptions, and, when misperceptions do occur, context may permit patients to recognize and repair the misperceptions. A reader who confuses *p* and *d* may misread the word *pen* as *den* when shown the word in isolation, but will read it correctly in a sentence such as, "A pen is used to sign important documents." For these patients the primary effects of scattered visual misperceptions are annoyance and slow reading rate. However, if misperceptions are very frequent, or if a patient's reading vocabulary and sentence comprehension skills are marginal, visual misperceptions may have more important effects.

> Sometimes patients are given practice in identifying inverted or reversed letters in isolation. For some patients this is a necessary preliminary to identifying them in context. However, the clinician should move into contextual stimuli as soon as possible.

Some aphasic patients can translate printed words into phonemic representations but are unable to attach meaning to the representations. They may repeat a troublesome printed word over and over but fail to deduce its meaning.

> Conventional . . . conventional . . . I should know this word. I've seen it before. I'm thinking "easy to get at" but that's not it . . . conventional . . . I'll need help on this one.

These patients may become better readers if they are taught to use context to deduce word meanings. Vocabulary drills and word-association exercises also may help these patients read better.

> These patients usually have similar problems recognizing spoken words. Treating auditory comprehension in tandem with reading comprehension may be appropriate for these patients.

Comprehension of Printed Sentences

Aphasic readers' comprehension of printed sentences usually is affected by many of the same variables that affect their comprehension of spoken sentences, as discussed previously (e.g., *length, syntactic complexity, redundancy*). Most aphasic patients' reading comprehension is worse than their comprehension of equivalent spoken materials. Many have difficulty converting printed words into their phonemic representations—a process that is important in reading but not in listening. The syntactic structure of printed texts tends to be more complex than that of spoken discourse, creating problems for many aphasic adults. Aphasic readers tend to overlook or misread function words such as *to, but,* and *by,* causing confusion or misinterpretation of the true meaning of printed sentences. Printed sentences have less extralinguistic support than spoken sentences. When a listener fails to comprehend a spoken sentence, the speaker may repeat, paraphrase, or simplify. The speaker's pauses, intonation, stress, reiteration, paraphrasing, and gestures all help facilitate listening comprehension. The time of day, the location of the interaction, the speaker's identity, and other situational characteristics of spoken interactions also reduce the listener's dependence on the linguistic content of the speaker's utterances.

Reading comprehension, like auditory comprehension, is largely a top-down process for competent readers. Competent readers use context to establish topic, infer the meaning of unfamiliar or unrecognized words, and bypass laborious syntactic analysis. Consequently, brain-injured patients who can read at the sentence level may comprehend sentences in paragraph contexts better than sentences in isolation, although their reading rate may be slow and their comprehension may be less than perfect.

Treatment with isolated free-standing sentences may be appropriate for some mildly impaired readers who struggle with complex syntax in printed sentences. These patients' reading comprehension may be enhanced by drills in which they are asked to interpret sentences with troublesome syntactic structures, such as passive sentences ("The woman was hugged by the man."), center-embedded sentences ("The dog the boy chased ran into the street."), and sentences expressing comparative relationships ("The policeman was shorter than the burglar."). These drills are most appropriate for mildly impaired readers whose primary complaint is failure to appreciate the meaning of syntactically complex sentences; whose word recognition, vocabulary, appreciation of text structure, and retention of information are reasonably well preserved; and for whom heuristic (top-down) processes still leave them puzzled about the meaning of syntactically complex sentences.

Reading drills with free-standing sentences also may be appropriate for patients whose comprehension of printed texts is so poor that the beneficial effects of context cannot operate. Improving the rate and accuracy with which these patients read and comprehend individual sentences may diminish these patients' workload enough to permit contextual influences to exert their beneficial effects.

Numerous workbooks containing sentence-level reading exercises appropriate for aphasic adults are on the market. Some require the patient to complete sentences that have missing words:

For breakfast, John likes bacon and ——— ——.

Others require the patient to choose a target word from a list of foils:

Brush is to teeth as comb is to —————.
ear hair brush rooster

Some require the patient to rearrange scrambled words into a sentence:

school is day most happy last the time for of a students

Scrambled-word sentences may challenge even patients with very mild impairments, and non-brain-damaged readers may find longer scrambled-word sentences a challenge. Creating a sentence from scrambled words requires knowledge of syntactic rules, analytic skills, attention, and good short-term memory.

Some are match-to-sample tasks, in which a printed sentence is presented along with several pictures, one of which matches the printed sentence, as in Figure 7-6.

Most patients who can read and comprehend at least some information from printed texts should be working with printed texts that challenge but do not exceed their reading ability. Reading passages should be selected so that the

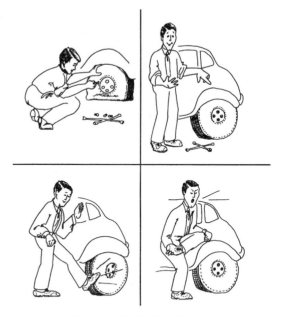

The man is kicking the tire.

Figure 7-6 ■ A response card for reading comprehension of the sentence "The man is kicking the tire."

patient can, at minimum, determine the overall topic of the passage, get most of the main ideas, and get at least some of the details. Clinicians can adjust the difficulty of reading materials by manipulating many of the variables that affect comprehension of spoken discourse *(familiarity, length, redundancy, cohesion and coherence, salience,* and *abstractness and directness)* plus variables that have a wider range in reading materials than in spoken discourse *(vocabulary* and *syntactic complexity).*

Stimulus Manipulations in Treating Reading

Familiarity The familiarity of reading material has strong effects on how easily a reader comprehends the material. Familiar material helps readers establish context, separate main ideas from details, and relate what they are reading to what they already know, all of which facilitates comprehension. Clinicians can exploit the effects of familiarity in treatment by using reading material that relates to a patient's knowledge, experience, and interests. As the patient's reading proficiency increases, less familiar material may be introduced to increase demands on lexical and semantic analysis, reasoning, intuition, and the ability to organize and retain information from texts.

Length Making reading passages longer increases their difficulty, provided the passages are made longer by adding new information and not by restating or paraphrasing old information. (Increasing a passage's length by restating or paraphrasing information actually may diminish passage difficulty by increasing the redundancy of the material and making its topic more obvious.) Making passages shorter does not always make them easier. When a passage is shortened drastically, it becomes more difficult for the reader to develop a sense of its topic and theme and to use context-based processes that permit top-down processing.

There is no absolute limit below which reading passages are too short to permit efficient use of top-down processes because a passage's

suitability for top-down processing depends on its structure as well as its length. As a general rule, passages less than about 100 words are likely to be too short to permit efficient use of top-down processes by most aphasic adults. Webb (1990) suggests that passages used in treating aphasic adults' reading should be at least 200 words long because it takes average readers that many words to develop a sense of the overall meaning of reading passages. Webb suggests that reading passages used in treating aphasic adults' reading should average about 500 words. However, 500-word passages may be too long for aphasic adults with retention and memory impairments.

Redundancy As is true for spoken discourse, redundancy (from *repetition, elaboration,* and *paraphrase)* in printed material makes it easier for readers to establish the overall sense of the material, organize it in memory, and recall its content. Repetition, elaboration, and paraphrase also contribute to the cohesion and coherence of printed material in the same way they contribute to the cohesion and coherence of information in spoken discourse (discussed previously).

Salience and Directness Salience and directness affect aphasic readers in the same way that they affect aphasic listeners' comprehension of spoken discourse. Aphasic readers, like non-brain-damaged readers, are better at comprehending and remembering main ideas than details, and aphasic readers, like non-brain-damaged readers, comprehend and remember stated information better than they comprehend and remember implied information.

Vocabulary Increasing the number of uncommon words in a reading passage usually increases its reading difficulty. Fortunately for readers with limited vocabulary, most newspapers, magazines, books, and similar materials written for the general public do not contain large proportions of uncommon words. According to Hayes (1989), 75% of the words in typical books for adult readers are within the 1000 most frequent words in English, and 88% are within the

T A B L E 7 - 3			
Percent of words that are within the 500, 1,000, 5,000, and 10,000 most frequent English words for various reading materials			

	Percent of words in the first:			
Material	**500**	**1,000**	**5,000**	**10,000**
Preschool books	73	81	94	97
Children's books	72	79	92	96
Comic books	68	75	89	93
Adult books	69	75	88	93
Popular magazines	62	69	85	91
Science abstracts	46	52	70	78

Data from Hayes, D. P. (1989). *Guide to the lexical analysis of texts.* (Tech. Rep. Series 89-96). Ithaca, NY: Cornell University Department of Sociology.

5000 most frequent English words. Table 7-3 provides frequency-of-occurrence estimates for various reading materials in the United States. Only specialized technical manuals and books contain many uncommon words. If a patient's goal is recreational reading, Hayes's data suggest that it makes little sense to belabor them with materials containing large numbers of uncommon words.

Syntactic Complexity The syntactic complexity of reading materials affects their reading difficulty, and, as noted earlier, aphasic adults often are tripped up by complex syntax. Most newspapers, magazines, and books are written with reasonably uncomplicated syntax. (The primary exceptions are some editorial and opinion pieces in newspapers or magazines and some novels.) Most recreational readers are unlikely to encounter syntactically complex materials, and when they do, context may permit them to substitute heuristic, top-down strategies for more laborious syntactic analysis. A reader who can handle passive sentences *(The cat was chased by the dog)*, cleft-object sentences *(It was the cat that the dog chased)*, dative sentences *(The banker gave the money to the robber)*, and conjoined sentences *(The dog barked at the cat and chased the rabbit)* should be able to handle the syntax of most commonly available reading materials, even when top-down processes cannot be substituted for syntactic analysis.

Readability Formulas Readability formulas attempt to quantify reading difficulty by measuring specific characteristics of printed texts and assigning a reading grade level to the result. Several dozen readability formulas have been published. (See Klare, 1984, for descriptions of the major ones.) Most readability formulas consider sentence length and vocabulary difficulty. Some count the number of long words (e.g., words of three or more syllables). Some consider grammatic characteristics such as number of prepositional phrases per 100 words. The most widely used readability formulas calculate readability by estimating syntactic complexity and vocabulary difficulty. Syntactic complexity is estimated by calculating the number of words per sentence, and vocabulary difficulty is estimated by calculating either the number of syllables per word (more syllables = greater vocabulary difficulty) or the number of low-frequency words in the passage.

Cloze procedures also have been used to measure readability. In cloze procedures, words are deleted from a text and readability is based on the number of errors normal readers make when they fill in the missing words.

Although there is some variability in how well each of the published procedures predict actual reading difficulty, no one procedure stands out as particularly accurate. Consequently, clinicians who wish to estimate the reading difficulty of printed materials might choose an easily calculated formula such as the *Dale-Chall formula* (Dale & Chall, 1948), the *Flesch Reading Ease Formula* (Flesch, 1948), or the *Fog Index* (Gunning, 1952).

The *Dale-Chall formula* is based on the average number of words per sentence and the number of words not in a 4000-word list of words known by most 4th-grade readers. The Flesch formula is calculated using the average number of words per sentence and average word length in syllables. The *Fog Index,* in addition to having one of the more interesting names, is easy to calculate. It is based on the average number of words per sentence and the number of words three or more syllables long.

It takes from 10 to 20 minutes to calculate readability for a 100- to 200-word text with even the simplest readability formulas. Some readability procedures have been computerized to lessen the time required to get a readability estimate, but the computerized procedures require that the text first be typed into an appropriately formatted computer text file, which may take longer than hand calculation.

Clinicians often bypass the time and effort of readability estimation by using commercially prepared materials with known readability, specified as a reading grade level. If their content is suitable for adult readers, these materials provide a convenient way for clinicians to obtain materials of predetermined reading difficulty for use in treatment of adults with reading impairments.

Commercial Reading Programs Commercial reading programs may be a good source of materials for treating patients' reading impairments. *Basal readers* commonly are used to teach reading comprehension in elementary schools. Basal readers provide an integrated approach to reading instruction, with teachers' manuals, stories, and expository passages for students to read and workbook exercises for students to complete. Most basal readers focus on specific reading and comprehension skills, but the number and type of skills differ from one basal reading program to another, and materials are not specific to any skill or subset of skills.

Objectives-oriented reading programs target specific reading skills (such as *getting main ideas* or *using context*) at several levels of reading difficulty and provide tests for measuring an individual's performance within each skill. Objectives-oriented programs differ in the number and kinds of skills addressed and in the reading levels for which they are appropriate. Most are designed for elementary-school use (Grades 1 through 6), so some may be inappropriate for use with adults because of their juvenile content. The *Specific Skills Series* of remedial reading materials (Boning, 1990), described in Chapter 5, is an objectives-oriented program that may be incorporated into treatment of aphasic adults' reading impairments.

Rosenshine (1980) divided the skills addressed by objectives-oriented reading programs into three categories: *locating details* (recognizing, paraphrasing, and matching specific information), *simple inferential skills* (understanding words in context, recognizing sequences of events, recognizing cause-and-effect relationships, comparing and contrasting), and *complex inferential skills* (recognizing main ideas or topics, drawing conclusions, predicting outcomes).

Carver (1973) has commented that only skills such as those subsumed under *locating details* are truly reading skills. He asserts that skills such as those subsumed under *simple* or *complex inferential skills* are not specific to reading but represent general reasoning ability. The implication is that one would not work on these skills only in reading if they represent general reasoning skills (or that working on them in reading might enhance performance on other activities that call on reasoning skills).

Treatment of aphasic patients' reading disabilities usually relies heavily on homework. Patients often work on reading assignments at home and bring the completed assignments to the clinic, where the clinician goes over the completed work, corrects errors and discusses them with the patient, and provides instruction and practice with new materials. Sometimes work on auditory comprehension is carried on simultaneously with work on reading to enhance generalization between the two skills.

GENERAL CONCEPTS 7-3

- Reading comprehension is a synergistic process, combining *word recognition, syntactic analysis,* and *semantic mapping.*

- *Surface dyslexia* and *deep dyslexia* are two patterns of reading impairment sometimes exhibited by brain-injured adults. Readers with *surface dyslexia* must use *phonologic analysis* to identify problem words. Readers with *deep dyslexia* must use *whole-word recognition* to identify problem words.

- Obtaining a *literary history* often is the first step in designing a program to treat acquired reading impairments.

- Aphasic adults who will not become recreational readers usually benefit from acquiring *survival reading skills,* which permit them to read simple everyday materials such as signs, bills, and medication instructions.

- *Word-recognition drills* may be appropriate for patients who cannot read at the sentence level and who exhibit signs of either surface dyslexia or deep dyslexia.

- Most patients who can read sentences should be working with sentences or paragraphs in treatment to permit top-down processes to operate.

- Patients who can comprehend simple texts generally should be working with texts that challenge their reading skills via manipulation of *familiarity, length, redundancy, cohesion, coherence, salience, directness, vocabulary,* and *syntactic complexity.*

- *Readability formulas* are a way to measure the reading difficulty of printed texts. Most readability formulas calculate reading grade levels based on vocabulary difficulty and sentence length.

- Commercial reading programs (*basal readers* and *objectives-oriented reading programs*) are useful sources of materials for clinicians who work with reading-impaired adults.

TREATMENT OF SPEECH PRODUCTION

Aphasic adults tend to be more troubled by impairments in speaking than by impairments in reading, writing, or listening comprehension, and aphasic adults' speech has important effects on how they are regarded by others in daily life. Accordingly, most speech-language pathologists give treatment of speech production an important place in their plans for aphasic adults. Which aspects of speech production get treated and how much speech production is emphasized relative to other communication modalities depends, of course, on the nature and severity of the patient's communication impairments. For patients who can produce few, if any, volitional words, drills requiring them to produce single words may be appropriate. For patients with some volitional speech, the emphasis may be on efficient and accurate production of phrases, sentences, or discourse.

Facilitating Volitional Speech

Sentence completion tasks can help get volitional speech from patients who on their own can produce little more than automatisms and stereotypic utterances. In sentence completion tasks, the clinician says a sentence in which the final word or the final few words are missing and the patient supplies the missing word or words. Highly constrained sentences containing word combinations that occur frequently in daily life (e.g., *A cup of _____.*) are the strongest facilitators of volitional speech. When a patient's responses to such highly constrained sentences are quick and accurate, treatment can move on to less constrained sentences (such as, *Put a stamp on the _____* or *We wear shoes on our _____.*). Stimulus sentences in which the missing elements are not constrained (*Today Joe bought a _____.*) do not elicit specific target words but may be incorporated into the late stages of sentence-completion treatment tasks to put more emphasis on volitional vocabulary search, word retrieval, and speech production.

Completing phrases or sentences representing overlearned everyday expressions is almost always easier for aphasic speakers than confrontation naming (Barton, Maruszewski, & Urrea, 1969; Podraza & Darley, 1977; Wyke & Holgate, 1973) or providing words in response to definitions given by the clinician (Barton, Maruszewski, & Urrea, 1969; Goodglass & Stuss, 1979). Highly constrained sentence-completion tasks can be used to facilitate subsequent confrontation naming; that is, a clinician might elicit a set of object names with highly constrained sentence completion stimuli, then follow with confrontation naming of the same objects. Confrontation naming usually improves when it follows sentence completion.

Unfortunately, the facilitating effects of sentence completion on confrontation naming are not very durable (Kremin, 1993). If the clinician waits a day or two and retests the patient's confrontation naming of items previously facilitated by sentence completion, they usually find that the patient's confrontation naming has returned to baseline. Less constrained sentence-completion items seem to have somewhat more durable effects.

> . . . the deblocking of a word via an automatic expression, although immediately very effective, leaves but a faint trace over time. On the other hand, the active search for a words within the semantico-syntactic framework of a neutral sentence induces less immediate success but guarantees nonetheless the same level of performance on naming tasks after 24 hours. (Kremin, 1993, p. 271)

It seems apparent that highly constrained sentence-completion tasks are best used as stepping stones to tasks in which volitional vocabulary search and word retrieval are required. If a patient cannot move from sentence completion to volitional word retrieval and speech production, sentence completion tasks are deadends and probably should be abandoned.

Word and phrase repetition provides a somewhat less powerful but fairly dependable way to get volitional speech from patients who produce little or no volitional speech in less constrained contexts. Repetition drills are common in treatment for patients with articulatory selection and sequencing impairments (apraxia of speech) and for patients with weakness, paralysis, or incoordination of muscle groups involved in speech (dysarthria). For these patients, the emphasis is on the mechanics of speech production. The use of repetition drills for these patients is discussed elsewhere.

Word and phrase repetition tasks sometimes are used early in treatment programs for some aphasic patients when the ultimate goal is to enhance linguistic or quasi-linguistic processes such as word retrieval and sentence formation. Repetition drills are used to get the patient started. Then the repetition drills gradually are replaced by activities that require vocabulary search and word retrieval, such as naming drills.

Confrontation naming drills require patients to name pictures (usually) or objects (sometimes) designated by the clinician. Confrontation naming drills can be used to move patients away from rote production of words and phrases toward more purposeful retrieval, encoding, and production of words and phrases. However, confrontation naming drills as an end in themselves may provide little lasting benefit to patients. Brookshire (1975) trained 10 aphasic adults to name pictures of common objects. Their naming improved within training sessions, but there was no evidence that the improvements carried over to the next day, and there was no generalization of improved naming from trained items to untrained items within training sessions.

Naming objects or pictures is not a very useful behavior, unless one is a child learning the names of things or an adult learning a new language. If the to-be-named item is present, naming it usually is unnecessary (and often inappropriate) because its presence creates shared knowledge between speaker and listener, making its name redundant. If an aphasic patient wishes to communicate the name of an object or picture in the immediate environment, the patient can do so by pointing rather than naming. Consequently, naming drills, like sentence completion and repetition drills, are best thought of as stepping stones to more advanced (and functional) speech communication.

Clinicians have known for decades that aphasic adults' retrieval and production of single words can be facilitated if the clinician provides prompts or cues to lead the patient in the direction of the target words. Weigl (1968) described what he called a "deblocking" approach to treatment, in which brain-damaged patients' inadequate responses to stimuli in one modality are facilitated by pre-stimulating the patient with cues delivered in another modality. For example, a clinician might provide the sound an object makes or a semantically related word prior to presenting each picture to be named. Users assume that the pre-stimulation primes the patient's response to the target stimulus.

Podraza and Darley (1977) studied the effects of four kinds of pre-stimulation on aphasic adults' picture naming: (1) pre-stimulation with the first sound of the name plus a neutral vowel (as in *buh* followed by a picture of a *bee*), (2) pre-stimulation with an open-ended sentence *(I got stung by a bumble————.)*, (3) pre-stimulation with the target word plus two unrelated foils *(line, bee, goat)*, and (4) pre-stimulation with three semantically related words *(sting, honey, hive)*. Podraza and Darley reported that three of the four pre-stimuli (first sound plus neutral vowel, open-ended sentence, and target word plus two foils) facilitated their participants' naming performance, with no clear differences

Podraza and Darley's procedures differ from those described by Weigl and his associates and, except for the open-ended-sentence condition, differ from deblocking procedures typically used in the clinic. Pre-stimulating with the target word plus several unrelated words seems strange because stimulation with the target word alone would be more effective in eliciting the target name. However, this changes the picture-naming task into a word-repetition task, which should be easy for most aphasic adults. That pre-stimulation with semantically related words worsened aphasic adults' naming performance is not surprising, given that aphasic adults' errors in confrontation-naming tasks often are related semantically to the target words, as Podraza and Darley mention.

among the three. Pre-stimulation with three semantically related foils worsened participants' naming performance, rather than helping it. The pattern of facilitation differed across participants, leading Podraza and Darley to conclude, "The emergence of a slightly different hierarchy of effectiveness for each of the participants in the study suggests that the use of these techniques or any other technique in language therapy must be based on a hierarchy determined individually for each patient" (p. 681).

Not all cues have equal power to facilitate aphasic adults' naming. Over the years numerous studies of the relative power of various cues have been reported (Barton, Maruszewski, and Urrea, 1969; Love and Webb, 1977; Pease and Goodglass, 1978; Weidner and Jinks, 1983), and several cueing hierarchies for clinical use have been proposed (Brown, 1972; Davis, 1993; Linebaugh & Lehner, 1977). Pease and Goodglass (1978) asked aphasic adults to name each of 174 pictures of common objects. When participants failed to name an item, they were prompted with one of six cues:

1. First sound/syllable ("It starts with *kuh,* or "It starts with *kof.*")
2. Sentence completion ("Pour me a cup of _____.")
3. Rhyme ("It rhymes with *toffee.*")
4. Function ("You drink it at breakfast.")
5. Location ("You drink it from a cup.")
6. Superordinate ("It's something you drink.")

The participants' success rates following each kind of cue were tabulated. The results are shown in Figure 7-7. The pattern of cue effectiveness was similar for participants with anomic aphasia, Broca's aphasia, and Wernicke's aphasia, although the magnitude of the effects differed across groups. Providing the first sound or syllable was most effective, followed by sentence-completion, rhyme, function, location, and superordinate cues.

Adding cues studied by others to Pease and Goodglass's list produces the following hierarchy, with cues arranged in approximate order of decreasing power:

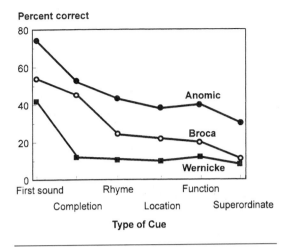

Percent correct

Figure 7-7 ■ **Effectiveness of cues in eliciting correct picture-naming responses from adults with anomic, Broca's, or Wernicke's aphasia.** (From Pease, D. M., & Goodglass, H. [1978]. The effects of cueing on picture naming in aphasia. *Cortex, 14,* 178-189.)

- Imitation ("Say _____")
- First sound/syllable
- Sentence completion
- Word spelled aloud
- Rhyme
- Synonym/antonym
- Function/location
- Superordinate

Standard hierarchies such as this can give clinicians a general idea of what to expect, on the average, from a group of aphasic patients, but exceptions for individual patients are common. Therefore clinicians typically do a test run to find the best cueing hierarchy for any given patient. They place the patient in a naming task and when the patient misnames or fails to name a target item the clinician provides a cue and observes its effect on the patient's naming. The clinician typically begins with the potentially most powerful cues and moves down the hierarchy to less powerful cues. The frequency with which each cue elicits target words then is used to arrange the cues into a personalized hierarchy for the patient.

A patient's cueing hierarchy is used in word-retrieval tasks as follows. When the patient fails to retrieve a target word, the clinician provides the least powerful cue in the hierarchy. If this cue elicits an accurate response, the patient and clinician move on to the next item. If the cue does not elicit an accurate response, the clinician delivers the next more powerful cue. This continues until a cue elicits an accurate response. When the patient produces the target word in response to a cue, the clinician reverses course through the hierarchy and presents the next less powerful cue, continuing until the patient either makes an error or makes accurate responses to all cues. If the patient makes it all the way through the hierarchy with accurate responses, the patient and clinician move on. If the patient makes an error somewhere along the way, the clinician once again reverses course and delivers progressively more powerful cues until the patient responds accurately, at which time the clinician and patient move on to the next item. This ensures that the patient's final attempt at naming an item is a successful production of the name.

When word-retrieval drills yield a corpus of words that the patient can dependably produce, treatment procedures may be modified to diminish the patient's reliance on clinician-supplied cues and substitute patient-generated cues or retrieval strategies. For example, patients whose word retrieval has been facilitated by the clinician's provision of a rhyming cue might be trained to think of a rhyme on their own, and patients whose word retrieval is facilitated when the clinician provides a synonym or an antonym might be trained to think of synonyms or antonyms on their own to elicit target words without the clinician's help. If patients' gestures help them produce the words they want, their use of gesture may be encouraged (or trained).

Behaviors Associated with Word-Retrieval Failure

What aphasic adults do when they fail to retrieve a word sometimes gives the clinician clues to the nature of the patient's word-retrieval troubles and may provide the clinician with indications of strategies the patient may be using to cope with word-retrieval failure. Marshall (1976) studied the spontaneous speech of 18 aphasic adults to determine what they did to cope with word-retrieval failures. Marshall described five such coping behaviors—*delay, semantic association, phonetic association, description,* and *generalization.*

- In *delay* the patient produces a filled or unfilled pause or "some stalling tactic to let the listener know they did not want to be interrupted and needed more time to produce the word" (p. 446).
- In *semantic association* the patient produces one or more words that are semantically related to the target word, including antonyms (front—*back*), class membership (fruit—*banana*), part–whole relationship (foot—*toe*), or serial relationship (Sunday—Monday—*Tuesday*).
- In *phonetic association* the patient produces words that are phonologically similar to the target word (hamper—clamper—*damper*).
- In *description* the patient describes characteristics of the target ("It's round and red and it grows on trees—it's an *apple.*").
- In *generalization* the patient produces general words and phrases without specific meaning ("It's one of those *things.* It's a *thing* that I know. It's a *spider.*").

Marshall reported that *semantic association* was the most frequently occurring behavior, followed by *description, generalization, delay,* and *phonetic association.*

Marshall evaluated the apparent success of these behaviors by calculating the percentage of times each behavior led to the target word. Delay was followed by successful production of the target word about 90% of the time. Semantic association and phonetic association preceded correct production of the target about 55% of the time. Description and generalization were followed by their intended targets only 35% and 17% of the time, respectively (Figure 7-8).

It is tempting to assume a cause-effect relationship between behaviors that precede suc-

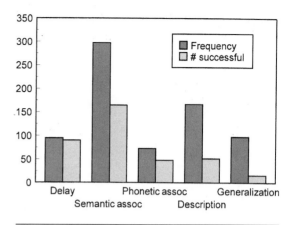

Figure 7-8 ■ Frequency of behaviors associated with aphasic adults' word-retrieval failures and the number of times each behavior preceded successful word retrieval.

cessful production of target words and the subsequent production of the target words. Although it may be that at least some of the behaviors described by Marshall represent purposeful strategies on the part of aphasic speakers, it seems likely that at least some are signs of word-retrieval problems, rather than strategies used to access words. This is a crucial difference

The behaviors Marshall describes simply may reflect how close patients are to the target word. Patients who delay then produce the target probably are on the verge of retrieving the target word at the beginning of the delay (the *tip of the tongue phenomenon*). Delay was the most "successful" behavior. Semantic and phonetic association behaviors suggest that the patient has some information about the word but not enough to retrieve the word. Semantic and phonetic association were moderately successful. Generalization and description suggest that the patient has failed to retrieve much beyond the semantic flavor of the word. Generalization and description were least likely to precede successful production of target words.

because if the behaviors represent strategies, one might wish to encourage the patients to engage in those that have the greatest success. If the behaviors are signs of unsuccessful retrieval strategies, one would probably not wish to increase their frequency and might even search for ways to eliminate them because they may diminish communicative efficiency.

Enhancing Word Retrieval in Speech

Rosenbek and associates (1989) described a three-part program for enhancing aphasic adults' word retrieval in connected speech. The program begins with diagnosis, moves on to strategy development and practice in controlled environments, and ends with the patient's internalization of strategies and generalization of strategy use across words and environments. The following program is modeled on that of Rosenbek and associates.

Part 1: Diagnosis Diagnosis involves two activities:

1. Generating a list of words and semantic categories (e.g., foodstuffs, tools, personal care items) that are especially important to the patient and family
2. Obtaining baseline measures of the patient's successful and unsuccessful word-retrieval strategies

The clinician interviews the patient and one or more family members to develop a list of important words representing several semantic categories. The clinician also observes the patient in unstructured interactions and in structured drill activities to determine how reliably the patient produces various categories of words (with special attention to those on the list), to identify strategies the patient may be using to cope with word-retrieval failure, and to get a sense of which strategies work and which do not.

Part 2: Strategy Development and Practice In this part of the program the patient receives structured practice to expand and strengthen word-retrieval strategies. If the patient already is using strategies to facilitate word retrieval, their use is reinforced. If the patient has few or no successful strategies, the clinician and

patient work together to develop some. The primary vehicle for strategy development is the patient's use of self-cueing (e.g., saying a related word, a rhyme, or the first sound of a word) to facilitate word retrieval. The patient then practices the selected strategies on words from the patient's list of important words in controlled drill activities. When retrieval of a word has been strengthened, the clinician may introduce other forms of the word. For example, if the patient's retrieval of the word *chair* has been enhanced and stabilized, practice with words and phrases such as *armchair, chairman, wheelchair, easy chair,* or *high chair* may follow. (Rosenbek and associates caution against introducing semantically related prompts—such as *table* or *couch* for *chair*—noting that semantically related words often interfere with retrieval of the previously stabilized target words.)

> As previously noted, Podraza and Darley (1977) found a negative effect when aphasic adults were pre-stimulated with spoken words in a word-retrieval task. They found that pre-stimulating with semantically related words worsened aphasic adults word retrieval.

Part 3: Stabilization and Generalization In this part of the program the focus is on helping the patient extend effective word-retrieval strategies to environments beyond the clinic and on moving the patient's word retrieval toward normalcy by replacing overt self-cueing strategies with covert ones. The emphasis is on self-correction and self-cueing by the patient and on extension of improved word retrieval from the tightly controlled elicitation conditions typical of the clinic to the less predictable conditions typical of daily life.

Activities to strengthen word associations and to enhance semantic representations may be incorporated into this phase of treatment. The patient may be asked to:

• Provide synonyms, antonyms, and rhymes for words presented by the clinician.

- Provide lists of words that are in categories specified by the clinician.
- Provide words to fill in blanks in sentences or narratives.
- Separate printed semantically-related words from unrelated words.
- Produce lists of words or word combinations with a common root (e.g., *wash, washer, washcloth, washing machine, car wash*).

As the patient's internal semantic associations and organization move toward normalcy, it is assumed that the patient's word retrieval will improve, diminishing the need for strategies to volitionally evoke words the patient wishes to say.

Sentence Production

Sentence-length utterances can be elicited in several ways. The simplest is *imitation,* in which the clinician says a sentence and the patient repeats it. Sentence-imitation drills are used most commonly to increase articulatory accuracy for patients with motor speech impairments or motor programming impairments, and sometimes they are used to increase auditory retention span for patients with aphasia. Sentence-imitation drills sometimes follow word-repetition drills for patients with speech production impairments. Imitation gets them talking. Then treatment moves them on to more difficult (and more natural) sentence production tasks.

Repetition-elaboration drill is used to move patients from repetition to less constrained responses. In repetition-elaboration drill, the clinician asks questions designed to elicit formulaic, stereotypic responses typical of those in social encounters and conversations:

Clinician: "How are you?"
Patient: "Fine. And how are *you?*"
Clinician: "What do you like for breakfast?"
Patient: "Bacon and eggs. What do *you* like for breakfast?"

Story completion elicits responses that are less constrained than those in repetition-elaboration drill. In story completion the clinician provides a two-sentence or three-sentence narrative and asks

the patient to provide a phrase or sentence to complete it:

Clinician: "It's ten o'clock and my children are still up. I want them to go to bed.
So I say to them. . . ."
Patient: "Go to bed."

Helm-Estabrooks (1982) developed a program for eliciting such utterances from aphasic adults, called the *Helm Elicited Language Program for Syntax Stimulation* (HELPSS).

Question-answer drill further diminishes response constraints. The clinician asks questions related to the patient's experiences, opinions, or general knowledge. The patient responds with a phrase or sentence:

Clinician: "What did you do last evening?"
Patient: "Watched TV and went to bed."
Clinician: "What's the most important difference between cats and dogs?"
Patient: "You don't have to walk a cat."

In *story elaboration* the clinician tells a short story and follows with a series of questions designed to elicit a phrase or sentence:

Clinician: "Fred and Ethyl decided to go out for dinner to celebrate Ethyl's birthday. They drove across town to a nice restaurant and had a nice meal. When the bill came, Fred reached for his wallet, only to discover that it was not there. What do you think Fred and Ethyl did next?"
Patient: "Maybe Ethyl paid the bill, if she had any money."
Clinician: "Where do you think Fred left his wallet?"
Patient: "At the bar, I suppose."

Story elaboration calls on several processes in addition to sentence formulation and production. The patient must comprehend the stories and retain the information long enough to produce the appropriate responses. The patient also must call on general knowledge, make inferences, and foresee consequences to formulate a response that is consistent with the story.

Picture-story elaboration is similar to story elaboration except that instead of telling the patient a story, the clinician shows the patient a picture depicting a situation with a salient theme and a predictable outcome (Figure 7-9) or a series of pictures depicting a sequence of events. Then the clinician asks the patient a series of questions to elicit phrase-length or sentence-length responses.

The clinician might ask the following questions about Figure 7-9:

- "What's the occasion?"
- "Why is the boy crying?"
- "What do you think will happen next?"

In *sentence construction* the clinician provides a spoken (or printed) word, phrase, or two or more related words and asks the patient to produce a sentence containing the words.

Clinician: "Give me a sentence containing the word *boy.*"

Patient: "The boy is happy."

Clinician: "Give me a sentence containing the words *man, drink,* and *coffee.*"

Patient: "The man drinks coffee."

Sentence production drills permit considerable flexibility in manipulating task difficulty. When the eliciting stimulus is a single word, task difficulty depends primarily on the part of speech and frequency in English of the stimulus

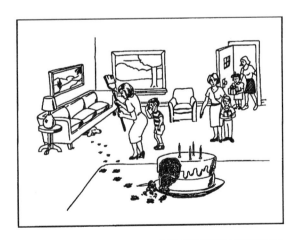

Figure 7-9 ■ A picture that might be used to elicit connected speech. The picture has a central theme and a predictable outcome and suggests events that happened before the events portrayed.

word. Nouns tend to be easiest for aphasic adults to incorporate into a sentence, followed by verbs, pronouns, adjectives, adverbs, and function words. ("Give me a sentence containing the word *man*" is easier than "Give me a sentence containing the word *before.*") Frequently occurring and concrete words are easier for most aphasic adults to incorporate into sentences than infrequently occurring and abstract words. When aphasic patients have to incorporate several words into a sentence, providing the words in noun-verb or noun-verb-noun order facilitates performance because the order of the words in the stimulus matches the subject-verb or subject-verb-object order of the two most common sentence structures. Scrambling the order of the words in the stimulus (noun-noun-verb or verb-noun-noun) increases task difficulty by requiring the patient to rearrange the words to create a syntactically correct sentence. Providing stimuli that represent common word combinations (such as *a piece of pie*) or express commonly encountered relationships (such as *man–drink–coffee*) makes the task easier for most aphasic patients.

Sentence production tasks sometimes can entice clinicians into thinking that grammaticality is what they and the patient should be seeking, when for most patients, communication, not grammaticality, is the answer. Ungrammatic utterances often do an adequate job of communicating an aphasic speaker's thoughts, wishes, and intentions. The patient who responds to "What did you do last evening?" with "TV—bed—sleep" has successfully, although not elegantly, communicated the essentials. Clinicians who insist on grammatic utterances run the risk of wasting their time and wasting the patient's time and energy. The principal exceptions are some high-level aphasic patients who, with a reasonable amount of coaching, are capable of speaking both informatively and grammatically.

Connected Speech

Connected speech is a generic label for speech in which a person produces several utterances in response to a stimulus, topic, or event. The utterances may be continuous, on a common topic, and not separated either by introduction of a new stimulus or by the contributions of another speaker *(monologue),* or the utterances may be separated by questions, comments, or contributions from another speaker *(conversation, interview).* Monologues are used more commonly in testing and treatment than conversation and interview, perhaps because monologues provide better control over the content and form of patients' responses and are easier to quantify.

Picture Description Picture description is one way of eliciting monologues. In picture description, target sentences are not constrained and the patient has free choice of the kinds of sentences produced and considerable latitude in word choice. However, the nature of the picture (or pictures) used to elicit descriptions may affect both the amount and kind of verbalizations elicited from the patient. Familiar occurrences or situations elicit more verbalization than unfamiliar ones. Pictures that suggest a past (events leading up to the situation or event depicted) and a future (events following the situation or event depicted) encourage those who describe them to go beyond the content of the pictures and talk about preceding and following events. Pictures depicting static situations often elicit enumeration (naming items in the picture) from patients, whereas pictures depicting dynamic interactions usually elicit more elaborate descriptions. Figure 7-10 shows two pictures. The one on the left is more likely to elicit enumeration than the one on the right.

Correia, Brookshire, and Nicholas (1990) empirically demonstrated that static speech elicitation pictures tend to elicit enumeration from aphasic adults. They had aphasic adults describe the speech elicitation pictures from the *Boston Diagnostic Aphasia Examination* (BDAE; Goodglass & Kaplan, 1983), the *Western Aphasia Battery* (WAB; Kertesz, 1982), and the *Minnesota Test for Differential Diagnosis of Aphasia* (MT-DDA; Schuell, 1972) (see Figure 5-22). The aphasic speakers' responses to the static WAB and MT-DDA pictures contained greater percentages of

Non-brain-damaged adults produce less story-like narratives when they talk about the MT-DDA picture than when they talk about the BDAE picture. Here is a transcript of what a graduate student said when asked to describe each picture:

The MTDDA picture. There's a house with a mailbox. The name on the mailbox is J. Smith. There's also a man flying a kite. There's another kite caught in a tree. There's a dog looking at the man. There's a woman pointing to the kite in the tree. There's a duck on a small pond. There's a house with smoke coming out of the chimney. That's about it.

The BDAE picture. There's a woman standing at a sink drying dishes. The water is on and running onto the floor, but she doesn't seem to notice. There are two kids behind the woman—probably the woman's son and daughter. The boy is standing on a stool which is about to tip over. He's in the act of getting . . . of stealing cookies from a cookie jar there in the cupboard. The stool is tipping and he's going to land on the floor. His sister is reaching up to get a cookie from him. The mother is completely oblivious to all that's going on. She's either asleep or on drugs.

enumerations (42% and 45%, respectively) than their responses to the more dynamic BDAE picture (38%), although only the difference between the MTDDA picture and the BDAE picture was statistically significant.

Prompted Story Telling Prompted story telling elicits stories by means of sequences of pictures that represent events in a story (Figure 7-11). The amount of speech a picture sequence elicits depends on the number of incidents pictured in the sequence, with more incidents generating longer speech samples. The picture sequence shown in Figure 7-11 elicited, on the average, slightly more than 80 words from aphasic speakers, but the range was substantial (23 words for a nonfluent patient to 164 words for a fluent patient).

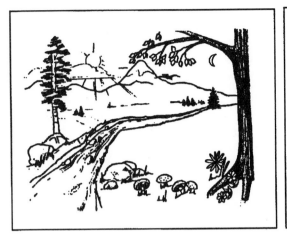
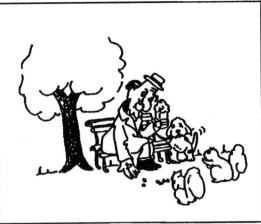

Figure 7-10 ■ Two pictures that might be used to elicit connected speech. The picture on the left is more likely to elicit enumeration than the picture on the right. When describing the left-hand picture a non-brain-damaged adult said, "Well there's a small stream running through a meadow. . . . Some toadstools or mushrooms in the foreground." When she described the right-hand picture she said, "There's an old man and his dog, probably in a park, because the man is sitting on a park bench and there are squirrels around. The man is feeding popcorn or peanuts to the squirrels. The dog is sitting by the bench wagging his tail. I wonder why he's not chasing the squirrels. That's a natural thing for dogs to do, you know." (Courtesy Howard E. Gardner, PhD.)

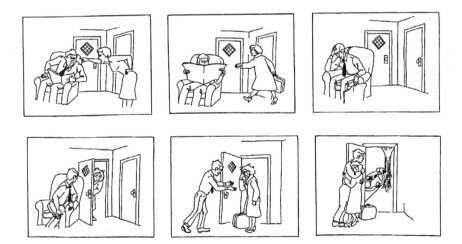

Figure 7-11 ■ A picture sequence that might be used to elicit prompted story telling in treatment activities.

Procedural Discourse Procedural discourse is connected speech made in response to requests such as "Tell me how you make pumpkin pie." When non-brain-damaged adults describe procedures such as making scrambled eggs, writing and mailing a letter, and doing dishes by hand they produce from 75 to 125 words per procedure, depending on the procedure (more complex procedures elicit longer samples). The range for aphasic speakers is great. Some nonfluent aphasic speakers may generate 25 to 30 words per procedure, and some fluent aphasic speakers may generate nearly 300.

Procedural discourse usually is not syntactically complex. Ulatowska and associates (1983) evaluated procedural descriptions produced by nonaphasic adults and aphasic adults and found that neither group produced many syntactically complex sentences. They commented that procedural descriptions do not require syntactically complex language, so even many patients with relatively severe aphasia produce syntactically adequate procedural descriptions (except, of course, those with Broca's aphasia who speak agrammatically).

Conversation Conversation sometimes is used to elicit speech from aphasic patients in treatment activities. However, these interactions often do not resemble natural conversations because the clinician does most of the talking and the patient's responses do not go beyond what the clinician requests, making the interaction more of an interview than a conversation, as in the sample on the right.

Unless carefully structured with pragmatic principles about conversational interactions firmly in place, such clinician–patient interactions are not very effective in eliciting connected speech from the patient. They are more appropriately used when the objective is to improve the patient's conversational behaviors (e.g., turn-taking, eye contact, and topic maintenance).

Clinician: "What kind of work did you do before your stroke?" Patient: "Foreman." Clinician: "A foreman. What company did you work for?" Patient: "Amurcan." Clinician: "Amurcan? Do you mean American? American what?" Patient: "Amurican Freight." Clinician: "American Freight. Is that a trucking company?" Patient: "Yeah." Clinician: "And you were a foreman. What kinds of workers did you supervise?" Patient: "Dock." Clinician: "People on the dock?" Patient: "Yeah." Clinician: "And what kind of jobs did they do?" Patient: "Oh—most ever'thing."

GENERAL CONCEPTS 7-4

- *Sentence-completion drills* may increase volitional speech for patients whose spontaneous speech is limited to automatic stereotypic utterances.

- *Confrontation-naming drills* are popular with clinicians but may not produce lasting effects or improve patients' daily life communication.

- *Cueing hierarchies* permit clinicians to manipulate the power of stimuli used to facilitate aphasic patients' performance in word-retrieval drills.

- Behaviors associated with word-retrieval failure may represent strategies used by a patient to retrieve words or may reflect a patient's unplanned response to word-retrieval failure.

- *Sentence-production drills* often proceed from tasks in which patients' responses are highly constrained (*imitation, story completion*) to open-ended tasks in which patients have considerable latitude in the nature of their responses (*story elaboration, sentence construction*).

- *Connected-speech drills* often proceed from tasks in which patients' responses are constrained (*picture description*) to less constrained tasks (*prompted story telling, procedural discourse, conversation*).

Writing

Many of the same cognitive processes used to produce spoken messages are used to produce written ones. It is only at the production stage that speaking and writing differ appreciably. Writers, unlike speakers, need a sense of how to spell. Writing requires enough visuomotor coordination and limb strength to produce written letters. Writers need better syntax than speakers because speakers can compensate for deficient syntax by providing prosodic clues to meanings, whereas writers do not have this option. Written style is more formal and more grammatically complex than spoken style. It should not be surprising that aphasic adults almost always write less well than they speak.

Aphasic patients' writing resembles their speech. Fluent speakers tend to be fluent writers. They write in cursive, produce well-shaped letters, and maintain horizontal and equally spaced writing lines. Nonfluent speakers tend to be nonfluent writers (partly because they are using their nonpreferred hand). They produce distorted letters, and their lines are uneven in contour and spacing. Nonfluent writers usually print, rather than write in cursive. Agrammatic speakers are likely to be agrammatic writers, and aphasic speakers who generate "empty" speech (devoid of meaning) are likely to generate "empty" written materials (Figure 7-12).

Treatment of Writing Impairments Most aphasic adults have disabilities in spelling and syntax that make it difficult or impossible for them to communicate effectively by writing. Consequently, most writing treatment programs for aphasic adults focus on spelling, syntax, and grammar, using didactic procedures and relying heavily on homework. Sometimes commercially available spelling and writing workbooks are used. Teaching written spelling and syntax to aphasic adults may be an exception to the general assumption that treatment involves *stimulation* or *reactivation* rather than *teaching*. In most cases, procedures used in teaching aphasic adults to spell and write do not differ from those used to teach beginning writers.

It may be fortunate that most aphasic adults do not really need advanced writing skills in daily life. If aphasic adults can write short notes, fill out forms, and write checks, they can probably get by in most daily life environments. Consequently, treatment programs that can get aphasic writers to this level are likely to be sufficient for many. Writing one's name is no doubt the most frequent single daily life writing act and often is the first treatment objective for patients who cannot write. Fortunately, writing one's name is a highly automatized writing activity. It is common to see adults with severe aphasia who can write their name when they can write nothing else.

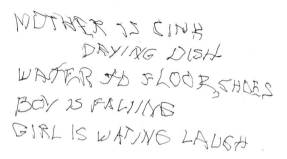

Figure 7-12 ■ **Written responses produced by an aphasic adult with nonfluent aphasia** *(left)* **and an aphasic adult with fluent aphasia** *(right)* **as they described the function of the 10 test stimuli in the** *Porch Index of Communicative Ability* **(Porch, 1981a).**

Most of the linguistic variables that affect how easy it is to produce spoken sentences (e.g., length, word frequency, syntactic complexity) also affect how easy it is to write them. Context affects aphasic persons' writing in the same way that it affects their speaking. If part of a sentence is provided and patients have only to complete the sentence, success rates are higher than if they have to produce the same words without contextual support. Cloze procedures, in which single words are deleted from printed passages, sometimes help patients get started. Most aphasic patients write single words better when they fill in blanks in a sentence or paragraph than when they have to write them in isolation.

Survival Writing Skills The concept of *survival writing skills* is a useful guide to treatment for patients with grossly impaired writing. The clinician and the patient (and sometimes family members) make a list of things that the patient would most like to be able to write. Treatment then is directed toward developing a core writing vocabulary and enough syntactic skills to enable the patient to perform the writing tasks on the list. The following list of writing skills was produced by a woman with moderately severe Broca's aphasia. The skills are listed in order of importance to the patient, from most important (top) to least important (bottom).

- Signing forms (which she could do)
- Writing shopping lists
- Writing checks
- Writing notes in greeting cards
- Writing personal letters

Treatment began with shopping lists. The patient brought several favorite recipes to each clinic appointment, and the patient and clinician used the recipes to make up a list of ingredients needed to prepare the recipes. The words in the ingredient list were incorporated into spelling drills, and the patient practiced writing problem words at home between clinic sessions. The patient also brought utility bills and check registers to clinic sessions. The patient and clinician used the bills and check registers to make up a list of words needed to write the checks. The words in the list were incorporated into check-

writing drills, and the patient practiced writing problem words at home between clinic sessions. When treatment moved on to note and letter writing, similar procedures were used to identify words the patient often misspelled when writing personal notes and letters. The word lists thus obtained were incorporated into spelling drills and spelling homework.

A Writing Treatment Program Haskins (1976) suggested a procedure for treating the writing impairments of aphasic patients who need more than survival writing skills. The procedure begins with auditory stimulation and progresses to production of written materials. A modified version of Haskins's progression follows:

- The patient points to letters after the clinician says the sound of the letter (not the letter name).
  1 letter—2 letters—3 letters, etc.
- The patient points to printed words after the clinician says the sound sequence for the word
  (e.g., /k/-/a/-/t/).
- The patient points to alphabet letters after the clinician names them.
  1 letter—2 letters—3 letters, etc.
- The patient points to printed words after the clinician spells them.
- The patient points to printed words after the clinician names them.
  1 word—2 words—3 words, etc.
- The patient traces letters of the alphabet.
- The patient copies letters of the alphabet.
- The patient writes letters of the alphabet to dictation.
  (a) In serial order
  (b) In random order
- The patient writes words to dictation.
  (a) The clinician spells words letter-by-letter and the patient writes each letter.
  (b) The clinician spells words, 1 second per letter and the patient writes the words.
  (c) The clinician says words and the patient writes them.
- The patient copies structured sentences (e.g., "I eat pie," "I eat cake," "I eat meat").

- The patient writes structured sentences to dictation.
  - (a) Word-by-word dictation
  - (b) Sentence dictation
- The patient writes sentences containing words provided by the clinician.

The earliest stages of Haskins's procedure likely would be needed only for severely aphasic patients (and one might question whether severely aphasic patients will ever become functional writers). Many patients will not need the auditory discrimination training provided in early steps (pointing to letters and words in response to the clinician's spoken directions). Patients who can write letters of the alphabet or simple words to dictation would not need the steps prior to *writing words to dictation.* Patients who need work at the single-letter level might profit more from filling in missing letters in lists of common words than from writing letters in isolation. (Context helps here, too.)

> Two principles governing treatment in general also are relevant to treating impaired reading. Exploit context whenever possible. Begin treatment at a level at which the patient is challenged but not overwhelmed.

It is unusual for an aphasic adult's overall treatment program to concentrate exclusively on writing. Treatment of writing impairments usually is an adjunct to other treatment, with considerable reliance on homework for the writing part of the program. If the clinician plans carefully, treatment of writing impairments can be coordinated with other treatment activities to create maximum generalization from writing to other communicative abilities, from other communicative abilities to writing, and from the clinic to daily life.

Spelling Intelligible writing requires reasonably good spelling. Aphasic patients are universally poor spellers. The severity of a patient's spelling troubles almost always parallels the severity of the patient's aphasia. Patients with se-

Figure 7-13 ■ Written responses produced by an aphasic adult in response to the command, "Write here what you do with each of these." ("These" are the 10 stimulus objects in the *Porch Index of Communicative Ability;* Porch, 1981a.)

vere aphasia rarely write well enough or spell well enough to become functional writers. Most patients with moderate aphasia can write comprehensible simple sentences, short notes, and personal letters, but frequent spelling errors make some words unintelligible and errors in syntax make some sentences unfathomable even to the most resourceful reader. Most patients with mild aphasia can write more complex sentences and longer texts, but frequent spelling errors may annoy both the patient and those who read what the patient has written. Figure 7-13 shows an aphasic person's performance when asked to write the function of each of the 10 test objects from the *Porch Index of Communicative Ability* (Porch, 1981a).

Computer-assisted spelling drills may be helpful to clinicians and patients who are working on spelling. A few such programs have been devised for aphasic adults (Katz & Nagy, 1984; Katz & associates, 1989; Seron & associates, 1980). Computer-based spelling programs designed for children also may be useful, although the juvenile themes of some programs may offend aphasic adults. Contemporary word-processing software can be of immense help to aphasic adults (and nonaphasic adults, too) who spell well enough to get close to the correct spelling of problem words. Most of these programs highlight misspelled words, and some provide a drop-down window in which the correct spellings of possible alternatives is given. (The word-processing program used to write this chapter gave *possible* and *possibly* as alternatives for *possilbe,* which I mistyped.) Many contemporary word-processing programs also include style-checking software, which may help aphasic adults identify syntactic miscues in sentences and text. Spell-checking and style-checking programs may be beneficial to higher-level aphasic adults who are at least mediocre spellers and who can write sentences with at least fair syntax.

GENERAL CONCEPTS 7-5

- Most of the linguistic variables that affect how easy it is for aphasic persons to produce spoken sentences (e.g., *length, syntactic complexity*) affect how easy it is for aphasic persons to write them.
- Aphasic patients with grossly impaired writing may benefit from acquiring *survival writing skills* that enable them to sign forms, make lists, write checks, and accomplish similar writing tasks.
- Aphasic patients who need more than survival writing skills may benefit from structured programs that progress from letter (grapheme) writing and word writing to sentence and paragraph writing.
- Published programs for treating aphasic persons' writing impairments usually must be modified to fit the needs of individuals.
- Commercially published spelling workbooks and computer-based spelling programs are suitable for many aphasic persons for whom work on spelling is an appropriate treatment focus.

GROUP ACTIVITIES FOR APHASIC ADULTS

Historically, group activities for aphasic adults have served multiple purposes. Some groups were organized to provide emotional and psychologic support to aphasic adults and family members. Some were organized to provide a more "natural" environment for aphasic adults' communication practice than that provided by one-to-one clinician–patient treatment activities. Some were organized to help aphasic adults prepare for reentry into familial, social, and commu-

nity roles. The purposes of group activities were not always clearly defined, and combinations of purposes were common. Kearns and Simmons (1985) surveyed 91 Veterans Administration Medical Centers to find out what kinds of group activities they offered to aphasic adults. Most respondents (84%) reported that the primary goal of their treatment groups was *language stimulation.* However, many respondents reported other goals—*emotional support* (59%), *carryover* (47%), and *socialization* (45%).

Family Support Groups

Participants in family support groups typically are family members or caregivers for aphasic adults. Most are spouses of aphasic adults. Often a spouse accompanies the aphasic partner to the speech and language clinic, and while the aphasic partner is in an individual or group treatment session, the spouse attends a family support group session. Family support groups serve several functions. They provide information to participants about the nature of aphasia and its effects on the aphasic person and family members. They permit participants to express feelings, share reactions, and discuss changes in family roles resulting from the presence of aphasia in the family. They help participants cope with the effects of aphasia on family members' social lives and recreation. They facilitate exploration and discussion of participants' attitudes toward rehabilitation and participants' expectations regarding outcome. They provide opportunities for cooperative problem solving. They provide strategies by which family members may facilitate communication between family members and aphasic persons. They help family members identify and practice ways to enhance the aphasic person's independence and self-sufficiency.

A clinical psychologist, a counseling psychologist, a social worker, a family therapist, or a professional who is trained to deal with emotional, psychologic, and familial problems usually moderates and facilitates family support groups. These professionals often team up with a speech-language pathologist to organize and conduct the support groups. The psychologist or family therapist takes the lead when the issue is emotional or psychologic; the speech-language pathologist takes the lead when the issue is communication.

> Kearns (1994) commented that few speech-language pathologists possess the requisite training to independently conduct support groups. "The speech-language pathologist's expertise in communicative disorders should be augmented by the input of a clinical psychologist or counselor if maximum benefit is to be derived from the group experience. Group counseling sessions are often very emotionally laden, and speech-language pathologists are seldom specifically trained to manage the psychological and emotional impact of disability." (p. 308)

Family support groups typically offer activities such as:

- Group discussions in which group members ask questions, exchange ideas and information, express attitudes, and discuss problems associated with aphasia and stroke
- Cooperative problem solving, in which participants help each other devise strategies for dealing with personal and familial issues created by the presence of aphasia in the family
- Role playing and group discussion, in which participants act out typical problem situations and interactions
- Lectures, demonstrations, or discussions about problems related to stroke and aphasia presented by resource persons

Psychosocial Groups

Psychosocial groups typically are comprised of aphasic adults. Some aphasic participants in psychosocial groups also may be receiving individual treatment for their communicative impairments. For other aphasic participants, a psychosocial group may be their only organized treatment.

> The primary purpose of psychosocial aphasia groups is to foster the development of emotional and psychological bonds that help members

cope with the consequences of aphasia. (Kearns, 1994, p. 305)

Psychosocial groups provide a supportive context in which participants may express feelings and get help in identifying and coping with the psychologic and emotional effects of aphasia. Psychosocial groups provide participants with social contact and the opportunity to interact with other aphasic adults who may be facing similar emotional, psychologic, and social issues. Psychosocial groups increase aphasic participants' self-esteem and capacity for independence. They also increase aphasic participants' motivation for social interaction and the confidence with which they communicate.

The group leader (a speech-language pathologist or other professional with appropriate training) organizes group activities, encourages appropriate interactions within the group, ensures that all group members have a chance to participate, and generally keeps group activities on track, while encouraging group members to assume increasing responsibility for initiating and carrying out group activities. Psychosocial group activities may include:

- Discussions in which participants express feelings and attitudes about personal, familial, or social issues
- Cooperative problem solving, in which the group helps individual participants analyze and find solutions to interpersonal and lifestyle issues and problems
- Role-playing in which participants act out troublesome daily life encounters, interactions, or situations
- Group activities such as games, competitions, field trips, sightseeing excursions, or attendance at theater or sporting events

Treatment Groups

Treatment groups provide aphasic adults with controlled experiences in communication in an environment in which they can try out new behaviors or new ways of communicating. Group treatment sessions may offer patients a more natural communication environment than individual treatment sessions with a clinician, but an environment that is better controlled and less threatening than everyday social interactions. Activities for treatment groups tend to be somewhat more controlled and task-oriented than psychosocial group activities. The group facilitator ensures that each group member receives stimulation appropriate to the group member's abilities and ensures that what happens in the group is consistent with the therapeutic objectives for each group member. Group activities range from didactic activities such as those typically seen in individual clinician–patient treatment to relatively freeform conversational interactions, with emphasis on communication among group members. Group treatment can provide patients with experiences that are not possible in one-to-one treatment activities. Group treatment is also cost-effective—more patients can be treated in groups than in one-to-one treatment. In practice, groups often have both psychosocial objectives and treatment objectives, and group activities often address both objectives.

Transition/Community Reintegration Groups

Transition/community reintegration group experiences help aphasic participants establish rewarding personal lifestyles and renew their participation in family and community activities. Transition/community reintegration groups prepare patients for participation in daily life activities by providing training and practice with strategies and problem-solving skills that enhance the aphasic person's confidence, independence, and competence in daily life. Transition/community reintegration groups also provide patients with information and advice about how to find and make use of community services such as adult day-care centers, visiting nurse services, and senior citizens' centers. Transition/community reintegration groups may have several objectives:

- To help aphasic persons accept persisting changes in their physical, cognitive, and communicative abilities

- To help aphasic persons develop and accept a realistic view of their current abilities and impairments
- To help aphasic persons develop a lifestyle consistent with their remaining abilities and interests
- To help aphasic persons discover and use appropriate social and community resources

Kagan and associates (Kagan & Cohen-Schneider, 1999; Kagan & Dailey, 1993) described a comprehensive volunteer-based psychosocial support-community reintegration program in which aphasic participants progress from an *introductory group* stressing psychosocial support in a context of freeflowing conversation to a *community aphasia program* in which participants can choose from a variety of groups, including *special-interest groups* (e.g., cooking, music), *skill-building groups* (e.g., reading, writing), *family support groups,* or *generic conversation groups.*

Volunteers recruited from the community are trained to serve as conversational partners, group leaders, and group facilitators; to rate participants' performance; to deal with participants' feelings of grief and loss; and to monitor and facilitate group evolution. The volunteers also are trained in conversational techniques "... that will help them better reveal the competence of those with aphasia" (Kagan & associates, 2001, p. 625). The groups progress through a preplanned sequence of activities. During the first group sessions, group members and volunteers share personal information and "tell their stories." These activities lead into group sessions in which the volunteers help group members discuss and better understand the nature of aphasia and its consequences for aphasic persons and their families. Following these educational sessions, group sessions focus on improving group members' communicative competence. Volunteers help group members devise, practice, and perfect strategies for successful communication. As the group moves toward closure the focus shifts to goal setting and life after the group. Members use group activities to establish personal goals and plan for a productive life following their group experiences. In the final sessions group members evaluate the effectiveness of the group, assess their personal progress, and say goodbye to other group members. Many group members then move on into a community aphasia program in which they explore special interests, enhance skills, or participate in social activities.

Kagan and Cohen-Schneider (1999) comment that by the time aphasic participants have completed the introductory program, they have become ". . . people who hold themselves differently, show genuine attachment to a new community of friends, and are beginning to see some kind of future for themselves" (p. 106). At this time no data-based evidence for the effectiveness of Kagan and associates' overall program is available, although Kagan and associates (2001) provide data supporting the effectiveness of their method of training volunteers.

Walker-Bastson & associates (1999) described a transition-reintegration program called the *Lifelink* approach—a weekly half-day program for aphasic adults designed to facilitate community re-entry and "participation in life." The program begins with individual treatment for each participant and progresses to community outings for groups of participants. Psychosocial support groups, led by a social worker, are provided for program participants and family members. Individual treatment is designed to (1) re-establish as much language as possible by systematic treatment, (2) establish at least one efficient modality for communication, and (3) prepare the aphasic person for success in group and community interactions. A personalized packet of material (e.g., vocabulary lists, outlines, pictures, articles, activities) is prepared for each aphasic person for use in individual and group treatment activities.

Lifelink group sessions begin with a review to ensure that all participants are aware of the group's overall goals and each participant's individual goals. Then participants engage in social conversation related to personal experiences (e.g., weekend activities, vacations, children). Then the group participates in a clinician-led discussion of current events, followed by theme-related group activities (discussions, debates, role-play activities, problem-solving exercises). A short wrapup, in which the group reviews the group's overall performance and discusses participants' use of communicative strategies and facilitators, ends the group session. No data to support the efficacy of the Lifelink program have been published.

Lyon (1989, 1992) described a program in which volunteers from the community are recruited and trained to serve as communication partners for aphasic adults. The communication partners are trained to help aphasic adults select, plan, and undertake daily life activities of their own choosing, either at home or in community settings. An aphasic adult, the aphasic adult's primary caregiver, and a communication partner make up a communicative triad. The communicative partners are trained and supervised by speech-language pathologists as the triads devise and test communication-participation strategies in mockups of real-life situations and settings. When the strategies have been perfected, the triads try them out in natural daily life settings. Strategies and settings are selected by the aphasic participant to reflect aspects of daily life community participation that are important to the aphasic participant—*ordering in a restaurant, making purchases in stores, visiting friends,* and so on. The communicative partner supports the aphasic person and the caregiver with advice and encouragement and may participate in community participation activities until the aphasic person and the caregiver have the confidence and skills needed for self-sufficient participation.

Lyon's program is not actually a group program in the traditional sense of the word, but its objectives resemble those of transition/community reintegration groups so closely that I have described it here.

A SHORT HISTORY OF GROUP TREATMENT FOR APHASIC ADULTS

Group treatment for aphasic adults became an important clinical concern during and after World War II with the arrival in military hospitals of large numbers of head-injured veterans. Only a few trained professionals were available to treat them, and group treatment permitted clinicians to provide treatment to large numbers of brain-injured veterans.

Although those who treated these brain-injured veterans called them aphasic, almost all the injured veterans had sustained traumatic brain injuries from bullets, shrapnel, or blows to the head. Of 696 "aphasic" patients seen in one army medical center, 681 had sustained traumatic brain injuries from external sources (Wepman, 1951). Their average age was 26 years. Contemporary practitioners would not call young patients with traumatic brain injuries aphasic. The cognitive-communicative impairments exhibited by individuals with traumatic brain injuries differ strikingly from those exhibited by patients with stroke (the primary cause of aphasia). Treatment objectives, treatment procedures, and patterns of recovery also differ between individuals who have experienced traumatic brain injuries and those who have experienced strokes.

One objective of the early group treatment programs was to "re-educate" brain-injured veterans by means of drill activities focused on speech, reading, writing, and mathematics. Psychotherapy and social and recreational activities provided psychologic and emotional support (Wepman, 1951). Few, if any, reliable tests were available to measure the effects of treatment, and practitioners typically provided testimonials, rather than data, about the effectiveness of their treatment programs.

We have felt it [treatment of brain-injured veterans] worthwhile. Some of the results are measurable enough, others show simply in the healthier and happier attitudes of those who leave us. We feel that we can conclude that we have been able to hasten the process of re-education; that we have pushed it far beyond the level usually obtained by the patient allowed to drift his own way without guidance (Sheehan, 1945, p. 153).

Group treatment for aphasic adults remained popular through the 1950s and early 1960s. Objectives typically included reducing group members' communicative impairments and providing social and psychologic support (Agranowitz & associates, 1954; Aronson, Shatin, & Cook, 1956; Backus & Dunn, 1952; Bloom, 1962; Corbin, 1951; and others).

In the group situation, it is possible to recreate and structure everyday situations with appropriate verbal behavior which was not only well established in the repertoire of the individual previous to his injury, but which occurs with great frequency in his daily immediate experience. Further, it is possible to reduce such verbal behavior to specific situational language units, which can be structured and repeatedly reinforced in the learning environment (Bloom, 1962, p. 13).

During the 1960s and 1970s the clinical emphasis in aphasia shifted away from group treatment and toward individualized one-to-one clinician–patient treatment. Those who wrote about aphasia advocated individual treatment and considered group treatment a sometimes useful adjunct to individual treatment.

We would argue that individual therapy and group therapy are entirely different classes of events, serve different purposes, and should not be confused . . . The clinician needs to judge when and how to facilitate a response, and when to give the patient time to produce one independently. He needs to adapt materials to individual needs and interests at successive stages of recovery. In short, treatment for aphasia must constantly be dovetailed to patient response. There are no mass methods, and none are possible. What reaches or helps one patient at one point in time loses another. For these reasons, we are unable to have confidence in group therapy as a basic method of treatment for aphasia . . . group therapy is wasteful, and sometimes deleterious, if used as a substitute for individual treatment (Schuell, Jenkins, & Jimenez-Pabon, 1964, pp. 343, 344).

Group therapy ... may be justified as an adjunct to individual therapy, providing that the adjunctive values can be achieved better in a group setting than on an individual basis and better in a "structured" arrangement than in some other informal social situation (Eisenson, 1974, p. 234).

We believe that one clinician and one aphasic person are the heart of successful treatment ... Groups replace individual treatment only if a patient has never responded or has stopped responding in individual work, but wants to continue treatment (Rosenbek, LaPointe, & Wertz, 1989, p. 184).

During the 1970s an emphasis on use of language in natural contexts (pragmatics) began to emerge, and some clinicians began to move away from traditional didactic stimulus-response drills toward activities in which aphasic patients were encouraged to get their message across using any means that worked. Clinicians began to incorporate elements of natural conversations into their treatment procedures, but the emphasis remained on individual treatment—group activities still were considered an adjunct to individual treatment by most practitioners.

During the 1980s and 1990s cost containment became a prominent focus within health care, and shortened hospital lengths of stay and restrictions on reimbursement for patient-care services contributed to speech-language pathologists' renewed interest in treatment groups for aphasic adults. Treatment groups became a way of maintaining the integrity of treatment in the face of declining reimbursement by those who pay for patients' health care.

We feel that it [group treatment] contributes in a very positive manner to the total rehabilitative process and is a solution to the "chronic stroke patient" syndrome. Group programs such as these are cost effective, both in dollars and in improved quality of life, because they integrate the patient into existing family and community structures. This reduces hospital dependency and focuses on health rather than disability (West, 1981, p. 151-152).

EFFICACY OF GROUP TREATMENT FOR APHASIA

In the 1980s and 1990s clinicians' belief in the worth of group treatment for aphasic adults was strengthened by the positive results of several studies of group treatment efficacy. Wertz and associates (1981) experimentally evaluated the efficacy of individual and group treatment for aphasic adults. Aphasic patients in *individual treatment* (Group A) received 8 hours of clinician-directed treatment per week for 44 weeks. Patients in *group treatment* (Group B) received 8 hours of group treatment and group recreational activities each week for 44 weeks. With minor exceptions, both groups made significant improvement on speech and language measures between 4 weeks post-onset (when they entered treatment) and tests at the end of 11, 22, 33, and 44 weeks of treatment. There were few significant differences between the two groups on any test occasion, although Group A almost always performed somewhat better than Group B (Figure 7-14). Both groups improved significantly be-

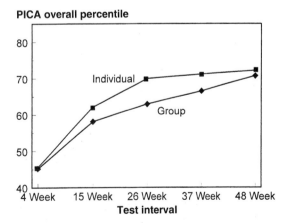

Figure 7-14 ■ Change in *Porch Index of Communicative Ability* (Porch, 1981a) overall percentile scores for participants who received individual treatment and for participants who received group treatment from intake into the study (4 weeks post onset of aphasia) to 15, 26, 37, and 48 weeks post onset.

tween 26 and 48 weeks post-onset (after 22 to 44 weeks of treatment, when, according to Wertz and associates, spontaneous recovery should no longer be taking place).

Wertz and associates concluded that both individual and group treatment of the kind provided in their study were efficacious.

> Our results indicate that individual treatment may be slightly superior to group treatment. However, the improvement displayed by our group-treated patients and the cost-effective advantages of group therapy should prompt speech-language pathologists to consider it for at least part of an aphasic patient's care. (p. 592)

In a study reported by Aten, Caligiuri, and Holland (1982) seven adults with chronic non-fluent aphasia received 2 hours of group treatment weekly. Treatment was directed toward improving the aphasic participants' functional communication by participation in simulated daily life activities such as shopping; giving and following directions; giving personal information; reading signs, labels, and posters; and expressing ideas. Aten and associates reported little change in participants' scores on the *Porch Index of Communicative Ability* (Porch 1981a) but reported significant improvement on the *Communicative Abilities in Daily Living* measure (Holland, 1980).

Holland and Beeson (1999) reported outcome data for 40 aphasic adults who joined aphasia treatment groups at various times post-onset, ranging from 3 months to 14 years. (The average was 2.8 years.) Each had participated in an aphasia group for at least 1 year, and each participant was tested yearly with the *Western Aphasia Battery* (WAB; Kertesz, 1982). Fifteen of the 40 participants made significant improvement, as measured by a gain of at least 5 points in the WAB aphasia quotient (AQ); 23 made no significant change in WAB AQ; and 2 significantly declined in WAB AQ. Holland and Beeson concluded that their results ". . . showed continued measurable language improvement during a period when they would be considered to have chronic aphasia" (p. 83). (We do not know, how-

ever, what percentage of these patients would have improved without participating in a group because Holland and Beeson had no control group with which to compare the group that participated in the treatment groups.)

Elman and Bernstein-Ellis (1999) evaluated the effects of group treatment on the communicative performance of 24 adults with chronic aphasia, which ranged from 7 months to 336 months in duration. Elman and Bernstein-Ellis randomly assigned participants to an *immediate-treatment group* and a *deferred-treatment group*. The immediate-treatment group received 5 hours of group treatment per week for 4 months. Treatment began as soon as participants were enrolled in the study. Group treatment focused on increasing participation in conversations and communicating information by whatever means possible.

The deferred-treatment group received immediate assessment but did not begin group treatment until the immediate-treatment group had completed its 4 months of treatment. To control for the effects of social contact, each participant in the deferred-treatment group attended 3 or more hours of social group activities of their choice (e.g., movement classes, art groups, church activities, support groups) while they waited for their 4 months of group communication treatment.

Several outcome measures, including a shortened version of the *Porch Index of Communicative Ability* (SPICA; Disimoni, Keith, & Darley, 1980), the *Western Aphasia Battery* (WAB; Kertesz, 1982), and *Communicative Abilities in Daily Living* (CADL; Holland, 1980) were administered at intake, after 2 and 4 months of treatment, and 4 to 6 weeks following cessation of treatment. The delayed-treatment group also was tested when they began group treatment. The test scores of the immediate-treatment group were significantly higher after 4 months of treatment than those of the delayed-treatment group (which had received only social stimulation). The delayed-treatment group did not change significantly on any measure from intake until the time at which they began group

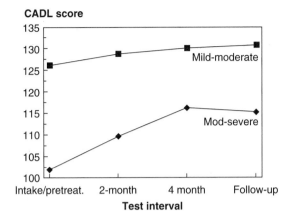

Figure 7-15 ■ **Communicative Abilities of Daily Living (CADL; Holland, 1980) scores for aphasic participants with mild-to-moderate aphasia and participants with moderate-to-severe aphasia at intake, after 2 months and 4 months of treatment, and at follow-up (4 to 6 weeks after treatment ended).** (Data from Elman, R. J., & Bernstein-Ellis, E. [1999]. The efficacy of group communication treatment in adults with chronic aphasia. *Journal of Speech, Language, and Hearing Research, 42,* 411-419.)

treatment, but after 4 months of delayed treatment their SPICA overall scores and their WAB AQ had increased significantly. Both groups maintained their improved test performance on follow-up testing after 4 to 6 weeks of no treatment. The CADL scores of participants with moderate-to-severe aphasia significantly increased after 2 and 4 months of group treatment, but CADL scores of participants with mild-to-moderate aphasia did not, perhaps as a result of a ceiling effect for the less severely aphasic participants (Figure 7-15). Elman and Bernstein-Ellis concluded that their treatment was efficacious: "The present study demonstrated that 5 hours per week of group communication treatment over 2- and 4-months duration provided efficacious treatment for adults with chronic aphasia" (p. 417).

Elman (1999) subsequently concluded a review of studies of the efficacy of group treatment for aphasia with the following statement:

What is encouraging about the research done to date is the growing consensus that group communication treatment holds real promise as a treatment method. Given the rapidly changing health care reimbursement environment, including the emergence and dominance of a managed care model, group communication treatment for individuals appears to provide an effective and economical option for delivering neurogenic communication treatment. (Elman, 1999, p. 6)

Some clinicians who had been pushed into group treatment by reimbursement considerations became convinced not only that group treatment could lead to meaningful changes in aphasic adults' communicative ability, but that group treatment might actually be superior to individual treatment in creating meaningful changes in aphasic adults' daily life communicative competence.

There was a time in the not-too-distant past when I [Holland] believed that group treatment was a useful adjunct to individual treatment for chronically aphasic adults. I have changed my mind. I now believe that individual treatment is a useful adjunct to group treatment for such patients (Holland & Ross, 1999, p. 116).

Notwithstanding Holland's dramatic change of attitude, there is at this time no compelling evidence to support the superiority of group treatment over individual treatment or vice versa. It is clear that at least some group treatment approaches significantly improve aphasic adults' communicative skills and daily life communicative competence. It is not clear that group treatment does this better than individual treatment, and it is not clear whether some combination of individual and group treatment might not be better than either approach by itself.

The current literature on group treatment suggests that a three-phase program, beginning with individual treatment, progressing to group treatment combined with group psychosocial support, and culminating in group maintenance-reintegration activities may be the best option for many aphasic adults. In the first phase *(individual treatment)* the aphasic person, the clinician, and family members identify and quantify the aphasic person's impairments, catalog the aphasic person's retained skills, and identify problems that the aphasic person and the family would like to resolve. The aphasic person and the clinician devise, test, practice, and refine strategies for dealing with the patient's impairments within controlled training conditions as the clinician provides advice, direction, and feedback.

When the aphasic person has perfected the strategies in individual treatment sessions, the focus of treatment moves to the second phase *(group treatment and psychosocial support),* wherein the aphasic person practices and refines the strategies within a supportive and controlled environment that resembles daily life settings. When the aphasic person has become a confident and competent communicator in the treatment-psychosocial support group, the aphasic person may move on to the third phase *(transition/reintegration),* wherein group activities help the aphasic person and family members adjust to changes in family relationships and lifestyle caused by the aphasic person's aphasia; help the aphasic person and family members identify social and community resources that may help them normalize their lifestyle; and help the aphasic person resume active participation in family, social, and community life. For some aphasic persons, participation in a transition/reintegration group may be a lifelong process. For others, a transition/reintegration group may provide the means by which they become independent and self-sufficient communicators in daily life, at which time the group experiences may no longer be needed.

Although empiric evidence clearly supports the efficacy of group treatment for aphasic adults, much work remains. Additional data-based research is needed to establish the efficacy of group treatment for aphasic adults, to determine which aspects of group treatment are responsible for any treatment effects observed, to formulate and test new approaches to group treat-

ment, and to evaluate the effects of multiple-component group treatment programs. The benefits of family support groups, psychosocial groups, and maintenance-reintegration groups for aphasic adults and family members are at this time undocumented, except for what Kearns (1994) calls "advocacy reports"—articles that declare the clinical value of aphasia groups without clearly describing treatment procedures or presenting data to support their claims. Data-based evidence for the effectiveness and efficiency of such groups is badly needed, as is development of reliable measurement instruments that will permit objective assessment of outcomes, which until now have been described using subjective measures of undocumented reliability and validity.

GENERAL CONCEPTS 7-6

- Groups for aphasic adults may serve several purposes, either individually or in combination. They include *family support, psychosocial support, treatment,* or *transition/community re-entry.*
- Group treatment for aphasic adults became important after World War II to meet the needs of large numbers of head-injured veterans.
- In the 1960s and 1970s group treatment fell out of favor, often replaced by one-to-one, didactic treatment activities.
- In the 1980s and 1990s group treatment regained popularity as concerns about *cost containment* and *functional communication* intensified.
- Several studies have shown that group treatment improves communicative abilities of adults with chronic aphasia. A few studies suggest that group treatment may be appropriate for adults in earlier stages of recovery from aphasia.
- A three-phase program consisting of *individual treatment* followed by *group treatment* and *group psychosocial support* and culminating in *transition/reintegration group* activities may be appropriate for many aphasic adults.

THOUGHT QUESTIONS

Question 7-1 A speech-language pathologist has completed his assessment of Mr. Murphy, an aphasic man, and is preparing to begin treatment of Mr. Murphy's comprehension impairments. Mr. Murphy's performance on spoken yes-no questions places him at the 25th percentile for aphasic adults. His performance on following-spoken-directions and sentence-verification comprehension tests places him at the 76th percentile for aphasic adults. What potential reasons do you see for the disparities in Mr. Murphy's test performance? What might the disparities suggest to you regarding treatment?

Question 7-2 You plan to begin treatment for Ms. Snyder, who is aphasic following a left-hemisphere stroke 2 months ago. Test results indicate that she has severe apraxia of speech and agrammatism, but listening comprehension and reading comprehension are relatively well preserved. You and Ms. Snyder agree that treatment will focus on improving her speech. The following transcript represents her description of the "cookie theft" picture (see Figure 5-22). Her description of the cookie theft picture is a good representation of her speech in daily life activities. What do you see as the most debilitating problems? What would you work on to make the greatest changes in Ms. Snyder's daily life communicative competence?

> Uh...uh...uh......moman....um........disses..........but ....no...uh...uh...and...and....waduh....um....floah....... and...and...and...um.....kidz.....and...and...and...er.... skool...no.......spool....but.....but....skool.....and...and .....and......tookies....no....but......turkies.....no ......and..and....kookus....um. ....and....um....fall.

Question 7-3 The following speech samples represent transcripts of Mrs. Bloom and Mr. Jones talking about the "birthday party" picture (Figure 7-9). They are typed without punctuation. The number of dots indicates the relative durations of pauses.

Mrs. Bloom produces the following speech sample. (She produces 105 words per minute.)

> and..um..what do you call it....but I guess the cat got into it and..uh he's hiding under the sitter and the mother is gonna......trying to get him out of there...and he cleaned up the rug and..uh the rest of the birthday cake...those ones there....children...boys and girls...are arriving and it's....um not too good a deal I'd say

Mr. Jones produces the following speech sample. (He produces 40 words per minute.)

> um...um...uh.....cake..and..um..and..and dog.....dog ate cake..and..and...trouble..... mom is mad....and..and..um..um..kid is crying...and..and... neighbors.....neighbors is coming

If you were to work with Mrs. Bloom and Mr. Jones to improve their speech, on what aspects of their speech would you focus your treatment?

Question 7-4 Mr. Osborne is moderately aphasic and wishes to regain enough reading ability for recreational reading (newspapers, magazines, novels). You evaluate his reading and find that his major problem is missing or misreading function words. His reading vocabulary and word-recognition skills are relatively well preserved. How might you go about improving his reading comprehension?

Right-Hemisphere Syndrome

HISTORICAL OVERVIEW

That the two hemispheres of the human brain serve different functions has been suspected since the mid 1800s. In 1836 Marc Dax, an obscure general practitioner in the wine-growing region of southern France, read a paper at a regional meeting of physicians. In the paper Dax asserted that the "memory for words" resides in the left brain hemisphere of right-handers. Dax died a year later, and his paper was generally ignored by the medical community. Then in 1861 Paul Broca, a French surgeon and amateur anthropologist, reported that he had seen eight patients with language disturbance secondary to brain injury and that all had lesions in the left hemisphere. He declared that the left hemi-

sphere of right-handers is responsible for "the faculty of articulate speech." Within the next few years Broca's claims were widely circulated, and the dominance of the left hemisphere for language became widely accepted.

Marc Dax's son, Gustave, also a physician, spent many years trying to force the medical community to recognize his father's precedence, claiming that Broca and others had ignored his father's 1836 report. He had little success, and Broca's place in the history of neurology was never seriously threatened.

During the next decade most physicians believed that the left hemisphere was dominant for almost all cognitive functions, with the right hemisphere responsible only for perceptual and motor functions and perhaps some rudimentary mental processes. Then, in 1874 John Hughlings Jackson, a British neurologist, asserted that the left hemisphere is responsible for language and that the right hemisphere is responsible for visual recognition, discrimination, and recall. Jackson thought that the right hemisphere might, however, play a minor role in language. He considered the left hemisphere the leader, responsible for creative uses of language, but allowed that the right hemisphere might participate in preprogrammed, automatic language functions.

During the next half century the right hemisphere's contribution to cognition and intellect was largely neglected as investigators, fascinated by Broca's findings, concentrated on exploring the allocation of responsibilities for language within the left hemisphere. It was not until the twentieth century that investigators began to explore the organization and function of the right hemisphere in any organized way.

The two world wars (1914-1917, 1941-1945) provided new insights into brain functions as physicians, psychologists, and others studied how missile wounds to the brains of battle-wounded veterans affected their behavior and cognition. These clinical studies provided new insights into how the two brain hemispheres collaborate.

In the 1960s neurosurgeons began performing commissurotomies (surgical disconnection of fibers in the corpus callosum) to control otherwise intractable seizures. Their patients, who now had brain hemispheres that could be tested independently of each other, provided a means for investigators to describe more explicitly the unique capabilities of the right hemisphere.

In the 1970s procedures were developed that enabled investigators to direct input to a single hemisphere in neurologically intact adults. The information provided by these procedures has enhanced substantially our knowledge of what the right hemisphere does and how it does it.

Although what we know is largely descriptive, with little sense of cause and effect, we slowly are becoming more sophisticated about the role of the right hemisphere in communication, cognition, and behavior.

> Statements about hemispheric specialization may be misleading unless the qualifier "in right-handed adults" is added. Few writers add the qualifier, and I will not belabor the reader with it. However, the reader should keep it in mind whenever reading descriptions of right-hemisphere-damaged adults.

Early theories of hemispheric function contended that the left hemisphere is specialized for language and reasoning and the right hemisphere is specialized for music and visual processes. This concept of hemispheric specialization gradually changed as investigators found that the two hemispheres appeared to operate in fundamentally different ways. Writers began to describe the left hemisphere as rational, analytic, and specialized for processing sequential, time-related material. They described the right hemisphere as intuitive, holistic, and specialized for processing nonlinear spatially distributed arrays of information.

Because auditory information often comes in time-ordered sequences (syllables in a word, words in a sentence) the left hemisphere may have greater responsibility for auditory events, and because visual information often comes in multidimensional arrays (pictures, scenes, faces) the right hemisphere may have greater responsibility for visual events. However, these hemispheric differences reflect the temporal or spatial nature of the information, rather than the modality through which the information enters the brain.

Contemporary neural network models of hemispheric specialization are moving away from such appealing but no doubt overly simplified concepts to emphasize the ways in which various brain regions collaborate to accomplish mental functions and produce and regulate behavior. These models conceptualize mental activity as the result of the spread of excitatory and inhibitory neural activation from place to place within the brain.

Regardless of how one chooses to explain the right hemisphere's contribution to cognition and behavior, it is clear that only about half of adults who sustain right-hemisphere brain injury develop communication impairments (Joanette & associates, 1983). The variables contributing to communication impairments following right-hemisphere brain injury are not well understood, although Joanette and associates suggest that patients with cortical lesions, a history of familial left-handedness, and low education levels are the most likely candidates. The relationship of the first two variables to right-hemisphere communication impairments makes intuitive sense. Because language and communication are cortical, rather than subcortical, processes it is not surprising that cortical lesions in the right hemisphere are more likely than subcortical lesions to produce communication impairments. (The same is true for left-hemisphere lesions.) Because familial left-handedness is likely to be related to right-hemisphere dominance for language, it is not surprising that left-handers with right-hemisphere lesions are more likely to develop communication impairments than left-handers without such a family history. There is no obvious logical relationship between low education level and the development of communication impairments by adults with right-hemisphere brain injury. It may be that low education levels are associated with other variables that actually account for the relationship (minimal brain injury, cognitive impairments, intellectual limitations, and similar variables that may lead an individual to drop out of school).

BEHAVIORAL AND COGNITIVE SYMPTOMS OF RIGHT-HEMISPHERE BRAIN INJURY

Descriptions in the clinical literature of the perceptual, cognitive, and behavioral consequences of right-hemisphere brain injury usually describe a stereotypic collection of impairments that by implication is exhibited by all adults with right-hemisphere brain injury. Adults with right-hemisphere brain injury are characterized as:

- Insensitive to others and preoccupied with self
- Oblivious to social conventions
- Unaware of or inattentive to physical and mental limitations
- Verbose, tangential, and rambling in speech
- Insensitive to the meaning of abstract or implied material
- Unable to grasp the overall significance or meaning of complex events

Some adults with right-hemisphere brain injury exhibit reduced overall level of arousal:

- They respond minimally to social or environmental stimuli.
- Their utterances are short and lack emotional inflection.
- They have difficulty maintaining attention for more than a few seconds.

Writers who describe the typical adult with right-hemisphere damage often do not mention that many adults with right-hemisphere brain injury do not exhibit the stereotypic collection of impairments, and they often pay little attention to variability in symptoms among right-hemisphere-damaged adults, although it is well known that not all right-hemisphere-damaged adults have the same impairments.

Group studies of adults with right-hemisphere brain injury contribute to misconceptions about the generality of stereotypic patterns of impairment. They do so by reporting test results for heterogeneous groups in which the location and severity of subjects' right-hemisphere brain injury have not been controlled for or reported. The results typically are reported as average group performance, with little consideration of how well individuals in the group conform to the group average. The validity of group studies of adults with right-hemisphere brain injury is further compromised by the failure of most to include control groups with left-hemisphere damage, which would permit readers to separate the effects of right-hemisphere brain injury from the effects of brain injury in general.

Group studies of right-hemisphere-damaged adults tend to include disproportionately large numbers of individuals with anterior brain injuries. This happens because right-hemisphere-damaged adults with posterior lesions usually are not paralyzed and consequently are discharged from the hospital within a few days of admission. This leaves the right-hemisphere-damaged adults with anterior brain injuries—who have left-sided paralysis and need physical therapy—in the hospital and accessible to investigators looking for participants. Individuals with posterior right-hemisphere damage who do make it into studies are likely to be in the immediate post-onset stage of recovery, when global effects of brain injury create symptoms attributable to brain injury in general, rather than to right-hemisphere brain injury.

> McDonald (1993) has pointed out the striking similarities between communicative and cognitive impairments of groups of patients with frontal lobe damage and the communicative and cognitive impairments of groups with right-hemisphere damage. McDonald comments that these similarities arise, at least in part, from the inclusion of large proportions of patients with frontal lobe damage in groups with right-hemisphere brain injury. Brownell and associates (2000) agree: "The catalogue of linguistic and cognitive impairments observed in RHD [right-hemisphere-damaged] patients could be substituted, usually without notice, into any review article on prefrontal impairments" (p. 321).

Tompkins (1995) alludes to the heterogeneity of symptoms in right-hemisphere-damaged adults as follows:

> One of the most important things to remember about adults with RHD is one of the most important characteristics of any "category" of people;

they are quite heterogeneous. Not all patients will have communicative impairments. Those who do will not have all symptoms, and individual patients will display different patterns of behavior. Complicating things further, it can be quite difficult to specify "disordered" status because normative information is almost nonexistent for abilities and performance broken down by age, education, socioeconomic status, and cultural variables. It is part of the clinical challenge in working with brain-damaged individuals to identify the presence and absence of the deficits that result from neurologic insult, as well as those that are not necessarily due to the brain injury. (pp. 15-16)

> Tompkins's comments relate equally well to all other categories of adults with brain injury.

The symptoms generated by right-hemisphere brain injury, like those generated by left-hemisphere injury, differ in their nature and severity depending on the location and magnitude of the brain injury causing the symptoms, although, as noted previously, our understanding of these relationships is imperfect. Although the relationships between damage in various regions of the right hemisphere and behavioral symptoms have yet to be dependably elucidated, many right-hemisphere-damaged adults exhibit distinctive cognitive and behavioral impairments. Some of the most striking are perceptual and attentional impairments.

Perceptual Impairments

Denial of Illness Denial of illness (anosognosia) is a common behavioral consequence of right-hemisphere brain injury, especially when individuals with right-hemisphere brain injury have parietal lobe damage. Denial takes several forms. Individuals with the lowest levels of denial acknowledge their disabilities but are indifferent to them. Those with moderate levels of denial acknowledge their disabilities but underestimate their severity and minimize their effects (a right-hemisphere-damaged individual with dense left hemiplegia repeatedly claimed that his paralyzed left arm and leg were "just a little weak" and gave him problems only when he attempted to climb stairs). Some individuals with severe denial disavow the existence of major disabilities such as paralysis, sensory loss, and visual field blindness, and some even deny ownership of their hemiplegic limbs. Those with severe denial sometimes claim to perform activities that clearly are beyond their physical abilities (a patient with left-sided paralysis claimed to be in training for the national speed-skating championships). Many right-hemisphere-damaged adults, even those with low levels of overt denial, ignore errors and may confabulate, argue, and justify their performance when someone calls attention to their miscues.

Neglect Right-hemisphere-damaged adults with *left hemispatial neglect* may fail to perceive tactile stimulation on the left side of the body and fail to notice visual or auditory stimuli in left-sided space. When individuals with left hemispatial neglect copy drawings or draw figures, objects, or scenes from memory, they tend to leave out left-side details. When individuals with left hemispatial neglect read printed materials, they may read only the material on the right side of the page and complain that the material makes no sense, as in the following transcript of a patient with right-hemisphere brain damage and left neglect who was asked to read a story from the *Discourse Comprehension Test* (Brookshire & Nicholas, 1993) (Box 8-1).

When individuals with hemispatial neglect read single words, they may ignore the leftmost letters in the words (e.g., reading *mistake* as *take*) or they may omit the left side of compound words (e.g., reading *blackboard* as *board*), provided that what they see represents a true word. When what they see does not represent a true word, individuals with hemispatial neglect may substitute or add initial letters to what they see to make a word (e.g., reading *chain* as *train* or *town* as *brown*). Longer words are more likely to be read incorrectly than are shorter words.

> When individuals with left hemispatial neglect substitute letters at the beginning of a word, their substitutions tend to contain the same number of letters as the substituted-for part of the target word, perhaps suggesting some sort of low-level awareness of the missed letters (Myers, 1999).

When individuals with left hemispatial neglect write sentences or texts they often displace what they write to the right side of the page, leaving an abnormally large margin on the left, which sometimes increases as the patient progresses down the page. Written lines produced by individuals with left hemispatial neglect tend to slant upward on the right, letters or words may be left out, and extra lines and strokes may be added to letters. Figure 8-1 shows a writing sample produced by a right-hemisphere-damaged patient who was describing the 10 test objects in the *Porch Index of Communicative Ability* (Porch, 1981a).

Individuals with left hemispatial neglect bump into objects on the left, and those in wheelchairs sometimes get trapped against the left side of doorways or other obstructions because they fail to perceive the obstruction and seem unaware of the obstruction even when trapped. Individuals with less severe neglect may attend to stimuli in their left hemispace if reminded, but they bump into objects on the left and may show other signs of inattention such as using only right-side trousers pockets or the right-side drawers and shelves of dressers, cupboards, and bureaus. Mild neglect may be detectable only with *simultaneous stimulation,* in which brief stimuli (such as flashes of light, gentle touches, or pinpricks) are presented simultaneously on both sides of the body. Individuals with mild neglect (sometimes called *hemispatial inattention*) do not perceive stimuli on the left when both sides are stimulated, but they perceive the stimuli when only the left side is stimulated.

Box 8-1. A Story told by a Patient with Right-Hemisphere Brain Damage

Stimulus Story

Fred and Ben were cousins who decided to go into business together painting houses. They put an ad in the paper and then spent all day Sunday getting their supplies organized. The next day, a woman named Mrs. Foster called and offered them their first job. She told them that she needed her house painted before Saturday because she wanted it to look nice for her daughter's wedding. Fred and Ben promised to work quickly and have the house painted by Thursday. They also offered to do the job at a reduced price because Mrs. Foster was their first customer. Mrs. Foster was pleased with their offer and told them to start painting whenever they were ready. Early the next morning, the men arrived at the Fosters' house and immediately went to work. By three o'clock they had finished the front of the house and were painting the trim on the upstairs windows. Then a man walked around the corner of the house and asked them what they were doing there. "Oh, you must be Mr. Foster," Ben responded. "I guess your wife forgot to tell you that she hired us to paint the house." The man frowned and replied, "But my name is Nelson. The Fosters live next door."

Transcript

(Patient comments and clinician responses are in italics.)

The patient begins: . . . went into business painting houses and then spent all day getting a woman named Mrs. Foster called . . . Mrs. Foster called . . . *Is this supposed to make sense?*

Clinician: *It should. Keep reading and we'll see if we can figure it out.*

Patient: *Well, all right. Should I start over?*

Clinician: *No, just keep reading from where you stopped.*

Patient: *Well, now I don't remember where I was.*

Clinician: *I think you had just finished reading this . . . Mrs. Foster called . . .*

Patient: *Okay* . . . Mrs. Foster called and told them she needed her house painted to look nice for her daughter's wedding. And have the house painted on Thursday . . . They had to have the house painted by Thursday at a reduced price because Mrs. Foster was pleased with their offer and told them they were ready . . . *Now it's not making sense again. What's going on here?*

Clinician: *Why not just keep reading and see what happens?*

Patient: *Well* . . . Early in the morning the men immediately set to work. By three o'clock they were painting the trim on the corner of the house. Then somebody came up and asked "Oh, are you Mr. Foster?" Ben responded . . . she hired us to paint the house . . . But my name is Nelson. The Fosters live next to me. . . . *So the guy painting the house was Ben . . .*

Clinician: *Well, what did you think of that?*

Patient: *I guess it's a story, but it doesn't make much sense. It could have been written a lot clearer.*

Comment

The patient fails to include material on the left side of the page, but when what he reads is grammatically and semantically unnatural, he realizes that something is wrong but attributes the problem to the printed material rather than to his reading of the material. As he reads he adjusts his starting place from line to line to maximize the grammaticality and meaningfulness of what he reads, but when the adjustment requires moving more than a few words he gets lost. As he progresses through the passage he begins changing words in the text to make it meaningful. When he finishes he knows that something was wrong in what he read, but he continues to believe that the problem is the material, rather than his reading.

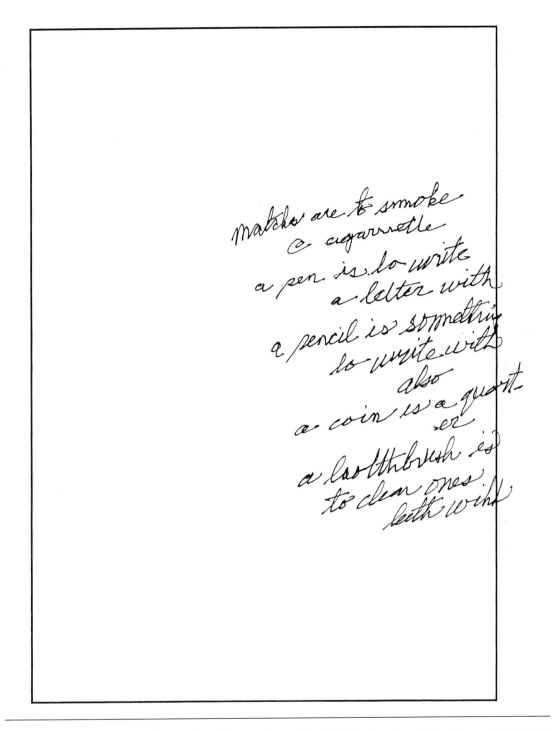

Figure 8-1 ■ A writing sample produced by a patient with right-hemisphere brain injury. The patient is describing in writing the 10 objects from the *Porch Index of Communicative Ability* (Porch, 1981a). The patient neglects the left-side test objects. The patient writes in cursive form, but what he writes is shifted rightward and sometimes crosses the right-side margin line. The patient begins writing partway down the page, and his written lines slant upward on the right. Several words contain extra strokes, and the patient fails to cross several *t*s (especially on the left).

Myers (1999) summarizes common symptoms of hemispatial neglect:

- Failure to respond to people, sounds, and objects to the left of the body midline
- Attending only to the right in self-care activities (e.g., dressing, shaving)
- Failure to move or attend to the left arm and leg
- Bumping into walls and doorways on the left
- Reading only the right-side parts of printed materials
- Displacing writing to the right side of the page
- Diminished awareness of physical and cognitive impairments
- Disinterest and lack of participation in rehabilitation

Neglect often affects right-hemisphere-damaged adults' use and placement of their arms and legs. Individuals with neglect often fail to use their left arm and leg to their full potential, although neurologic examination yields no evidence of left-sided weakness or sensory loss. This phenomenon sometimes is called *motor neglect.* When questioned, these individuals may claim that the left-side limbs are dead, useless, or do not belong to them. Wheelchair-bound individuals with neglect may allow their left arm to hang down beside the wheelchair, risking injury if fingers or hand become entangled in the wheel, and these individuals may allow their left foot to drag, rather than placing it on the footrest.

Neglect seems more than a perceptual or motor problem. Clinical reports and experimental investigations suggest that neglect may represent disrupted mental representations of external space, diminished ability to direct attention to left-sided space, or both. There are several accounts in the literature of right-hemisphere-damaged adults who, when they are asked to describe familiar spaces or scenes from memory, describe only right-sided space or describe right-sided space in greater detail than left-sided space. For example, a right-hemisphere-damaged woman who was asked to describe her home while mentally walking through it from the front to the back provided an elaborate description of the rooms on the right but ignored the rooms on the left. When she was asked to describe the same living space while mentally walking through it from the back to the front, she described the rooms on the previously neglected side and ignored those she previously had described.

Several theories have been proposed to explain why and how neglect happens. *Representational theories* (Bisiach & associates, 1981) propose that neglect is caused by disturbed internal representation of external space. Representational theories can explain the omission of left-side information when adults with neglect are asked to describe familiar scenes from memory. *Arousal theories* (Heilman, Schwartz, & Watson, 1978; and others) propose that right-hemisphere-damaged individuals' perceptual systems are less responsive to stimuli in the neglected space. *Attentional engagement theories* (Arguin & Bub, 1993) propose that individuals with neglect have difficulty directing attention to the neglected space, and *attentional disengagement theories* (Posner & associates, 1987) propose that these individuals' attention is captured and held by stimuli in non-neglected space, preventing them from redirecting it to stimuli on the neglected side.

Individuals with right-hemisphere brain injury and left neglect often exhibit signs of engagement and disengagement in everyday life. When sitting quietly, these individuals often lean toward the right and turn their head to the right, regardless of the surrounding environment. If sitting next to a blank wall on the right, these individuals will lean toward and look at the wall rather than attending to what is happening in the world away from the wall.

Support for attentional theories of neglect comes from studies showing positive effects of cueing, in which individuals with neglect are instructed to attend to left-sided space, and from studies showing that individuals with neglect tend to neglect the left side of *ipsilesional* space. (That is, they exhibit reduced sensitivity to visual stimuli in the left half of visual displays presented completely within the right visual field.) As this is written, there is no empiric evidence that clearly favors any of these theories.

Neglect may be caused by damage in either hemisphere, but neglect usually is more severe and persistent following right-hemisphere damage (Cummings, 1983). Although exact statistics are unknown, the literature suggests that two thirds or more of adults with right-hemisphere brain injury exhibit neglect, but less than one fifth of adults with left-hemisphere brain injury do so (Ogden, 1985; Schenkenberg, Bradford, & Ajax, 1980). Neglect can occur following injury in any cortical region, but it is most common and most severe after right parietal lobe injury (Mesulam, 1982; Watson & Heilman, 1979), especially following injuries affecting posterior and inferior regions of the right parietal lobe. Neglect occasionally follows subcortical injury (most often in the thalamus and basal ganglia), but the incidence of subcortical neglect is far lower than the incidence of cortical neglect (Ferro, Kertesz, & Black, 1987; Rafal & Posner, 1987; Vallar & Perani, 1986; Watson & Heilman, 1979; and others). Individuals with left-sided neglect often exhibit left visual field blindness, but individuals with no demonstrable visual field blindness may exhibit neglect (Willanger, Danielsen & Ankerhus; 1981). Neglect sometimes resolves either partially or completely in the first days or weeks after brain injury.

Constructional Impairment Many brain-injured adults perform poorly when they are asked to draw or copy geometric designs, create designs with colored blocks, reproduce two-dimensional stick figures, or reproduce three-dimensional constructions using wooden blocks. Deficient performance on such tasks, in the absence of visual perceptual or motor impairments that could cause it, is called *constructional impairment* (sometimes erroneously called *constructional apraxia*).

Apraxia is a disorder in which planning and execution of volitional sequential movements are disrupted. Constructional impairments represent visuospatial perceptual and organizational impairments, rather than motor-planning impairments.

Constructional impairments appear following injury in either brain hemisphere but are more frequent and more severe following right-hemisphere injury, especially injuries affecting the right parietal lobe or the right parieto-occipital region. Adults with left-hemisphere brain injury also make errors on constructional tests, and counting the number of errors made does not discriminate between those with left-hemisphere brain injury and those with right-hemisphere brain injury (Gainotti & Tiacci, 1970). Adults with right-hemisphere injury and adults with left-hemisphere injury do not, however, make the same kinds of errors.

Adults with right-hemisphere damage tend to respond quickly and impulsively. They make mistakes that they often try to correct by adding more lines to their drawings or by aimlessly rearranging stick or block designs. Adults with right-hemisphere damage tend to leave out details on the left side of drawings or constructions. Those with severe neglect reproduce only the right side. When adults with right-hemisphere brain injury copy drawings they may add extraneous lines, rotate and fragment the drawings, and render three-dimensional drawings in two dimensions. Their drawings look fragmented, disorganized, and crowded, and they often are misplaced to the right side of the page.

Adults with left-hemisphere damage tend to respond slowly and cautiously, with false starts, hesitations, and self-corrections, but they tend not to make gross mistakes that must be corrected by redrawing or adding lines to drawings or that require the individual to completely restructure stick or block designs. Adults with left-hemisphere damage simplify figures or constructions and produce drawings in which proportions and dimensionality are accurate but angles and lines are distorted (Lezak, 1983). Their drawings look incomplete and clumsy but coherent. Adults with left-hemisphere brain injuries benefit from having a model to copy, whereas those with right-hemisphere injuries do not (Hecaen & Assal, 1970). Many of these differences are apparent in Figure 8-2, which shows a set of figures copied by an adult with left-hemisphere brain injury and the same set of figures copied by an adult with right-hemisphere brain injury.

Topographic Impairment Individuals with topographic impairment (sometimes called *topological disorientation*) have difficulty relating to extrapersonal space. They have difficulty following familiar routes, reading maps, giving directions, and performing other tasks that depend on internal representations of external space. Myers (1994) has suggested that at least some of right-hemisphere-damaged adults' problems in this domain may arise from failure to recognize familiar landmarks or to learn new landmarks because they fail to attend to visual cues. Some individuals with topographic impairment compensate for the impairment by talking themselves through a sequence of directions. One right-hemisphere-damaged patient reported that he found his way

back to his room by talking himself through the following sequence:

> I go to the end of the hall and look both ways. I find the hall with the window at the end. I go down that hall. The first door past the nurses' station is my room.

Right-hemisphere-damaged adults' ability to talk themselves through a route sets them apart from individuals with disorientation and confusion, who also get lost easily but have no idea where they are or how they got there.

Geographic Disorientation Geographic disorientation is less common than topographic impairment, but the two often occur together (Tompkins, 1995). Individuals with geographic disorientation recognize at least the general nature of their surroundings but are mistaken about their geographic location. (A patient at a medical center in Minnesota believed that he was in a medical center in South Africa. Another patient at the same medical center believed that he was in a school in South Dakota.) Geographic disorientation, in its pure sense, is distinct from orientation to time and person. Individuals with geographic disorientation know the day, month, and year, and they know who they are and have at least a general sense of who those around them are but are confused about where they

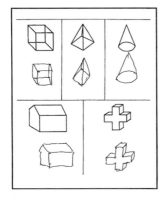 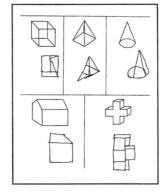

Figure 8-2 ■ **Performance on a figure-copying test by a patient with left-hemisphere brain injury** *(left)* **and a patient with right-hemisphere brain injury** *(right).*

are. The reasons for geographic disorientation are unknown. Geographic disorientation may arise from the affected individual's inability to construct a mental representation of geographic locations based on cues available from their immediate surroundings (Tompkins, 1995).

> Many hospitalized adults, non-brain-injured as well as brain-injured, lose track of what day it is after several days in the hospital because there are few reminders of what day it is in most hospitals, but most hospitalized adults know where they are geographically.

An unusual disturbance called *reduplicative paramnesia* occasionally follows right-hemisphere brain injury. Individuals with reduplicative paramnesia believe in the existence of duplicate persons, places, body parts, or events. One patient with reduplicative paramnesia claimed that there were two identical hospitals in his home city, another claimed to have two left legs, and a third claimed that she was living with two identical husbands. The causes of reduplicative paramnesia are not known, but its presence may be related to disturbed spatial perception and impaired visual memory. Reduplicative paramnesia is strongly related to injury in the right brain hemisphere, but a more precise localization within the right hemisphere has not been suggested.

Visuoperceptual Impairments Right-hemisphere-damaged adults typically have little difficulty identifying real objects or recognizing pictures or drawings of objects when they are portrayed naturalistically in prototypic views. Visuoperceptual impairments become apparent when right-hemisphere-damaged adults are asked to identify objects, pictures, or drawings that are incomplete, distorted, or otherwise changed from their traditional prototypic form (Myers, 1994). Right-hemisphere-damaged adults typically have difficulty identifying line drawings

of objects when one drawing is superimposed on another, and they typically fail to recognize familiar objects depicted in incomplete or fragmented form, shown in unusual orientation, or depicted with unusual size relationships (Figure 8-3). Right-hemisphere-damaged adults' visuospatial impairments seem less perceptual than organizational—they have no difficulty describing the visual characteristics of stimuli they fail to recognize. When visual stimuli are simple, clear, and unambiguous right-hemisphere-damaged adults respond normally, but when the stimuli are incomplete, degraded, or distorted, right-hemisphere-damaged adults are inclined to misinterpret them.

Facial Recognition Deficits Some adults with right-hemisphere brain injury are unable to recognize otherwise familiar persons by their facial features. They also perform poorly on other tasks that depend on perception and integration of facial features, such as identifying famous people from photographs and choosing pictures of people previously shown to them from a group containing previously seen pictures and previously unseen foils. This impairment is called *prosopagnosia* (from the Greek words for *face* and *knowledge*). These individuals' facial recognition deficits usually affect perception of cartoons and line-drawn faces as well as actual

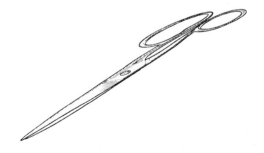

Figure 8-3 ■ **A drawing of a common object depicted in an unusual orientation. Patients with right-hemisphere brain injury often find it difficult to identify drawings that depict familiar objects in unusual orientations, with unusual size relationships, or in distorted form.**

faces and photographs, and they may extend beyond human faces—for example, accounts of a bird watcher who no longer recognized different species of birds and a farmer who no longer recognized his cows following right-hemisphere strokes (Albert & associates, 1981). Individuals who fail to recognize others by their facial features usually recognize them when they speak or by other features such as clothing, hair color and style, body type, or gait.

> Presumably the bird watcher still could tell different birds by their songs, and perhaps the farmer could tell his cows apart by the sound of their voices, their coloring, or the way they walked.

Some individuals with prosopagnosia have difficulty distinguishing between male and female faces, old and young faces, or human and animal faces. Facial recognition deficits are common following posterior right-hemisphere brain injury (Hecaen & Angelergues, 1962; Warrington & James, 1967; Whitely & Warrington, 1977), but persisting prosopagnosia probably requires bilateral damage (Albert & associates, 1981; Cohn, Neumann, & Wood, 1977; Damasio, 1985; Damasio & Damasio, 1983; Meadows, 1974). Facial recognition deficits seem to be independent of disordered visuospatial perception (McKeever & Dixon, 1981) and recognition of emotion (Cicone, Wapner, & Gardner, 1980; Ley & Bryden, 1979). Occasionally, a right-hemisphere-damaged patient with prosopagnosia claims that relatives and friends have been abducted and replaced by impostors—a condition called *Capgras' syndrome*.

Recognition and Expression of Emotion

Our experience of emotion is mediated by the limbic system, but our appreciation of others' emotions and our expression of personal emotions appear to be mediated in large part by the right hemisphere in right-handed adults (Tucker & Frederick, 1989). Right-hemisphere-damaged adults' impairments in appreciating emotions generally are attributed to deficiencies in three domains—*appreciating prosodic cues to emotion in others' speech, appreciating the emotional implications of facial expressions,* and *appreciating the emotional tone associated with stereotypic emotional situations* such as weddings or funerals.

> The limbic system includes phylogenetically old portions of the cerebral cortex, subcortical structures, and pathways connecting them to the diencephalon and brain stem. The functions of the limbic system are related to survival of the individual and continuation of the species, including eating behavior, aggression, expression of emotion, and endocrinal aspects of the sexual response.

Many right-hemisphere-damaged adults seem not to appreciate the significance of prosodic indicators of emotion. Whether this deficit actually represents an underlying disturbance of emotional competence is not clear. There is some evidence that right-hemisphere-damaged adults' insensitivity to prosodic indicators of emotion is caused by failure to perceive, discriminate, and process the acoustic information related to pitch and intonation patterns, rather than by failure to attach emotional significance to accurately perceived acoustic information. Patients who fail to attach appropriate meanings to prosodic indicators of emotion nevertheless can identify upward and downward vocal intonation patterns (Robin, Tranel, & Damasio, 1990).

Many investigators have reported that adults with right-hemisphere brain injury fail to correctly interpret facial expressions indicative of emotion (Blonder, Bowers, & Heilman, 1991; Cicone, Wapner, & Gardner, 1980; DeKosky & associates, 1980; and others). Right-hemisphere-damaged adults' interpretation of facial expression typically has been tested by presenting still photographs of people producing static representations of feigned emotions. Because movement cues to the expressions are not available, identification of the emotions portrayed in the photographs depends completely on analysis of visuospatial information (e.g., narrowing of eyes, mouth curvature). Because adults with right-hemisphere brain injury have difficulty analyzing visuospatial information and integrating individual features into a composite whole, it may be that what seems to be a problem in interpreting facial expression actually reflects an underlying impairment in the analysis and integration of visuospatial information (Myers, 1999).

Myers (1999) has commented that patients with right-hemisphere brain injury rarely complain about impaired recognition of facial expressions, perhaps because they are unaware of it.

Several studies have reported that adults with right-hemisphere brain injury perform poorly when asked to match the emotional tone of short stories with pictured scenes (Cicone, Wapner, & Gardner, 1980), identify emotions portrayed in pictured scenes (Bloom & associates, 1992; Cancelliere & Kertesz, 1990), or identify emotions portrayed in isolated spoken sentences (Blonder, Bowers, & Heilman, 1991). However, some contradictory evidence has been reported. Tompkins and Flowers (1985) reported that adults with right-hemisphere brain injury performed comparably to adults with left-hemisphere brain injury when asked to identify the emotions conveyed by spoken sentences. Myers (1994) has asserted that determining the emotional tone of situations, sentences, and narratives requires that individuals recognize that emotional tone is present, discriminate cues that signal emotions, and integrate the cues into an overall representation of an emotion—all of which characteristically are problems for adults with right-hemisphere brain injury.

In summary, many adults with right-hemisphere brain injury appear to have diminished appreciation of emotions conveyed by speech prosody, facial expression, narratives, or pictorial representations, at least when they are asked to identify the emotional tone of such materials presented in a test environment. However, it is not clear that their abnormal performance on these tasks actually reflects impaired appreciation of emotions and not impairment of some other cognitive process or processes. Regardless of the underlying reasons, many adults with right-hemisphere damage seem deficient in recognizing and expressing emotion in daily life interactions. They are insensitive to emotional tone conveyed by others' facial expression and tone of voice, and when they do assign emotional significance to spoken materials, facial expressions, body language, or situations, they often choose the wrong emotion.

Attentional Impairments

Attentional impairments are common in brain-injured adults, and adults with right-hemisphere brain injury are no exception. In fact, it is possible that many of the surface manifestations of right-hemisphere brain injury represent, at least in part, disturbances of underlying attentional processes. Many adults with right-hemisphere damage have difficulty focusing, maintaining, and shifting attention. These impairments make them distractible in treatment activities and interfere with many daily life activities. Attentional impairments make it difficult for these individuals to determine the overall meaning of situations and events, separate what is important from what is not, identify relationships among elements of information, maintain appropriate patterns of interactions with conversational partners, and maintain coherence in their speech and writing. Attentional impairments often make it difficult or impossible for right-hemisphere-damaged adults to maintain focus in treatment activities.

Attention no doubt represents the interaction of several cognitive processes, and some investigators have divided attentional processes into multiple components, which they believe represent different underlying skills. Adults with right-hemisphere brain injury may exhibit impairments in any or all of these attentional processes:

- *Arousal* denotes the physiologic and behavioral readiness to respond.
- *Vigilance* denotes ongoing sensitivity to stimulation.
- *Orientation* denotes direction of attention toward a stimulus.
- *Sustained attention* denotes maintenance of attention over time.
- *Selective attention* (sometimes called focused attention) denotes maintenance of attention in the presence of competing or distracting stimuli or attending to individual stimuli within an array.
- *Alternating attention* denotes moving attention from stimulus to stimulus in response to changing task requirements or changing intentions.
- *Divided attention* denotes performing more than one activity simultaneously (e.g., driving an automobile while carrying on a conversation).

GENERAL CONCEPTS 8-1

- Contemporary theories of hemispheric function depict the left hemisphere as better at processing *sequential, time-related* material that is suitable for linear processing and depict the left hemisphere as better at processing *nonlinear, spatially distributed* arrays.
- About one half of adults with right-hemisphere injury develop significant communicative impairments. Right-hemisphere-damaged adults with *cortical lesions* and *familial history of left-handedness* are most likely to develop communicative impairments.
- Patients with right-hemisphere brain injury are described in the literature as *insensitive to others and preoccupied with self; oblivious to social conventions; unconcerned about physical and mental impairments; verbose, tangential, and rambling in speech; insensitive to the meaning of implied or abstract material;* and *unable to grasp the overall significance of complex events.*

- The literature on right-hemisphere brain injury is biased toward patients with *anterior right-hemisphere* injuries because they are likely to be hospitalized longer than patients with posterior right-hemisphere injuries.
- Several perceptual abnormalities may follow right-hemisphere brain injuries. The perceptual abnormalities appear to be related to *disturbed or incomplete mental representations of visuospatial relationships, impaired attention,* or *a combination of the two.*
- *Denial of illness (anosognosia)* and *left hemispatial neglect* are common consequences of right-hemisphere brain injuries. Visual field blindness does not cause neglect, although patients with left hemispatial neglect often have left *homonymous hemianopia.*
- Several theories have been offered to explain neglect. *Arousal theories* propose that right-hemisphere-damaged adults are less sensitive to stimuli in neglected space. *Attentional engagement theories* propose that right-hemisphere-damaged adults have difficulty directing attention to neglected space. *Attentional disengagement theories* propose that right-hemisphere-damaged adults' attention is caught and held by stimuli in non-neglected space.
- *Topographic impairment* and *geographic disorientation* sometimes follow right-hemisphere brain injury. Patients with topographic impairment appear to have *distorted internal representations* of external space. Patients with geographic disorientation *confuse the geographic location* of familiar people, places, or things, perhaps because of difficulty inferring location from cues provided by the patient's surroundings.
- *Visuoperceptual impairments* (difficulty recognizing objects, pictures, or drawings presented in unusual formats) and *facial recognition deficits (prosopagnosia)* are common consequences of right-hemisphere brain injuries. These impairments may represent failure to integrate elements of visual informa-

tion into a coherent representation of the perceived stimulus.

- Many patients with right-hemisphere brain injuries appear *insensitive to the emotional tone* of facial expression, body language, situations, and verbal materials. Some patients with right-hemisphere brain injuries *fail to communicate emotional tone* by speech prosody, facial expression, and body language. It is not clear that these impairments are truly emotional in nature and not the result of impairment in some other cognitive processes.
- Attentional impairments are common following right-hemisphere brain injury. The impairments may affect *arousal, vigilance, orienting, sustained attention, selective attention, alternating attention,* and *divided attention.* Directly treating attentional impairments may prove more beneficial to patients than treating the surface manifestations of attentional impairments.

COMMUNICATIVE IMPAIRMENTS ASSOCIATED WITH RIGHT-HEMISPHERE DAMAGE

In addition to perceptual, affective, and attentional impairments, many adults with right-hemisphere damage have communicative impairments that make it difficult for them to communicate emotion; express themselves coherently and efficiently; comprehend humor, sarcasm, and nonliteral material; and interact appropriately in conversations.

Diminished Speech Prosody

The speech of many right-hemisphere-injured adults lacks normal variability in vocal pitch and loudness, making their speech monotonous and seemingly devoid of emotion. Many adults with right-hemisphere brain injury also exhibit reduced spontaneity and variety in the nonverbal movements that typically accompany speech (e.g., head nods, gestures). Although prosodic disturbances are most obvious in right-hemisphere-damaged adults' expression of emotion, they frequently affect their nonemotional utterances as well. These prosodic disturbances include:

- Slower-than-normal speech rate, with uniform spacing between sounds, syllables, and words, giving speech a robot-like quality
- Reduced emphatic stress in phrases and sentences (e.g., *George* wrecked Linda's car versus George wrecked *Linda's* car)
- Diminished pitch variability, leading to restricted intonation and failure to distinguish between questions (upward pitch change) and assertions (downward pitch change)

It is not clear which right-hemisphere-damaged adults are most likely to have prosodically flattened speech. Bryden and Ley (1983) and Shapiro and Danly (1985) attributed this phenomenon to damage in the right frontal lobe. Colsher, Cooper, and Graff-Radford (1987) subsequently challenged this conclusion, claiming that adults with right-hemisphere frontal lobe injury have essentially normal variability in vocal pitch. Myers (1994) and Tompkins (1995) comment that some right-hemisphere-damaged adults' reduced speech prosody may be caused by muscle weakness (dysarthria) rather than by an underlying affective impairment. Tompkins also noted that diminished speech prosody sometimes follows brain injury outside the right hemisphere.

Some right-hemisphere-damaged adults seem aware that their voice does not communicate their emotional state to listeners, and they compensate by communicating their emotional state with propositional speech (e.g., the right-hemisphere-damaged adult who, in the middle of a challenging treatment activity, said to the clinician [in a monotone], "You don't seem to realize it, so I guess I have to tell you that I'm tired of this and I wish you'd get lost."). That some right-hemisphere-damaged adults verbally compensate for their lack of prosody suggests that their prosodic deficiencies do not necessarily signify an underlying affective impairment. However, it is true that many of the same individuals who fail to communicate emotion via speech prosody also fail to appreciate emotions conveyed by others' speech prosody and facial expression, lending credence to the assumption that they have an underlying affective impairment.

Anomalous Content and Organization of Connected Speech

One of the most striking communicative impairments of right-hemisphere-damaged adults is their excessive, confabulatory, and sometimes inappropriate connected speech. These anomalies become apparent when right-hemisphere-damaged adults are placed in narrative production tasks in which they tell (or retell) stories in response to pictures, picture sequences, or stories told to them by another. The speech they produce under these conditions has been de-

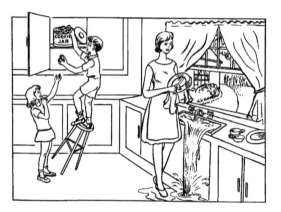

Well, this is a scene in a house. It looks like a fine spring day. The window is open. I guess it's not Minnesota, or the flies and mosquitoes would be coming in. Outside I see a tree and another window. Looks like the neighbors have their windows closed. There's a woman near the window wearing what appears to be an inexpensive pair of shoes. She's holding something that looks like a plate. On the counter there, there's a hat and two caps that look like they would fit on a child's head. The woman is looking out the window, and the water's on, and it's running on the floor. Looks like she needs to call the plumber. *(Clinician: "Is there anything over here?" Points to left side of picture.)* Well, I see two people... children... a boy and a girl. The boy is getting cookies from the cupboard and the girl is laughing and waving. There's also a stool. Perhaps the boy is stealing cookies and perhaps the girl...or the stool is going to fall. There's a window beside the cookie jar, but it doesn't have any curtains.

Figure 8-4 ■ **A right-hemisphere-damaged patient's description of the "cookie theft" picture from the *Boston Diagnostic Aphasia Examination.*** (From Goodglass, H., Kaplan, E., & Barresi, B. [2001]. *The assessment of aphasia and related disorders* [3rd ed.]. Philadelphia: Lippincott Williams & Wilkins.)

scribed as *excessive* and *rambling* (Gardner & associates, 1983); *repetitive* and *irrelevant* (Tompkins & Flowers, 1985); and *tangential, digressive,* and *inefficient* (Myers, 1994). They use more words but produce less information than either non-brain-injured adults or adults with left-hemisphere brain injury (Diggs & Basili, 1987; Myers, 1979; Rivers & Love, 1980). Their narratives tend to be fragmented and lack cohesion and an overall theme or point because they tend to focus on incidental details, fail to establish relationships among events, insert tangential comments, and permit personal experiences and opinions to intrude into their narratives. The transcript in Figure 8-4 shows several of these characteristics.

The patient begins by making three inferences. One is correct and relevant ("the scene is in a house"); the other two are potentially correct, but irrelevant ("it looks like a spring day, it must not be Minnesota"). The patient then continues on to enumerate elements on the right side of the drawing, with occasional interjection of irrelevant comments. After misinterpreting the plate and two cups shown on the counter as a hat and two caps (but inferring, from their size, that they must be for children), the patient begins to appreciate the problem with the overflowing sink. When the clinician directs the patient to the left side of the drawing, the patient begins by enumerating pictured elements, then eventually arrives at the appropriate interpretation. He ends by misinterpreting a cupboard door as a window, but correctly perceives that the "window" has no curtains. This patient's narrative contains many characteristics of right-hemisphere syndrome. He focuses on the right-hand side of the picture. He begins by enumerating pictured elements and slowly develops interpretations expressing relationships among the elements. He adds irrelevant and tangential comments. He misinterprets visual information. He makes inferences that may be consistent with his interpretation of visual information or underlying relationships but are inconsistent with the true sense of what is portrayed.

Impaired Comprehension of Narratives and Conversations

Adults with aphasia comprehend discourse better than their performance on tests of single-sentence comprehension suggests that they should, but the converse seems true for most adults with right-hemisphere damage (Brownell, 1988). Right-hemisphere-damaged adults' impairments in discourse comprehension reflect many of the same underlying disabilities that compromise both their production of narratives and their ability to get along in daily life—insensitivity to relationships among events, failure to judge the appropriateness of events or situations, and making premature assumptions based on incomplete analysis of events and situations. Many adults with right-hemisphere brain injury have particular difficulty comprehending implied meanings in narratives and conversations (Brownell & associates, 1986) and are seemingly unable to get beyond literal interpretations of what they hear or read. They interpret idiomatic expressions, figures of speech, and metaphors literally. They fail to identify incongruous, irrelevant, or absurd statements and offer confabulatory or bizarre reasons for accepting them as true. They are unable to judge the appropriateness of facts, situations, or characterizations in stories or conversations and cannot extract morals from stories. These deficiencies in discourse comprehension carry over into their comprehension of conversations. Right-hemisphere-damaged adults ". . . often seem to lack a full understanding of the context of an utterance, the presuppositions entailed, the affective tone, or the point of a conversational exchange. They appear to have difficulties in processing abstract sentences, in reasoning logically, and in maintaining a coherent stream of thought . . ." (Gardner & associates, 1983, p. 172). They respond to conversations in piecemeal fashion without making connections between related items of information, and they fail to appreciate situational variables that denote the nature of a conversation (Myers, 1999).

Right-hemisphere-damaged adults' difficulties with nonliteral language are not always complete.

Sometimes they fail to appreciate nonliteral meanings in one context but get them in another. For example, some right-hemisphere-damaged adults who cannot select pictures representing the implied meanings of nonliteral statements can explain them orally, some who cannot choose the best punch lines for printed jokes nevertheless choose endings that are surprising, and some who do not choose the appropriate printed responses to indirect requests such as "Can you open the door?" respond appropriately to their nonliteral meaning in daily life interactions (Tompkins, 1995). Some who misperceive or misinterpret elements of narratives in test situations perceive and interpret similar elements appropriately when narratives occur in daily life situations with more contextual support. Like adults with left-hemisphere damage, those with right-hemisphere damage tend to perform better in natural situations that provide situational context than in testing or treatment activities that limit that context.

Brownell and associates (1986) have suggested that right-hemisphere-damaged adults actually do make inferences suggested by discourse but that their inferences are premature and incorrect. According to Brownell and associates, these individuals are trapped by their erroneous inferences and are unable to reject or revise them when subsequent material shows their erroneous inferences to be incorrect. The problem for these individuals seems not to be that they cannot *make* inferences but that they are too readily led into inappropriate ones, from which they cannot escape.

Results reported by Nicholas and Brookshire (1995b) support Brownell and associates' suggestion that right-hemisphere-damaged adults can make inferences. Nicholas and Brookshire evaluated the *Discourse Comprehension Test* performance of 20 adults with right-hemisphere damage. The group of right-hemisphere-damaged adults correctly answered 80% of the questions that required inferences based on information given in short narratives. The right-hemisphere-damaged adults performed as well on questions related to implied information as either aphasic adults with left-hemisphere damage or traumatically brain-injured adults.

Tompkins and her associates offer a *suppression deficit hypothesis* to explain right-hemisphere-damaged adults' inability to escape from inappropriate inferences in discourse comprehension (Tompkins & associates, 1997; Tompkins & Lehman, 1998; Tompkins & associates, 1996; Tompkins & associates, 2001). The suppression deficit hypothesis assumes (1) that right-hemisphere-damaged adults activate multiple meanings when they interpret materials that are conducive to multiple interpretations and (2) that right-hemisphere-damaged adults are impaired in their ability to suppress interpretations that are initially activated but later prove irrelevant or incompatible.

> RHD [right-hemisphere-damaged] patients do generate inferences and hold on too long to those that become inappropriate to a final, integrated interpretation. (Tompkins & Lehman, 1998, p. 41)

Tompkins and Lehman (1998) offer the results of several studies of right-hemisphere-damaged adults' performance in on-line language processing tasks as support for a suppression deficit hypothesis. However, a study by Tompkins and associates (2001) failed to confirm the existence of suppression deficit specific to right-hemisphere-damaged adults. Under the conditions of the study both normal elderly adults and adults with right-hemisphere damage failed to suppress initial inferences that subsequently were shown to be inappropriate. As this is written, the suppression deficit hypothesis awaits definitive confirmation.

A suppression deficit hypothesis conceivably could explain other prototypic right-hemisphere-damage impairments such as impulsivity; tangentiality in speech; social inappropriateness; and difficulty with idioms, metaphor, and humor, although Tompkins and her associates make no such claims.

Brownell and his associates have asserted that right-hemisphere-damaged adults' problems in comprehending discourse may be attributable to impaired *theory of mind* (Brownell & Friedman, 2001; Brownell & associates, 2000; Happe, Brownell, & Winner, 1999; Winner & associates, 1998). *Theory of mind* denotes the ability to appreciate ". . . the contents of other people's minds—their beliefs and emotions—to understand their actions and utterances" (Brownell & Friedman, 2001, p. 197). Brownell and associates base their assertions concerning adults with right-hemisphere brain injury on the results of several studies in which right-hemisphere-damaged adults performed tasks in which they were asked to distinguish lies from jokes (Winner & associates, 1998), evaluate speakers' choice of terms with which to refer to people who were not present (Brownell & associates, 1997), or comprehend stories that depend on appreciating story participants' beliefs (Happe, Brownell, & Winner, 1999). According to Brownell and his associates, accurate performance in these tasks requires that those doing the tasks appreciate others' mental states, emotions, knowledge, and beliefs.

Right-hemisphere-damaged adults as a group performed poorly on tasks that depended on "theory of mind," whereas their performance on tasks that required comprehension of material that did not depend on "theory of mind" approximated that of normal elderly adults. The results of their studies led Brownell and his associates to consider impaired theory of mind a possible explanation for other characteristic signs of right-hemisphere brain damage such as anosognosia:

> . . . it may be fruitful to think of acquired RHD [right-hemisphere damage] as (in some cases) a syndrome of impaired theory of mind. (Happe, Brownell, & Winner, 1999, p. 230)

Group performance did not, however, always represent the performance of individuals in the groups:

> Not all of our RHD patients were equally impaired, a few were not measurably impaired at all. Some-

what more surprising is that some control subjects consistently performed poorly. An impaired ability to conceptualize others' mental states may thus be a non-specific marker for various conditions, including but not limited to focal right-hemisphere damage. (Winner & associates, 1998, p. 101)

Although a theory-of-mind explanation for right-hemisphere-damaged adults' impairments may be intuitively appealing, definitive evidence for its centrality in right-hemisphere-damaged adults' impairments is not currently available. The studies in which apparent theory-of-mind impairments in right-hemisphere-damaged adults have been demonstrated have used *metalinguistic tasks* in which participants make after-the-fact interpretations or judgments about printed or spoken situations or vignettes. They have not shown theory-of-mind deficits when right-hemisphere-damaged adults are called on to exercise theory of mind in natural situations. Tompkins and Lehman (1998) have commented that in metalinguistic tasks:

> . . . the mental effort and conscious awareness of stimulus properties that are required by these kinds of tasks render them inappropriate for assessing the relatively automatic operations that are integral to language processing and other aspects of cognitive functioning. (p. 31)

Also, it is not clear that right-hemisphere-damaged adults' differential performance on theory-of-mind tasks and non-theory-of-mind tasks uniquely depends on theory of mind because the tasks in which right-hemisphere-damaged adults exhibit theory-of-mind impairments appear to require more effortful cognitive processing than non-theory-of-mind tasks. What appears to be impaired theory of mind actually may reflect the increased processing demands of theory-of-mind tasks relative to control (non-theory-of-mind) tasks.

Pragmatic Impairments

Pragmatic impairments affect the social and interactional aspects of language, such as turn-taking, topic maintenance, social conventions, and eye

In a study by Winner and associates (1998), right-hemisphere-damaged adults and normal controls listened to short stories that ended either with an ironic joke or a lie by one character. Participants in the study answered questions about story characters' mental states. First-order mental states represented one character's knowledge (X knows . . .). Second-order mental states represented one character's knowledge of what another character knew (X knows that Y knows . . .). Right-hemisphere-damaged adults' appreciation of first-order mental states approximated that of the control group, but their appreciation of second-order mental states was impaired significantly. Winner and associates attributed the right-hemisphere-damaged adults' impaired performance to impaired theory of mind. However, inferring second-order mental states seems a more demanding task in terms of processing workload, making the source of the right-hemisphere-damaged adults' impaired performance unclear.

contact. Pragmatic impairments are common consequences of right-hemisphere brain injury. Many right-hemisphere-damaged adults begin and end conversations abruptly; are poor at maintaining eye contact with conversational partners; talk excessively and without regard for their listener; have difficulty staying on topic; interject irrelevant, tangential, and inappropriate comments into conversations; and fail to make needed conversational repairs. Many right-hemisphere-damaged adults also are insensitive to rules governing conversational turn-taking, especially those related to "yielding the floor" to conversational partners.

Not all right-hemisphere-damaged adults are pragmatically inappropriate in conversations. Prutting and Kirchner (1987) evaluated the conversational behavior of right-hemisphere-damaged adults while they engaged in a 15-minute conversation with another adult. Prutting and Kirchner tabulated the occurrence of 30 categories of appropriate or inappropriate behaviors. As a group the right-hemisphere-damaged adults failed to maintain adequate eye contact, produced speech with diminished emotional tone, were slow in responding to the conversational partner's utterances, deviated from conversational topics, and talked too much. However, not all exhibited this pattern. Of 9 right-hemisphere-damaged subjects, 2 had violations in only 1 category (eye contact), whereas 1 subject had violations in 13 of the 30 categories. Prutting and Kirchner's results at the group level are consistent with descriptions of right-hemisphere-damaged adults' conversational behavior found in the literature, but it is clear that not all adults with right-hemisphere brain injury fit the stereotypic description.

Clinician: "Well, Mr. Spencer, what are you planning to do this afternoon?"
Patient: "Well, I have OT." (occupational therapy)
Clinician: "What are you doing in OT?"
Patient: "Yesterday they were having us bake a cake. From a mix in a box. White cake with pink icing. It looked awful and it tasted worse."
Clinician: "Why were you baking a cake?"
Patient: "It wasn't just me. There were a couple or three other people in on it. I don't have the foggiest why they were there or what planet they came from. How come you're wearing that scarf around your neck? Are you cold?"
Clinician: "No, it's what you call a fashion accessory. It adds some color. Do you like it?"
Patient: "Maybe if you were sitting on a horse."

Kennedy & associates (1994) evaluated 12 right-hemisphere-damaged adults' conversational behaviors as they conversed with non-brain-injured adults. They divided the conversational behaviors into two categories. One category represented *topic-related skills* (introducing topics, maintaining topics, elaborating on topics, and terminating topics). The other represented *turn-taking skills* (making assertions, requesting information or action, communicating emotion, acknowledging the other's contributions, and committing to a future action).

The two groups did not differ significantly in topic-related skills but differed in turn-taking. The right-hemisphere-damaged group made significantly more assertions than the non-brain-injured group, but they also made significantly fewer requests for information. The right-hemisphere-damaged group took more conversational turns but said fewer words in each turn (which, as Kennedy and associates commented, may be one reason that they took more turns). Kennedy and associates commented that several right-hemisphere-damaged subjects spent most of their turns talking about themselves and rarely asked their conversational partners for information. They also commented that some right-hemisphere-damaged adults introduced new topics after their conversational partner had indicated the conversation was over, suggesting that they were insensitive to their conversational partner's intent. (*Clinician:* "I've really enjoyed talking with you. Perhaps we can do this again someday soon." *Patient:* "Tonight I'm going to the football game with my brother.")

There was great variability among the right-hemisphere-damaged participants in Kennedy and associates' study, with some participants exhibiting severely impaired conversational skills and others appearing essentially normal, leading Kennedy and associates to comment that right-hemisphere-damaged adults' premorbid conversational style should be considered when evaluating their postmorbid conversational skills.

In combination, the results reported by Kennedy and her associates and by Prutting and Kirchner show that not all adults with right-hemisphere damage have significant pragmatic impairments, and they also show that those who are pragmatically impaired do not necessarily exhibit the same impairments. Consequently, treatment of right-hemisphere-damaged adults'

This could be said for all aspects of communication and related skills for all categories of brain-injured adults.

pragmatic impairments must be based on careful analysis of the performance of individuals.

TESTS FOR ASSESSING ADULTS WITH RIGHT-HEMISPHERE BRAIN INJURY

Objective assessment of right-hemisphere-damaged adults' linguistic, cognitive, and communicative abilities received little attention before the mid 1970s and consequently it is considerably less sophisticated than assessment of aphasic adults, which has been going on for more than 50 years. At the time this is written, three standardized procedures for evaluation of adults with right-hemisphere brain injury have been published and several nonstandardized procedures have been reported in the literature.

Standardized Procedures

The *Right Hemisphere Language Battery* (RHLB; Bryan, 1989) contains seven subtests:

1. The *metaphor picture subtest* assesses comprehension of spoken metaphors such as *under the weather* or *keep it under your hat* by requiring the patient to choose a picture that represents the metaphor from a set of four pictures.
2. The *written metaphor subtest* assesses comprehension of similar metaphors in printed form by requiring the patient to choose a sentence that expresses the meaning of a printed metaphor from a set of four sentences.
3. The *comprehension of inferred meaning subtest* assesses appreciation of implied meanings expressed by short, spoken narratives.
4. The *appreciation of humor subtest* assesses the patient's ability to choose, from four printed sentences, the correct humorous punch line for printed jokes.
5. The *lexical semantic subtest* is a spoken-word-to-picture-matching subtest in which the patient points to pictures named by the examiner from among foils representing semantic, phonologic, or visual similarities to the target picture.
6. In the *production of emphatic stress subtest* the examiner reads the first clause of a two-clause sentence aloud, and the patient reads

the second, which is designed to elicit certain patterns of emphatic stress (e.g., *Clinician:* "He sold the *large* car and . . ." *Patient:* ". . . bought a *small* one.").

7. The *discourse analysis rating* permits the examiner to rate a patient's cumulative performance during the test, while in conversation with the examiner, and while doing a picture-description task. Ratings are assigned in 11 categories (such as *humor, variety,* and *turn-taking*) using a four-point scale for each rating.

The RHLB manual provides a general description of hemispheric specialization for language, the major behavioral consequences of right-hemisphere brain injury, and a summary of some literature on language processing by the right hemisphere. The manual also provides administration and scoring instructions for RHLB subtests, a summary of studies using the RHLB, a section on test interpretation and applications, plus appendices containing a rating scale for discourse and a table for converting RHLB raw scores to T scores.

The RHLB is standardized on 30 adults with vascular right-hemisphere damage, 10 adults with nonvascular right-hemisphere damage, 30 adults with vascular left-hemisphere damage, 10 adults with nonvascular left-hemisphere damage, and 30 neurologically normal adults. Means and standard deviations for right-hemisphere-damaged, left-hemisphere-damaged, and normal groups on each subtest are provided. Significant and nonsignificant differences among the three groups on each subtest (measured by analysis of variance) are reported. Test-retest reliability (evaluated by *t*-tests and correlation coefficients) is reported for each subtest, and correlations among the subtests of the RHLB are provided.

The RHLB provides a reasonably comprehensive look at the major communicative functions likely to be affected by right-hemisphere brain injury. However, as Tompkins (1995) has noted, the RHLB has several fairly serious deficiencies in reliability and validity and an inadequate normative sample.

The *Mini Inventory of Right Brain Injury* (MIRBI; Pimental & Kingsbury, 1989) is a standardized test that, according to the authors, can be used to identify the presence of right-hemisphere brain injury, determine the severity of right-hemisphere brain injury, identify the strengths and weaknesses of right-hemisphere-damaged adults, guide treatment, and document progress.

The MIRBI contains 27 test items divided among 10 categories: *visual scanning* (2 items), *integrity of gnosis* (finger identification, tactile perception, two-point tactile discrimination—3 items); *integrity of body image,* including neglect (1 item); *reading and writing* (5 items); *serial 7s* (e.g., subtracting 7 from 100, subtracting 7 from the remainder—1 item); *clock drawing* (1 item); *affective language* (repeating sentences with happy intonation and sad intonation—2 items); *appreciation of humor, incongruities, absurdities, figurative language* (8 items); *similarities* (8 items); and *affect and general behavior* (observation and rating by examiner—4 items).

The test manual contains sections on administration, scoring, and test interpretation and a summary of MIRBI results for 30 adults with right-hemisphere brain injury, 13 adults with left-hemisphere brain injury, and 30 non-brain-injured adults. Correlations between MIRBI scores and age, education, and time post-onset are reported. Comparisons of overall MIRBI scores and scores on each item are reported for the three groups. Sections on the reliability and validity of the MIRBI are also included. Because it contains only 35 items spread across 10 categories, the MIRBI seems best used as a screening test to identify individuals who may have communication impairments that may be assessed in greater detail by additional testing.

The *Rehabilitation Institute of Chicago Evaluation of Communicative Problems in Right-Hemisphere Dysfunction-Revised (RICE-R)* (Halper & associates, 1996) includes:

- An interview with the patient
- Observation of the patient in interactions with family members and hospital staff
- Ratings of attention; eye contact; awareness of illness; and orientation to place, time, and person

- Ratings of facial expression, speech intonation, and topic maintenance in conversation
- Four tests of visual scanning and tracking
- Ratings of written expression
- A scale for rating pragmatic communication skills
- A story-retelling task
- A metaphoric language test

Cut-off scores for assigning a severity rating to an individual's level of impairment are provided for each subtest. The RICE-R is standardized on 40 adults with right-hemisphere brain injury and 36 non-brain-damaged adults.

Nonstandardized Procedures

Gordon and associates (1984) described an extensive nonstandardized protocol for evaluation of adults with right-hemisphere damage. The protocol provides for assessment of:

- *Visual scanning and visual inattention* (neglect and visuospatial abilities)
- *Activities of daily living skills* (arithmetic, reading, copying)
- *Sensorimotor integration* (tactile perception, estimation of body midline, manual dexterity)
- *Visual integration* (face recognition, visual assembly, figure-ground discrimination, and copying geometric forms)
- *Higher cognitive and perceptual functions* (verbal and performance subtests from the *Wechsler Adult Intelligence Scale*)
- *Linguistic and cognitive flexibility* (analogies, auditory comprehension, generative naming, and logical memory)
- *Affective state* (comprehension of affect, plus depression and mood ratings made by the examiner)

Gordon and associates tested 385 right-hemisphere-damaged adults with their protocol, but the number of participants tested differed across subtests. They provide numerous statistics for each subtest. For many subtests the data are subdivided according to patient variables such as age, education, or presence of visual field deficit. Although not standardized, the protocol describes materials and procedures for numerous tests of linguistic, cognitive, perceptual, and affective functions and provides a large corpus of data about how adults with right-hemisphere damage perform on those tests. It should prove useful to clinicians who are looking for assessment materials or need information about how adults with right-hemisphere damage perform on tests such as those in the protocol. The protocol includes some standardized tests as subtests, many of which have been revised since the Gordon and associates report, so the norms provided will not be usable with current versions of the standardized tests (Tompkins, 1995).

Adamovich and Brooks (1981) described a procedure for evaluating the communicative deficits of adults with right-hemisphere brain injury. Their procedure includes tests of auditory comprehension, oral expression, and reading from the *Boston Diagnostic Aphasia Examination* (Goodglass & Kaplan, 1983); the *Revised Token Test* (McNeil & Prescott, 1978); the *Hooper Visual Organization Test* (Hooper, 1983); the *Boston Naming Test* (Kaplan, Goodglass, & Weintraub, 1983); the *Word Fluency Task* (Borkowski, Benton, & Spreen, 1967); and portions of the verbal absurdities, verbal opposites, and likenesses and differences subtests of the *Detroit Tests of Learning Aptitude-2* (Hammill, 1985).

The Adamovich and Brooks procedures are unstandardized, do not have adequate norms, and do not have documented reliability or validity. However, they may prove useful as a source of materials and ideas for locally constructed protocols for evaluation of adults with right-hemisphere brain injury.

Tests of Pragmatic Abilities

Right-hemisphere-damaged adults' pragmatic abilities typically are assessed with rating scales, not all of which were designed for use with right-hemisphere-damaged adults. The RHLB and the RICE each contain short scales for rating pragmatic behaviors. The RHLB provides a scale for rating discourse that addresses several categories of pragmatic behavior:

* *Supportive routines* (e.g., greetings, thanks)

* *Assertive routines* (e.g., complaining, demanding, criticizing)
* *Formality* (formality of language and behavior)
* *Turn-taking* (taking and yielding the conversational "floor")
* *Meshing* (pace, timing, and pauses)

The RICE-R scale provides for rating 12 pragmatic behaviors divided among four categories:

1. *Nonverbal communication* (intonation, facial expression, eye contact, gestures, and movements)
2. *Conversational skills* (initiation, turn-taking, verbosity)
3. *Use of linguistic context* (topic maintenance, presupposition)
4. *Referencing skills* (organization and completeness of a narrative)

The RHLB's coverage of truly pragmatic behaviors is limited. The scale in the RICE-R has enough detail to make it useful as a screening measure or as a quick assessment of changes in pragmatic behaviors as a consequence of treatment.

The *Pragmatic Protocol* (Prutting & Kirchner, 1987) permits assessment of pragmatic behaviors in conversational interactions. Users score the occurrence of inappropriate pragmatic behaviors while the patient engages in 15 minutes of conversation with a familiar partner. Inappropriate pragmatic behaviors are assigned to one of 30 categories, representing *verbal aspects* such as speech acts, topic maintenance, turn-taking, and communicative style; *paralinguistic aspects* such as vocal intensity and quality, prosody, and fluency; and *nonverbal aspects* such as physical proximity, posture, and eye contact (Figure 8-5).

The scoring procedures for the *Pragmatic Protocol* overemphasize violations because any occurrence of inappropriate behavior in a category causes that category to be marked deficient, even though the person being evaluated may have had several occurrences of appropriate behavior in the same category. Consequently, the person being evaluated is penalized for a single occurrence of inappropriate behavior in a category but gets no credit for appropriate be-

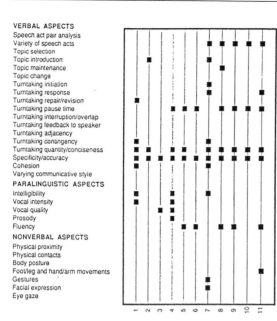
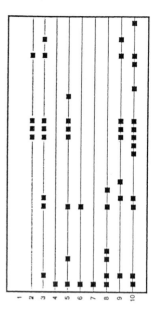

Figure 8-5 ■ **Patterns of performance on the *Pragmatic Protocol* for adults with left-hemisphere brain injuries and adults with right-hemisphere brain injuries. Adults with left-hemisphere damage** *(left)* **tend to be deficient in pause time, quantity/conciseness, specificity, accuracy of speech, and speech fluency. Adults with right-hemisphere damage** *(right)* **tend to be deficient in adjacency; contingency; and quantity/conciseness of turns, prosody, and eye gaze.**

haviors in the same category, even when the appropriate behaviors outnumber the inappropriate ones.

In its published form, the *Pragmatic Protocol* seems best used as a screening instrument to identify problem areas that then can be evaluated in greater detail by counting both appropriate behaviors and inappropriate behaviors in problem categories. Prutting and Kirchner apparently agree because they suggest that a patient's performance on the *Pragmatic Protocol* should lead to detailed assessment of the patient's pragmatic performance, focusing on inappropriate pragmatic behaviors identified by the *Pragmatic Protocol*. They also recommend that clinicians use the results of the detailed assessment to determine the probable impact of the inappropriate behaviors on daily life interactions.

The *Communicative Effectiveness Index* (CETI; Lomas and associates, 1989) is a rating scale designed to assess severely aphasic adults' functional communication, but it may be useful for some in assessing severely impaired right-hemisphere-damaged adults' functional communication. The CETI is described in Chapter 3.

Communication Activities in Daily Living-2nd Edition (CADL-2; Holland, Frattali, & Fromm, 1998), like the CETI, was designed to assess aphasic adults' functional communication, but it may be used to assess the communicative effectiveness of adults with right-hemisphere damage. Because CADL-2 samples communicative behavior in a number of contexts other than conversational interactions, using it together with a conversationally oriented instrument such as the *Pragmatic Protocol* may provide a more comprehensive picture of right-hemisphere-damaged adults' pragmatic strengths and weaknesses than use of either instrument by itself. CADL-2 is described in Chapter 3.

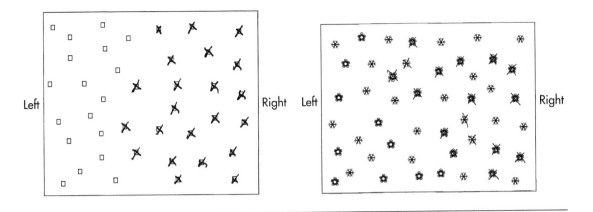

Figure 8-6 ■ A simple cancellation test for neglect *(left)* and a more complex one *(right)* completed by a patient with right-hemisphere brain injury. The patient was instructed to cross out all the boxes on the page on the left and to cross out only the flowers on the page on the right. The patient shows evidence of neglect on both tests. The patient also erroneously crossed out several snowflakes on the page on the right.

Tests of Visual and Spatial Perception, Attention, and Organization

Adults with right-hemisphere brain injury often have difficulty in tasks requiring perception of complex visual stimuli and appreciation of spatial relationships. These difficulties appear to reflect attentional and integrational impairments, such as inattention to visual stimuli (especially on the side contralateral to the patient's brain injury), diminished ability to perceive or discriminate complex stimuli, and inability to integrate or synthesize individual elements of complex visual stimuli into a meaningful whole. Consequently, tests of visual attention and organization are an important part of the assessment protocol for adults who may have right-hemisphere damage.

Most tests for visual inattention *(neglect)* are paper-and-pencil tests. *Cancellation tests* are the most common. In cancellation tests the patient is asked to mark, circle, or cross out lines, letters, or figures (e.g., stars, crosses) printed at various locations on a printed page. Individuals with neglect tend to miss stimuli on the side of the page contralateral to their brain injury. Albert's (1973) *Test of Visual Neglect* is typical. The patient is given a sheet of paper on which

short lines have been drawn in random locations and is asked to cross out each line. A variation on these simple cancellation tests is provided by the *Bells Test* (Gauthier, Dehaut, & Joanette, 1989). In the *Bells Test* the test-taker is required to circle drawings of bells that are scattered across the page and interspersed with drawings of other objects. Because test-takers must selectively circle only the drawings of bells, the *Bells Test* is more difficult than straight cancellation tasks and may be a more sensitive test of inattention than straight cancellation tasks (Gauthier, Dehaut, & Joanette, 1989).

Figure 8-6 *(left)* shows a simple cancellation test in which a patient with left neglect was asked to cross out small squares. Figure 8-6 *(right)* shows a more complex cancellation test in which a patient with left neglect was asked to cross out flowers and ignore snowflakes.

Line bisection tests provide another way to test for visual neglect. The patient is given a page on which several horizontal lines of different lengths are printed, and he or she draws a short vertical line on each line to divide it into two equal halves. Individuals with neglect tend to divide the lines so that the segment in the

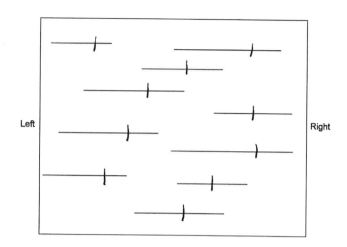

Figure 8-7 ■ A right-hemisphere-damaged patient's performance on a line-bisection test. The patient's line bisection marks are displaced to the right, toward non-neglected space.

Left

Right

neglected visual field is longer than the segment in the intact field—the bisecting line is displaced into the non-neglected half of the visual field, as in Figure 8-7. Displacement of the patient's dividing mark toward the non-neglected half-field tends to increase as lines move farther into the neglected visual field.

> Myers (1999) suggests that the lines in line bisection tasks should be about 1 inch (25 cm) long. According to Myers, shorter lines are too easy to bisect and longer lines create too much variability in non-brain-damaged adults' line bisection performance to make them a reasonable test for right-hemisphere-injured adults.

Copying and drawing tests are yet another way to test for visual neglect. In copying tests the patient is given a drawing to copy. (Often the drawing is of a symmetric object with more or less mirror image properties on each side of the drawing's midline—for example, a clock face, a daisy, or a human figure.) Individuals with neglect tend to omit detail from the side of the drawing contralateral to their brain injury (Figure 8-8). Myers (1999) recommends that drawings used to test neglect should have a midline with an equal number of objects on each

side of the midline and an equal number of lines on the left side and right side of each object.

In *drawing from memory tests* the patient is asked to draw familiar objects or simple scenes from memory. Individuals with neglect tend to leave out detail on the side of the drawing contralateral to their brain injury (Figure 8-9).

Scanning tests are still another way to test for visual neglect. In scanning tests the patient is given a page on which a horizontal array of numbers, letters, or (less frequently) objects is printed and the patient is asked to circle or cross out every occurrence of a target item (e.g., all occurrences of the letter B in a line of randomly arranged alphabet letters). Scanning tests resemble cancellation tests, except that in scanning tests the stimuli are in horizontal linear arrays, rather than random arrays, and in scanning tests there are more distractors (stimuli not to be marked).

The *Behavioural Inattention Test* (Wilson, Cockburn, & Halligan, 1987) is a standardized test battery for assessing neglect. It is unique among neglect tests in its inclusion of subtests to assess performance in daily life activities that might be affected by neglect (e.g., reading maps, dialing telephones, or reading menus and newspaper articles) in addition to traditional paper-and-pencil tests.

Horner and associates (1989) suggested that it may take more than one test of neglect to identify the presence of neglect in many right-hemisphere-

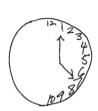
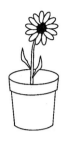
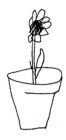

Figure 8-8 ■ A clock face drawn from memory and a flower copied by a patient with right-hemisphere damage and neglect.

Figure 8-9 ■ A scene copied by a patient with right-hemisphere damage and neglect. The stimulus drawing is on top and the patient's reproduction is on the bottom. (Courtesy Penelope Myers, Ph.D.)

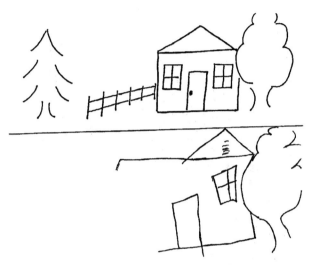

damaged adults' test performance. They administered tests of line bisection, drawing from memory, copying simple drawings, reading, and writing to 106 adults with right-hemisphere brain injury and reported that no single test identified the presence of neglect in all who had neglect.

Myers (1999) concurs and recommends that combinations of neglect tests be administered to ensure that neglect, when present, is detected. She also suggests that a patient's combined score on several tests of neglect may give the best estimate of the overall severity of neglect. Myers recommends the following combination of tasks for assessing neglect:

- A simple cancellation task
- Copying a drawing
- Drawing from memory (e.g., a clock, a human figure)
- Line bisection

Myers recommends calculating a left–right ratio for each of these tests (*elements missing in the left half of the drawing versus elements missing in the right half of the drawing*). According to Myers, ratios greater than 1 denote the presence of left neglect, with larger ratios denoting more severe neglect.

Tests of Component Attentional Processes

Although attentional processes implicitly are tested in many of the tests described previously, clinicians sometimes supplement them with tests that assess specific attentional processes in more detail.

Sustained attention may be assessed with cancellation and scanning tests or with *trail-making tasks* and *mazes*. In *trail-making tasks* the patient is given a sheet of paper on which sequences of letters, numerals, or a combination of letters and numerals are printed in a quasi-random array (Figure 8-10). The patient is asked to draw lines connecting the letters or numerals in sequence, according to a rule (e.g., 1-A-2-B, and so on). In *maze tasks,* the patient is asked to draw a continuous line to trace a path from the beginning to the end of the maze (Figure 8-11). Both tasks require the patient to maintain a mental representation of the appropriate path as they draw. Making the paths longer and more complex increases the difficulty of the tasks.

Some *visual sustained-attention tests* may be presented by means of a personal computer. Visual stimuli (colored squares, dots, flashes of light, and similar stimuli) appear on the computer monitor screen at unpredictable times and at unpredictable locations. The patient presses a key on the computer keyboard to report the occurrence of each stimulus. The computer keeps a record of hits, misses, reaction times, and the overall time taken to complete the test. Some *auditory sustained-attention tests* may be presented via audiotape recordings, and a few may be presented by means of a personal computer. Auditory sustained-attention tasks require the person doing the task to maintain attention to mixed strings of auditory stimuli and report the occurrence of designated targets (e.g., clicks, tones).

Selective attention customarily is assessed with tasks like those used to test sustained attention but with competing or distracting stimuli added. For example, an auditory sustained-attention test in which the patient signals when they hear a designated tone can be made into a selective attention test by embedding the designated tones in a series of competing or distract-

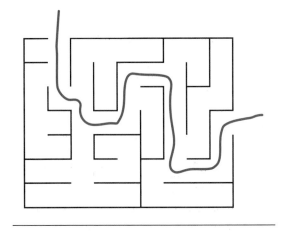

Figure 8-11 ■ **A simple maze.**

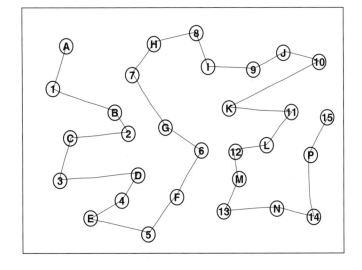

Figure 8-10 ■ **A trail-making test. The test-taker creates a path by alternately connecting letters and numerals.**

ing sounds. A sustained-attention test in which the patient is expected to report the occurrence of a single target stimulus (e.g., a chirp or a tone with a given frequency) becomes a selective attention test when the target sounds are embedded in strings of nontarget sounds and the patient is expected to report only the target sounds.

Some paper-and-pencil cancellation tests also qualify as selective attention tests if the patient must identify and mark stimuli meeting a certain criterion and pass over those that do not or if distracting material is included with or overlaid on the test stimuli. The *Stroop Test* is a widely used test of selective attention. In the *Stroop Test* the test-taker is shown a set of color names printed in ink colors that conflict with the color names (e.g., the word *red* printed in blue ink). The speed with which the tested individual reads the printed words is compared with the speed at which the individual names the colors in which the words are printed. Typically it takes longer to read words printed in conflicting colors than to identify ink colors. Large differences between the two are considered indicators of impaired selective attention.

The distinction between sustained attention and selective attention is in some respects an artificial one because even in simple sustained-attention tasks the patient must selectively attend to the visual or auditory stimuli and not to some other aspect of the task such as the label on the computer monitor, the background noise on the auditory stimulus tape, or the pattern on the wallpaper.

Tests of *alternating attention* require the tested individual to refocus attention in response to changing task requirements. Most are sustained-attention tests in which response requirements periodically are changed. A patient may be placed in a cancellation task that begins with the patient crossing out the odd numbers in a random list of numbers. When the patient's performance has stabilized, the examiner says *even,* and the patient is expected to cross out only the even numbers. The test continues with the examiner periodically changing the target

response each time the patient's performance stabilizes. In a more challenging alternating attention test, the patient begins a serial calculation task by subtracting 5 from a specified number, subtracting 5 from the remainder, and so on. When the patient's performance stabilizes, the examiner says *add,* and the patient reverses direction and begins adding by 5. The task continues with the examiner changing from addition to subtraction or vice versa each time the patient's performance stabilizes.

Divided-attention tests come in two formats. One format requires test-takers to participate in two tasks simultaneously and to make different responses in each task. For example, the tested individual may be required to perform a paper-and-pencil cancellation task by crossing out all occurrences of the letter *b* in randomly arranged letter strings and simultaneously listen to a list of randomly arranged spoken numbers and say *yes* whenever the number *5* occurs. (This is sometimes called a *dual-task* format.)

Another divided-attention format requires the tested individual to retain several bits of information in immediate memory while performing mental operations on the information. The *digits backward* test is one of the easier tests in this format. In the digits backward test the examiner says a string of randomly arranged single-digit numbers and the patient repeats them in reversed order. Some other relatively easy tests in this format are counting; saying the alphabet, days of the week, or months of the year in reverse order; and counting forward by 2s, 3s, 4s, or 5s. More difficult tests include orally spelling words backwards, doing serial subtractions (beginning with a number provided by the examiner, the test-taker subtracts a specified number then subtracts the specified number from the remainder, and so on, as in *100-93-86-79—*), and saying letters and words alternatively in sequence *(A-1-B-2—)*. The *Paced Auditory Serial Addition Test* (PASAT; Gronwall, 1977) is a challenging divided-attention test in which strings of single-digit numbers are presented orally at a predetermined rate, and the test-taker is required to add each digit to the immediately preceding one and say the result (e.g., the string *3-6-5-1-9* requires the response *9-11-6-10.*). Lezak (1995) has commented that the PASAT is a difficult and stressful task even for non-brain-injured adults, who experience great pressure and a sense of failure even when they are doing well. Consequently, Lezak reserves the PASAT for detection and demonstration of very subtle attentional impairments.

Tests of Visual Organization

Tests of visual organization usually require the patient to identify *incomplete visual stimuli,* identify *fragmented visual stimuli,* or discriminate pictured objects from their background *(figure-ground discrimination). Incomplete figure tests,* as the name implies, contain drawings of familiar objects with missing elements. The patient is asked to say or write the name of each test item. Figure 8-12 shows an example of an incomplete figure test item.

In tests of *fragmented visual stimuli* the patient is shown drawings of common objects that have been divided into parts, and the parts have been rearranged to disguise their identity (Figure 8-13). Tests with fragmented stimuli usually are more sensitive to visual organization impairments than tests with incomplete stimuli (Lezak, 1995). The *Object Assembly* subtest of the *Wechsler Adult Intelligence Scale* (WAIS; Wechsler, 1981) requires identification of fragmented visual stimuli, as does the *Hooper Visual Organization Test* (Hooper, 1983). In the *WAIS Object Assembly* subtest, the patient is given cut-up pressboard figures of familiar objects (a human figure, a human head in profile, a hand, or an elephant) and is asked to assemble them. In the Hooper test, the patient is presented with a series of pictures depicting cut-up line drawings of common objects and is asked to say or write the name of the object depicted in each item.

Visual figure-ground tests contain stimuli in which test figures are embedded in more complex figures (as in the *Hidden Figures Test;* Thurstone, 1944), stimuli in which test figures overlap (Poppelreuter, 1917), stimuli in which

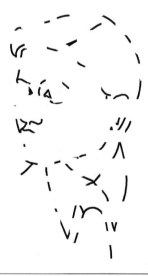

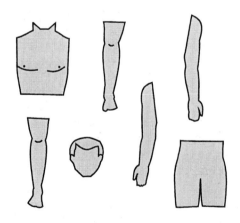

Figure 8-12 ■ **An example of an incomplete figure test item.**

Figure 8-13 ■ **An example of an object assembly test item. The components of the figure are made of heavy paperboard or fiberboard. The test-taker assembles them as he or she would assemble a jigsaw puzzle.**

lines are drawn over test figures, or stimuli in which test figures are partially occluded by masks (Luria, 1965). Figures 8-14, 8-15, and 8-16 give examples of items that may be found in visual figure-ground tests.

GENERAL CONCEPTS 8-2

- Several communicative impairments may follow right-hemisphere brain injury:
  - —*Diminished speech prosody* and *reductions in movements that accompany speech*
  - —*Excessive, confabulatory,* tangential, and sometimes *inappropriate* connected speech

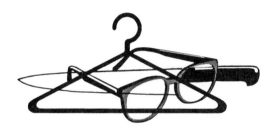

Figure 8-14 ▪ An example of an overlapping-figures test item.

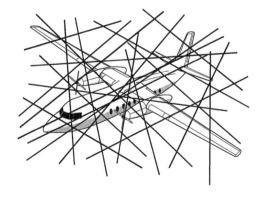

Figure 8-15 ▪ An example of a figure-ground test item in which lines have been drawn over a drawing of an object that the test-taker is asked to identify.

  - —*Impaired comprehension of narratives and conversations* attributable to insensitivity to relationships, premature assumptions, failure to judge the appropriateness of events and situations, and failure to appreciate implied meanings
  - —*Pragmatic impairments* related to turn-taking, topic maintenance, social conventions, and eye contact
- Tompkins and her associates have offered a *suppression deficit hypothesis* to account for right-hemisphere-damaged adults' impaired discourse comprehension. The suppression deficit hypothesis suggests that right-hemisphere-damaged adults cannot suppress initially activated assumptions or inferences, which are later shown to be inappropriate or irrelevant.
- Brownell and his associates have suggested that right-hemisphere-damaged adults' impaired discourse comprehension may be caused by impaired *theory of mind*—the ability to appreciate the content of other people's minds, including their knowledge, intentions, and emotions.
- Several standardized and nonstandardized tests for measuring cognitive and communicative impairments of patients with right-hemisphere brain injury are available and may provide an overview of a right-hemisphere-damaged

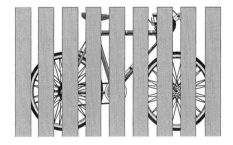

Figure 8-16 ▪ An example of a figure-ground test item in which the test stimulus is partially occluded by a mask.

patient's communicative and cognitive strengths and weaknesses. Detailed assessment often requires administration of supplemental tests of pragmatics, communication, visuospatial abilities, and attention.

- Right-hemisphere-damaged adults' pragmatic abilities typically are assessed with *rating scales.* Some rating scales are part of larger test batteries for assessing right-hemisphere-damaged adults such as the *Right Hemisphere Language Battery* or the *Rehabilitation Institute of Chicago Evaluation of Communicative Problems in Right-Hemisphere Dysfunction.* Others are free-standing rating scales such as the *Pragmatic Protocol* or the *Communicative Effectiveness Index,* which are not designed exclusively for right-hemisphere-damaged adults.

- The presence and severity of neglect may be assessed with *cancellation tests, line-bisection tests, copying and drawing tests,* or *scanning tests.* A combination of several tests may be required to detect subtle signs of neglect.

- The *Behavioural Inattention Test* is designed to measure the effects of neglect on everyday activities.

- Comprehensive assessment of right-hemisphere-damaged adults' attentional abilities requires assessment of *sustained attention, selective attention, alternating attention,* and *divided attention.*

- Right-hemisphere-damaged adults' visual organization may be assessed with tests that require them to *identify incomplete or fragmented visual stimuli* or to *discriminate visual stimuli from a background.*

TREATING ADULTS WITH RIGHT-HEMISPHERE BRAIN INJURY

We know less about treatment of right-hemisphere-damaged adults than we do about treatment of left-hemisphere-damaged (aphasic) adults, in part because the communication impairments of right-hemisphere-damaged adults largely were unrecognized and untreated until about 20 years ago and in part because focal right-hemisphere damage seems to produce

more diffuse effects on behavior than focal left-hemisphere damage. Consequently, identifiable (and treatable) right-hemisphere syndromes are not as well described as left-hemisphere aphasic syndromes.

Within the last few years a treatment literature on right-hemisphere-damaged adults has begun to develop, although most is anecdote and opinion without much empiric support. Nevertheless, we now know that many right-hemisphere-damaged adults exhibit communicative impairments that can be objectively described and that treatment can help at least some of them compensate for their impairments. However, there are several major differences between right-hemisphere-damaged adults and left-hemisphere-damaged aphasic adults that affect both the nature of treatment and its probable outcome. These differences largely are attributable to the fact that left-hemisphere brain injury tends to produce focal effects on specific linguistic and communicative abilities, whereas right-hemisphere brain injury tends to produce diffuse effects that are not readily reducible to specific communicative abilities.

Communicative impairments of adults with left-hemisphere damage are relatively discrete and can be classified and quantified with reasonable reliability. The communicative failures of adults with left-hemisphere brain injury usually are relatively obvious and can be counted (e.g., misnaming pictures, missing the last two parts of a three-part command). The relationships between left-hemisphere-damaged adults' performance on diagnostic tests and their underlying communicative impairments tend to be straightforward—for example, the relationship between errors on tests of confrontation naming and impaired word retrieval.

The communicative impairments of adults with right-hemisphere damage are less discrete and tend to be less amenable to simple counts of errors because they represent more diffuse failures, such as treating serious situations as humorous or failing to follow conversational rules. The relationships between right-hemisphere-damaged adults' performance on diagnostic tests and their underlying communicative impairments usually are less straightforward and require more assumptions—for example, the relationship between errors on tests requiring correct interpretations of idioms or metaphors and failure to make inferences.

Criteria for what constitutes normal performance are somewhat better defined for the impairments exhibited by adults with left-hemisphere brain injury and aphasia than for adults with right-hemisphere brain injury. Reasonably comprehensive and valid norms for communicative abilities such as listening comprehension, reading comprehension, vocabulary, naming, and speech production (likely to be affected by left-hemisphere brain injury) are available but not for most of the cognitive and communicative abilities likely to be affected by right-hemisphere brain injury. When the focus is on pragmatic appropriateness, conversational style, appreciation of nonliteral material, and the like, intuition, judgment, and consultation with patient, family, and caregivers often replace standardized norms in determining what is "normal" for a particular patient.

Treatment of right-hemisphere-damaged adults' communication impairments may target a variety of deficits affecting receptive and expressive aspects of communication—difficulty organizing and synthesizing information, difficulty separating what is important from what is not, inability to use contextual cues to ascertain meanings, interpreting figurative language literally, overpersonalization, reduced sensitivity to pragmatic or extralinguistic aspects of communication, or tangentiality and excessive detail in speech. Right-hemisphere-damaged adults' communicative impairments often are magnified by cognitive and behavioral abnormalities such as denial of illness, indifference to and denial of impairments, distractibility, problems maintaining attention, impulsivity, and impaired reasoning and problem-solving.

Cognitive and Behavioral Abnormalities

Indifference and Denial Indifference to impairments and denial of errors can be important obstacles to treatment of right-hemisphere-damaged adults' communicative impairments. Indifference and denial usually diminish with neurologic recovery, but some individuals remain oblivious to their impairments for months and years, and some may be at risk when denial combines with poor judgment regarding daily life activities such as driving, hunting, or solo trekking. (Hereafter I will use *indifference* in a broad sense to entail both *indifference* and *outright denial.*)

Most right-hemisphere-damaged adults are compliant and willingly participate in treatment programs, although their participation is more likely to be passive than active. If asked to participate in making decisions about the content and focus of treatment, they often talk a good game but fail in its execution. They tend not to do more than is specifically required and may resist, either overtly or covertly, even doing what is specifically required. They often fail to carry out assignments unless closely supervised. Homework assignments are likely to be neglected unless someone in the patient's living environment provides supervision and direction. When confronted about their failure to carry out assignments, they may confabulate or offer implausible reasons for not doing the assignments.

According to Tompkins (1995) right-hemisphere-damaged adults who remain uncritical of their poor performance and unconcerned about their impairments are poor treatment candidates, and she recommends that treatment be deferred until denial resolves. While the clinician waits for resolution, Tompkins suggests that the clinician establish baselines, identify impairments, and select potential treatment approaches. For patients who are neurologically recovered but still remain indifferent to their impairments, Tompkins recommends simplifying treatment goals, modifying the patient's living environment to limit the negative effects of indifference, and teaching compensatory strategies to family members and associates.

Clinicians can compensate for the effects of indifference by making treatment activities highly structured, defining a clear set of treatment goals, and communicating the treatment goals to the

A right-hemisphere-damaged patient is taking a written spelling test. The clinician gets the patient started and watches as the patient completes the first 10 of 30 items in the test.

Clinician: "You're doing fine, Mrs. Perkins. Do you think you can finish by yourself?"

Patient: "Of course I can. This is not really very hard, after all."

Clinician: "O.K. I'll come back in about 10 minutes and see how you're doing."

(Leaves. Ten minutes later the clinician returns and looks at the test.)

Clinician: "What happened? You're still on number 10."

Patient: "Well, for goodness sake. You left, you know."

Clinician: "But you said you could finish by yourself."

Patient: "When you left, you didn't say anything about me going on. So I assumed that we'd finished this. Are we finished, or not?"

patient and family. Indifference sometimes can be treated indirectly, in the context of activities directed toward other goals, by giving the patient immediate feedback after erroneous or inappropriate responses, by confronting the patient when the patient denies errors, and by improving the patient's self-monitoring first in highly structured activities and later in less structured ones.

Clinicians may work on indifference by having the patient (or the patient and family) collaborate in making a list of the patient's strengths and weaknesses. Entries in the list then may be singled out for attention in treatment activities. Sometimes videotaping treatment activities and reviewing them with the patient improve patients' awareness of errors and inappropriate responses. For patients with extreme denial, the clinician may begin by reviewing, with the patient, videotapes of social interactions involving others or videotapes of staged interactions in which one participant makes errors or inappropriate responses resembling those made by the patient. When the patient becomes adept at identifying errors and inappropriate responses in the behavior of others, videotapes in which the patient is a participant may be introduced.

Many right-hemisphere-damaged adults who deny their own errors are quick to spot errors when others make them.

Finally, a few words of caution. Many right-hemisphere-damaged adults can, with help, make lists describing their own pattern of errors and inappropriate responses, talk constructively about the lists, and even identify their errors and inappropriate responses in carefully structured treatment activities, but they fail to anticipate them or do much about them either in less structured treatment activities or in daily life. The transition from identifying and talking about errors and inappropriate responses to doing something about them may be arduous, requiring carefully programmed generalization procedures and the active participation of the patient's family members and daily life associates. It is crucial that family members and caregivers participate in treatment programs for patients with denial to ensure that the patient and family understand the relationship between treatment activities and goals, to ensure that homework assignments are completed, and to facilitate transfer of treatment gains from the clinic to the patient's daily life.

Attentional Impairments and Distractibility Tompkins (1995) commented that attentional impairments may cause or exacerbate communication impairments following right-hemisphere brain injury. She noted that sustained attention is crucial for comprehension and production of discourse and that selective attention is important for maintaining coherent interpretations of printed and spoken materials, establishing referential relationships, and making inferences. According to Tompkins, control of attention is important in keeping track of plots in movies and television shows, revising interpretations, and resisting distractions (and no doubt in other daily life communicative activities). She suggests that working on attentional capacity and control may provide a greater clinical payoff than working on their surface manifestations.

Treatment of attentional impairments takes many forms, ranging from paper-and-pencil or computer-presented attention drills to activities requiring patients to focus and maintain attention in natural contexts. A sampling of these activities follows.

Sustained Attention Drills to improve sustained attention range from paper-and-pencil tasks such as letter cancellation and solving mazes to vigilance drills that require the patient to monitor a visual display or strings of auditory stimuli and press a key when a target stimulus occurs. The easiest visual and auditory sustained-attention tasks are those in which a single target stimulus appears against a constant background. Increasing the time between stimuli, making the intervals between stimuli less predictable, and increasing the overall duration of the task all serve to make sustained-attention tasks more difficult. Patients with attentional impairments often do well as sustained-attention tasks begin but have increasing difficulty as the task progresses and the load on sustained attention increases.

The *starry night* task (Rizzo & Robin, 1990) is a computerized visual sustained-attention task that permits manipulation of task difficulty across a wide range. A pattern of dots (which resembles a starry night sky) is displayed on the monitor screen, and dots appear and disappear at unpredictable times and locations. The patient presses a key when he or she sees a dot appear or disappear. The computer keeps a record of the patient's hits, misses, and reaction times. The density of the dots, the rate at which they appear or disappear, and the duration of the task can be adjusted to manipulate task difficulty.

Paper-and-pencil sustained-attention tasks usually are less challenging than computer-based tasks because paper-and-pencil tasks do not require a constant level of sustained attention across the task. Patients can slow down or stop when their attention lags and resume when their level of attention increases, thereby minimizing errors, although the time it takes them to finish the task increases.

Selective Attention Treatment of selective attention usually relies on drills in which the patient performs sustained-attention tasks in the presence of competing or distracting stimuli. A common way to treat impairments in selective attention is to place the patient in a sustained-attention task and play a tape recording of distracting sound (e.g., conversations, radio programs, popular music) in the background. Choosing distractions that the patient is likely to encounter in daily life (e.g., a radio playing, background conversations) helps prepare the patient for resisting these distractions in daily life and helps ensure that improvements in selective attention obtained in treatment activities carry over to the patient's daily life.

Alternating Attention Almost any sustained-attention task can be modified to create an alternating-attention task by periodically changing stimulus characteristics or response requirements during the task. For example, a patient might practice shifting attention from one conversational partner to another in recorded conversational interactions. Alternating-attention tasks also can be created by combining two different tasks and alternately switching between them. For example, a patient might practice alternating between doing a paper-and-pencil sustained-attention task and participating in a conversational interaction.

Divided Attention Treatment to improve attention to two or more aspects of a task may consist of drills in tasks similar to those used to test divided attention. Tompkins (1995) commented that one objective of divided-attention treatment for patients with right-hemisphere damage might be to give them training in volitional allocation of mental resources. According to Tompkins, this is necessary because some patients can no longer perceive which aspects of a task are most important and should receive the most attention. Tompkins recommends training these patients to systematically analyze tasks and situations to decide which aspects are most important, and then giving them practice in volitional allocation of attention.

Attention tasks no doubt fall along a continuum. At one end are simple cancellation or vigilance tasks, which demand attentional stamina but do not put much strain on the patient's ability to ignore distracting or competing stimuli. At the other end are the most challenging sustained-attention tasks, which demand both attentional stamina and the ability to ignore distracting or competing stimuli.

There is no strong empiric evidence that right-hemisphere-damaged adults' improved performance on attention drills generalizes to naturalistic contexts, although anecdotal reports suggest that such generalization occurs, at least for some of them. Clinicians sometimes attempt to ensure generalization to daily life contexts by working on attention in contexts that resemble those the patient will encounter in daily life. Patients may be placed in conversational interactions in which they must maintain eye contact, stay on topic, respond appropriately to changes in topic, and get and retain a reasonable amount of specific information. For patients who can handle such interactions in quiet and nondistracting environments, noise, movement, or interruptions gradually may be introduced to increase the patients' resistance to distraction. (See Chapter 9 for more on treating attentional impairments.)

Impulsivity Impulsivity can have major effects on many right-hemisphere-damaged patients' performance in treatment and in daily life. In treatment, many right-hemisphere-damaged patients respond before the clinician has finished delivering task instructions or stimuli, interrupt treatment activities with tangential and irrelevant comments, begin tasks before they understand what is expected, and stop working on tasks before finishing them. In daily life they fail to anticipate task requirements as they begin

tasks; take on tasks and enter situations that are beyond their abilities; fail to complete activities; and respond to their first impressions of messages, events, or situations, creating mistakes, misinterpretations, and social blunders.

Clinicians sometimes manage right-hemisphere-damaged patients' impulsiveness by incorporating distinctive stimuli as *stop* and *go* signals for patient responses. For example, patients might be taught to monitor a clinician-controlled signal light as an indicator of when they are permitted to respond. If the light is off, the patient cannot respond but must wait until it comes on. As the patient's impulsive responses diminish under the control of the light, the light gradually may be replaced by verbal or gestural cues from the clinician (spoken *wait* or a *stop* hand gesture). The clinician's cues then gradually may be reduced and control gradually may be transferred to patient self-cueing.

Impaired Reasoning and Problem-Solving Right-hemisphere-damaged patients' impaired reasoning and problem-solving can have important effects on the conduct of treatment and its outcome. Right-hemisphere-damaged patients tend to get lost in the details of treatment activities and lose track of general goals and objectives. They are not very good at anticipating when a treatment task is likely to give them trouble, and when they do get into trouble, their responses are likely to be impulsive, inappropriate, and ineffective. Their impaired reasoning and problem-solving makes them of little help to the clinician in deciding on treatment objectives and choosing the ways in which the objectives are to be reached.

Treatment of reasoning and problem-solving impairments entails structured practice in a variety of tasks that require reasoning, foresight, and problem-solving, such as role-playing situations in which problem-solving skills are needed (e.g., getting a refund for defective merchandise); proposing solutions to problems posed by the clinician (e.g., "You are at a shopping mall and you come upon a 3-year-old boy standing alone and crying. What would you do?"); and planning activities such as vacations, field trips, and picnics. A formal, prescriptive, and highly structured approach to problem-solving should help most right-hemisphere-damaged patients get started:

- Identify the problem.
- Think of several possible solutions.
- Evaluate the feasibility and potential consequences of each solution.
- Choose the best solution.
- Apply it.
- Evaluate the results.

With extensive practice, some right-hemisphere-damaged patients can move away from a highly structured and prescriptive problem-solving strategy toward a less formal and less laborious one. Few, however, progress to the point at which problem-solving becomes automatic and instinctive.

Communicative Impairments

Reading Impairments Right-hemisphere-damaged patients' visual neglect is a common target of treatment because neglect has important effects on their ability to read and comprehend printed materials. Numerous procedures for treating neglect have been described in the literature, but little is known of their effectiveness or generalizability.

Diller and Weinberg (1977) described a comprehensive treatment program for treating visual neglect. The program teaches patients to scan both sides of visual space, with emphasis on left-side space. Patients in Diller and Weinberg's program receive systematic practice in visual tasks such as visually tracking a moving target across visual fields, detecting flashing lights in various locations in both visual fields, letter cancellation, or reading printed paragraphs projected on a wall so they encompass both visual fields. The primary objectives of Diller and Weinberg's program are to make patients aware of their neglect, force patients to view visual stimuli systematically, and make newly acquired skills automatic by means of massed repetition.

Several techniques for getting patients with left neglect to attend to the left side of printed text have been reported in the literature. Typically, salient markers (such as colored vertical lines, colored dots, or rulers) are placed at the left margin of printed material. The patient is instructed to scan leftward until the patient sees the marker whenever beginning a new line of text. Sometimes the patient is instructed to keep one finger on the marker and to scan back to it when beginning each new line. The patient's dependence on the markers gradually is reduced by making the markers less salient and by eventually replacing them with the patient's internal monitoring of whether or not the material makes sense.

Stanton and associates (1981) described a comprehensive approach to treating neglect in reading. Their treatment program includes several tasks designed to enhance patients' awareness of, and attention to, the neglected side. In one task, patients match printed letters, numbers, and words from a column in the right visual field with numbers, letters, and words printed in a column in the left visual field. In another task they read aloud printed sentences, beginning with large-print sentences and large blank spaces between sentences and progressing to single-spaced small-print sentences. In another task they read printed paragraphs aloud, progressing from paragraphs printed in large letters with double spacing between lines to standard books, magazines, and newspapers, some in double-column format.

Stanton and associates use verbal cues to remind patients to attend to the left side of the materials. They begin with the clinician instructing the patient, "Tell yourself out loud—look to the left," at the end of each line and progress to self-initiated verbal cues by the patient, who vocalizes (or subvocalizes) "Look to the left" at the end of each line. As the patient progresses, overt verbal cues gradually are eliminated and are replaced by covert cues. Stanton and associates recommend that clinicians take advantage of right-hemisphere-damaged patients' good verbal skills by having them ask themselves, "Does that make sense?" at the end of each sentence or periodically while they read.

Myers (1994) suggests that the most effective techniques for treating neglect are those in which patients internalize the need to look to the left, rather than depending on external cues or self-cueing. One such procedure was described by Myers and Mackisack (1990). The procedure is built around two techniques, called *edgeness* and *bookness*. The edgeness technique requires the use of a work space (a rectangular board or grid) with a raised border. First the patient becomes familiar with the spatial boundaries for a task by tracing the perimeter of the work space with one finger. Then the clinician places colored cubes at various locations on the work space. The patient is told how many cubes are on the work space and that they are to find and remove all of them. The clinician does not tell the patient where to look but simply encourages him or her to continue looking until all the cubes are found. The difficulty of the task is determined by the number of cubes (more cubes = greater difficulty), their placement (more cubes in neglected space = greater difficulty), and the presence of foils (cubes may be in two colors, only one of which the patient is to find and remove). To extend improved scanning from this task to other tasks, Myers and Mackisack suggest that patients be encouraged to extend the edgeness technique to other tasks by tracing the boundaries of other appropriate surfaces, such as writing tablets and books.

The bookness technique resembles the edgeness technique and is specific to reading. The patient first orally describes a closed book placed in front of him or her at the visual midline, then traces its perimeter with a finger. Then the patient opens the book and traces its perimeter, again describing what he or she sees. Reading tasks printed in the book then are administered, beginning with matching tasks that require the patient to match stimuli on the left and right sides of the book. Patients trace the perimeter of the book before each trial. The clinician in-

creases the difficulty of the reading tasks by increasing the number of stimuli and adding foils. As the patient's attention to the left side of the book improves, the requirement that the patient trace the perimeter of the book gradually is eliminated. Myers (1994) sees two advantages to the edgeness and bookness techniques. First, they teach the patient to search to the left without the need for external cues, which increases the likelihood of generalization to other tasks. Second, they help maximize the patient's overall level of attention, which may generalize to other treatment tasks.

Myers (1999) suggests that manipulating the meaningfulness of the right and left sides of printed materials may help neglect patients attend to the left side of the materials. To encourage leftward search, information that permits interpretation of printed materials should be distributed from left to right so that the patient must attend to the left side to make sense of the material. This means that lists of single words should be controlled so that reading only the right half of the words does not yield a real word. Words such as *cavalry, lemonade,* and *conversation* encourage leftward search; words such as *pancake, everything,* and *attend* do not.

The characteristics of printed sentences may be manipulated in similar fashion to encourage leftward search. A sentence such as:

Everett hid the key to his aunt's house under a rock.

does not yield a complete and unambiguous meaning without the information provided by the words on the left. A sentence such as:

When she saw the rattlesnake in the garage Emma screamed and ran to the phone to call 911.

in contrast, yields a complete and unambiguous idea without the words to the left. (Its length also increases the probability that a patient with neglect will see only the portion on the right of the latter sentence.)

Several reports have suggested that neglect patients' performance on tests of left hemispatial neglect may be improved by requiring them to perform active left-limb movements in left hemispace before the tests of neglect are administered (Halligan, Manning, & Marshall, 1991; Joanette & associates, 1986). Several explanations have been offered for the effects of left-sided limb movements on neglect, including increased activation of the right hemisphere, visual cueing toward left hemispace, and motor cueing toward left hemispace. At present no one knows how long the facilitating effects of left-limb movements last or whether they affect neglect in tasks other than those used to test neglect. (Robertson and North [1993] assert that passive limb movements have no effect on neglect.) Myers (1999) suggests priming attention to left hemispace by requiring that the patient perform purposeful left-limb movements such as tracing the border of the workspace with the left hand, moving the left arm up and down, or tapping with the left foot before starting tasks requiring attention to left hemispace.

Many patients with right-hemisphere brain damage have paralyzed left limbs, making it impossible to prime attention to the left hemispace via left limb movements.

Treating right-hemisphere-damaged adults' attentional impairments is thought by many investigators and clinicians to have positive effects on their neglect. Myers (1994) suggests that treatment for neglect might include tasks to increase right-hemisphere-damaged patients' overall level of arousal, their capacity to sustain attention, and their capacity to selectively attend to certain stimuli while ignoring others. Because many models of neglect attribute a prominent role to attentional abnormalities, indirect treatment of neglect by direct treatment of attention seems intuitively reasonable, although verification of the relationship between attentional skills and neglect awaits empiric results.

Pragmatic Impairments Treating right-hemisphere-damaged patients' pragmatic impairments may be facilitated by calling on their preserved verbal skills. Clinician coaching and clinician–patient strategy development alternate with structured practice. Videotapes provide feedback to patients regarding their pragmatic behaviors in conversational interactions. The videotapes also serve as a record of patients' progress (or lack thereof) in improving their pragmatic appropriateness. The approach proceeds roughly as follows.

At the beginning of treatment, one or more 15-minute to 20-minute conversations between the patient and another person (the clinician or someone chosen by the clinician and patient) are recorded on videotape. These videotapes provide baseline measures of the patient's conversational behaviors.

After the baseline videotapes are made, the clinician leads the patient through a short general discussion of language pragmatics. When the patient has a good sense of what language pragmatics are and how pragmatic behaviors function to maintain and regulate communication, the clinician and patient jointly view several videotapes of conversations not involving the patient (e.g., television talk shows, excerpts from movies, or videotapes made specifically for this purpose). During the viewing they evaluate the occurrence and appropriateness of pragmatic behaviors, with special attention to violations of pragmatic rules and conventions (e.g., interruptions, tangentiality, monopolizing the conversation).

When the patient has demonstrated some facility at identifying violations of pragmatic and conversational rules in interactions involving others, the clinician and patient jointly view the baseline videotape(s) and identify instances in which the patient engages in appropriate or inappropriate pragmatic behaviors. The clinician and patient use the results of their evaluation of the patient's performance to select pragmatic behaviors to be targeted in treatment. They formulate immediate and long-term goals and set up a plan for reaching the goals. The plan usually includes structured conversational interactions between the patient and clinician in which the patient practices agreed-on strategies for improving a targeted behavior, alternating with videotaped conversational interactions in which the patient uses the strategies either with the clinician or with others. These videotapes provide the patient with documentation of progress and provide the clinician and patient with indications of pragmatic behaviors that should be attended to in the next phase of treatment. The process is repeated for successive pragmatic behaviors until all behaviors selected for treatment have been addressed.

Eye contact, turn-taking, and *topic maintenance* are frequent targets for treatment because they often are a problem for patients with right-hemisphere damage and because improving them can have striking effects on a right-hemisphere-damaged patient's conversational appropriateness. Increasing a patient's eye contact may require only that the clinician say, "look at me" at appropriate times in treatment interactions. When the patient responds consistently to the clinician's cues, the cues gradually may be faded and eventually replaced with patient self-cues. Giving the patient specific points at which to make eye contact may be helpful if the patient has difficulty making the transition from clinician cues to self-cues. Teaching the patient to make eye contact when the patient begins and ends each utterance and then extending eye contact to the beginning and end of the conversational partner's utterances may provide a structured way for patients to maintain reasonably appropriate eye contact in conversations.

Teaching right-hemisphere-damaged patients to follow conversational turn-taking rules typically is approached in stepwise fashion. The clinician explains turn-taking rules and talks about how conversational participants know when to take or yield conversational turns. Then the clinician and the patient engage in structured practice in which the patient concentrates on turn-taking without being concerned about other

aspects of communication such as message formulation or inferential reasoning. The structured practice may include (1) watching videotapes of conversational interactions (such as television talk shows) and discussing how the participants knew when to talk and when to let the other person talk; (2) preparing a script for a conversational interaction with appropriate conversational turns, videotaping it, then critiquing it; and (3) videotaping a free conversation, viewing it, and identifying appropriate and inappropriate turn-taking behavior. When the patient begins to exhibit reasonably good appreciation of normal turn-taking, turn-taking may be incorporated into other treatment activities and into free conversation with the clinician.

Teaching right-hemisphere-damaged patients to maintain conversational topics usually requires some instruction and much structured practice. The instruction involves pointing out to the patient that conversations usually have a central theme or topic that lasts through several conversational turns and includes convincing the patient that he or she often strays from the topic during conversations. Structured practice may involve activities such as (1) identifying topics in printed materials such as newspaper or magazine articles; (2) watching videotapes of conversational interactions and identifying topics, identifying when the topic changes, and discussing how the topic change was brought about by the participants; and (3) engaging in structured conversations with the clinician while maintaining a specified topic for a given length of time or a given number of conversational turns.

Some of what appear to be pragmatic impairments, such as failure to observe social conventions, failure to appreciate a speaker's implied intent, verbosity, tangentiality, and responding inappropriately to figurative language, actually may represent problems in attending to subtle cues, organizing and interpreting complex information, or making inferences. These impairments may be more effectively and efficiently treated, at least in the initial stages of treatment, by treating the underlying cognitive impairments than by working on conversational interactions. In later stages of treatment, direct work on conversational interactions may be appropriate.

Inference Failure and Communication Impairments Myers (1991) has asserted that many right-hemisphere-damaged patients' communication impairments can be accounted for by a central impairment in making inferences. She called this impairment *inference failure.* According to Myers, inference "requires an interaction between two types of recognition—the recognition of key elements and the recognition of their relationship to one another and to other contextual cues" (p. 4). Also according to Myers, general failure to go beyond the superficial meaning of events or situations to their deeper (implied) meanings may explain right-hemisphere-damaged patients' tendency to interpret metaphor, humor, idioms, and indirect requests literally; their pragmatic deficits in conversations; their impaired expression of emotion; their impulsivity and denial of illness; their facial recognition deficits; their verbose, tangential, and inefficient speech; and their failure to produce integrated stories and descriptions.

As noted earlier, Brownell and associates (1986) have reported that right-hemisphere-damaged adults make inferences—but make the wrong ones—based on their initial surface interpretations and fail to revise their initial inferences based on subsequent information. The transcript of a right-hemisphere-damaged adult earlier in this chapter is striking not so much because the patient failed to make inferences but because he made incorrect ones. These findings somewhat weaken Myers's arguments for inference failure as a general explanation for right-hemisphere-damaged adults' impairments.

If Myers is correct, treatment of right-hemisphere-damaged patients' communicative impairments would be most efficient and effective if it focused on teaching them to make inferences. As their ability to make inferences improves, the surface impairments that depended on making inferences should improve. Tompkins (1995) comments, however, that Myers's explanation is "underspecified," that other impairments may masquerade as inference failures, and that inference failure may be related to a more general concept—that of *mental effort.* Myers's hypothesis has yet to be validated, but if the existence of inference failure as a central process were to be confirmed, clinicians would have a promising alternative to current treatment-by-symptom approaches for remediating right-hemisphere-damaged patients' communicative impairments.

The following short list of tasks contains examples of activities that would be appropriate for treatment that focuses on teaching patients to make inferences.

Appreciation of humor. The patient is given a printed joke, minus its punch line, and chooses the humorous punch line from a set containing a humorous punch line and nonhumorous foils. The patient is given a cartoon minus its caption and chooses the humorous caption from a set containing a humorous caption and nonhumorous foils.

The quack was selling a potion, which he claimed would make men live to a great age. He claimed he himself was hale and hearty and over 300 years old. "Is he really as old as that?," asked a listener of the youthful assistant. "I can't say," replied the assistant.

"I don't know how old he is." (*Nonhumorous ending*)

"I've only worked for him 100 years." (*Humorous ending*)

"There are over 300 days in a year." (*Nonsequitur*)

(From Molloy, R., Brownell, H.H., & Gardner, H. [1990]. Discourse comprehension by right-hemisphere stroke patients: deficits of prediction and revision. In: Y. Joanette & H. Brownell [Eds.], *Discourse ability and brain damage: Theoretical and empirical perspectives.* New York: Springer-Verlag, pp. 113-130.)

Appreciation of the implied meanings of metaphors and idioms. The patient hears (or reads) a common metaphor or idiomatic expression then chooses the correct interpretation from a group containing the correct interpretation plus foils that include a literal interpretation of the metaphor or idiom.

Frank didn't go to work because he felt *under the weather.*
Frank got caught in the rain. *(Literal interpretation)*
Frank felt ill. *(Correct idiomatic interpretation)*
Frank was afraid of storms. *(Related response)*
Frank lived in the city. *(Unrelated response)*

Identification of verbal and pictorial absurdities. The patient is shown pictures containing absurd or unlikely relationships (e.g., a rabbit chasing a dog), identifies the absurd or unlikely relationships, and explains why they are absurd or unlikely. The patient listens to a short spoken narrative in which there are absurd or inconsistent statements, identifies the absurd or inconsistent statements, and explains why they are absurd or inconsistent.

Mrs. Jones took her daughter Hannah to the doctor. She said to the doctor, "I brought her in because she's had a fever for two days and has been coughing and sneezing. *I want you to tell me if her shoes are too tight.*"

Comprehension of implied information in discourse. The patient listens to spoken discourse, answers questions testing implied information, and tells the main point or moral for the discourse. The patient reads printed discourse and does the same things.

Retelling stories. The patient listens to a story, then retells it by paraphrasing and interpreting it, rather than repeating it verbatim. The presence of main ideas and the presence of implied information in the retellings is evaluated to determine the extent to which the patient organizes information from the story and makes the appropriate inferences.

Perceiving relationships. The patient categorizes items according to similarities and differences or class membership (e.g., telling why scissors and a saw are alike, listing things that one might find at a picnic, naming ferocious animals). The patient analyzes familial relationships (e.g., "How is your son's uncle related to you?"). The patient generates lists of divergent functions (e.g., telling the clinician all the ways in which one could use a brick) (Chapey, 1994).

Divergent tasks may exacerbate some patients' tendency toward tangentiality. If carefully controlled, divergent tasks may provide ways of working on tangentiality. If not carefully controlled, they may reinforce it.

Resource Allocation and Right-Hemisphere Brain Injury Tompkins (1995) has proposed that many right-hemisphere-damaged patients' impairments and anomalous behaviors can be explained by limitations on the availability of mental resources. She notes that right-hemisphere-damaged patients' performance varies with the processing demands placed on cognitive resources, that right-hemisphere-damaged patients can use context to facilitate problematic performance, that right-hemisphere-damaged patients' performance in conditions of high processing load covaries with their functional working memory, and that right-hemisphere-damaged patients' partially correct performance is consistent with limitations in processing resources.

Tompkins cautions that a resource-allocation explanation of behavior after the fact "can be made to fit almost any outcome, and, as such, runs the risk of explaining nothing" (p. 85). She recommends that investigators test specific predictions to validate (or disprove) resource allocation as an explanation of right-hemisphere-damaged adults' cognitive and behavioral aberrations.

Joanette and Goulet (1994) offered a hypothesis similar to that of Tompkins, namely that right-hemisphere-damaged patients' performance may be governed by task complexity—the more complex the task, the more difficulty right-hemisphere-damaged patients have with it. Task complexity and resource allocation explanations of right-hemisphere-damaged patients' impairments may offer equivalent explanations using different labels because more complex tasks should require more cognitive resources and vice versa. Both explanations await experimental validation, and it remains to be seen if resource allocation and task difficulty actually represent different concepts.

Generalization Generalization of improved performance from level to level within treatment tasks, from one treatment task to another, and from treatment tasks to the patient's daily life is an important issue for right-hemisphere-damaged patients, their clinicians, and their families. As a group, right-hemisphere-damaged adults tend not to spontaneously generalize responses or strategies from one context to another. Their progress through successive levels of treatment tasks may be slowed by failure to apply skills and strategies learned at one level to the next level. Transitions between treatment tasks may be compromised by the patient's failure to generalize what is learned in one task to related tasks. Finally (and perhaps most importantly), generalization of gains made in the clinic to the patient's daily life may be compromised by the patient's failure to apply what is learned in the clinic to daily life interactions. Consequently, successful treatment of right-hemisphere-damaged adults requires that clinicians give careful attention to procedures for enhancing generalization, both within treatment activities and from treatment activities to daily life.

Generalization Across Treatment Tasks
The generalization procedures described in Chapter 6 provide some methods by which clinicians can build generalization into their treatment procedures for right-hemisphere-damaged patients. These procedures may be modified or elaborated on as needed to account for the behavioral and cognitive impairments exhibited by right-hemisphere-damaged patients (e.g., impaired attention, impaired inferencing, impulsiveness, indifference). Because of right-hemisphere-damaged patients' behavioral and cognitive impairments, generalization procedures for them tend to be more prescriptive and more carefully structured than generalization procedures for patients with left-hemisphere damage.

One way of dealing with right-hemisphere-damaged patients' stimulus boundedness and impaired inferencing abilities is to make the steps between treatment levels small. Making the steps small and minimizing changes in stimulus characteristics and response requirements between levels helps right-hemisphere-damaged patients by diminishing the need for making inferences and changing response sets. Yorkston's (1981) description of a program to teach a right-hemisphere-damaged patient to transfer from his wheelchair to his bed dramatically underscores the need for small-step transitions for some patients with right-hemisphere brain injury. Yorkston began with a seven-step procedure, which proved completely beyond the patient's capacity. She then expanded it to 17 steps, then 27 steps, and eventually added the self-cue "Have you finished this step?" at the end of each step before the patient eventually learned to transfer. Yorkston cautioned that clinicians should never assume that a right-hemisphere-damaged patient will make logical transitions from one step to another and commented that, "Rarely, if ever, does one err in the direction of breaking a task into too many steps" (p. 283).

Generalization from task to task within treatment activities can be enhanced by making the source task (the one in which the patient has learned a set of responses or a strategy) resemble the target task (the one to which generalization is intended). Similarity between tasks can be manipulated by adjusting the task stimuli, the responses required in the task, or the context in which the task is presented (e.g., paper-and-pencil versus computer presentation). Requiring new responses to new stimuli in a new context maximizes between-task differences and works against generalization, whereas maintaining consistency of stimuli, responses, and context minimizes between-task differences and increases the probability that learning will generalize. (For related information, see "Programming Common Stimuli" in Chapter 6.)

Loose training (see Chapter 6) is another way in which clinicians can enhance right-hemisphere-damaged patients' generalization across tasks. By allowing stimulus conditions, response requirements, and reinforcement contingencies to vary within a controlled range, the clinician prevents the patient's performance from becoming too tightly bound to a restricted set of conditions and thereby increases the probability that learned responses and strategies will transfer across treatment tasks.

> Many clinicians routinely begin treatment in a task under tightly controlled conditions, and when the new learning has stabilized, they gradually loosen the training conditions, regardless of the source and nature of a patient's cognitive or communicative impairments.

Generalization from the Clinic to Outside Environments Right-hemisphere-damaged patients' tendency not to generalize from task to task or from level to level within tasks in the clinic is mirrored in their tendency not to generalize what they acquire in the clinic to outside environments. However, clinicians are not powerless. Tompkins (1995) identifies several ways in which clinicians can ensure or enhance generalization across settings.

- *Provide enough training trials to consolidate and stabilize responses so that patients can produce them in novel or stressful contexts.* Poorly consolidated and incompletely

learned responses or strategies tend not to generalize from the context in which they are acquired to other contexts, although some disciplined and motivated patients may, with careful coaching by the clinician, volitionally make such generalizations. However, few patients with right-hemisphere damage have the discipline and motivation to generalize from one context to another volitionally because of indifference and difficulty sustaining effort and attention. Usually it is necessary to bring these patients' responses to an over-learned, automatic level to ensure that they generalize what they learn in the clinic to the outside.

- *Train a variety of related responses (e.g., eye contact, turn-taking and relevance in conversations), rather than single responses.* This resembles loose training. The idea behind this principle is that training several related responses both provides the patient with alternatives when the primary response is not available and creates a network of associations that raises the overall probability of appropriate responses in the target contexts.

- *Train responses and strategies in a variety of tasks and present the tasks in a variety of contexts (e.g., role-playing, simulated natural environments, and natural environments).* This principle incorporates elements of *programming common stimuli* and *sequential modification* (see Chapter 6). Training responses or strategies in a variety of tasks helps stabilize and consolidate responses and diminishes the patient's dependence on the exact conditions under which responses are acquired. Presenting treatment tasks in a variety of contexts increases the patient's tolerance for changes in context and increases the probability that the treated responses or strategies will generalize from the treatment setting to other settings. In incorporating stimuli from other settings (topics, situations, people) into treatment tasks also enhances generalization from the treatment setting to the other settings.

- *Incorporate aspects of the target environment (topics, stimuli, contingencies, people, situations) into treatment activities.* This principle is related to the preceding one and speaks more directly to how clinicians enhance generalization from clinic activities to the patient's daily life environment. Topics, situations, response contingencies, and sometimes people can be transplanted from the patient's daily life environment to the clinic, where they are incorporated into treatment activities. Their presence in treatment activities imbues them with power to elicit, maintain, and control the patient's strategies.

- *Train self-instruction and verbal mediation.* Self-instruction and verbal mediation can be important adjuncts to other generalization procedures for patients with right-hemisphere brain injury. Clinicians can exploit right-hemisphere-damaged patients' well-preserved verbal skills by teaching them self-instructional or self-cueing strategies that are (overtly or covertly) verbally mediated. For example, a patient with neglect might be taught to compensate while reading by saying (or thinking), "Find the left-hand side of the page at the beginning of every line of text."

- *Enlist the help of family members, friends, and caregivers.* Family, friends, and caregivers can be a powerful force for generalization of responses and strategies from the clinic to the patient's daily life. In many respects family, friends, and caregivers can function as surrogate clinicians by manipulating stimuli, arranging situations and experiences, and administering response contingencies under the direction of the speech-language pathologist. Family, friends, and caregivers also can monitor the patient's daily life performance and provide the clinician with information about how much generalization actually is taking place.

Generalization is one of the most challenging components of treatment for clinicians who work with right-hemisphere-damaged adults. Unless generalization specifically is targeted and systematically trained, what the right-hemisphere-damaged patient learns in the clinic is likely to stay there. Fortunately, procedures to enhance and ensure generalization are available, and their systematic application can help ensure that improvements in right-hemisphere-damaged adults' communication transfer to their daily life.

GENERAL CONCEPTS 8-3

- Left-hemisphere damage tends to produce *focal impairments* that may be quantified relatively easily, whereas right-hemisphere damage tends to produce *diffuse impairments* that are less amenable to quantification.

- Treatment of right-hemisphere-damaged patients' cognitive and communicative impairments may be complicated by one or more of several cognitive and behavioral abnormalities:
  —*Denial and indifference,* which sometimes may be amenable to direct or indirect intervention
  —*Attentional impairments* and *distractibility,* which may be treated with paper-and-pencil or computer-based tasks that target *sustained attention, selective attention, alternating attention,* or *divided attention*
  —*Impulsivity,* which may be treated with external *stop* and *go* signals that are progressively shaped into patient-generated self-cues
  —*Impaired reasoning and problem-solving,* which may be treated with structured activities such as role-playing and prescriptive problem-solving strategies
  —*Neglect* in reading, which may be treated by external cues to the left side of printed materials, by treatment activities that heighten patients' awareness of left hemispace, or by treatment activities that enhance general attentional processes
  —*Pragmatic impairments,* which may be treated by calling on right-hemisphere-damaged adults' intact verbal skills, together with coaching and structured practice with compensatory strategies

- Some right-hemisphere-damaged adults' apparent pragmatic impairments actually may represent problems in attending to subtle cues, problems in making inferences, or problems organizing and interpreting complex information.

- Myers has suggested that a central impairment called *inference failure* causes many right-hemisphere-damaged patients' communicative and cognitive impairments and recommends that treatment focus on enhancing these patients' ability to make inferences.
- Tompkins has suggested that many of the cognitive, communicative, and behavioral abnormalities exhibited by patients with right-hemisphere brain injuries are caused by *limitations in the availability of the resources* required to carry out the mental operations required in tasks that are sensitive to right-hemisphere brain injury. Joanette and Goulet offer a similar explanation, phrased in terms of *task difficulty.*
- *Generalization* is a crucial issue for patients with right-hemisphere damage because they tend not to spontaneously generalize new learning from the clinic to daily life, from one task to another, or from level to level within treatment tasks. Consequently, procedures to enhance and maintain generalization are an important part of treatment for most patients with right-hemisphere brain damage.
- Tompkins has suggested several ways to enhance right-hemisphere-damaged adults' generalization of behavior across settings:
    - —Provide enough training trials to consolidate and stabilize responses.
    - —Train a variety of related responses.
    - —Train responses across a variety of tasks and contexts.
    - —Incorporate aspects of the target environment into treatment.

- —Train self-instruction and verbal mediation.
- —Involve right-hemisphere-damaged adults' family members, friends, and caregivers in treatment.

THOUGHT QUESTIONS

Question 8-1 Fred Bicep is a 26-year-old man who experienced sudden headache and left-side arm and leg weakness shortly after bench-pressing 350 pounds at his fitness center. He was taken to his local hospital's emergency room, where the examining physician recorded the following findings:

Alert and cooperative, but seemed confused
Complains of severe headache
Speech intelligible, but rambling and incoherent
Left-side hemiparesis, arm greater than leg
Exaggerated reflexes, left arm and leg; plantar extensor reflex (Babinski), left
Left homonymous hemianopia
Left neglect

What do you think caused Fred's signs and symptoms? What do you think the physician will do after she finishes examining Fred? What would you predict regarding Fred's potential recovery? How might Fred's recovery differ from someone who had a right-hemisphere occlusive stroke?

Question 8-2
Sophia Snyder, a right-handed woman with right-hemisphere damage and moderately severe left hemispatial neglect is shown the three arrays *(A, B, C)* several times each in random order and asked to point to the squares in each array. What pattern of responses would you expect from Ms. Snyder in this task? Which squares would you expect her to consistently identify? Which ones would you expect her to consistently miss? Are there squares that you would expect her to identify only part of the time? What do you think

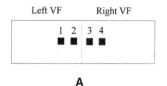

A

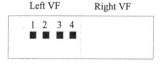

B

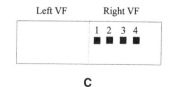

C

would happen if you gave her a large number of trials (50 or more) with these stimuli (presented in random order) in one session?

Question 8-3 Consider the following excerpt from an interview with Glenda Glindon, a hospitalized 67-year-old right-handed woman who is 3 days post-onset of a stroke in the posterior branch of the middle cerebral artery in her right brain hemisphere.

Clinician: "What brings you to the hospital?"

Patient: "Well, they say I'm having trouble walking."

Clinician: "Why is that?"

Patient: "I guess I'm having trouble with my legs. They put me in physical therapy every day."

Clinician: "Why are you in physical therapy? What kind of trouble are you having with your legs?"

Patient: "They say it's my left leg."

Clinician: "What happened to your left leg?"

Patient: "They say it's not working because I had a stroke, but I don't know about that."

Clinician: "Are you having any other problems?"

Patient: "Just being in this place and putting up with all the doctors."

What behavioral characteristics of right-hemisphere brain injury are reflected in the interview? What does the interview suggest regarding potential issues that might arise during evaluation and treatment of this patient? (Assume that reimbursement issues and access to the patient will not be problems. Someone will pay for rea-sonable services and the patient will be available to you for assessment and treatment.)

Question 8-4 You receive a referral on Mr. Blanding, a 58-year-old right-handed man who had a posterior right-hemisphere stroke 3 days ago. The referring neurologist asks you to evaluate the patient to determine if Mr. Blanding is a candidate for cognitive-communicative therapy. If you determine that he is a candidate for such treatment, Mr. Blanding will be transferred to a long-term care ward for the duration of the treatment for up to 6 weeks. If you determine that he is not a treatment candidate, he will be discharged to his home in northern Minnesota in 2 days. (He lives in a small town in a rural area. Treatment there is not an option.) You can schedule Mr. Blanding for no more than 4 hours of testing in the next 2 days.

What tests would you administer? You do not have access to a "right-hemisphere test battery," such as those described in the textbook. You must choose individual tests that address specific impairments. Consider how you can fit your selections into a 4-hour period, and choose tests that are most likely to indicate Mr. Blanding's potential as a treatment candidate.

Question 8-5 How would the risks for an individual with left neglect who elects to drive an automobile in England differ from those for an individual with left neglect who elects to drive an automobile in the United States?

Traumatic Brain Injury

Traumatic brain injuries are caused by abrupt external forces acting on the head. These forces are generated when a moving object (e.g., a bullet, a club, or a baseball) strikes the head or when the moving head strikes a stationary object (e.g., an automobile windshield, a tree, or a sidewalk). If the skull is fractured or perforated and the meninges are torn or lacerated, the injury is called a *penetrating head injury* or *open-head injury.* If the skull and meninges remain intact, the injury is called a *nonpenetrating head injury* or, more frequently, a *closed-head injury* or *closed-head trauma.* Penetrating injuries often are caused by missile wounds or blows to the head by sharp objects. Closed-head injuries often are caused by motor-vehicle accidents and falls.

INCIDENCE AND PREVALENCE OF TRAUMATIC BRAIN INJURIES

Traumatic brain injury is a significant social, economic, and medical problem in contemporary society. Each year about 1.25 million U.S. residents receive medical attention for traumatic brain injuries (Guerrero, Thurman, & Sniezek, 2000). About one in four are hospitalized (Thurman & Guerrero, 1999). Of those who are hospitalized, about one in six die from their injuries. Of those who survive hospitalization, about one in three are left with permanent disabilities (Thurman & associates, 1999; Figure 9-1). Thurman and associates (1999) estimate that in the United States there are about 5.3 million survivors of traumatic brain injury living with disabilities related to their brain injuries.

Estimates of the incidence of traumatic brain injury vary widely, from 95 per 100,000 (Centers for Disease Control and Prevention, 1997) to 200 per 100,000 (Kraus, 1993; Rosenthal & associates, 1990). The reported incidence of traumatic brain injury has declined gradually during the past decade, perhaps because of declining rates of hospitalization for less severe traumatic brain injuries together with newer counting methods that focus on hospitalized cases and cases ending in death. The true incidence of traumatic brain injury is not known, but it probably lies between 100 per 100,000 and 250 per 100,000 in the United States.

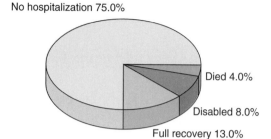

Figure 9-1 ■ Outcome for adults who sustain traumatic brain injuries in the United States. Twenty-five percent are hospitalized because of their injuries. Of all adults who sustain traumatic brain injuries, about 4% die before leaving the hospital, about 8% leave the hospital with permanent communicative or cognitive disabilities, and about 13% recover with no substantial communicative or cognitive disabilities (although many will exhibit subtle impairments if carefully tested). (Based on data reported by Thurman, D. J., Alverson, C. A., Dunn, K. A., & associates. [1999]. Traumatic brain injury in the United States: A public health perspective. *Journal of Head Trauma Rehabilitation, 14,* 602-615.)

Most traumatic brain injuries (approximately 90%) are closed-head injuries. About two thirds of all traumatic brain injuries are caused by motor-vehicle accidents. Falls and assaults account for most of the rest. Males are more likely than females to receive traumatic brain injuries (Figure 9-2). About twice as many males than females receive head injuries, but the difference is larger for young adults. For young adults between 15 and 25 years old three to five males are traumatically brain injured for every female so injured; for 20-year-olds the ratio of males to females is approximately 4:1 (Annegers & associates, 1980).

Toddlers and older adults are less likely to experience traumatic brain injuries than 15- to 25-year-olds, but they are more likely to experience them than the general population (Finlayson &

Cases Per Year Per 100,000 Population

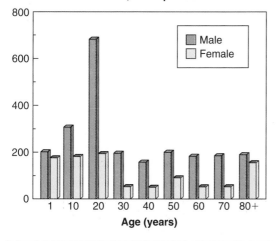

Figure 9-2 ■ The frequency of traumatic brain injuries in males and females according to age. (Data from Annegers, J. F., Grabow, J. D., Kurland, L. T., & associates. [1980]. The incidence, causes, and secular trends of head trauma in Olmsted County, Minnesota. *Neurology, 30,* 912-919.)

Garner, 1994). Falls account for most traumatic brain injuries in toddlers and the very old, whereas motor-vehicle accidents account for most traumatic brain injuries in young adults (Finlayson & Garner, 1994; Van Houten & associates, 1994). Traumatic brain injury is the leading cause of neurologic disability in persons under the age of 50 (Finlayson & Garner, 1994).

RISK FACTORS

Several variables other than age and sex affect the probability of traumatic brain injury. One of the most conspicuous is substance abuse. About half (40% to 60%) of patients admitted to hospitals following traumatic brain injuries are intoxicated at the time of admission (Brismar, Engstrom, & Rydberg, 1983; Rutherford, 1977). Motor-vehicle accidents, falls, and assaults, in that order, cause most of the traumatic brain injuries sustained by intoxicated adults. Many assault-related injuries are related to the use of alcohol, drugs, or both by the aggressor, the vic-

tim, or both (Giles & Clark-Wilson, 1993). Hillbom and Holm (1986) estimate that the incidence of brain injury in alcoholic adults is two to four times greater than the incidence of brain injury in the general population.

School adjustment and *social history* also are related to the probability of traumatic brain injury. Haas, Cope, and Hall (1987) reported that 50% of a large group of severely brain-injured patients had a history of poor academic performance (failure in two or more subjects, diagnosed learning disability, or school dropout). Giles and Clark-Wilson (1993) comment that poor academic performance may be related to underlying neurologic impairments causing distractibility, attentional impairments, lowered frustration tolerance, impulsivity, rebelliousness, egocentrism, sociopathic behavior, and substance abuse, all of which increase the probability of head injuries from motor-vehicle accidents, assaults, and falls.

Socioeconomic status also affects the probability of traumatic brain injury. Individuals with low income, especially those who live in areas with high population density (central cities), have a higher probability of traumatic brain injury (primarily from assaults and falls) than do individuals with higher income who live in areas of low population density (Macniven, 1994).

The divorce rate for traumatically brain-injured adults in the United States is approximately four times that of those divorced in the general U.S. population (Kerr, Kay, & Lassman, 1971). However, the high divorce rate for traumatically-brain-injured adults may be related to other variables such as substance abuse, social maladjustment, and personality.

The influence of *personality type* on the probability of traumatic brain injury has received a fair amount of attention. The general conclusion is that *Type A* personalities (characterized by competitiveness, impulsivity, belligerence, and hostility) are more likely to sustain traumatic brain injuries than are *Type B* personalities (characterized by cooperativeness, deliberateness, and helpfulness) (Evans, Palsane, & Carrere, 1987).

A *history of traumatic brain injury* increases the probability of additional traumatic brain injury. The probability of a second traumatic brain injury is three times greater for individuals who have sustained a previous traumatic brain injury than for the general population. The probability of a third traumatic brain injury for an individual who has had two traumatic brain injuries is eight times greater than the probability of traumatic brain injury for an individual with no previous brain injury (Annegers & associates, 1980).

Participation in high-risk sports increases the risk of traumatic brain injury. Professional and amateur boxers have a particularly high rate of diffuse brain injury, which gradually increases in severity throughout the boxer's career, presumably because of repeated mild brain trauma. Motorcycling, bicycling, snowmobiling, and rock climbing are associated with increased risk of traumatic brain injury, although wearing appropriate safety helmets significantly diminishes the risk of head injury.

> Bicycle riders wearing helmets have an 88% reduction in risk of traumatic brain injury (Thompson, Rivara, & Thompson, 1989), and comparable reductions in injury are no doubt associated with use of helmets in other sporting activities in which participants' heads receive sudden acceleration or deceleration, strike unyielding surfaces, or are struck by moving objects.

Although each of the foregoing variables affects the probability of traumatic brain injury, many interactions among variables certainly exist, making it difficult or impossible to isolate the effects of any single variable. For example, alcohol and drug abuse are likely to be related to socioeconomic status, school adjustment, educational achievement, and personality variables, and each of the latter variables is likely to interact with one or more of the others. Consequently, it

is impossible to estimate the amount by which the presence of any single variable increases the probability of traumatic brain injury. However, it seems clear that adding risk factors adds to the probability that an individual will sustain a head injury.

> Most young head-injured adults are unmarried, unemployed males of low socioeconomic status (Barber & Webster, 1974).

PATHOPHYSIOLOGY OF TRAUMATIC BRAIN INJURY

Information about what happens inside the skull in traumatic brain injury comes from two sources—post-mortem studies of the brains of animals with laboratory-induced brain injuries and post-mortem studies of the brains of humans who have succumbed to traumatic brain injuries. Because the human brains available for post-mortem study belong to patients who die from their injuries, most of what we know about traumatic brain injury comes from patients who have sustained severe brain injuries. Post-mortem studies of patients with mild or moderate traumatic brain injuries are extremely limited. Consequently, the neuropathology of mild or moderate traumatic brain injury is based more on extrapolation and intuition than on empiric evidence.

Penetrating Brain Injuries

Most penetrating brain injuries are caused by missiles (e.g., bullets, stones, artillery shell fragments, other projectiles). Some are caused by blunt instruments (e.g., clubs, baseball bats), and some are caused by falls in which the head strikes a sharp object.

The amount and nature of brain damage caused by missiles depends on the velocity of the missile. High-velocity missiles (e.g., rifle bullets, military projectiles) usually create more physical damage to cranial contents than low-velocity missiles. High-velocity missiles perforate the skull and pierce the brain substance, often exiting through the skull opposite the point of entry. Their high kinetic energy creates a pressure wave that has an explosive impact on the skull and brain, destroying tissue on both sides of the projectile's track and causing diffuse bleeding and tissue disruption throughout the brain and brain stem. The missile carries foreign material (hair, skin, and bone fragments) into the brain, increasing the risk of infection. High-velocity missile wounds to the brain almost always are fatal, usually within minutes to hours after injury (Grafman & Salazar, 1987).

Low-velocity missile wounds (e.g., bullets from handguns, shrapnel) are less often fatal but are nevertheless dangerous. The missile penetrates the skull and travels into the brain, carrying foreign material with it. The missile tunnels through the brain, causing tissue destruction along the missile's track but not in more remote regions. If the missile has sufficient velocity to strike the skull opposite the point of entry, it may ricochet and cause additional brain injury opposite the entry point.

Some low-velocity impacts (e.g., being struck on the head with a club or striking the head on a table edge in a fall) may cause penetrating injuries if the force of the impact is concentrated in a small area. Such low-velocity impacts fracture, rather than perforate, the skull. If the fracture is severe, bone fragments may be pushed into the brain beneath the fracture, and brain tissue beneath the impact site may be cut, torn, and bruised. Damage to the brain following such low-velocity impacts may be surprisingly slight because most of the energy of the blow to the head is spent in fracturing the skull and comparatively little is transmitted to the brain.

Between 20% and 40% of low-velocity penetrating injuries cause the patient's death (Grafman & Salazar, 1987), although mortality is greater (up to 90%) for penetrating injuries caused by handguns. If the patient survives the first day after a penetrating brain injury, infection, bleeding, and increased intracranial pressure (either from swelling of the brain or from hydrocephalus) become important threats to the patient's survival. Penetrating injuries in the brain stem usually are fatal because of damage to structures that regulate respiration, heart rate and blood pressure, and other vital functions.

Adults who survive penetrating head injuries and their physiologic consequences almost always are left with physical, cognitive, and linguistic impairments. These impairments (except those caused by high-velocity missiles) usually are focal, rather than diffuse, and reflect loss of functions served by the brain regions destroyed by the injury.

Nonpenetrating Brain Injuries

In nonpenetrating brain injuries (closed-head trauma) the meninges remain intact and foreign substances do not enter the brain. Nonpenetrating injuries can be divided into two general categories: *acceleration injuries* and *nonacceleration injuries.*

Acceleration injuries (sometimes called *moving-head injuries*) are produced when the unrestrained head is struck by a moving object or the moving head strikes a stationary object. Nonacceleration injuries (sometimes called *fixed-head injuries*) are produced when the restrained head is struck by a moving object (the patient is lying on a hard surface or sitting with his or her head against an unyielding surface when the head is struck). Acceleration injuries also may occur when the rapidly moving head abruptly changes direction without striking a surface, as in whiplash injuries in motor-vehicle accidents.

Nonacceleration Injuries Nonacceleration injuries usually produce less severe traumatic brain injury than acceleration injuries. Blows to a moveable head are estimated to be 20 times more devastating than blows to a fixed head (Pang, 1989). The primary consequences of nonacceleration injuries are related to deformation of the skull by the impact of the moving object. The skull is rigid but slightly elastic, so a blow to the head deforms the skull at the point of impact and drives it against the brain surface, causing localized damage to the meninges and brain cortex at the point of impact—damage called *impression trauma* (Figure 9-3). It is not clear if impression trauma is caused by the impact of the depressed skull against the brain or by negative pressure that develops when the skull snaps back to its original shape.

If a nonacceleration injury is caused by a slow-moving object with a large surface area, *ellipsoidal deformation* of the skull may occur (see Figure 9-3). When the skull is forced from its customary oval shape to a more circular one, its volume increases. This change in volume creates a pressure gradient that causes brain tissue to expand outward from central structures (the ventricular walls, corpus callosum, and basal ganglia). The outward movement stretches and shears brain tissue, causing it to bleed and swell.

Some nonacceleration brain injuries cause skull fractures. Fractures at the base of the skull are more serious than fractures higher up because basal skull fractures may damage cranial nerves or the carotid arteries. Regardless of its site, any skull fracture is dangerous if the meninges beneath the fracture are torn because of bleeding from damaged meningeal blood vessels and the potential for infection by bacteria penetrating the damaged meninges. At one time the severity of closed head injuries was measured by whether or not the skull was fractured. However, it is now clear that the presence (or absence) of skull fracture does not predict the severity of brain damage.

Acceleration Injuries When traumatic brain injury is caused by sudden acceleration or deceleration of the head, the brain and brain stem often suffer diffuse damage caused by their movement within the skull. The movement is caused by inertial forces generated either when the head is moving rapidly through space and comes to a sudden stop (as when it strikes the floor after a fall) or when the head is at rest and is suddenly accelerated (as when it is struck by a blunt object). Acceleration injuries can in turn be subdivided into two categories—*linear acceleration injuries* and *angular acceleration injuries.*

Linear acceleration injuries occur when the head is suddenly accelerated by an outside force moving along a linear path aligned with the center axis of the head (see Figure 9-3). Because resting bodies tend to stay at rest, the head and its contents resist acceleration, but within a few milliseconds the skull begins to move parallel with the direction of the outside force. However, the brain is not firmly anchored within the skull, and it has its own resting inertia, which keeps it at rest for a few milliseconds after the skull begins to move. The inertial lag causes the brain to be compressed against the inner surface of the skull at the point of impact. This compression may cause bruises and abrasions on the surface of the brain where it strikes the skull. Such injuries are sometimes called *coup injuries* (*coup* is a French word, pronounced *coo*, which means *blow* or *impact*).

Within a few milliseconds after the skull begins to move, the brain also begins to move and quickly accelerates to the rate at which the skull is moving. Then the movement of the head is stopped abruptly, either by the tethering action of the vertebrae and neck muscles or by striking a surface or object. Because a moving mass tends to keep moving, the contents of the skull resist deceleration. Therefore, it takes a few milliseconds for the brain to stop moving after the skull stops moving. The mismatch in deceleration compresses the brain against the inner surface of the skull opposite the point of impact. This compression causes localized injury to the surface of the brain on the opposite side from the blow that first started the head moving. These opposite-side injuries are called *contrecoup* (pronounced *contra-coo*) injuries.

Coup and contrecoup injuries cause focal damage to the meninges, brain cortex, and nearby subcortical brain tissue where the brain is compressed against the skull. Coup and contrecoup injuries are sometimes called *translational trauma* (Teasdale & Mendelow, 1984) and only occur as a consequence of linear acceleration and deceleration of the head. Translational trauma is more likely following blows to the front or back of the head than

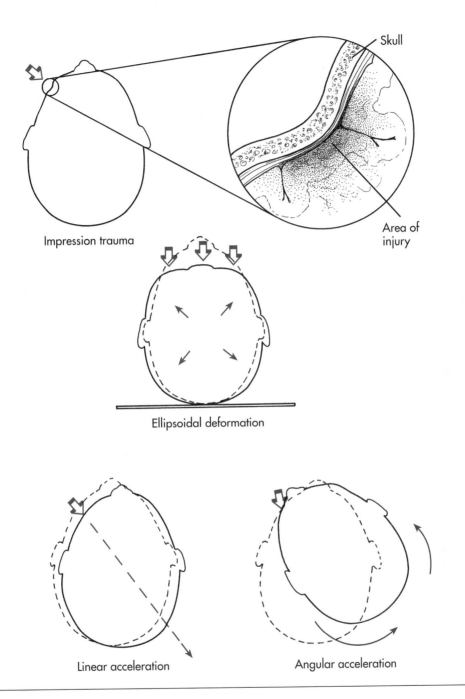

Skull

Area of
injury

Impression trauma

Ellipsoidal deformation

Linear acceleration

Angular acceleration

Figure 9-3 ■ Physical consequences of blows to the head. Impression trauma is caused by blunt force applied to a small area of the skull. The skull is depressed at the point of impact with consequent injury to meninges and brain tissue beneath the point of impact. Ellipsoidal deformation is caused by blunt force applied to a large area on the restrained head. The skull is forced from its usual ellipsoidal shape to a more nearly circular shape. Linear acceleration of the skull and its contents is caused by blunt force applied on a line through the central axis of the unrestrained head. Angular acceleration of the skull and its contents is caused by blunt force applied at an angle to the central axis of the unrestrained head, causing the head to rotate away from the point of impact.

blows to the side of the head. This is because the space between the brain and the skull (the epidural space) is greater at the front and back than at the sides. Consequently, the potential for linear brain movement within the skull is greater when the head moves front-to-back than when it moves side-to-side.

The same physical processes operate when the head is moving at a constant rate of speed in a linear path and suddenly is stopped. The consequences for the skull and brain are equivalent to those generated by sudden acceleration of the head. Shaken baby syndrome (shaken impact syndrome) is the medical label for a collection of brain injuries in infants and toddlers caused by violent shaking (usually intentional, by an angry caregiver). The combination of violent shaking and the child's weak neck muscles cause the child's head to bounce to and fro, causing diffuse acceleration injuries to the child's fragile brain tissue. Whiplash injuries in motor-vehicle accidents also sometimes cause acceleration injuries to the brain.

Blows that strike the head off-center propel it at an angle from the direction of the blow and cause the head to rotate away from the blow (Figure 9-3). This causes what is called *angular acceleration* of the skull and its contents. Inertial forces are generated by angular acceleration, but the forces are rotational rather than linear. Within a few milliseconds of impact the skull begins to rotate and move at an angle away from the point of impact. The brain's inertia causes it to remain at rest for a few milliseconds after the skull begins to move, generating twisting and shearing forces that are concentrated in axial structures (the midbrain, basal ganglia, brain stem, and cerebellum). Then the brain begins to move away from the point of impact and to rotate in the same direction as the skull. Within a few more milliseconds the tethering action of the vertebrae and neck muscles abruptly stop the move-

ment of the head and cause it to rebound in the opposite direction. The brain's inertia causes it to continue rotating in its original direction for a few milliseconds, causing a second episode of twisting and shearing forces concentrated in axial structures. (The twisting forces in the second episode move in the opposite direction to those in the first episode.)

Shearing forces tend to be concentrated at the boundaries between gray matter (supportive tissue) and white matter (fiber tracts). For this reason, shearing forces and associated bleeding and swelling tend to be more severe around major white fiber tracts, especially the internal capsule, the corpus callosum, and the brain stem. Angular acceleration of the head and rotation of cranial contents within the skull usually produce more severe brain injuries than linear acceleration of the head, wherein cranial contents are not subjected to twisting forces (Ommaya, Grubb, & Naumann, 1971).

Cranial nerve injuries are common following acceleration injuries to the brain. Front-to-back acceleration injuries (e.g., falling and striking the back of the head) may stretch and tear the olfactory nerve (CN 1) leading to loss of the sense of smell *(anosmia)*. Injuries to nerves controlling the extraocular muscles (CN 3, CN 4, CN 6) may compromise eye movements and cause double vision *(diplopia)* because of misalignment of the eyes. Injury to CN 8 may cause ringing or buzzing in the ears *(tinnitus)* or vertigo.

The twisting and shearing forces created within the brain by angular acceleration, or the stretching and tearing forces created by linear acceleration, cause damage to nerve-cell axons diffusely scattered throughout the brain substance—a condition called *diffuse axonal injury*. Diffuse axonal injury is a common consequence of traumatic brain injury and is assumed to be responsible for many of the diffuse cognitive and behavioral impairments that follow traumatic brain injury. Some diffuse axonal injury probably occurs whenever consciousness is lost following head injury (Giles & Clark-Wilson, 1993), and widespread diffuse axonal injury is considered to be a common cause of *vegetative state,* in which the patient has sleep-wake cycles but makes no purposeful movements, does not talk, cannot follow instructions, and does not track visual stimuli. Vegetative state is the result of severe diffuse damage to cortical and subcortical regions with relative preservation of the brain stem.

> Diffuse brain damage also may be caused by other conditions, such as cerebral anoxia or bacterial or viral infections.

The twisting and shearing forces associated with acceleration injuries do not cause immediate disconnection of axons from their neural cell bodies. The twisting and shearing forces stretch, rather than tear, nerve axons. Within 2 to 3 hours after injury the stretched axons swell, and within the next several hours (sometimes up to 24 hours) the axons separate at the site of the swelling. The disconnected axonal segments then deteriorate—a process that may not be complete until 2 days post-injury. Axonal degeneration following moving-head injury is a diffuse process, affecting some axons in a region of injury and leaving others untouched, creating a spotty pattern of deafferentation (loss of input to a neuron from other neurons). This means that neurons in the region of injury may lose only part of their synaptic inputs from other neurons.

Intact axon terminals adjacent to regions of limited deafferentation may send fibers into the regions of deafferentation (a process called *collateral sprouting* or *dendritic proliferation*). This repair process may at least partially explain physiologic recovery in patients with mild to moderate traumatic brain injury. (Patients with severe brain injuries may have lost too many axons to permit meaningful recovery as a consequence of such reafferentation.) Focal lesions, such as those associated with stroke and tumor, cause dense regions of deafferentation, which no

doubt severely limits the role of reafferentation in physiologic recovery from such focal injuries.

In addition to twisting and shearing, rapid acceleration and deceleration of the head causes abrasions and lacerations of cortical tissues as the brain moves within the cranial vault. As the brain moves, it scrapes against the inner surface of the cranial vault. Because the floor of the cranial vault is uneven and irregular and the walls and roof are relatively smooth (Figure 9-4), abrasions and lacerations tend to concentrate on the bottom surfaces of the frontal lobes and the anterior temporal lobes. Abrasions and lacerations in the parietal lobes, occipital lobes, and the convexities of the frontal lobes are uncommon because the walls and roof of the cranial vault in those regions are comparatively smooth and featureless (Figure 9-5).

Traumatic Hemorrhage Cuts and bruises on the brain surface and twisting and shearing within the brain cause bleeding *(hemorrhage)* and accumulations of blood *(hematomas).* There are four major categories of traumatic hematoma, depending on where the blood accumulates—*epidural hematoma, subdural hematoma, subarachnoid hematoma,* and *intracerebral hematoma.*

Epidural hematomas, as the label suggests, are accumulations of blood between the dura mater and the skull. They are caused by lacerations of the middle meningeal artery, middle meningeal vein, or a dural venous sinus. Automobile accidents are the most common cause of epidural hematoma, but trivial events such as falls and sports injuries sometimes cause them. Of epidural hematomas 90% are associated with skull fracture (Teasdale & Mendelow, 1984). About 20% to 30% of patients with epidural hematoma die as a consequence of their head injuries. Mortality from epidural hematoma is strongly related to whether the bleeding is from an artery (death in about 85% of cases) or a vein (death in about 15% of cases). Arterial bleeding usually is marked by massive hemorrhage, with symptoms progressing rapidly, often culminating in death within a few hours. Venous bleeding usually follows a less dramatic

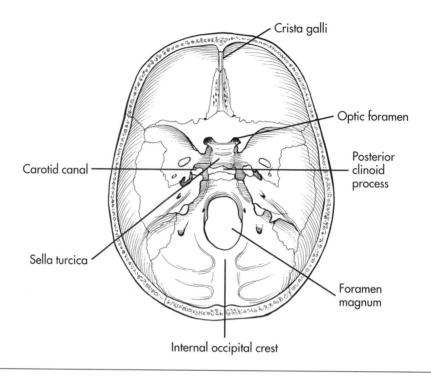

Crista galli

Optic foramen

Posterior clinoid process

Carotid canal

Sella turcica

Foramen magnum

Internal occipital crest

Figure 9-4 ■ **The floor of the skull. The crista galli, the posterior clinoid process, and the sella turcica are ridges in the skull floor. These and other prominences on the skull floor contribute to contusions and abrasions on the bottom surface of the brain in acceleration injuries.**

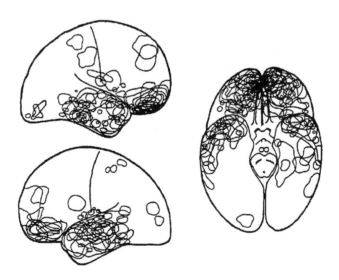

Figure 9-5 ■ **The location of brain contusions in a series of 40 traumatically-brain-injured adults. The most frequent location for contusions is the bottom surface of the frontal lobes, followed by the bottom surface of the anterior temporal lobes.** (From Courville, C.B. [1937]. *Pathology of the central nervous system.* Mountain View, CA: Pacific.)

course, with slow progression of symptoms. Small venous hemorrhages may ooze blood so slowly that they produce no overt symptoms, and the bleeding may be detected only with imaging scans of the head during routine evaluation of the patient.

The magnitude of the symptoms caused by epidural hemorrhages depends to some extent on the location of the hemorrhage. Bleeding into the posterior inferior epidural space can cause compression of the brain stem, leading to respiratory distress, decreased heart rate, and increased blood pressure. Bleeding into the frontal and superior epidural space is likely to be less serious because centers for vital functions are far away and because there is more epidural space to accommodate the hematoma before it begins to displace brain structures. The most common treatment for epidural hematomas is surgical removal, which usually is relatively easy because of the hematoma's accessibility just beneath the skull.

Subdural hematomas, as the name suggests, are accumulations of blood beneath the dura— between the dura and the arachnoid. Subdural hematomas are twice as common as epidural hematomas and twice as deadly, with 60% (or greater) overall mortality. Motor-vehicle accidents are the most common cause of subdural hematoma, and about half are associated with skull fractures. The source of most subdural hematomas is laceration of cortical blood vessels caused by abrasions and contusions on the brain surface. Acute subdural hematomas usually develop within a few hours and almost always within a week of the injury. The combination of increasing pressure and displacement of brain tissue by the expanding hematoma, if not controlled, may lead to coma and death within a few hours. Surgical removal of the hematoma is the most common treatment for acute subdural hematomas.

Chronic subdural hematomas are common in older patients and in patients with long-term alcoholism, both of whom have increased risk of falling and "who usually have some degree of brain atrophy with a resultant increase in the size of the subdural space" (Friedman, 1983, p. 10). Often the injury that precipitates the hematoma is relatively trivial (usually a fall with a bump on the head). The hemorrhage gradually fills the subdural space, and within a few weeks a membrane forms around the hematoma. Eventually the hematoma may reach a size at which it produces symptoms, which often wax and wane. Headache and tenderness in the affected area are the most common symptoms, although progressive dementia and decreasing levels of consciousness may develop. Surgical evacuation of the hematoma was for many years the treatment of choice, but mortality rates were distressingly high. In the last decade or so, a more conservative procedure has been successful. In this procedure, a catheter is inserted into the hematoma through an opening in the skull. The fluid then is continuously drained into a container below the level of the head.

Subarachnoid hematomas, caused by rupture of pial vessels within the subarachnoid space, are a common consequence of traumatic brain injuries and often are associated with subdural hemorrhages. Little is known about the long-range consequences of slowly accumulating blood in the subarachnoid space, although it is known to contribute to *cerebral vasospasm* (discussed later in this chapter). Rapid accumulation of blood following massive subarachnoid hemorrhage is, however, associated with massive headache and rapid neurologic deterioration, often ending in death.

Intracerebral hematomas are caused by rupture of blood vessels within the brain *(intracerebral hemorrhage).* Intracerebral hemorrhages usually develop in subcortical white matter, the basal ganglia, and the brain stem. Occasionally a large intracerebral hematoma bleeds into the ventricular system, creating a secondary subarachnoid hematoma, usually with devastating effects on the patient. A pattern of multiple small intracerebral hemorrhages sometimes occurs in combination with diffuse axonal injury caused by translational trauma—a combination that often leads to coma and death of the patient (Adams, Graham, & Scott, 1980).

The foregoing consequences of traumatic brain injury are the result of the forces exerted on the brain at the time of injury. They are accounted for by the mechanical effects of compression, stretching, shearing, abrasion, and laceration of the brain and meninges. For this reason they are sometimes called *primary consequences.* The primary consequences usually generate *secondary consequences,* which represent the brain's responses to trauma or to the failure of other somatic functions (e.g., cardiac output or pulmonary function). These secondary consequences often are more devastating than the primary consequences. Although no statistics are available, it is likely that more patients with traumatic brain injuries die from the secondary consequences of their injuries than from the physical damage to the brain suffered at the time of the accident. (Death rates from traumatic brain injuries are highest in the first 3 days, with 50% to 75% of deaths occurring within 72 hours.)

Secondary Consequences of Traumatic Brain Injury

Cerebral Edema Accumulation of fluid is the brain's generic response to a wide variety of conditions, such as trauma, anoxia, infection, and inflammation. The fluid may accumulate between the brain and skull, within the ventricles, or within brain tissues, causing tissues to swell—a condition called *cerebral edema.* Cerebral edema almost always develops around the primary site of brain injury, but it can occur far from the primary injury site. Cerebral edema often follows diffuse injuries, such as those caused by translational trauma, and is an important cause of increased intracranial pressure. The effects of cerebral edema on intracranial pressure usually become significant within 4 to 6 hours post-injury and peak in 24 to 36 hours.

Traumatic Hydrocephalus Swelling of brain tissues (especially in midbrain regions) sometimes compresses the passages through which cerebrospinal fluid circulates between the ventricles and into the subarachnoid space. The trapped cerebrospinal fluid exerts pressure on the walls of the ventricles, causing the ventricles to expand, compressing brain structures, and elevating intracranial pressure.

Elevated Intracranial Pressure Perhaps the most dramatic (and deadly) consequence of traumatic brain injury is buildup of pressure within the cranial vault. The pressure buildup may be a secondary consequence of cerebral edema, traumatic hydrocephalus, or hemorrhage. The elevated pressure compresses and displaces brain tissues, and the patient exhibits inexorably increasing neurologic impairment as intracranial pressure increases. Increased intracranial pressure is the most frequent cause of death from traumatic brain injury; monitoring and controlling intracranial pressure is one of the primary concerns in medical management of traumatically-brain-injured patients.

Generalized pressure on brain tissue may cause neurologic impairments but only if the pressure becomes very great. The brain seems reasonably tolerant of modest increases in pressure, provided the pressure is distributed equally throughout the cranial vault. Unfortunately, traumatic brain injuries produce pressure gradients in which pressure is greatest at and around the site of injury and decreases with increasing distance from the injury. These pressure gradients displace brain tissues away from regions of high pressure into regions of low pressure. The tissues are distorted, stretched, compressed against the skull, and forced against projections and partitions within the skull, usually with ominous consequences because the brain is as intolerant of displacement and distortion as it is tolerant of moderate increments in generalized intracranial pressure.

As intracranial pressure increases, injured cell walls leak fluid into extracellular space. Damaged blood vessels leak blood into brain tissue or adjacent spaces. The brain swells, increasing the forces that displace and distort brain tissues. If uncontrolled, this sequence of events quickly leads to coma and brain death.

The most dangerous consequence of regional increases in intracranial pressure is *herniation,* in which cerebral structures are pushed around rigid partitions in the cranial vault or extruded through cranial orifices. Herniation is discussed in Chapter 1.

Prolonged high levels of intracranial pressure inevitably cause irreversible brain damage, often culminating in coma and death. Fortunately, intracranial pressure can be monitored and controlled. Physicians may directly monitor intracranial pressure by inserting a pressure transducer into the cranial vault. Several procedures are available for controlling intracranial pressure. The patient may be hyperventilated to increase blood oxygen levels. Increased blood oxygen causes cerebral arteries to constrict, decreases cerebral blood volume, and provides at least temporary reductions in intracranial pressure. Steroids (antiinflammatory medications) may be administered to reduce cerebral edema. The patient's body temperature may be lowered *(hypothermia)* to diminish brain swelling. Diuretics (medications that increase the body's excretion of fluids) may be administered. If these treatments are unsuccessful, the patient may be put into a barbiturate coma to decrease cerebral metabolism and constrict cerebral blood vessels. Sometimes surgical removal of swollen brain tissue may be needed to control increased intracranial pressure if less radical measures to manage brain swelling fail.

Ischemic Brain Damage In addition to the impairments caused by the effects of tissue destruction, swelling, and tissue displacement, most traumatically-brain-injured patients sustain at least some ischemic brain damage. Graham, Adams, and Doyle (1978) reported ischemic damage in 91% of patients who had died of head injuries. Ischemic brain damage can occur for several reasons. Injury to cardiovascular and pulmonary systems may compromise respiratory and cardiac output, leading in turn to diminished blood oxygenation and reduced blood supply to the brain. Elevated intracranial pressure may squeeze blood vessels and reduce the volume of blood reaching the brain. Cerebral vasospasm (discussed in next section) may decrease the carrying capacity of the cerebral vessels, especially when cardiac output is reduced.

Severe head injury may disrupt autoregulation of blood pressure, making cerebral blood flow dependent on arterial pressure (Lewelt, Jenkins, & Miller, 1982). For these patients, elevated blood pressure causes excessive cerebral blood flow. Lowered blood pressure (more common following traumatic brain injury) causes diminished cerebral blood flow with consequent impairments attributable to cerebral ischemia.

Severe head injury also may disrupt vascular responsiveness to blood gas levels (Marion, Darby, & Yonas, 1991). Ordinarily, above-normal carbon dioxide levels in the blood (as with pulmonary obstruction or hypoventilation) trigger dilation of cerebral blood vessels to increase blood oxygenation, and below-normal carbon dioxide levels trigger constriction of cerebral blood vessels to diminish blood oxygenation. Disruption of vascular responsiveness to blood gas levels in brain-injured patients with diminished pulmonary function may contribute to cerebral ischemia, with consequent negative effects on the patient's physical, cognitive, and behavioral condition.

Cerebral ischemia and its effects are far more prominent in patients with severe head injuries than in patients with mild to moderately severe head injuries, but it seems likely that some patients with moderate head injuries (and perhaps a few with mild head injuries) may be affected in subtle ways by brain ischemia. The distribution of damage from these ischemic processes varies, but damage is most common in the basal ganglia and surrounding structures and in the watershed cortical regions adjacent to the distributions of the three major cerebral arteries.

Cerebral Vasospasm Cerebral vasospasm (contraction of the muscular layer surrounding blood vessels) occurs in 15% to 20% of head injuries. Cortical arteries that are inflamed by the presence of blood from a subarachnoid hemorrhage are most frequently affected by vasospasm, although any artery can be affected, especially if it is in or near the site of primary injury. Other causes of cerebral vasospasm include stimulation of cerebral blood vessels by chemical or metabolic disruptions and injury to control centers that regulate dilation and constriction of cerebral arteries. Cerebral vasospasm alone rarely is responsible for major neurologic complications. However, when vasospasm is inflicted on a system already compromised by other consequences of brain injury, it may contribute to significant worsening of a patient's condition.

Alterations in the Blood-Brain Barrier
In addition to the tissue destruction, neural disorganization, and vascular changes already described, traumatic brain injury also induces changes in the blood-brain barrier (Povlishock & associates, 1978). The blood-brain barrier normally regulates the movement of various substances from the blood into the tissues of the brain. Brain injury may disrupt this regulation, allowing normally excluded substances (proteins, neurotransmitter chemicals) to enter brain tissue. More severe brain injuries are more likely to disrupt the blood-brain barrier than less severe injuries. (This relationship between severity of injury and magnitude of secondary consequences is, of course, true for all secondary consequences.) The passage of normally excluded substances into the brain may contribute to accumulation of fluid within brain tissues and swelling of the tissues *(cerebral edema)*.

Severity of Brain Injury and Physiologic Consequences

Not surprisingly, the nature and severity of neuropathology caused by traumatic brain injury determines the nature and severity of patients' symptoms and also determines, in large part, the extent of patients' recovery. Patients with mild traumatic brain injury typically have damaged axons scattered throughout the brain, with diffuse and spotty neural degeneration primarily in the brain stem. Relatively good physiologic recovery usually

occurs, no doubt aided by neuroplasticity (collateral axonal sprouting, dendritic proliferation).

Patients with moderate traumatic brain injury have diffuse axonal damage spread throughout the brain and brain stem. Lacerations and contusions on the surface of the brain, primarily in the temporal and frontal lobes, destroy brain tissue, creating focal lesions. Lacerated and torn blood vessels may leak, creating hematomas. Neuroplasticity usually contributes to moderate amounts of physiologic recovery.

Patients with severe traumatic brain injuries typically have extensive axonal damage throughout the brain and brain stem. Hemorrhages are common and may be life-threatening. Vascular ischemic changes also are common in the first few days following injury. Hypotension from blood loss or from compromised autoregulation of blood pressure may add to brain ischemia. Hypoxia from pulmonary obstruction or hypoventilation may further diminish the brain's oxygen supply. Neuroplasticity typically contributes little to physiologic recovery because the density of axonal damage throughout the brain precludes important beneficial effects from collateral axonal sprouting and dendritic proliferation.

The primary and secondary physical consequences of traumatic brain injury are important determinants of traumatically-brain-injured patients' eventual level of recovery, but they are not the only determinants. Patient variables such as age, gender, and personal history also can affect recovery, although their influence is not as strong as that of physical consequences. In the following section we consider how some of these variables relate to recovery from traumatic brain injury and to each other.

GENERAL CONCEPTS 9-1

- Head injuries can be classified as *penetrating* or *nonpenetrating,* depending on whether the skull is fractured or perforated and the meninges are torn or cut. Most *penetrating brain injuries* (in which the skull and meninges are compromised) are caused by *missiles* (bullets or other projectiles).

- *Nonpenetrating* (closed-head) injuries are more common than penetrating head injuries. Most are caused by *motor-vehicle accidents*.

- The risk of traumatic brain injury is greatest for young males between the ages of 15 and 25 years of age, especially those who abuse alcohol or other substances.

- Closed-head injuries may occur when the restrained head is struck by a moving object *(fixed-head injury or nonacceleration injury)* or when the moving head strikes a stationary object or abruptly changes direction *(moving-head injury or acceleration injury)*. Acceleration injuries usually produce more severe brain trauma than nonacceleration injuries.

- *Linear acceleration injuries* are caused by sudden acceleration of the head by a force that moves through the midline of the head. *Angular acceleration injuries* are caused by sudden deflection and rotation of the head by a force that strikes the head at an angle.

- *Coup* and *contrecoup brain trauma* are most common following *linear acceleration* of the head, and *rotational trauma* is most common following *angular acceleration*. Angular acceleration usually produces more severe brain trauma than does linear acceleration.

- Both linear acceleration and angular acceleration cause stretching and shearing of brain tissues, which in turn cause *diffuse axonal injury* within the brain. Movement of the brain within the cranial vault causes *abrasions* and *lacerations* on the surface of the brain.

- Movement and deformation of the brain within the cranial vault may cause bleeding *(traumatic hemorrhage)* within the brain *(intracerebral hemorrhage)* or on the surface of the brain *(extracerebral hemorrhage)*. Extracerebral hemorrhages may be *epidural, subdural,* or *subarachnoid* hemorrhages.

- *Cerebral swelling* (edema) is an important secondary consequence of traumatic brain injury. Cerebral swelling can cause *traumatic hydrocephalus* or *elevated intracranial pressure*. Elevated intracranial pressure is an important cause of death within the first hours after brain injury. Death often occurs because of *herniation,* in which brain tissues are pushed against cranial partitions or through openings in the skull by localized regions of increased pressure within the cranial vault.

- Head trauma often causes disruption of blood supply to the brain, may disrupt autoregulation of blood pressure, and may cause cerebral vasospasm, all of which may contribute to *brain ischemia* (insufficient oxygen supply to brain tissues).

PROGNOSTIC INDICATORS IN TRAUMATIC BRAIN INJURY
Duration of Coma

Not surprisingly, patients who have severe brain injuries recover less well than patients with milder injuries. This relationship has been recognized for more than 100 years, and investigators have worked not so much to confirm the relationship between severity of brain injury and outcome as to ascertain reliable indicators of the severity of brain injury that do not require post-mortem examination of the brain.

One of the most reliable indirect indicators of the severity of brain injury is the magnitude and duration of alterations in consciousness (Macniven, 1994). Deeper and longer-lasting unconsciousness *(coma)* is associated with poorer eventual recovery (Carlsson, Svardsudd, & Welin, 1987; Gilchrist & Wilkinson, 1979; Jennet & associates, 1977; Ruesch, 1944; and others). Katz and Alexander (1994) reported outcomes based on length of coma for 119 traumatic-brain-injury patients with diffuse axonal injury. Outcomes were progressively worse as the duration of coma increased (Figure 9-6).

Until the 1970s, investigators' understanding of the relationship between the magnitude and duration of altered consciousness and outcome was compromised because different investigators measured the level and duration of unconsciousness in different ways and used different measures of outcome, which prevented comparisons across studies. Then, in the early 1970s,

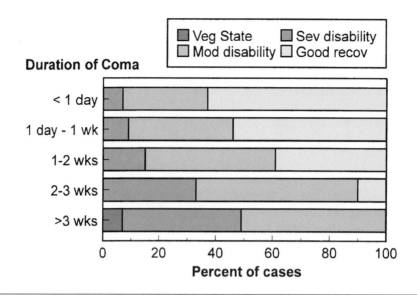

Figure 9-6 ■ **The relationship between the duration of coma following severe traumatic brain injury and eventual recovery. Longer durations of coma are associated with poorer eventual recovery.** (Data from Katz, D. I., & Alexander, M. P. [1994]. Traumatic brain injury. In D. C. Good & J. R. Couch, *Handbook of neurorehabilitation* [pp. 493-549]. New York: Dekker.)

investigators began to develop standardized measures of consciousness and outcome.

Teasdale and Jennett (1974) helped bring uniformity to how levels of consciousness were measured with the *Glasgow Coma Scale* (GCS), which provided a consistent way of rating a patient's level of consciousness based on eye opening, verbal responses, and motor responses observed during the immediate post-injury period (Table 9-1). To arrive at a GCS score, the examiner determines the patient's highest level of eye-opening, motor behavior, and verbal responses and sums the scores for the three levels. GCS total scores can range from 3 to 15, and *coma* is operationally defined as a GCS total score of 8 or less (Eisenberg & Weiner, 1987). Practitioners routinely divide patients into three levels of severity based on GCS score. Scores of 3 to 8 denote *severe head injury,* scores of 9 to 12 denote *moderate head injury,* and scores of 13 to 15 denote *mild head injury.*

A normal adult would score 15 on the Glasgow Coma Scale, but the GCS rating follows a known head injury; hence 15 = mild head injury.

Initial GCS scores have been shown to predict traumatically-brain-injured patients' eventual recovery, if the patient is assessed during the early stages of recovery but long enough after injury that nonneurologic contributors to the patient's impairments (such as alcohol intoxication) have dissipated (Bowers & Marshall, 1980; Jennett & associates, 1976; Katz, 1992; Langfitt, 1978; and others). Most studies of the relationship between GCS scores and outcome have used the GCS score at 6 hours post-accident as the reference value for predicting outcome.

The GCS has been shown to best predict eventual recovery for patients at the two ends of the severity continuum—patients who eventu-

	TABLE 9 - 1	
	The Glasgow Coma Scale	
Category of behavior	Description	Value
Eye opening	Opens eyes spontaneously	4
	Opens eyes to verbal command	3
	Opens eyes in response to pain	2
	No response	1
Motor responses	Obeys verbal commands	6
	Attempts to pull examiner's hand away during painful stimulation	5
	Moves limb away from painful stimulus	4
	Flexes body in response to pain	3
	Extends limbs, becomes rigid in response to pain	2
	No response	1
Verbal responses	Converses and is oriented	5
	Converses but is disoriented	4
	Utters intelligible words but does not make sense	3
	Produces unintelligible sounds	2
	No response	1

Data from Teasdale, G., & Jennett, B. (1974). Assessment of coma and impaired consciousness. *Lancet, 2,* 81-84.

ally "die or walk away" (Segatore & Way, 1992). For traumatically-brain-injured patients at middle severity ranges (the ones for whom clinicians typically are most concerned with predicting recovery) the GCS has been shown not to reliably predict patients' eventual level of independence (Segatore & Way, 1992; Shatz & Chute, 1995).

The *Glasgow Coma Scale* has been shown to be highly reliable (Teasdale & Jennett, 1976) but relatively insensitive because a wide range of behaviors must be reduced to a small number of possible scores. However, experience with the GCS apparently counts—experienced users are more reliable than inexperienced users (Rowley & Fielding, 1991). Because no exceptions are made for untestable categories of behavior, the GCS may overestimate the severity of impairment for some patients, such as intubated patients who are verbally competent but cannot talk because of intubation, patients with facial injuries whose eyes are swollen shut, or patients with paralyzed or immobilized limbs for whom motor responses are difficult or impossible. The timing of assessment also can affect the predictive reliability of the GCS. Some patients with traumatic brain injuries are alert and clear-headed in the first few hours post-injury and then deteriorate, so GCS scores obtained at the standard 6 hours post-injury may give an unduly optimistic estimate of recovery for these patients.

The *Comprehensive Level of Consciousness Scale* (CLOCS; Stanczak & associates, 1984) was designed to compensate for some of the deficiencies of the Glasgow Coma Scale by assessing a broader range of responses. The CLOCS provides for measurement of posture, resting eye position, spontaneous eye opening, ocular movements, pupillary reflexes, motor functioning, responsiveness, and communicative effort. Behaviors in these eight categories are subjectively rated using 5-point to 9-point scales. Table 9-2 shows the rating scales for two behavioral

T A B L E   9 - 2

The General Responsiveness and Best Communicative Effort Scales from the Comprehensive Level of Consciousness Scale

Scale 7: General Responsiveness

8   The patient is fully aroused and alert or, if asleep, arouses and attends to the examiner following only mild or moderate stimulation. The arousal outlasts the duration of the stimulus.

7   The patient is aroused by mild or moderate stimulation, but on cessation of stimulation returns to his or her former state, or the patient displays marked psychomotor agitation shortly after stimulus onset.

6   The patient is aroused only by noxious stimulation.

5   In response to noxious stimulation, the patient displays a purposeful withdrawal or a typical facial grimace. There is no arousal.

4   In response to noxious stimulation, the patient displays gross, disorganized withdrawal. There is no facial grimace or arousal.

3   In response to noxious stimulation, the patient displays only a feeble, disorganized withdrawal or flexion. There is no arousal or facial grimace.

2   Any decorticate rigidity.*

1   Any decerebrate rigidity.*

0   Total absence of discernible motor activity, even in response to noxious stimulation.

Scale 8: Best Communicative Effort

7   Normal communication is possible through speech, writing, gesturing, and so on.

6   Profuse spontaneous or elicited verbalizations (signs, gestures). The communication is intelligible but may be bizarre, jargonistic, and/or perseverative.

5   The patient responds to verbal, written, or signaled instructions with spontaneous but unintelligible or poorly articulated verbalizations (signs, gestures) or in a coded manner such as eye blinking, finger tapping, or hand squeezing. If intubated, the patient responds appropriately to commands.

4   The patient spontaneously vocalizes, verbalizes, or makes signs or gestures but gives no indication that he or she comprehends any form of receptive language.

3   The patient visually tracks an object passed through his or her visual field and/or turns his or her head toward the examiner as if wishing to communicate, or the patient generates spontaneous moaning or muttering coupled with reliable eye contact or searching behaviors.

2   Spontaneous, random muttering or moaning only.

1   Muttering or moaning in response to noxious stimulation.

0   No elicited or spontaneous vocalizations, searching behaviors, or eye contact.

Data from Stanczak, D. E., White, J. G., Gouview, W. D., & associates. (1984). Assessment of level of consciousness following severe neurological insult. *Journal of Neurosurgery, 60,* 955-960.

Decorticate rigidity, Upper limbs are flexed at the elbows, wrists, and fingers and are adducted (drawn toward the midline) at the shoulders. The lower limbs are extended and rotated inward and the feet are flexed downward. (This appears with damage in subcortical white matter, thalamus, and internal capsules bilaterally.) *Decerebrate rigidity,* Upper limbs are extended, drawn toward the midline, and rotated inwardly. The lower limbs are extended and rotated inward and the feet are flexed downward. The head and heels are bent backward and the body is bowed forward. The patient's jaw may be clenched. (This appears with temporal lobe herniation and midbrain compression.)

categories—*general responsiveness* and *communicative effort*. Similar scales are used to rate behaviors in the other six behavioral categories.

The CLOCS is more sensitive to subtle changes in patients' responsiveness than the *Glasgow Coma Scale*. Stanczak and associates (1984) have shown that CLOCS scores at discharge from the hospital reliably predict the recovery of traumatically-brain-injured patients. Although the CLOCS is a more sensitive instrument, it takes longer than the *Glasgow Coma Scale* to score, and the GCS remains the most widely used measure for assessing traumatically-brain-injured patients' level of consciousness in the immediate post-injury period.

anterograde amnesia

Duration of Post-traumatic Amnesia

The duration of post-traumatic amnesia (the time following coma during which the patient is unable to store new information and experiences in memory) has been considered an indirect indicator of the severity of brain injury and a fair predictor of outcome. Several studies have shown that the duration of post-traumatic amnesia is inversely related to a patient's eventual level of recovery from traumatic brain injury (Bond, 1976; Levin & associates, 1979; Katz, 1992; and others). Katz (1992) reported Glasgow outcome scores for 114 consecutive patients with diffuse axonal injury. Post-traumatic amnesia lasting less than 2 weeks was associated with good recovery in 80% of cases, whereas no patient with post-traumatic amnesia lasting longer than 12 weeks made a good recovery.

In the late 1970s investigators began to question the reliability of the retrospective estimates of post-traumatic amnesia that were being used in studies that related post-traumatic amnesia to recovery. Consequently, efforts were made to replace subjective estimates of post-traumatic amnesia with standardized procedures to permit more detailed and more reliable assessment.

The *Galveston Orientation and Amnesia Test* (GOAT; Levin, O'Donnell, & Grossman, 1979) was designed to track recovery of orientation and memory by traumatically-brain-injured pa-

tients who are emerging from coma (Table 9-3). The GOAT consists of 10 questions that assess the patient's ability to remember and produce biographic information (orientation to person), the patient's orientation to place and time, and the patient's memory for events immediately preceding or following the patient's injury.

The patient begins the GOAT with 100 points, and points are subtracted for each failed test item. Scores from 80 to 100 are considered average, scores from 66 to 79 are considered borderline, and scores from 0 to 65 are considered impaired. Scores on the GOAT have been found to correlate with the severity of brain injury as indicated by CT scans and *Glasgow Coma Scale* scores (although the correlations are not strong enough to permit accurate predictions of recovery for individual patients), and also have been found to correlate with traumatically-brain-injured patients' eventual level of recovery (Levin, O'Donnell, & Grossman, 1979).

The GOAT can be a useful screening test for getting a general idea of a patient's level of cognitive functioning and responsiveness, although orientation is weighted more heavily than amnesia and memory. Because it requires spoken responses, the GOAT may overestimate the severity of impairment for patients with focal language-dominant-hemisphere pathology superimposed on the diffuse damage typical of traumatic brain injury.

The *Glasgow Coma Scale* and the *Comprehensive Level of Consciousness Scale* were designed to measure patients' responsiveness in the immediate post-injury period, and the *Galveston Orientation and Amnesia Test* was designed to measure memory and orientation in the immediate post-injury period. Not surprisingly, practitioners also began using them to predict traumatically-brain-injured patients' eventual recovery, but it soon became apparent that these measures did not reliably predict the eventual recovery of individual patients—which, in fairness to their designers, these measures were not designed to do. These measures were developed to allow comparisons of patients across

retro = pretraumatic

T A B L E   9 - 3

Galveston Orientation and Amnesia Test (GOAT)

Question	Point value
What is your name?	2
When were you born?	4
Where do you live?	4
Where are you now? (city)	5
Where are you now? (hospital)	5
On what date were you admitted to this hospital?	5
How did you get here?	5
What is the first event you can remember *after* the injury?	5
Can you describe in detail (e.g., date, time, companions) the first event you can recall *after* the injury?	5
Can you describe the last event you recall *before* the accident?	5
Can you describe in detail (e.g., date, time, companions) the first event you can recall *before* the injury?	5
What time is it now?	(A)
What day of the week is it?	(B)
What day of the month is it?	(C)
What is the month?	(D)
What is the year?	(E)

(A), 1 for each half hour removed from correct time to maximum of 5
(B), 1 for each day removed from correct one
(C), 1 for each day removed from correct date to maximum of 5
(D), 5 for each month removed from correct one to maximum of 15
(E), 10 for each year removed from correct one to maximum of 30

institutions; they were not intended as a tool to describe the recovery of individual patients.

In 1975 Jennett and Bond proposed a standardized procedure for characterizing recovery in traumatic brain injury, called the *Glasgow Outcome Scale* (GOS; Table 9-4). The GOS was a substantial improvement over the poorly defined measures of outcome previously used and has good within-examiner and good examiner-to-examiner reliability. The GOS does not have sufficient sensitivity to predict small but important differences in outcome, but it provides a standardized and reliable procedure for quantifying gross differences in outcome among brain-injured patients.

Several attempts to expand the *Glasgow Outcome Scale* to make it more sensitive have run into problems of unreliability. As a general rule, the more choices judges are given in rating any phenomenon, the less they will agree on their ratings. The simplest way to ensure the reliability of a rating scale is to keep the number of possible ratings small. Unfortunately, rating scales with small numbers of possible ratings tend to be insensitive to small differences in the phenomenon being rated. There is almost always a trade-off between sensitivity and reliability when one develops a rating scale.

T A B L E   9 - 4

The Glasgow Outcome Scale

Rating	Definition
1	*Death.* Includes death clearly attributable to indirect or secondary effects of brain injury, such as pneumonia.
2	*Persistent vegetative state.* The patient displays sleep-wake cycles but makes no organized responses to stimulation during periods of wakefulness.
3	*Severe disability (conscious but disabled).* The patient is dependent on others for daily care by reason of mental or physical disabilities or a combination of both.
4	*Moderate disability (disabled but independent).* The patient can travel by public transportation and work in a sheltered workshop. The patient may have motor impairment, language impairment, intellectual and/or memory impairment, and personality disruption.
5	*Good recovery.* The patient resumes normal life but may have minor neurologic and psychologic impairments. Return to work is not a prerequisite for this rating.

Data from Jennett, B., & Bond, M. (1975). Assessment of outcome after severe brain damage: a practical scale. *Lancet, 1,* 480-484.

The *Rancho Los Amigos Scale of Cognitive Levels* (RLAS; Hagen & Malkamus, 1979) provides a standard set of eight categories to which clinicians can assign brain-injured patients according to their cognitive and behavioral characteristics (Table 9-5). The eight RLAS levels characterize patients in terms of their arousal, responsiveness, restlessness, attention, memory, and executive ability. Many clinicians assume that the time-course of individual patients' recovery follows RLAS levels. (Many do, although the length of time spent at each level differs across patients.)

There is some evidence that the length of time spent at lower RLAS levels is related to eventual outcome (Hagen & Malkamus, 1979). The longer a patient remains at Levels 1 through 4, the poorer the prognosis for recovery, but the relationship is not perfect, and sizeable errors in prediction can occur. The three highest RLAS levels are more sensitive to language impairments than the five lowest levels. Consequently, higher-level patients with focal damage in the language-dominant hemisphere tend to be rated somewhat lower on the RLAS than patients with diffuse but symmetric damage or patients with foci of damage in the non-language-dominant hemisphere.

Sbordone (1991) developed a scale that has fewer levels but covers a greater range of recovery than the *Rancho Los Amigos Scale.* However, the Sbordone scale (Table 9-6) takes longer to complete, is less reliable, and is a relative newcomer. Consequently, the *Rancho Los Amigos Scale* continues to be more widely used. The RLAS is a better choice if ease of use and reliability across examiners and institutions is a concern. The Sbordone scale is a better choice if sensitive measurement is important and reliability across examiners or institutions is less important.

The *Disability Rating Scale* (DRS; Rappoport & associates, 1982) was created to provide a more sensitive measure of progress and measure a wider range of recovery than the *Glasgow Outcome Scale,* from which the DRS is derived. The DRS permits observers to rate a patient's level of function in eight areas: *eye opening, verbal response, motor response, feeding, toileting, grooming, dependence on others,* and *employability,* using rating scales that depend on the functional area being rated (Table 9-7). Possible

T A B L E   9 - 5
The Rancho Los Amigos Scale of Cognitive Levels

Level	Definition
1. No response	No response to pain, touch, sound, or sight.
2. Generalized response	Inconsistent, nonpurposeful, nonspecific responses to intense stimuli. Responds to pain, but response may be delayed.
3. Localized response	Blinks to strong light, turns toward or away from sound, responds to physical discomfort. Inconsistent responses to some commands.
4. Confused-agitated	Alert, very active, with aggressive and/or bizarre behaviors. Attention span is short. Behavior is nonpurposeful, and patient is disoriented and unaware of present events.
5. Confused-nonagitated	Exhibits gross attention to environment. Is highly distractible, requires continual redirection to keep on task. Is alert and responds to simple commands. Performs previously learned tasks but has great difficulty learning new ones. Becomes agitated by too much stimulation. May engage in social conversation but with inappropriate verbalizations.
6. Confused-appropriate	Behavior is goal-directed, with assistance. Inconsistent orientation to time and place. Retention span and recent memory are impaired. Consistently follows simple directions.
7. Automatic-appropriate	Performs daily routine in highly familiar environments without confusion but in an automatic robot-like manner. Is oriented to setting, but insight, judgment, and problem-solving are poor.
8. Purposeful-appropriate	Responds appropriately in most situations. Can generalize new learning across situations. Does not require daily supervision. May have poor tolerance for stress and may exhibit some abstract reasoning disabilities.

Data from Hagen, C., & Malkamus, D. (1979). *Interaction strategies for language disorders secondary to head trauma.* Paper presented at the annual convention of the American Speech-Language-Hearing Association, Atlanta, GA.

DRS scores range from 0 to 29, with higher scores indicating greater disability.

The *Disability Rating Scale* has been shown to be more sensitive to change than the *Glasgow Outcome Scale* (Hall, Cope, & Rappoport, 1985) and to have greater reliability than the *Rancho Los Amigos Scale of Cognitive Levels* (Gouvier & associates, 1987). The DRS, like the *Glasgow Outcome Scale,* is relatively insensitive to change for patients with mild traumatic brain injuries.

Livingstone and Livingstone (1985) described another procedure for measuring outcome, called the *Glasgow Assessment Schedule* (GAS;

Table 9-8). The GAS permits users to rate outcome in six domains *(physical condition, subjective complaints, personality change, cognitive functioning, occupational functioning, and proficiency in activities of daily living).* Overall scores on the GAS range from 0 to 81, with higher scores representing more severe impairment. Like the DRS, the GAS is more sensitive to changes in performance than the *Glasgow Outcome Scale.* However, the *Glasgow Outcome Scale* continues to be more widely used despite absence of evidence for its validity and reliability, perhaps because it is shorter and simpler and

TABLE 9 - 6

Cognitive and behavioral stages of recovery from traumatic brain injury

Stages of recovery	Characteristics
Stage 1	In coma
Stage 2	Opens eyes
	Severe agitation-restlessness or vegetative state
	Severe confusion
	Disoriented to space and time
Stage 3	Oriented to place but not time
	Moderate confusion
	Denial of cognitive deficits
	May complain of somatic problems
	Fatigues very easily
	Poor judgment
	Marked to severe attention deficits
	Severe memory deficits
	Severe social difficulties
	Severe problem-solving difficulties
Stage 4	Oriented to place and time
	Becoming aware of cognitive deficits
	Mild confusion
	Mild to moderate attention difficulties
	Marked problem-solving difficulties
	Moderate to marked memory deficits
	Early onset of depression-nervousness
	Unsuccessful attempts to return to work or school
	Poor endurance
	May appear relatively normal
	Moderate to marked social difficulties
Stage 5	Significant depression-nervousness
	Mild to moderate memory deficits
	Mild to moderate problem-solving difficulties
	Frequent comparison to premorbid self
	Given little hope of additional recovery
	Has returned to work or school
	Mild to moderate social difficulties
Stage 6	Mild memory impairment
	Mild problem-solving difficulties
	Acceptance of residual deficits
	Improving social relationships
	Return of most premorbid responsibilities
	Generally positive self-image

From Sbordone, R. J. (1990). Psychotherapeutic treatment of the client with traumatic brain injury: a conceptual model. In J.S. Kreutzer & P.H.Wehman (Eds.), *Community integration following traumatic brain injury* (pp. 144-145). Baltimore: Paul H. Brookes.

The Disability Rating Scale

Category	Patient characteristic	Rating
Arousability, awareness, responsivity	Eye opening	0 = spontaneous 1 = to speech 2 = to pain 3 = none
	Communication ability	0 = oriented 1 = confused 2 = inappropriate 3 = incomprehensible 4 = none
	Motor responses	0 = obeying 1 = localizing 2 = withdrawing 3 = flexing 4 = extending 5 = none
Self-care activities	Feeding	0 = complete 1 = partial 2 = minimal 3 = none
	Toileting	0 = complete 1 = partial 2 = minimal 3 = none
	Grooming	0 = complete 1 = partial 2 = minimal 3 = none
Dependence on others	Level of functioning	0 = completely independent 1 = independent in special environment 2 = mildly dependent 3 = moderately dependent 4 = markedly dependent 5 = totally dependent
Psychosocial adaptability	Employability	0 = not restricted 1 = selected jobs 2 = sheltered workshop (noncompetitive) 3 = not employable

Disability rating total score	Level of disability
0	None
1	Mild
2-3	Partial
4-6	Moderate
7-11	Moderately severe
12-16	Severe
17-21	Extremely severe
22-24	Vegetative state
25-29	Extreme vegetative state

Data from Rappoport, M., Hall, K. M., Hopkins, K., & associates. (1982). Disability rating scale for severe head trauma: coma to community. *Archives of Physical Medicine and Rehabilitation, 63,* 118-123.

TABLE 9 - 8

The Glasgow Assessment Schedule

Patient characteristic	Scoring*	Patient characteristic	Scoring*
Personality Change		**Cognitive Functioning**	
Emotional lability	a	Immediate recall	a
Irritability	a	2-minute recall	a
Aggressiveness	a	Attention, concentration	a
Other behavioral change	a	Orientation	a
		Current intelligence	a
Subjective Complaints			
Sleep disturbance	a	**Physical Examination**	
Incontinence	a	Dysphasia	a
Family stress	a	Dysarthria	a
Financial problems	a	Abnormal tone: right leg	a
Sexual problems	a	Abnormal tone: left leg	a
Alcohol: excess, poor tolerance	a	Abnormal tone: upper limbs	a
Reduced leisure, sporting activities	a	Walking	a
Headache	a	Cranial nerves	a
Dizziness, loss of balance	a	Seizures	a
Parasthesia	a		
Reduced sense of smell	a	**Activities of Daily Living**	
Reduced hearing	a	Cooking	b
Reduced vision	a	Other domestic tasks	b
		Shopping	b
Occupational Functioning		Traveling	b
Working: same job	0	Personal hygiene	b
Working: similar job	0	Feeding	b
Working: less skilled job	1	Dressing	b
Not working: employable	2	Mobility	b
Not working: not employable	3		

Data from Livingstone, M. G., & Livingstone, H. M. (1985). The Glasgow assessment schedule: clinical and research assessment of head injury outcome. *International Rehabilitation Medicine, 7,* 145-149.
*a, normal (0), moderate (1), severe (2); b, on own (0), with help (1), unable to do (2).

perhaps because it arrived first and developed a cadre of users before the GAS and the DRS arrived on the scene.

Although the severity of traumatic injury plays the most prominent part in determining patients' eventual recovery, the nature of the injury also plays a part. Focal injuries usually have a better prognosis than diffuse injuries. Neurologic recovery following focal traumatic brain injuries proceeds faster and plateaus earlier (but usually at a higher level) than recovery from diffuse injuries (Katz & Alexander, 1994). However, when focal injuries are superimposed on diffuse injuries the prognosis for recovery suffers (Filley & associates, 1987). The presence of diffuse axonal injury is associated with poor outcome (Uzzell & associates, 1987), as is the presence of secondary brain damage caused by increased intracranial pressure, cerebral edema, anoxia, or hypoxia (Andrews & associates, 1990; Miller & associates, 1978). Patients with diffuse hypoxic injury have a particularly ominous prognosis, especially those who remain comatose for 1 week or more. These unfortunate patients are virtually certain to remain severely disabled for the rest of their lives (Katz, 1992).

Patient-Related Variables

Of several patient-related variables, *age* is the most important predictor of outcome following traumatic brain injury. Older patients with traumatic brain injuries have higher mortality than younger patients. The mortality of traumatically-brain-injured patients age 60 and older is approximately twice that of patients age 20 or younger (Wilson & associates 1987). Older patients are more likely to sustain hemorrhages than younger patients, and the hemorrhages are likely to be larger (Katz & Alexander, 1994). Older traumatically-brain-injured patients recover less rapidly and are more likely to exhibit persistent confusion, attentional impairments, and memory impairments than younger patients (Jennett & Teasdale, 1981). For these reasons older patients are more likely than younger patients to remain dependent on caregivers.

Substance abuse also has negative effects on outcome following traumatic brain injury. Alcoholic traumatically-brain-injured patients have longer periods of coma, lower levels of consciousness after emerging from coma, longer hospitalizations, and greater impairments of memory and verbal learning than nonalcoholic patients (Alfano, 1994). These relationships may be explained, at least in part, by the physiologic consequences of alcohol intoxication at the time of brain injury. Patients who are alcohol-intoxicated at time of injury are more likely to experience cerebral hypoxia, hemorrhage, or cerebral edema than their nonintoxicated counterparts (Alfano, 1994). The effects of substance abuse other than alcohol abuse on recovery from traumatic brain injury have received little empiric study, although presumably chronic drug abuse would have similar negative effects.

Several other patient-related variables have been shown to have minor effects on recovery from traumatic brain injury. *Intelligence* and *socioeconomic status* apparently have some effect on outcome. More intelligent individuals and those with higher socioeconomic status seem to recover better than less intelligent individuals or those with lower socioeconomic status. *Premorbid personality disorders and emotional disturbances* also may negatively affect recovery. Patients with maladaptive personality characteristics and premorbid emotional instability have a somewhat poorer prognosis than those without such disturbances (Humphrey & Oddy, 1981; Rutter, 1981).

The effects of individual patient-related variables on outcome are weak and easily overwhelmed by other more potent variables such as the severity and nature of brain injury. Additionally, many patient-related variables are correlated and tend to occur in combination (e.g., low intelligence, low socioeconomic status, and substance abuse), making determination of the effects of individual variables intimidating, if not impossible. Finally, even the most dependable prognostic variables are best at predicting average outcomes for groups of patients and are less reliable when applied to individual patients. Experienced clinicians give the greatest prognostic weight to the most robust indicators (severity and nature of brain injury) but recognize that outcome for individual patients may not replicate group findings, even for the most robust indicators.

Behavioral and Cognitive Recovery

The general course of recovery following traumatic brain injury is one of improvement, but the pattern of improvement differs from that seen following vascular accidents. Recovery from vascular accidents usually is curvilinear across time, with rapid recovery immediately after onset and gradually slowing recovery thereafter.

Recovery from traumatic brain injuries often proceeds in stepwise fashion. Intervals of little or no change alternate with periods of rapid improvement. The relationship between the severity of patients' impairments in the first few weeks post-onset and their permanent level of impairment is much stronger for vascular accidents than it is for traumatic brain injury, making it more difficult to predict traumatically-brain-injured patients' permanent level of impairment in the first weeks post-onset than to make the same prediction for vascular patients.

Traumatically-brain-injured patients typically progress through a fairly predictable sequence of stages during recovery. Patients with moderate to severe brain injury invariably lose consciousness immediately after the accident. The interval of unconsciousness can last from a few seconds to weeks or, rarely, months. Return to consciousness begins a period of undifferentiated activity, in which the patient is awake but responds indiscriminately and purposelessly to the environment. The patient does not maintain focused attention for more than a few seconds and the patient's overall level of arousal fluctuates unpredictably from moment to moment. During this time the patient is hyperresponsive to stimulation, agitated, and irritable. Repetitive stereotyped movements (rocking, thrashing) are common, as are striking out, shouting, biting, and emotional lability. As recovery continues the patient becomes more lucid and behavior becomes more purposeful, but restlessness, agitation, and irritability persist, although at lower levels.

Eventually the patient becomes oriented to time and place and begins to respond appropriately to simple requests, although the patient's attention span is short and distractibility is high. With the passage of time the patient begins to perform daily routines with supervision and direction, but judgment, memory, and abstract reasoning remain impaired. With continued recovery the patient begins to function independently in familiar situations, but problems with memory and abstract reasoning remain. A few patients eventually resume premorbid activities, although almost always with subtle but important impairments in memory, abstract reasoning, and tolerance for noise and distractions.

The *Rancho Los Amigos Scale of Cognitive Levels* provides a convenient way to characterize traumatically-brain-injured patients' cognitive and behavioral status at various stages of recovery, although not all traumatically-brain-injured adults spend time at each RLAS level. Some with mild brain injuries skip the early levels or pass through them so quickly that intervention at those levels is not an issue. Some with severe brain injuries do not make it to the higher levels. The rate at which individuals pass through each level varies across individuals. Some linger at a given level longer than others, and some pass through levels very rapidly or skip levels entirely. The reader should keep in mind that RLAS levels are better used as an index of the severity of brain injury than as a timetable for recovery. A severely injured patient still may be at RLAS level 3 at 3 weeks post-injury, whereas a patient with a less severe brain injury may be at RLAS level 6 at the same time post-injury.

Comatose and Semi-Comatose (Rancho Los Amigos Levels 1 and 2). RLAS Level 1 and Level 2 patients are bedbound, usually in an intensive-care unit or long-term care facility. Most are comatose or minimally responsive. Many have tubes in place to maintain an open airway, assist breathing, and provide for removal of secretions. Most have intravenous lines and urinary catheters in place. Some are attached to sensors used to monitor intracranial pressure, heartbeat, and respiration. Some have nasogastric tubes in place for administration of liquid nutrition, and a few have gastrostomies (openings into the stomach through which liquid diets are administered). Level 1 patients are unresponsive or minimally responsive to all external stimulation. Level 2 patients may respond intermittently and inconsistently and in a generalized manner to intense stimulation (especially painful stimulation).

Responsive and Agitated (Rancho Los Amigos Levels 3 and 4). Patients at RLAS levels 3 and 4 are awake and responsive, but their responses are inconsistent and may be nonpurposeful. RLAS level 3 and 4 patients are agitated, restless, impulsive, and highly distractible, and they inevitably exhibit massive impairments in attention, memory, reasoning, and problem-solving. Patients at levels 3 and 4 are not oriented to person, place, or time. Patients at level 3 do not interact with their environment in a purposeful way. Patients at level 4 interact with their environment, but their behavior is primitive and socially inappropriate, and they are not sensitive to environmental or social cues that normally regulate behavior. Level 4 patients have little tolerance for stress or frustration, which can lead to explosive emotional outbursts, including physical aggression. Level 4 patients do not monitor their own behavior, do not notice mistakes, and may deny the existence of impairments.

Restless and Distractible (Rancho Los Amigos Level 5). Patients at RLAS level 5 are restless, distractible, and impulsive but are not generally agitated. Some are oriented to place but not to time. (Orientation to time seems to be particularly impervious to the effects of recovery.) Most are aware that they have been injured but are unaware of the nature of their impairments and do not notice errors and inappropriate responses. RLAS level 5 patients customarily exhibit profound impairments in attention, memory, reasoning, judgment, and problem-solving.

RLAS level 5 patients do not tolerate long or challenging tests or treatment tasks. They fatigue easily and have short attention spans, which prevents them from participating meaningfully in tasks that require sustained attention and effort. Their interactions with others are at a less primitive level than is true for patients at earlier stages of recovery, although their impulsivity and impaired judgment may contribute to frequent episodes of inappropriate behavior. They are inconsistently responsive to social cues and observe basic social conventions with occasional lapses. They can perform familiar tasks but are unable to learn new ones. Stressful or challenging situations often provoke these patients into emotional outbursts, which are striking in their intensity and equally striking in how quickly and completely they dissipate. Patients at RLAS level 5 remain highly controlled by their immediate environment, exhibit little capacity for independent thought or behavior, and generally carry out daily life activities in a robot-like manner.

Confused, Purposeful (Rancho Los Amigos Level 6). Patients at RLAS level 6 are not strikingly restless, distractible, or impulsive. Most are inconsistently oriented to person, place, and time, although time sense usually remains impaired. Most patients at RLAS level 6 know that they have been injured but do not have good understanding of the specifics of their injuries. Patients at RLAS level 6 usually have a general sense of their impairments and are aware of at least some errors, although they tend not to correct them. They behave appropriately in most interpersonal interactions, although the content of what they say may not be consistent with the conversational context. Most have compromised word retrieval and verbal fluency, and most have striking problems in the pragmatic aspects of communication. These patients' performance on simple structured tasks may be acceptable, but their performance breaks down in unstructured settings, on more complex tasks, or when they are faced with challenging or stressful situations. RLAS level 6 patients invariably have extreme difficulty dealing with abstraction, implication, and inference.

Dependent (Rancho Los Amigos Level 7). Patients at RLAS level 7 typically have moderate attentional, memory, and problem-solving impairments and obvious communication impairments (word-retrieval failures, excessive repetition and filler, false starts and circumlocutions, and impaired conversational turn-taking and topic maintenance), although their communication in conversations that do not last more than a few minutes may appear normal. The self-monitoring skills of patients at RLAS level 7 are better than those of patients at lower levels, but lapses still occur. Patients at RLAS level 7 continue to have moderate problems with abstractions, implications, and inferences. They tend not to get beyond surface interpretations of nonliteral material, situations, and events. They have moderate ability to control their immediate environment and limited ability to work independently if given highly structured assignments and substantial coaching, although insight, judgment, and problem-solving are problematic. They often get lost in details and fail to grasp the overall meaning of events, situations, or communications. Depression and anger often become prominent for patients at RLAS level 7 as it becomes obvious that complete recovery of premorbid abilities is unlikely or impossible.

Semi-Independent (Rancho Los Amigos Level 8). Patients at RLAS level 8 function independently in structured and familiar situations, but most need supervision and direction in unfamiliar and unstructured ones. Almost all exhibit subtle cognitive impairments, although communication and interpersonal skills usually are close to normal. Patients at RLAS level 7 perform well in structured tasks in which instructions and response requirements are clear and unambiguous, and they are capable of generalizing what they learn in one context to similar contexts, but their performance deteriorates when they encounter unanticipated challenging or stressful situations. Many patients at RLAS level 8 can invoke compensatory strategies to cope with new or unusual situations. However, when they become fatigued or feel stressed, their performance deteriorates. Some patients at RLAS level 8 may return to school or work or assume other preinjury responsibilities, although usually at a reduced level.

GENERAL CONCEPTS 9-2

- Deeper and longer-lasting unconsciousness *(coma)* following head injury is associated with poorer eventual physical and cognitive recovery.
- The *Glasgow Coma Scale* (GCS) is a popular scale for rating head-injured patients' level of consciousness. *Glasgow Coma Scale* scores assigned a few hours after head injury reliably predict head-injured patients' recovery, but GCS scores are too coarse to capture small but important patient characteristics.
- The *Comprehensive Level of Consciousness Scale* is more sensitive than the Glasgow Coma Scale because it samples a broader range of responses, but it is not as widely used as the GCS.

- The duration of *post-traumatic amnesia* is an indirect indicator of the severity of brain injury and is inversely related to degree of recovery. The *Galveston Orientation and Amnesia Test* (GOAT) is designed to track recovery of orientation and memory by traumatically-brain-injured patients who are emerging from coma.
- The *Glasgow Outcome Scale* provides a standardized and reliable procedure for quantifying gross differences in recovery among brain-injured patients.
- The *Disability Rating Scale* provides a more sensitive measure of progress and measures a wider range of recovery than the *Glasgow Outcome Scale.*
- The *Rancho Los Amigos Scale of Cognitive Levels* is a widely used scale that provides a set of eight categories to which clinicians can assign brain-injured patients based on their cognitive and behavioral characteristics.
- *Age* is the most important patient-related variable for predicting recovery from traumatic brain injury. Other patient-related variables include substance abuse, intelligence, personality, and socioeconomic status. Many patient-related variables are correlated and occur in combinations.
- Traumatically-brain-injured patients typically progress through a fairly predictable sequence of stages as they recover. The *Rancho Los Amigos Scale of Cognitive Levels* provides a reasonably accurate chronology for this sequence of stages.
- As brain-injured patients progress through the levels of the *Rancho Los Amigos Scale of Cognitive Levels* their behavior progresses from *unresponsive* to *responsive*, from *agitated* to *nonagitated*, from *confused* to *oriented*, from *inappropriate* to *appropriate*, and from *automatic* to *purposeful.*

ASSESSING ADULTS WITH TRAUMATIC BRAIN INJURY

Assessing traumatically-brain-injured adults is an evolutionary process. As a patient's physical, cognitive, and behavioral characteristics change with recovery, what happens in testing also changes. For example, tests that are appropriate for patients in the immediate post-injury period, when confusion and agitation are prominent, may be irrelevant for patients in later stages of recovery, when subtle cognitive impairments are the primary concern.

Level of Consciousness and Responsiveness to Stimulation

The speech-language pathologist's primary concerns with comatose and semi-comatose patients (RLAS levels 1 to 3) are to determine the patient's level of consciousness, to get a sense of the nature and severity of the patient's injuries, and to learn something about the progression of the patient's physical, behavioral, and cognitive status since the time of injury. This information comes from the patient's medical record, from discussion with other professionals involved in the patient's care, and from direct observation of the patient.

Assessment of comatose and semi-comatose patients focuses on establishing their alertness and responsiveness to stimulation. Standard rating scales such as the *Glasgow Coma Scale* or the *Glasgow Assessment Schedule* provide a general subjective estimate of these characteristics, but clinicians usually augment the impressions provided by rating scales with objective measurement of the patient's alertness and responsiveness to stimulation. The clinician often gets a sense of the patient's sleep-wake cycles, either by direct observation of the patient or by consulting the patient's medical chart, family members, or patient-care personnel. The clinician usually finds out how much of the day the patient spends sleeping, what parts of the day the patient typically is awake, and the times of day during which the patient is most alert and responsive.

The clinician also determines how easily the patient is aroused from sleep. The most easily aroused patients awaken to environmental sounds or verbal commands. More difficult to arouse patients may require light touch, shaking,

or even painful stimulation (squeezing, pinching) to awaken them.

> Comatose and semi-comatose patients who do not respond to neutral or pleasant stimuli often respond to unpleasant or noxious stimuli, usually by some sort of avoidance response (withdrawing a limb, averting the head, closing the eyes).

Finally the clinician assesses the patient's responsiveness to stimulation. The clinician observes the patient when the patient is awake and alert. The clinician records the patient's responsiveness to environmental stimuli (e.g., a television or radio playing; people entering and leaving the patient's room; being talked to, touched, and moved by nursing personnel). Then the clinician systematically evaluates the patient's responsiveness to selected stimuli.

The patient's *responsivenes to speech* may be assessed by greeting the patient, talking to the patient, and noting whether the patient looks toward the speaker, changes facial expression, attempts to speak, or responds motorically. For patients who respond to such general speech stimulation, the clinician may get a sense of the patient's comprehension by requesting simple responses that are known to be within the patient's physical ability (such as "open your eyes," "look at the ceiling").

The patient's responsiveness to *visual stimulation* may be assessed by introducing lights or brightly colored objects into the patient's field of vision and noting whether the patient looks toward them and by moving a light or a brightly colored object through the patient's visual field and noting whether the patient visually tracks them. For patients who do not orient to or track moving objects, the clinician may rapidly move a hand or some other object toward the patient's eyes and note whether a protective eye-blink response occurs.

The patient's responsiveness to *tactile stimulation* may be assessed by lightly touching and stroking the patient's limbs. For patients who do not respond to light touch and stroking, the clinician may assess their response to pressure (pinching, squeezing), hot and cold, or rough and smooth tactile stimulation.

Assessment of the patient's responsiveness to *olfactory stimuli* may include pleasant odors such as cologne, vanilla extract, or almond extract and unpleasant odors such as ammonia or rubbing alcohol. Finally the clinician may assess the patient's responsiveness to pleasant *taste sensations* such as fruit juice or honey and unpleasant tastes such as lemon juice or vinegar.

> Taste and smell are phylogenetically more primitive senses and may elicit responses from brain-injured patients when visual and auditory stimuli do not.

During the assessment the speech-language pathologist watches the patient for subtle responses to stimulation, such as changes in respiration rate, changes in muscle tone, subtle movements, changes in facial expression, eye blinks, or brief vocalizations contingent on stimulation. The clinician records the nature, magnitude, and consistency of the patient's responses to each stimulus.

A few organized protocols for assessing severely impaired patients with traumatic brain injuries have been described in the literature (Ansell & Keenan, 1989; Helm-Estabrooks & Hotz, 1991; Rader & Ellis, 1994; and others). Although they differ in specifics, all provide for assessing patients' arousal; attentiveness; and responses to auditory, visual, tactile, and olfactory stimulation. Most are sensitive to changes in arousal, attention, and responsiveness, and some have acceptable reliability.

The information from the assessment of the patient's responsiveness to stimulation serves as a baseline against which the rate and magnitude of the patient's subsequent recovery may be evaluated. During the days that follow, the clinician periodically observes the patient's responsiveness and documents the results, providing the treatment team with important information regarding the patient's progression through the early stages of recovery.

Orientation

As traumatically-brain-injured patients return to consciousness and begin responding to environmental stimuli, they enter a state of profound disorientation, confusion, and agitation (RLAS levels 4 and 5). When this happens, the clinician becomes concerned with getting baseline measures of orientation and memory. However, administering long or difficult tests of cognition, language, or communication is out of the question because of these patients' behavioral and cognitive impairments. Objective assessment of these patients usually is limited to brief tests that provide a limited sample of performance representing basic levels of communication and cognition.

Screening tests of orientation, memory, and amnesia such as the *Mini Mental Status Examination* (Folstein, Folstein, & McHugh, 1975) or the *Galveston Memory and Orientation Test* (Levin, O'Donnell, & Grossman, 1979) often suffice to track patients' progress during this stage of recovery. Performance data obtained with such tests can be supplemented with subjective ratings, using any of several rating scales designed for use with traumatically-brain-injured adults. The simplest rating scales (such as the *Glasgow Coma Scale*), which are intended for frequent ratings (daily or more often) are too insensitive to be of much value for tracking traumatically-brain-injured adults' performance at this stage of recovery. Consequently, the clinician usually chooses a more detailed rating scale, such as the *Glasgow Assessment Schedule* (Livingstone & Livingstone, 1985), the *Disability Rating Scale* (Rappoport & associates, 1982), or subsections of the *Comprehensive Level of*

Consciousness Scale (Stanczak & associates, 1984) to track these patients' recovery.

Orientation (awareness of self and appreciation of how one relates to others or to the environment) is a major problem in the post-coma phase of recovery. Clinicians customarily divide orientation into orientation for *person* (who one is and who others in one's environment are), *place* (where one is), and *time* (what year, month, day, and hour it is plus a sense of the passage of time). A few standardized procedures for assessing orientation have been reported in the literature, but most clinicians rely on the orientation items from screening examinations of mental status such as the *Mini-Mental Status Examination* (Folstein, Folstein, & McHugh, 1975) or the *Galveston Orientation and Amnesia Test* (Levin, O'Donnell, & Grossman, 1979) plus questions asked during the patient interview.

Most mental status screening examinations contain items that test basic orientation to time, place, and personal information, such as the patient's name, age, and marital status. The clinician can gather supplementary information about a patient's orientation to place by asking questions to assess the patient's concepts of direction and distance during an interview. For example, the clinician might ask the patient to indicate the direction of various locations (including the patient's home) from the place of the interview and to estimate distances between the place of the interview and those locations. To assess the patient's sense of time beyond the standard questions relating to day, hour, month, year, and season, the clinician may ask questions about what time of the day certain events happen (e.g., meals, group meetings, visits by family). The clinician can test the patient's sense of elapsed time by asking questions such as, "How long have you been in this medical center?" or "How long has it been since your family last came to visit?"

Cognitive and Communicative Abilities

Patients at RLAS levels 5 and above tolerate testing, although those at level 5 may not tolerate long or challenging tests. By the time patients reach these stages, their agitation and confusion have substantially resolved and underlying cognitive and communication impairments become more prominent. Cognitive and communication impairments become a major focus of assessment with RLAS levels 5 and 6 patients, and it is at these stages that patients first receive detailed assessment of *alertness, attention, visual perceptual abilities, memory, language and communication,* and *reasoning and problem-solving.*

Patients at RLAS levels 7 and 8 tolerate challenging tests and do not have the profound and pervasive cognitive impairments typical of traumatically-brain-injured patients at lower stages. Their cognitive performance in some domains may be within normal limits, although islands of substantial impairment usually remain. For many it may be apparent that restitution of remaining cognitive impairments is not in the cards, leading to a shift in clinical focus away from retraining cognitive abilities and toward providing the patient with strategies to compensate for cognitive impairments that cannot be repaired.

The scope and pattern of testing depends, of course, on each patient's tolerance for testing and each patient's particular pattern of impairments. However, most clinicians assess alertness, attention, visual perceptual abilities, memory, language and communication, and reasoning and problem-solving for patients at RLAS levels 7 and 8 with follow-up testing to explore more carefully impairments identified in the initial tests.

Alertness and Attention

Alertness Van Zomeren, Brouwer, and Deelman (1984) described two categories of alertness: *tonic alertness* and *phasic alertness. Tonic alertness* refers to an individual's ongoing, continuing receptivity to stimulation. Tonic alertness changes slowly and reflects the individual's overall state of arousal. Diurnal rhythms, increasing drowsiness in monotonous tasks, and the "mid-afternoon slump" are examples of changes in tonic alertness. Most traumatically-brain-injured patients appear to have lower-than-normal resting levels of tonic alertness, but the magnitude of their cyclic changes in tonic alertness does not seem greater than normal. Brain-injured patients who drift off or fall asleep during testing or treatment do so because of lowered tonic alertness.

Phasic alertness refers to momentary, rapidly occurring changes in receptivity to stimulation. Changes in phasic alertness occur within milliseconds. Phasic alertness is strongly affected by the individual's intentions and interests. Increased alertness in response to warning signals or significant events are examples of changes in phasic alertness.

Lowered tonic alertness is an inconvenience for the patient and may slow the patient's progress in treatment, but disturbed phasic alertness usually is more disruptive, both in treatment activities and in daily life. In treatment activities patients with diminished phasic alertness tend to make errors on initial stimulus items, and their performance deteriorates when treatment tasks change. They may fail to perceive short-duration stimuli unless given a warning signal, and they may fail to perceive subtle changes in instructions or treatment stimuli. In daily life they may miss key elements in conversations and they may respond slowly or erroneously to rapidly occurring events or stimuli, such as traffic signals.

Attention Attentional impairments are a universal consequence of traumatic brain injury, and assessment and treatment of traumatically-brain-injured patients' attentional impairments is an important concern of most treatment programs. Most traumatically-brain-injured patients have impaired *selective attention,* which means that they are distractible and have difficulty maintaining attention in the face of competing stimuli. In figure-ground tasks (both visual and auditory) these patients have difficulty discriminating foreground figures from backgrounds and may be distracted by irrelevant aspects of stimuli, such as the border around a picture or irrelevant details in stories or events. Traumatically-brain-injured patients with impaired selective attention typically perform poorly on visual figure-ground tests (embedded figures, overlapping figures, masked or occluded figures), and they may have difficulty separating what is important from what is not important in spoken and printed materials.

Impairments in *sustained attention* are not clearly separable from impairments in selective attention because impaired selective attention is certain to disrupt performance on tasks that require sustained attention. However, there are traumatically-brain-injured patients who perform well on selective attention tasks but do poorly on tests requiring sustained attention. These patients' performance deteriorates as the time during which they must maintain attention increases. They do poorly on tests such as digits backward, backward spelling, oral arithmetic, and challenging vigilance tasks.

Most traumatically-brain-injured patients have difficulty in quickly shifting attentional focus from one stimulus to another or from one aspect of a task or situation to another (called *alternating attention*). They perform poorly in tasks in which response requirements change or in which they are required to transfer attentional focus from one characteristic of task stimuli to another.

Divided attention tasks create major problems for most traumatically-brain-injured patients, who typically cannot maintain attentional focus on two aspects of a task. Traumatically-brain-injured patients usually have great difficulty with dual-task divided attention tasks in which they must maintain attention to two different tasks simultaneously. (More information on attention and its assessment can be found in Chapter 8.)

Alertness and attention are without a doubt strongly related, and it may be that alertness and attention are different labels for the same mental processes. Patients with diminished tonic alertness seem likely to have difficulty sustaining attention over time, and patients with diminished phasic alertness seem likely to have difficulty focusing attention or quickly changing attentional focus in response to changes in the environment. It also seems likely that heightening a patient's level of alertness and arousal (e.g., with medications) would have positive effects on the patient's attentional processes. Nevertheless, it may be useful for clinicians to differentiate between alertness and attention because there may be some patients who exhibit dissociations between the two.

Visual Processing Visual processing impairments are most common in traumatically-brain-injured patients who are in the early stages of recovery, although some patients (especially those with posterior brain injury) continue to have significant problems processing visual information in the middle and late stages of recovery. These patients perform poorly on tests that require identification of incomplete or fragmented visual stimuli or partially occluded stimuli and on visual figure-ground tests such as those described in Chapter 8.

Memory

Retrospective Memory and Prospective Memory Impaired memory is an important early consequence of traumatic brain injury, and memory disturbances plague most traumatically-brain-injured patients throughout the course of their recovery. Memory has been divided in many ways by different writers. Those who are concerned with traumatically-brain-injured adults find it useful to divide memory into *retrospective* and *prospective* memory.

Retrospective memory is memory for past events and experiences and for information acquired in the past. Most traumatically-brain-injured patients have problems with retrospective memory. They fail to remember conversations, events, people, or situations from minute to minute or, more often, from hour to hour or day to day. Most standardized memory tests are designed to assess retrospective memory.

Prospective memory is the ability to remember to do things at specific times—keep an appointment, prepare dinner, or feed the cat. Some writers (including Lezak, 1995) suggest that impaired prospective memory is not an impairment of the memory system itself, but results

from failing to recognize contextual cues that ordinarily would trigger specific memories *(remembering to remember)*. A traumatically-brain-injured person might, for example, see an empty cat-feeding dish on arising in the morning and not recall that the cat customarily is fed first thing in the morning. (Presumably the hungry cat would provide stronger and more salient reminders on finding the dish empty.)

Declarative Memory and Procedural Memory Retrospective memory can be divided into *declarative memory* and *procedural memory* (Tulving, 1983). Declarative memory can be loosely characterized as *what we know about things,* and procedural memory can be loosely characterized as *what we know about how to do things.* Knowledge of who we are, our parent's names and birthdays, the capital city of Poland, how many eggs make a dozen, the composition of a protein molecule, the names of the cranial nerves, and other such material is stored in declarative memory. Information in declarative memory can be brought to conscious awareness and verbally reported. Declarative memory almost always is compromised by traumatic brain injury.

Remembering how to perform previously learned behavioral routines (driving an automobile, making a tuna salad sandwich, repairing a television set, doing a neurologic examination) calls on information in procedural memory. Information in procedural memory cannot be brought to conscious awareness but must be accessed via performance of the activity to which the information relates.

Procedural memory has been described as "a collection of habits which can be applied automatically without having to think about new response strategies" (Garner & Valadka, 1994, p. 92). Traumatic brain injury apparently affects procedural memory less than declarative memory, and there are reports of traumatically-brain-injured patients who learn and use newly trained procedural routines, although they are not aware of learning them and cannot verbally describe them (Ewert & associates, 1989; Parkin, 1982; Verfaelli, Bauer, & Bowers, 1991).

One's memory of having performed a procedure can be brought into consciousness, and the steps in the procedure can be reported verbally. However, one's knowledge of the exact sequence, timing, amplitude, and other characteristics of the behaviors in the procedure only can be accessed by performing the procedure. Every good mechanic can tighten a nut on a bolt tightly enough so that it will not loosen but not so tightly that it breaks the bolt or the nut, but none can tell a novice how to do it, and a novice can only learn how by doing it many times.

Episodic Memory and Semantic Memory

We are not finished chopping memory into smaller pieces because declarative memory can be divided into *episodic memory* and *semantic memory* (Tulving, 1972). Episodic memory can be loosely characterized as memory for personally experienced events. Experiences stored in episodic memory are time-specific and place-specific. Our knowledge of who we were with and what we were doing at certain points in time comes from episodic memory as does our sense of relationships between events that took place at different points in time. In many respects our sense of who we are comes largely from information in episodic memory.

Semantic memory contains our organized knowledge of the world, including most of what

However, some information in semantic memory, such as the knowledge that some barking dogs do bite, may be based on one incident stored in episodic memory, which illustrates the interactions and overlap between episodic memory and semantic memory. It also shows that some of what we "remember" in semantic memory may be constructed from incidents stored in episodic memory, but that is another (too long) story. In everyday life, exchanges of information between episodic and semantic memory are no doubt common.

we learned in educational settings (e.g., facts, dates, names, places). Semantic memory contains information that permits us to report that John Quincy Adams was the sixth President of the United States, that there are 12 eggs in a dozen, that gasoline stations usually are found on busy highways, or that some barking dogs do bite.

Pre-Traumatic Memory Loss and Post-Traumatic Memory Loss

One more chop, and our cutting up of memory will be complete. Impairments of retrospective memory in adults with traumatic brain injuries have been divided into two categories, called *pre-traumatic memory loss* and *post-traumatic memory loss*.

The concepts of pre-traumatic and post-traumatic memory loss were developed by Russell and his associates (Russell, 1971; Russell & Espir, 1961; Russell & Nathan, 1946) based on their studies of traumatically-brain-injured British armed forces personnel during and after World War II. Russell and his contemporaries called pre-traumatic memory loss *retrograde amnesia* and post-traumatic memory loss *anterograde amnesia*. Over the years these difficult-to-keep-straight labels gradually have been replaced by the more descriptive and easier-to-remember labels *pre-traumatic memory loss* and *post-traumatic memory loss*. However, some contemporary writers still use the original labels.

Both pairs of labels refer to a period for which a traumatically-brain-injured patient has no recollection of experiences that happened during the period—hence the terms *amnesia* and *memory loss*. As the labels suggest, *pre-traumatic memory loss* is loss of memory for experiences that happened before the patient's brain injury and *post-traumatic memory loss* is loss of memory for experiences that happened after the injury (Figure 9-7).

Pre-traumatic memory loss may have two components. Loss of memory for the short interval (seconds to minutes) immediately preceding the patient's injury apparently is caused by disruption of the neurochemical processes responsible for incorporating information into long-term memory. Loss of memory for the hours (or

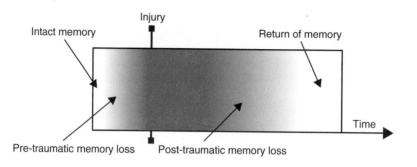

Figure 9-7 ▪ **A schematic representation of memory loss associated with traumatic brain injury. Pre-traumatic memory loss is loss of memory for experiences preceding the injury and post-traumatic memory loss is loss of memory for experiences following the injury. Post-traumatic memory loss almost always covers a longer time interval than pre-traumatic memory loss.**

days) preceding the injury apparently is caused by disrupted access to information incorporated into long-term memory prior to the patient's injury. Events occurring in the seconds to minutes preceding injury are not encoded into memory, whereas the events happening hours or days before injury are in memory but cannot be accessed and retrieved. Pre-traumatic memory loss usually shrinks as the patient recovers, and most patients eventually recover memory for all but the last few minutes before their brain injury, presumably because experiences in the last few minutes never made it into long-term memory.

Corkin and associates (1987) reported the duration of pre-traumatic memory loss for 121 cases of traumatic brain injury in veterans of the Korean conflict. About one third of the patients experienced no pre-traumatic memory loss, and for most that did the interval of memory loss was less than 1 hour (Figure 9-8). The duration of pre-traumatic memory loss was not significantly related to whether the injuries were penetrating or nonpenetrating. These results are consistent with results reported by Russell and Nathan (1946), who studied the duration of pre-traumatic memory loss in 973 traumatically-brain-injured survivors of World War II. Of Russell and Nathan's subjects, 86% experienced pre-traumatic memory loss, but only 14% experienced loss for time intervals of more than 30 minutes.

Post-traumatic memory loss is "inability to retain new information in the minutes, hours, days, or weeks following the injury" (Corkin & associates, 1987, p. 318). Post-traumatic memory loss generally is considered to represent failure to incorporate experiences into long-term memory. Post-traumatic memory loss usually begins at the time of injury, but some patients may have brief intervals of memory for events that happened immediately after their injury, with loss of memory for later-occurring events. Russell's (1971) original definition of post-traumatic memory loss included both the period of coma and the period following it in which the patient fails to remember experiences. Most contemporary writers exclude the period of coma and assume that post-traumatic memory loss coincides roughly with the period of confusion and disorientation following the patient's emergence from coma (Baddeley & associates, 1987). Post-traumatic memory loss almost always lasts longer than pre-traumatic memory loss. Figure 9-9 summarizes results reported by Corkin and associates (1987) for Korean conflict survivors. Whereas pre-traumatic memory loss rarely spanned more than seconds to minutes, post-traumatic memory loss often spanned days or weeks. Russell (1971) and Jennett (1976) have reported similar results.

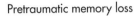

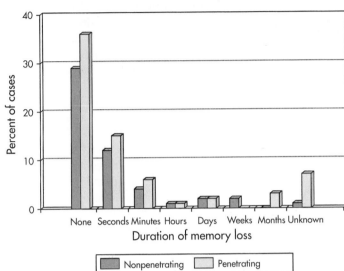

Figure 9-8 ■ The duration of pretraumatic memory loss in 121 cases of penetrating or nonpenetrating traumatic brain injuries from the Korean conflict. (Data from Corkin, S. H., Hurt, R. W., Twitchell, T. E., & associates. [1987]. Consequences of penetrating and nonpenetrating head injury: posttraumatic amnesia, and lasting effects on cognition. In H. S. Levin, J. Grafman, & H. M. Eisenberg [Eds.], *Neurobehavioral recovery from head injury* [pp. 318-329]. New York: Oxford University Press.)

Figure 9-9 ■ The duration of posttraumatic memory loss in 121 cases of penetrating or nonpenetrating traumatic brain injuries from the Korean conflict. (Data from Corkin, S. H., Hurt, R. W., Twitchell, T. E., & associates. [1987]. Consequences of penetrating and nonpenetrating head injury: posttraumatic amnesia, and lasting effects on cognition. In H. S. Levin, J. Grafman, & H. M. Eisenberg [Eds.], *Neurobehavioral recovery from head injury* [pp. 318-329]. New York: Oxford University Press.)

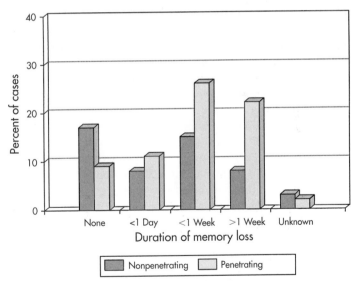

As mentioned earlier, the problem in post-traumatic memory loss is getting information into long-term memory. Patients with post-traumatic memory loss may participate in conversations, take tests, and carry out activities of daily living but have no subsequent recollection of those experiences. They do not remember meetings, conversations, or people from hour to hour or from morning to afternoon. Post-traumatic memory loss has far more serious consequences for the patient than pre-traumatic memory loss and causes greater disruption in the patient's daily life.

According to Lezak (1983) traumatically-brain-injured patients are most troubled by post-traumatic memory loss because of its effects on daily life, whereas their lawyers are most troubled by pre-traumatic memory loss because of their failure to remember events leading up to the accident.

The duration of post-traumatic memory loss is moderately related to the duration of coma and may be a better predictor of eventual recovery than duration of coma (Levin, Benton, & Grossman, 1982), with longer post-traumatic memory loss suggesting greater residual impairments. Patients with post-traumatic memory loss of 1 month or more are likely to have permanent memory deficits, and if post-traumatic memory loss lasts 3 months or more, the patient is likely to have permanent and severe impairments of cognition, learning, and memory (Brooks, 1989; Katz & Alexander, 1994).

Most measures of the duration of pre-traumatic and post-traumatic memory loss are actually retrospective estimates based on patients' accounts of when they first began remembering experiences after their accidents, and there are no standard procedures for obtaining these estimates. Consequently, it seems likely that considerable unaccounted-for variability exists in the measures. (For example, it is difficult, and perhaps impossible, to separate what a patient actually remembers about the time immediately following the accident from what family members, staff, or others have told the patient about that period.) Even so, there is sufficient consistency of results across studies of pre-traumatic and post-traumatic memory loss to give us reasonable confidence about the relative duration and time-course of these memory impairments.

For patients who can tolerate the testing, clinicians are likely to administer a comprehensive retrospective/declarative memory assessment battery that includes tests of *retention span, retention and recall of new information, retrieval of information from remote memory,* and *visual memory.*

Testing Retention Span   *Retention span* refers to the number of bits of information an individual can store in memory given a single exposure to the information. Retention-span testing may assess *immediate retention,* in which the test-taker's memory for information is tested immediately after the information is presented. Retention-span testing also may assess *short-term retention,* in which the test-taker's memory for the information is tested following a delay interval of a few seconds to a minute.

The most common way of testing immediate retention span is *digit span testing,* in which the examiner reads lists of single-digit numbers aloud and the patient repeats each list when the examiner finishes reading it. Immediate retention-span tests typically begin with two-digit or three-digit lists, with the number of digits in successive lists increasing until the patient can no longer repeat a list without error. Digit span tests are found in several memory assessment batteries and in most general intelligence tests such as the *Wechsler Adult Intelligence Scale-Revised* (Wechsler, 1981) and the *Stanford-Binet Intelligence Test* (Terman & Merrill, 1973). Lists of random letters or lists of unrelated words sometimes are used to measure immediate retention span. Normal spans for digits, letters, and words are similar and range from five to seven items.

Digit-span, letter-span, and word-span tests are auditory-verbal tests, in that the patient must comprehend and retain strings of spoken words long enough to repeat them. A few immediate retention span tests with nonverbal stimuli have been described in the literature. The most common of these tests are *block-tapping* tests, in which a set of blocks is placed before the patient and the examiner taps some of them in prearranged order. The patient then is asked to tap the blocks in the same order the examiner tapped them. As in digit-span tests, the number of blocks in the sequence increases until the patient can no longer duplicate the examiner's tapping patterns without error. The *Knox Cube Test* (Arthur, 1947) is the most well-known block-tapping test. However, the cubes in the *Knox Cube Test* are arranged in a row, permitting test-takers to mentally number them, thus using a verbal strategy to perform the test. The *Corsi Block-Tapping Test* (Milner, 1971) eliminates this possibility by arranging the blocks in a random array.

Short-term retention customarily is assessed by administering a retention-span test and imposing a delay between the examiner's presentation of test items and the patient's opportunity to respond. The delay interval usually lasts for only a few seconds and rarely exceeds 1 minute.

Test-takers typically help themselves remember the items in short-term retention span tests by mentally rehearsing the information until they are permitted to respond (most often by subvocally repeating the digits, letters, or words in the test items). Some short-term retention span tests prevent such rehearsal by requiring that the test-taker count backward or say the alphabet backward during the delay interval. The intervening activity is called *interference.* Normal adults whose retention performance is errorless with unfilled delays of up to 30 seconds only recall about 60% to 75% of items after a 10-second delay with interference (Lezak, 1995). The performance of adults with traumatic brain injuries is even more strongly affected by interference. For some patients, imposing a 3-second filled delay is sufficient to completely disrupt short-term retention.

Testing Recall of New Information Recall tests come in two forms. In the *subspan format* the examiner repeats a three-word or four-word list until the patient can repeat them back. Then the examiner goes on with other activities and after 5 minutes or so asks the patient to recall the list. In some variants, the examiner prompts the patient for unremembered words at the time of recall testing by giving a related word or category, and sometimes the examiner provides recognition trials for items the patient fails to remember after the prompts. In recognition trials the examiner provides several words, one or more of which are words the patient has failed to remember, and the patient is asked if any of the words were those that were to be remembered.

In the *supraspan format* the examiner reads a list of words that exceeds the patient's immediate retention span. (Lists usually contain 15 or more words.) After the first reading the examiner asks the patient to repeat as many of the words as the patient can remember. The examiner writes down the words produced by the patient and the order in which they were produced. Then the examiner repeats the list and again asks the patient to say as many as the patient can remember. This procedure continues until the patient has learned the entire list or for a predetermined number of trials (usually four or five). In some tests, a recognition trial is provided after the final recall trial for patients who have not learned the list in the prescribed number of trials. The *Auditory-Verbal Learning Test* (Rey, 1964) and the *California Verbal Learning Test* (Delis & associates, 1987) are frequently administered supraspan tests.

Testing Retrieval of Information from Remote Memory In retrieval tests the examiner asks the patient questions related to biographic information, such as the place and time of the patient's school attendance, the nature of the patient's first employment, and so on. It is not always necessary to administer a separate test of remote memory because some items in most screening tests of mental status test remote memory. Biographic information also may be obtained during the patient interview or as part of routines for gathering patient information when filling out test forms.

Testing Visual Memory In typical tests of visual memory the examiner shows the patient cards on which geometric designs (such as the one shown in Figure 9-10) are printed and asks the patient to draw them from memory. Many such tests are available, but the *Memory for Designs* subtests from the *Stanford-Binet Intelligence Scale* (Terman & Merrill, 1973), the *Memory for Designs Test* (Graham & Kendall, 1960), the *Visual Reproduction Test* (Wechsler, 1987), the *Rey Complex Figure Test* (Rey, 1941), and the *Benton Visual Retention Test* (Benton, 1974) are among the most popular with clinicians who work with traumatically-brain-injured adults. The Benton test differs from the others in that its designs are designed to be sensitive to the presence of hemispatial neglect (see Figure 9-10).

If a patient fails a drawing-from-memory test, the clinician may administer a visual memory test in which the patient is asked to recognize, rather than draw, previously presented visual stimuli. Some of these tests resemble visual reproduction tests, in that the stimuli are geometric designs—for example, the *Recurring Figures Test* (Kimura, 1963) and the *Visual Retention Test* (Warrington & James, 1967). In others the stimuli are drawings of real objects, as in the *Continuous Recognition Memory Test* (Hannay, Levin, & Grossman, 1979), in which the stimuli are plants, sea creatures, and animals. In most recognition memory tests the patient is shown a series of cards, each containing a different drawing or picture. Then a second set of cards, which contains the previously seen items plus additional foils, is shown to the patient and the patient indicates the items previously seen.

Testing Prospective Memory The foregoing tests focus on retrospective memory. Impaired retrospective memory is an important consequence of traumatic brain injury, but so is impaired prospective memory. Impaired prospective memory prevents many traumatically-brain-injured pa-

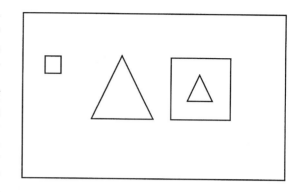

Figure 9-10 ■ **A plate from the *Revised Visual Retention Test*. The inclusion of smaller figures in the periphery make these designs sensitive to visual inattention.** (From Benton, A. L. [1992]. *The revised visual retention test*, ed 5. San Antonio: The Psychological Corporation.)

tients from functioning independently in daily life social, vocational, or educational activities. Tests of retrospective memory are not sensitive to impaired prospective memory (Sunderland, Harris, & Baddeley, 1983). In response to these concerns, Wilson, Cockburn, and Baddeley (1985) developed the *Rivermead Behavioural Memory Test* (RBMT) to test the functional effects of memory impairments by measuring performance in tasks that mimic everyday situations. The RBMT contains 14 items, some of which test retrospective memory and some of which test prospective memory in situations resembling situations likely to be encountered in daily life (Box 9-1).

The RBMT can be scored in two ways. A *screening score* can be calculated based on pass-fail scoring of each item. A more sensitive *profile score* can be calculated by more detailed scoring of each item. The RBMT manual and two supplements provide administration instructions, scoring guidelines, information on reliability and validity, and norms for adults aged 16 to 64 years. The RBMT takes, on average, about 30 minutes to administer.

A second version of the RBMT with greater sensitivity to mild memory impairment, called the *Rivermead Behavioural Memory Test-*

Box 9-1. The Rivermead Behavioural Memory Test

- The examiner shows the patient a photograph, and tells the patient the pictured person's name (e.g., *Catherine Taylor*).
- The examiner borrows a possession from the patient and, in view of the patient, hides it in a drawer or cupboard, then tells the patient to ask for the belonging at the end of the session and to tell the examiner where it is hidden.
- The examiner sets a timer to sound an alarm in 20 minutes and tells the patient to ask about his or her next appointment when the alarm sounds.
- The examiner shows the patient 10 line drawings of common objects and asks the patient to name each one.
- The examiner reads aloud a short narrative and asks the patient to retell it.
- The examiner shows the patient the 10 line drawings the patient named earlier together with 10 new drawings, and asks the patient to identify the ones the patient has seen before.
- The examiner shows the patient pictures of five faces, one at a time, and asks the patient to tell the examiner whether the person is male or female and older or younger than 40 years old. The examiner tells the patient that the patient will be expected to remember them later.
- The examiner walks a short route in the room (e.g., to the door, bookshelf, sink, desk, chair)

and leaves an envelope at one place on the route while the patient watches. The examiner then gives the envelope to the patient and asks the patient to walk the same route and leave the envelope in the same place as the examiner did.
- The examiner shows the patient the five pictures of faces seen before together with five new ones and asks the patient to identify the ones the patient has seen before.
- The examiner asks the patient 10 questions that assess orientation to person, place, and time.
- The examiner asks the patient to again retell the story previously read aloud by the examiner and retold by the patient.
- The examiner asks the patient to retrace the route demonstrated earlier and to put the envelope in the same place as it was put earlier.
- The examiner shows the patient the picture presented at the beginning of the examination and asks the patient to provide the person's name.
- The examiner announces that the test is over. If the patient does not spontaneously ask for the hidden possession, the examiner prompts the patient. ("You were going to remind me to give you something of yours.")

Extended, was published in 1999 (Wilson, Cockburn, & Baddeley). The RBMT-E doubles the amount that must be remembered, but test items and administration are similar to the original RBMT. The results of two studies conducted by the test's publisher suggest that the extended version is more sensitive to mild memory impairments than the original RBMT.

GENERAL CONCEPTS 9-3

- The primary objectives of assessment with comatose and semi-comatose patients with traumatic brain injury are to *estimate the nature and severity of the patients' injuries,*

evaluate the progression of the patients' status since their time of injury, and *determine their responsiveness to stimulation.*
- Assessment of patients who have returned to consciousness and begun responding to stimuli usually focuses on determining their *orientation* (to person, place, and time) and assessing their *mental status.* The *Galveston Orientation and Amnesia Test* and the *Mini-Mental Status Examination* often are used for these purposes.
- Alertness sometimes refers to *tonic alertness*—an individual's ongoing receptivity to stimulation—and sometimes to *phasic alertness*—an

individual's momentary, rapidly occurring receptivity to stimulation. Impaired phasic alertness usually is a greater problem for adults with traumatic brain injury than is impaired tonic alertness, although both may be diminished by brain injury.

- Several varieties of attention have been described in the literature: *focused attention, selective attention, sustained attention, alternating attention,* and *divided attention.* Adults with traumatic brain injuries often are impaired in all, although focused attention typically recovers relatively soon after the patient's return to consciousness.

- *Visual processing impairments* usually resolve soon after traumatically-brain-injured patients' return to consciousness, unless a patient has sustained extensive posterior brain trauma.

- *Retrospective memory* is memory for the past—events, experiences, and information previously acquired. Most patients with traumatic brain injury have compromised retrospective memory. *Prospective memory* is remembering to do things at specific times— remembering to remember. Most patients with traumatic brain injury have impaired prospective memory, which can drastically compromise their independence in daily life activities.

- Retrospective memory can be divided into *declarative memory* and *procedural memory.* Declarative memory contains what we know about things, and procedural memory contains what we know about how to do things. Declarative memory usually is more affected by traumatic brain injury than is procedural memory.

- Declarative memory can be divided into *episodic memory* and *semantic memory.* Episodic memory contains memory for personally experienced events. Semantic memory contains our organized knowledge of the world.

- Memory impairments of individuals who have traumatic brain injury can be characterized as *pre-traumatic memory loss* (loss of memory for events happening before the injury) or *post-traumatic memory loss* (loss of memory for events happening after the injury). Pre-traumatic memory loss usually spans a shorter time interval than post-traumatic memory loss, although both tend to shrink as patients recover.

- *Retention span* denotes the number of new bits of information one can hold in immediate memory given a single exposure to the information. Retention-span testing usually includes a test of *immediate retention span,* in which the test-taker reproduces the information immediately after it is presented, and a test of *short-term retention,* in which the test-taker must wait for a prescribed time interval before reproducing the information.

- *Recall of new information* usually is tested with lists of unrelated words that are read aloud to the test-taker until the test-taker can repeat the list. Then, after a delay interval, the examiner asks the test-taker to say the words in the list.

- *Retrieval of information from remote memory* usually is tested by asking the patient questions related to biographic information, such as where and when the patient went to school and where the patient has worked.

- *Visual memory* usually is tested by showing the patient cards on which geometric patterns are printed and asking the patient to draw them from memory.

- The *Rivermead Behavioural Memory Test* tests the functional effects of impaired prospective memory by measuring performance in tasks that resemble everyday situations.

LANGUAGE AND COMMUNICATION

Most traumatically-brain-injured adults at Rancho Los Amigos Level 5 and above produce speech that is phonologically, syntactically, and semantically within normal limits. (The primary exceptions are those with brain stem, cerebellar, or peripheral nervous system damage who are dysarthric. Assessment of these patients follows the same pattern as assessment of patients with dysarthria from other causes. See Chapter 11.)

Traumatically-brain-injured patients at Rancho Los Amigos Level 5 and above often make errors on tests of confrontation naming, but most of their naming errors reflect visual misperceptions or the patient's inability to inhibit competing responses, rather than word-retrieval impairments. Word-retrieval failures in spontaneous speech sometimes occur, but unless they are very frequent they do not seriously compromise communication in everyday activities. This is not true for relevance and efficiency. Most traumatically-brain-injured adults, except for those with mild head injuries, produce speech that is intermittently (at least) irrelevant, confabulatory, circumlocutory, tangential, fragmented, and noncohesive but (usually) linguistically acceptable. Add to this their faulty appreciation and observance of pragmatic rules and conventions, and the stereotypic picture of the traumatically-brain-injured speaker emerges. On the comprehension side, most traumatically-brain-injured adults do well if the material to be comprehended is structured and literal, but their comprehension often deteriorates when they are confronted with unstructured material or when appreciation of the meaning of the material depends on appreciation of indirect meanings such as metaphor, humor, or sarcasm.

> The speech and comprehension performance of traumatically-brain-injured adults has much in common with that of patients with right-hemisphere brain damage. One reason for this commonality may be the large proportions of patients with frontal-lobe damage in groups of right-hemisphere-damaged adults and the high probability that traumatically-brain-injured adults will have frontal lobe damage (McDonald, 1993).

Few traumatically-brain-injured adults exhibit patterns of language impairment that justify calling them aphasic, although many exhibit mild word-retrieval problems, diminished auditory and reading comprehension for complex materials, and occasional literal or verbal paraphasias. The communication impairments seen following traumatic brain injuries usually are secondary consequences of underlying impairments in attention, memory, reasoning, and problem-solving. Consequently, standard aphasia tests usually are not suitable for assessing the language and communication impairments of traumatically-brain-injured adults. Standard aphasia tests highlight skills such as word retrieval, syntactic processing, and comprehension of literal material (skills that usually are preserved following traumatic brain injury) and downplay or ignore skills such as organization and integration of complex information and appreciation of nonliteral and implied meanings (skills that are most likely to be compromised by traumatic brain injury). As a result, performance on an aphasia test usually overestimates traumatically-brain-injured adults' actual communicative competence.

Ylvisaker and Urbanczyk (1994) describe the reasons why aphasia tests may not be appropriate for traumatically-brain-injured patients:

> To the extent that communication is negatively affected by attentional, perceptual, organizational, and executive system dysfunction, language testing by its very nature may compensate for the underlying weakness. For example, the controlled testing environment reduces attentional challenges; clear instructions and well defined tasks help to ensure orientation to task and reduce the effects of cognitive inflexibility; test items that include only relatively small amounts of language compensate for organizational weakness; the deliberate rate at which information is presented compensates for difficulties with speeded performance; the supportive and encouraging manner of the examiner may compensate for an inability to cope with interpersonal stress; and commonly used tests fail to measure the individual's ability to learn new information and skills and to generalize new skills from one setting or task to another. (p. 174)

> Ylvisaker and Urbanczyk's last sentence gets the award for the longest sentence in this book.

> The conversational sample should represent a true conversation and not an interview (sometimes called "semi-structured conversation") in which the examiner asks questions and the patient answers them. Such "conversations" do not discriminate traumatically-brain-injured adults from adults without brain injuries (Snow, Douglas, & Ponsford, 1995).

Ylvisaker and Urbanczyk's comments do not mean, however, that tests used to evaluate aphasic adults have no place in the evaluation of adults with traumatic brain injuries. Selective testing of reading, writing, speaking, and listening focused on the perceptual and processing impairments likely to be affected by traumatic brain injury may be useful in quantifying traumatically-brain-injured patients' language and communication abilities. Depending on the severity of the patient's brain injury and the pattern of the patient's impairments, some or all of the following tests may be appropriate for traumatically-brain-injured adults who are cooperative and can attend well enough that their test performance is a valid indication of their true ability level.

- A receptive vocabulary test such as the *Peabody Picture Vocabulary Test* (Dunn & Dunn, 1981) to estimate usable listening vocabulary
- A test of spoken discourse comprehension to assess the patient's comprehension of stated and implied main ideas and details from spoken narratives
- A test of reading vocabulary and reading comprehension such as the *Gates-MacGinitie Reading Test* (Gates & associates, 2000)
- A test of generative naming such as the *Word Fluency Measure* (Borkowski, Benton, & Spreen, 1967) to assess the patient's ability to produce conceptually related words under time pressure
- A sample of connected speech elicited by picture description or story narration to assess the content, organization, and efficiency of the patient's connected speech
- A sample of conversation in which the presence and appropriateness of pragmatic aspects of the patient's communication may be evaluated

A test of naming or word retrieval may be appropriate for patients who appear to have word-retrieval problems.

- A general test of word finding such as the *Test of Adolescent/Adult Word Finding* (German, 1990) to assess word finding in a variety of contexts
- A confrontation naming test such as the *Boston Naming Test* (Kaplan, Goodglass, & Weintraub, 2001) to assess the patient's ability to retrieve and produce words on demand
- A test of generative naming, such as the *Word Fluency Test,* (Borkowski, Benton, & Spreen, 1967) or a category naming test.

A sentence comprehension test may be appropriate for patients who have difficulty with items in a test of discourse comprehension.

- The *Token Test* (DeRenzi & Vignolo, 1962) to assess the patient's short-term auditory retention span and comprehension of spoken sentences with high information density
- The *Test for Auditory Comprehension of Language* (Carrow-Woodfolk, 1999) to assess comprehension of grammatic morphemes and to assess comprehension of phrases and sentences with differing syntactic structures

Tests of written spelling, arithmetic, and higher-level reading comprehension, plus challenging language-production tests such as proverb interpretation tests, may be appropriate for traumatically-brain-injured adults with mild cognitive or communicative impairments. For traumatically-brain-injured adults with dysarthria, a motor speech examination and a measure of speech intelligibility would be appropriate.

Depending on the patient's pattern of communication impairments, other tests of speech, language, and communication may be appropriate. Comprehensive testing of spelling and reading comprehension may be important for high-level patients concerned with return to school or work. Extended evaluation of pragmatic skills may be important for patients who are contemplating return to environments that require interactions with others. Comprehensive evaluation of verbal planning and problem-solving may be important for patients who intend to return to jobs in which those skills are required.

ABSTRACT THINKING

Impaired abstract thinking is almost a universal consequence of brain damage. Lezak (1995) describes it as "... inability to think in useful generalizations, at the level of ideas, or about persons, situations, events not immediately present (past, future, or out of sight)" (p. 602). Lezak comments that tests of other cognitive processes such as planning, organizing, problem-solving, and reasoning also supply information about abstract thinking.

Adults with moderate to severe traumatic brain injuries do poorly on tests of abstract thinking regardless of the modality in which test items are presented or the nature of the responses required. Those with less severe injuries may perform well on some tests and poorly on others, depending on the complexity of the test and whether the test addresses an impaired stimulus or response modality (Lezak, 1995).

Commonly administered verbal tests to assess abstract thinking include *proverb interpretation tasks,* in which the patient tells the meaning of common proverbs such as "Don't put the cart before the horse" (Delis, Kramer, & Kaplan, 1988; Gorham, 1956); and *similarities and differences tasks,* in which the patient tells how two words are similar *(orange/banana)* or different *(bird/dog)* (Terman & Merrill, 1973; Tow, 1955; Wechsler, 1981).

Commonly administered nonverbal (visual) tests to assess abstract thinking include the *Progressive Matrices* (Raven, 1960, 1965) and *categorization and sorting tasks.* Raven's *Standard Progressive Matrices* (1960) and *Coloured Progressive Matrices* (1965) are tests of intelligence and reasoning with low verbal loadings, making them useful for estimating the intellectual and reasoning skills of patients with language impairments. Both matrices tests are multiple-choice tests in which the patient is shown visual patterns in which a part is missing. The patient is asked to choose from a set of six or eight choices the one that completes the stimulus (Figure 9-11). The *Standard Progressive Matrices* consists of 60 items divided into five sets of 12 items each. The

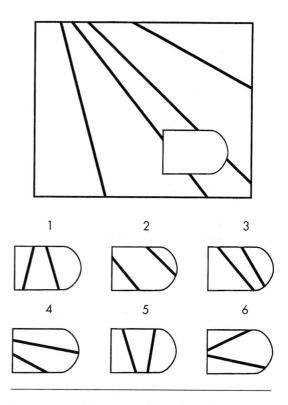

Figure 9-11 ■ **An example of a *Progressive Matrices* task. The person taking the test chooses the pattern segment at the bottom that best completes the overall pattern at the top.**

Coloured Progressive Matrices consists of 36 items, is easier, and is for testing children and for testing adults 65 years old or older. The *Standard Progressive Matrices* has numerous difficult items that may require verbal reasoning for their solution. For most brain-injured patients, the *Coloured Progressive Matrices* are appropriate. However, for patients with mild brain injuries, the standard (more difficult) version may be appropriate.

In *categorization and sorting tests,* the patient must determine the rules for assigning stimuli to categories by means of a trial-and-error process in which the examiner tells the patient only "right" or "wrong" following correct or incorrect assignments (Mahurin & Pirozzolo, 1986; Reitan & Wolfson, 1993). The *Wisconsin Card Sorting Test* (WCST; Grant & Berg, 1948) is a widely used categorization and sorting test. In the WCST the test-taker is given a deck of cards, each of which contains one to four symbols *(triangle, cross, star, circle).* The symbols on each card are printed in one of four colors *(red, green, yellow, blue).* The test-taker is instructed to sort the cards into four stacks according to the examiner's feedback.

The test-taker begins sorting the cards and the examiner says "right" or "wrong" after each placement. When the test begins, color is the principle governing the sort, and the examiner says "right" whenever the patient sorts a card by its color. When the test-taker has deduced the color-sorting principle (10 consecutive correct placements), the principle for sorting changes to form. (The only signal of the change to the test-taker is a change in the feedback provided for sorting responses.) When the test-taker has deduced the form-sorting principle, the principle changes to number, and so on, for two cycles of color-form-number. Performance on the WCST can be scored in several ways, but most users score the number of runs of 10 consecutive correct sorts and the number of perseverative errors (failure to change sorting responses to match changes in the sorting principle).

REASONING

According to Lezak (1995), tests of reasoning assess an individual's capacity for logical thinking,

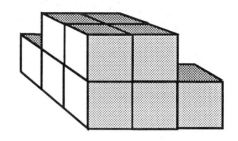

Figure 9-12 ■ An example of a block-counting test stimulus. The difficulty of a block-counting test item depends on the number of blocks and the number of blocks hidden from view.

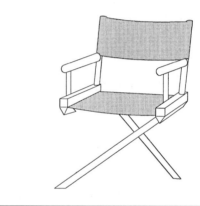

Figure 9-13 ■ An example of a picture-completion test stimulus. The person taking the test tells what is missing from the test stimulus.

appreciation of relationships, and practical judgment. Reasoning tests can be divided into three categories: *verbal reasoning tests, arithmetic and numeric reasoning tests,* and *visual-spatial reasoning tests.*

Verbal reasoning tests include:

- *Tests of reasoning and judgment* such as items in the *Wechsler Intelligence Scale* (Wechsler, 1981) in which the patient is asked to respond to questions (e.g., "What would you do if you find an unmailed letter on the street?").
- *Verbal absurdities tests* such as items in the *Stanford-Binet Intelligence Scale* (Terman & Merrill, 1973) in which the patient is asked to

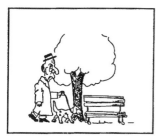 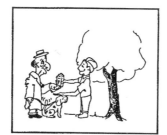 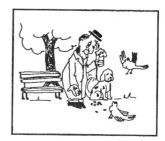

Figure 9-14 ■ **An example of a picture-arrangement test stimulus. The person taking the test rearranges the pictures to tell a story. The pictures are shown in story order. The examiner gives them to the person taking the test in scrambled order.**

identify the logical inconsistencies in items (e.g., "Bill Jones's feet are so big that he has to pull his trousers on over his head.").

- *Logical relationship tests* such as *Verbal Reasoning* (Corsini & Renck, 1992) in which the patient must arrive at a conclusion based on analysis of logical relationships presented in a short narrative (e.g., "Fred is taller than Bill but shorter than Oliver. Helen is taller than Oliver and shorter than Bill . . .").

Arithmetic and numerical reasoning tests include:

- Arithmetic story problems (Walsh, 1985; Wechsler, 1981) in which the patient is asked to solve story problems (e.g., "Bill has 8 pencils. Frank has 4 times as many pencils as Bill. How many pencils do they have together?").
- *Block-counting tests* (McFie & Zangwill, 1960; Newcombe, 1969; Terman & Merrill, 1973) require the patient to count how many blocks are depicted in drawings of three-dimensional stacks of blocks (Figure 9-12). The difficulty of items in these tests depends on the number of blocks depicted and the number of blocks in the stack that are hidden from view.

Visual-spatial reasoning tests include:

- Picture-completion tests such as those in the *Wechsler Intelligence Scale* (Wechsler, 1981) in which the patient tells what is missing from drawings of common objects, human figures, or animal figures drawn with missing parts (Figure 9-13).

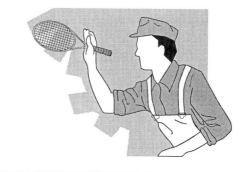

Figure 9-15 ■ **A picture-absurdities test item. The person taking the test tells what is wrong with the picture.**

- Picture-arrangement tests (Wechsler, 1981) in which the patient arranges scrambled pictures to portray a story-like sequence of events (Figure 9-14).
- Pictured-absurdities tests (Terman & Merrill, 1973) in which the patient tells what is wrong with pictures depicting bizarre or impossible relationships or situations (Figure 9-15).

PLANNING AND PROBLEM-SOLVING

Planning and problem-solving call into play several abilities, including thinking ahead, understanding the future consequences of present actions, considering alternatives, and making choices. Impairment of any of these skills can dis-

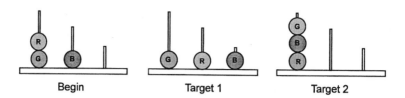

Begin   Target 1   Target 2

Figure 9-16 ■ **A tower test. The test-taker starts with the blocks arranged in a pattern by the examiner** *(Begin)*. **Then he or she is given a drawing that shows the blocks rearranged in a new pattern and is asked to move the blocks to create the new pattern with the smallest number of moves possible. The number of moves the test-taker makes to create the new pattern is recorded.** *Target 1* **can be accomplished in two moves.** *Target 2* **cannot be accomplished in less than five moves.** (From Shallice, 1982).

rupt or devastate planning and problem-solving. There are few standardized tests designed exclusively to measure planning and problem-solving skills, although most construction tests involve some degree of planning and maze tests require both planning and problem-solving. Two less well-known tests that require planning and problem-solving for successful performance are the *tower tests* (Shallice, 1982; Glosser & Goodglass, 1990; Saint-Cyr & Taylor, 1992) and the *Tinkertoy test* (Lezak, 1995).

In the *tower tests* the test-taker must rearrange colored rings, beads, or blocks on upright dowels to end with a specified arrangement (Figure 9-16). Performance is scored as the number of moves required to get from the starting position to the specified final arrangement.

In the *Tinkertoy test* 50 pieces of a standard Tinkertoy set are placed in front of the patient, who is told to "make whatever you want with these." The patient then is given 5 minutes to plan and execute the construction, after which the examiner asks, "What is it?" and writes down the patient's response. The final construction is scored with a seven-category system that takes into account the number of elements in the construction, whether it has moving parts, whether it is freestanding and three-dimensional, the appropriateness of the name given by the patient, and errors (misfits, incomplete fits, failed fits). According to Lezak, the *Tinkertoy test* allows pa-

tients to initiate, plan, and structure a potentially complex activity and carry it out independently.

> Tinkertoys are collections of small dowels of various lengths and colors, plus connectors, wheels, and other parts that can be assembled into constructions of considerable complexity, complete with moving parts.

TEST BATTERIES USEFUL IN EVALUATION OF TRAUMATICALLY-BRAIN-INJURED ADULTS

Several test batteries for assessment of traumatically-brain-injured adults' cognition and language have been published, but most have weaknesses in coverage, norms, reliability, or standardization that compromise their value as stand-alone instruments for traumatically-brain-injured adults. However, some may be useful as screening instruments to identify gross impairments, which then can be evaluated in more detail with follow-up tests. Brief descriptions of some of the major test batteries follow. Because there is considerable variability in their psychometric properties, potential users should examine a test's validity, reliability, norms, and coverage before adopting it for routine clinical use.

The *Brief Test of Head Injury* (BTHI; Helm-Estabrooks & Hotz, 1991) is a screening test for evaluating adults with severe impairments following traumatic brain-injury. The BTHI contains 31 items in seven sections: *orientation-attention, following commands, linguistic organization, reading comprehension, naming (pictures, objects), memory (immediate, recent, remote), and visual-spatial skills.* Section scores and BTHI total score can be converted into percentile rankings and standard scores for comparison with the norm group. Clinicians may find the BTHI a useful supplement to (or replacement for) rating scales such as the *Rancho Los Amigos Scale of Cognitive Levels* (Hagen & Malkamus, 1979) for establishing baseline performance and tracking recovery of severely impaired traumatically-brain-injured patients.

The *Ross Information Processing Assessment-Second Edition* (RIPA-2; Ross, 1996) contains 10 subtests to assess *immediate memory, recent memory, remote memory* (two subtests), *spatial orientation, orientation to the environment, recall of information, problem-solving and reasoning, organization of information,* and *auditory comprehension and retention.* The RIPA-2 test manual provides normative information for a group of 126 traumatically-brain-injured adults.

The *Scales of Cognitive Ability for Traumatic Brain Injury* (SCATBI; Adamovich & Henderson, 1992) contains 41 subtests divided among five sections: *perception and discrimination, orientation, organization* (categorization, association, sequencing), *recall,* and *reasoning.* The total score for each section can be converted to a percentile rank and a standard score, and the overall score on the SCATBI can be converted to a severity rating. The percentiles and standard scores are based on the performance of a norm group of 244 traumatically-brain-injured adults and 78 non-brain-injured adults. The SCATBI has a greater range of item difficulty than most tests for traumatically-brain-injured adults. (It contains some items that non-brain-damaged adults are likely to find difficult.) Because of its length (it takes approximately 2 hours to administer the

entire SCATBI) and the range of difficulty of test items, clinicians are unlikely to administer the entire test on any single test occasion. It is practical for clinicians to administer individual sections because normative information is provided for individual sections. The SCATBI appears to be a reasonable general-purpose test battery for higher-level traumatically-brain-injured adults, although clinicians may wish to supplement information provided by the SCATBI with the results of other tests that provide more detailed information about areas of impairment identified with the SCATBI.

Although not normed on traumatically-brain-injured adults, the *Woodcock-Johnson Psycho-educational Battery-Revised* (WJR; Woodcock & Johnson, 1989) includes several tests that are appropriate for assessing specific cognitive abilities of higher-level patients with traumatic brain injuries. The WJR has two components—the *Woodcock-Johnson Tests of Cognitive Ability-Revised* (WJR-COG) and the *Woodcock-Johnson Tests of Achievement-Revised* (WJR-ACH). The range for most of the subtests in the WJR is from age 2 to adult, and norms are provided for ages 2 to 90. The design and standardization of the WJR permit use of most subtests in isolation. For these reasons, the WJR-COG can provide a valuable set of tests for assessing a broad range of abilities across a wide range of ability levels, and performance of traumatically-brain-injured patients can reliably be compared with that of non-brain-damaged individuals of equivalent age.

The *Woodcock-Johnson Tests of Cognitive Abilities* are divided into two sections (batteries). The *standard battery* contains seven subtests:

1. *Memory for names:* the patient must remember nonsense names (such as *jawl, kiptron*) for cartoon figures.
2. *Sentence recall:* the patient repeats words and sentences, ranging from a one-syllable word to a 33-syllable sentence.
3. *Visual matching:* the patient searches an array of numbers for a designated target.
4. *Incomplete words:* the patient identifies spoken words with missing sounds.

5. *Visual closure:* the patient identifies common objects represented by incomplete drawings or by photographs taken from unusual angles.
6. *Picture vocabulary:* the patient says the names of pictured items, from high-frequency names to low-frequency names.
7. *Analysis-synthesis:* the patient solves puzzle-like problems by applying symbolically represented rules.

The *supplemental battery* of the WJR-COG contains 12 supplemental subtests that relate to the subtests in the standard battery.

1. *Visual-auditory learning:* the patient must learn real-word names for nonrepresentational symbols.
2. *Memory for words:* the patient recalls word lists ranging from one word to eight words.
3. *Cross-out:* the patient crosses out target symbols in a linear array of targets and foils.
4. *Sound blending:* the patient identifies fragmented spoken words.
5. *Picture recognition:* the patient chooses drawings from an array containing previously seen items and foils.
6. *Oral vocabulary:* the patient gives synonyms and antonyms for familiar words.
7. *Concept formation:* the patient learns rules that determine the placement of large and small colored forms.
8. *Delayed-recall names:* the patient is given a delayed-recall trial (2 to 4 days later) of the *memory for names* subtest in the standard WJR-COG battery.
9. *Delayed-recall–visual-auditory learning:* the patient is given a delayed version of the *visual-auditory learning* subtest in the supplemental battery.
10. *Sound patterns:* the patient tells whether pairs of nonsense words are *same* or *different.*
11. *Spatial relations:* the patient chooses jigsaw-puzzle-like forms that combine to form a more complex figure.
12. *Listening comprehension:* the patient provides a missing word to complete a sentence.

Achievement test batteries provide another important resource for clinicians who wish to evaluate the performance of higher-level traumatically-brain-injured patients in tasks that provide an indication of potential success in school or other activities that depend on mathematics, reading, writing, spelling, and vocabulary skills. The *Woodcock-Johnson Tests of Achievement-Revised* (WJR-ACH; Woodcock & Johnson, 1989) are divided into two sections. The standard battery contains 12 tests to assess reading, mathematics, and written language. The supplemental battery contains two reading subtests and two writing subtests.

The *Peabody Individual Achievement Test-Revised* (PIAT-R; Markwardt, 1989) contains six subtests:

1. *Mathematics:* the patient works out multiple-choice problems ranging from number and symbol recognition to complex algebra and geometry problems.
2. *Reading recognition:* the patient reads single-letter and word-recognition items, plus items in which the patient reads aloud printed words ranging from familiar to unfamiliar.
3. *Reading comprehension:* the patient chooses from a set of four pictures the one described by a printed sentence.
4. *Spelling:* a multiple-choice test in which the patient identifies printed letters and words and chooses correctly spelled words from sets containing a correctly spelled word and three incorrect spellings.
5. *Written expression:* the patient writes a short narrative related to a picture stimulus.
6. *General information:* a question-answer test of information gained in daily life, reading, or school.

The PIAT-R manual provides norms for each subtest, so the PIAT-R subtests, like the WJR subtests, can be administered and interpreted individually. Subtest scores can be converted into percentile ranks for ages from 5 to 18 years and into grade equivalents and age equivalents.

GENERAL CONCEPTS 9-4

- The speech of most traumatically-brain-injured adults is *irrelevant, confabulatory, circumlo-*

cutory, tangential, fragmented, and *noncohe-sive* but *linguistically acceptable.* Most often fail to recognize and follow *pragmatic rules and conventions.*

- Most traumatically-brain-injured adults comprehend well-structured and literal spoken or printed language, but their comprehension deteriorates when they must deal with unstructured material or nonliteral material such as metaphor, humor, or sarcasm.

- *Standard aphasia tests* are not usually appropriate for assessing traumatically-brain-injured adults' language and communication because they focus on skills that usually are not much affected by traumatic brain injury (e.g., word retrieval, comprehension of literal material) and neglect skills that are affected by traumatic brain injury (e.g., organization of complex information, appreciation of non-literal meanings, language pragmatics).

- Tests of *receptive vocabulary, naming* (especially generative naming), *sentence comprehension, discourse comprehension, picture description,* and *pragmatic appropriateness* are likely to be appropriate for adults with traumatic brain injury, depending on the severity of their injury.

- Most adults with traumatic brain injury exhibit impaired *abstract thinking.* Verbal abstract thinking may be assessed with *proverb interpretation tests* or *similarities and differences tests.* Nonverbal abstract thinking may be assessed with the *Progressive Matrices* or *categorization and sorting tests.*

- *Impaired reasoning* (logical thinking, appreciation of relationships and judgment) is a common consequence of traumatic brain injury. Comprehensive assessment of reasoning includes tests of *verbal reasoning, arithmetic and numeric reasoning,* and *visual-spatial reasoning.*

- *Impaired planning and problem-solving* are common following traumatic brain injury and continue to be problematic even for well-recovered individuals. Construction and maze tests require planning and problem-solving. *Tower tests* and the *Tinkertoy test* permit as-

sessment of high-level planning and problem-solving.

- Several test batteries for assessing traumatically-brain-damaged adults have been published and may be used to identify gross impairments that can be evaluated in greater detail with follow-up tests.

- Subtests of the *Woodcock-Johnson Psychoeducational Battery* may be useful for evaluating specific cognitive abilities of higher-level individuals with traumatic brain injuries. Subtests from achievement test batteries such as the *Woodcock-Johnson Tests of Achievement* or the *Peabody Individual Achievement Test* also may be used to evaluate the performance of higher-level traumatically-brain-injured patients, especially those who may return to school.

TREATMENT OF TRAUMATICALLY-BRAIN-INJURED ADULTS
Approaches to Treatment

Treatment of traumatically-brain-injured adults requires the collaboration of many professionals, including physicians, nurses, neuropsychologists, speech-language pathologists, occupational therapists, physical therapists, clinical psychologists, social workers, and vocational counselors. Interdisciplinary collaboration is especially important in the early stages of the patient's recovery, when medical, physical, and behavioral impairments are most severe. The physical, cognitive, and behavioral impairments exhibited by traumatically-brain-injured patients cross professional boundaries and require a unified, integrated program of treatment that extends from the clinic to the patient's daily environment.

According to Kay and Silver (1989), "... rehabilitation [of traumatically-brain-injured patients] must be interdisciplinary in the truest sense of the word. There must be ongoing communication among team members (not just with a central leader), care planning that cuts across disciplines, and coordination by a professional who is an expert in the cognitive and behavioral problems of head-injured persons" (p. 147).

The first programs for treatment of traumatically-brain-injured adults did not arise out of any particular theoretic rationale and were not based on careful analyses of traumatically-brain-injured adults' performance. The practitioners who designed and carried out these first treatment programs generally were operating under the assumption that stimulation of mental processes is the key to improving traumatically-brain-injured adults' performance. Consequently, the early treatment programs immersed patients in drill activities that were designed to stimulate and restore mental processes.

These early treatment programs usually used a *teach-to-the-test* approach, in which tests of generic skills (reading, reasoning, problem-solving) were administered, deficient performance in specific skills was identified, and treatment consisted of drills to stimulate the patient with activities that targeted the deficient skills. The treatment activities often resembled the tests that were used to identify the patient's deficient skills, and treatment frequently relied on workbooks and computer-based programs designed for remedial education in the schools. Sohlberg and Mateer (1989) call this treatment approach the *general stimulation* approach. General stimulation approaches to rehabilitation of traumatically-brain-injured adults largely have been abandoned in favor of theory-driven or model-driven approaches.

One early reason for clinicians' disenchantment with stimulation approaches to traumatic brain injury rehabilitation was their recognition that stimulation treatment had little effect on traumatically-brain-injured adults' daily life. Immersing patients in a program of general stimulation sometimes produced favorable changes in their test scores but rarely led to improvements in their ability to get along in daily life. This realization led some clinicians to abandon stimulation treatment in favor of a *functionally oriented* approach to treatment. Functionally oriented treatment programs focused on improving patients' daily life competence by training them to perform specific everyday tasks in situations that resembled daily life. For example, a patient might be trained to plan a meal, make a shopping list, and go to a market and purchase the items on the list, either in a real-life market or in a mock-up in the rehabilitation facility.

Those who believe in functionally oriented treatment assume that traumatically-brain-injured adults' rehabilitation is most efficient and effective when treatment is carried out in contexts that replicate the daily life contexts to which improved performance is to generalize. Treatment activities typically consist of structured experiences in mock-ups of real-life settings and situations, in which patients are coached in the skills and behaviors needed for successful performance.

Functionally oriented treatment proved a quick way to train traumatically-brain-injured adults to operate with maximum success in specific activities of daily life, producing "individuals who can perform particular activities under the conditions in which they were taught" (Sohlberg & Mateer, 1989, p. 20). A major drawback of most functionally oriented treatment is that generalization across tasks and situations often is limited or absent, which means that patients must be trained in a very large number of daily life tasks to function independently in an everyday environment.

Cognitive rehabilitation approaches to treatment of traumatically-brain-injured adults seek to promote patients' capacity for independent function in daily life by focusing on remediation of specific cognitive processes such as *attention, memory,* and *language.* Cognitive rehabilitation treatment typically consists of hierarchically organized drills. The choice of cognitive processes and the hierarchical arrangement of drills are based on a theoretic rationale that may be explicitly or implicitly defined. Improvements in a cognitive process are assumed to create improved performance in a broad range of activities that depend on the process. For example, improving a patient's sustained attention would be expected to improve the patient's performance in all tasks that require sustained attention. Cognitive rehabilitation sometimes is called *component* training because it focuses treatment on specific components of a patient's overall pattern of impairment.

Behavior therapy represents yet another approach to rehabilitation of traumatically-brain-injured adults. Behavior therapy focuses on direct modification of abnormal behaviors, using procedures based on learning principles. Behavior therapy emphasizes direct, objective measurement of target behaviors and the use of stimulus control, reinforcement, and punishment to modify the frequency of target behaviors, the form of target behaviors, or both. Behavior therapy is not necessarily (or usually) a stand-alone treatment. It is a part of many functionally oriented treatment programs and often is a central focus for residential treatment programs and transitional living programs for traumatically-brain-injured adults.

Most contemporary treatment programs for traumatically-brain-injured adults include a mix of functionally oriented treatment, cognitive rehabilitation, and behavior therapy. Behavior therapy usually plays a prominent role in the immediate post-coma phase of treatment when control and modification of aberrant behaviors are major concerns. Cognitive rehabilitation usually plays a prominent role in the middle stages of treatment when restoration of cognitive abilities is the primary focus. Functionally oriented treatment becomes more prominent as traumatically-brain-injured patients move into the later stages of recovery, when preparation for life after the rehabilitation facility and the patient's reintegration into society become primary concerns.

Treatment goals and procedures for traumatically-brain-injured adults are intimately related to the traumatically-brain-injured adults' responsiveness and capacity for goal-directed behavior. Treatment of comatose or semi-comatose patients (Rancho Los Amigos Scale, Levels 1 to 3) consists primarily of sensory stimulation, and the purposes of treatment are to increase the patient's responsiveness to the environment and to facilitate the patient's return to consciousness.

Comatose: The patient exhibits neither arousal or awareness of surroundings. The patient's eyes are closed and the patient shows no evidence of sleep-wake cycles. *Semi-comatose* (sometimes called vegetative state): The patient has sleep-wake cycles, may open eyes in response to stimulation, and may inconsistently orient to the source of stimulation but neither comprehends nor produces language or gesture and makes no purposeful motor responses. If vegetative state lasts longer than 1 month, it may be called persistent vegetative state.

Treatment of confused and agitated patients (Rancho Los Amigos Scale, Level 4) usually combines environmental control to reduce the patient's confusion and disorientation and to control maladaptive behavior, response contingencies to directly manage and modify inappropriate or maladaptive behavior, and (sometimes) pharmacologic management to reduce the patient's agitation and facilitate new learning or relearning.

Treatment of confused and nonagitated patients (Rancho Los Amigos Scale, Level 5) focuses on increasing the patient's control over the immediate environment, stimulating the patient's basic cognitive skills, and increasing the patient's appropriateness in interactions with others. The overall treatment objectives for patients at this stage of recovery are to stimulate basic motor and sensory functions, to reestablish basic self-care skills (feeding, dressing, toileting, grooming), to improve orientation, and to reestablish functional communication.

Treatment of Rancho Los Amigos Scale, Level 6 (confused, appropriate) patients usually is strongly oriented toward cognitive skills. Treatment objectives for Level 6 patients include improving attention and memory, facilitating organized thinking, and practicing organized use of knowledge.

As patients reach Rancho Los Amigos Scale, Level 7 (automatic, appropriate), treatment of cognitive skills (*attention and memory, plan-*

ning and foresight, organized thinking, and *organized use of knowledge*) continues. For many patients at Level 7 it becomes apparent that some cognitive impairments will not yield to direct treatment, and the emphasis of treatment shifts to providing the patient with compensatory strategies for dealing with chronic cognitive impairments.

For patients whose recovery takes them to Rancho Los Amigos Scale Level 8 (purposeful, appropriate), treatment focuses on consolidating gains in cognitive and communicative skills obtained at previous stages of treatment, firming up previously trained compensatory strategies, and facilitating the patient's reentry into family, community, school, and work environments.

Sensory Stimulation

Treatment of comatose and semi-comatose patients depends primarily on *sensory stimulation,* in which the patient is repeatedly stimulated in auditory, visual, tactile, olfactory, and taste modalities. Comatose patients often receive several short (10-minute to 15-minute) intervals of stimulation every day, together with passive range-of-motion activities to prevent muscle deterioration. The purposes of sensory stimulation are "... to increase the patient's alertness/arousal and responsiveness to the environment and to prevent sensory deprivation . . . to facilitate changes in responsiveness such as increased consistency and specificity of response and/or decreased latency of response" (Cherney, Halper, & Miller, 1991, p. 59).

Many practitioners believe that sensory stimulation hastens traumatically-brain-injured patients' emergence from coma, but there is no empiric evidence supporting this belief. Nevertheless, the idea makes intuitive sense, and as Kay and Silver (1989) point out, "It would seem to make sense on rational grounds that it is better to provide regular, gentle sensory input to comatose patients than to let them lie unattended and unstimulated (physically and sensorially) for long periods of time" (p. 149).

There is some indirect evidence for the benefits of sensory stimulation from studies of animals. Some studies have shown that animals with experimenter-induced brain damage who then are placed in a stimulating environment recover their ability to learn new behaviors to a greater degree than animals with equivalent brain damage kept in a nonstimulating environment. Other studies have shown that animals raised under conditions of sensory deprivation are less active and learn less well than animals raised under normal conditions. (The relevance of the latter research to traumatically-brain-injured adults depends on the assumption that their comatose or semi-comatose state causes sensory deprivation.)

Sensory stimulation is an uncomplicated procedure and most adults of average intelligence can learn it in two or three training sessions. Consequently, many speech-language pathologists train caregivers to provide the stimulation and keep a record of the patient's responses. After they are trained, the caregivers provide the stimulation. The speech-language pathologist periodically reviews the response records to determine if changes in the patient's responsiveness are taking place and also periodically (usually weekly) personally assesses the patient's responsiveness to the stimuli used in the stimulation program.

The nature of sensory stimulation depends on the patient's general level of arousal. Stuporous and lethargic patients may be stimulated with intense stimuli to increase their level of arousal. Excitable and restless patients may receive gentle, rhythmic stimulation to calm them. Some practitioners stimulate phylogenetically older senses (touch, movement, olfaction) first, and stimulate phylogenetically younger senses (vision, audition) later. Most change the form and modality of stimuli frequently to avoid habituation on the part of the patient. Many practitioners believe that familiar voices, touches, and activity are intrinsically more effective than unfamiliar ones, but there is no evidence to confirm this belief.

Environmental Control

Environmental control refers to procedures by which confused and agitated patients' confusion and agitation are abated by controlling how the patient's environment is arranged and what happens in it. The objective of environmental control is to alter the patient's daily life environment to create maximally stable and predictable surroundings, thereby minimizing the patient's confusion and agitation and maximizing the patient's successful performance. Significant events (e.g., therapy appointments, meals, or visits from family members) are organized into a consistent routine, so that they happen at the same time, in the same place, and with the same people each day.

As the patient's agitation and confusion diminish, the controls over the patient's environment gradually are loosened and the salience of cues and reminders gradually is modulated. These changes permit the patient gradually to assume responsibility for some daily routines while keeping challenges and stresses manageable.

Behavior Management

Behavior management complements environmental modification by directly targeting certain behaviors to increase the frequency of adaptive behaviors and diminish the frequency of maladaptive behaviors. Environmental modification controls and shapes behavior and facilitates successful performance by reducing or eliminating stimuli that produce agitation and confusion and replacing them with stimuli that help the patient cope with the environment despite cognitive limitations and alterations in emotions and personality. These manipulations of the environment control what behaviorists call *antecedent stimuli* (stimuli that function to elicit or maintain certain behaviors). Another, more di-

rect, way of managing traumatically-brain-injured patients' behavior is by manipulation of *response contingencies.*

In Chapter 6, two main categories of what is called *feedback* were identified. *Incentive feedback* denotes a class of stimuli that can maintain (or eliminate) behaviors whose only function is to elicit (or avoid) the feedback stimuli. *Information feedback* denotes a class of stimuli that provides information about the appropriateness, correctness, or accuracy of the responses that elicit the feedback.

Traumatically-brain-injured patients who are in the early stages of recovery usually are not affected by intangible consequences (*information feedback*) such as verbal praise or reproof. Tangible, primary consequences (*incentive feedback*) are needed. Tangible consequences include positive consequences, such as sweets, music, touching, massaging, or other pleasurable stimuli, and negative consequences, such as noise, bright light, or painful stimuli.

> Traumatically-brain-injured patients in the early stages of recovery do not meet the conditions under which intangible consequences (information feedback) are effective. They are not internally motivated to get better. Much of their behavior is primitive and unmodulated by cortical control mechanisms. Consequences that depend on interpretation by the cerebral cortex and appreciation of others' intentions and desires are unlikely to affect these patients' behavior.

Four procedures for directly managing behavior by means of manipulation of response contingencies are available to clinicians. In *positive reinforcement* pleasurable stimuli are delivered contingent on desired responses. In *negative reinforcement* aversive stimuli are removed contingent on desired responses. In *punishment* aversive stimuli are delivered contingent on undesired responses. In *extinction* selected responses elicit neither pleasurable nor aversive stimuli.

When response contingencies are used to modify or maintain the behavior of confused and agitated traumatically-brain-injured patients, the stimuli used as response contingencies must have incentive value and they must be delivered consistently following each occurrence of the target behavior(s). Positive reinforcement can increase the frequency of some target behaviors, provided that the behaviors do not require great effort and do not lead to conditions that the patient finds aversive (such as the clinician asking the patient to repeat or elaborate on a behavior).

Negative reinforcement sometimes can be a surprisingly powerful tool for modifying the behavior of severely agitated and confused patients, who prefer being left alone to being harassed by the clinician to make effortful responses that have no immediate payoff. Sometimes a clinician may turn a confused and agitated patient's desire to be left alone to clinical advantage by making termination of a treatment activity contingent on the patient's performance. Initially only one or two simple responses are required to terminate the activity ("If you tell me the year you were born, I'll go away and leave you alone."). Then the clinician gradually changes the criteria so that more responses, or more effortful responses, are required to terminate the activity. As the patient's agitation and confusion diminish, treatment activities (and the clinician's presence) usually become less unpleasant to the patient and response contingencies shift from negative reinforcement to positive reinforcement.

> A subtle side effect of such negative reinforcement procedures is that they give severely disabled patients an opportunity to control what happens in their environment— control that is not often afforded patients at this stage of recovery.

Punishment has a limited role in managing the behavior of confused and agitated patients. Physical punishment (e.g., slapping, pinching) is morally and legally impermissible. Milder forms of punishment, such as the sound of a buzzer or loud verbal reproof, sometimes may help suppress a confused and agitated patient's inappropriate behavior. However, the suppressive effects of punishment usually are temporary because the behavior usually reappears as soon as the punishment is discontinued. More durable changes in behavior usually can be obtained by other forms of reinforcement and by controlling the patient's environment to minimize undesirable behavior.

Sometimes caregivers unintentionally provide positive reinforcement for undesirable behaviors by paying attention when the patient behaves unacceptably and ignoring the patient at other times. Extinction (ensuring that a behavior receives no reinforcement) may help eliminate unacceptable behaviors, especially if extinction is combined with positive reinforcement of alternative behaviors. Extinction may not be very effective at modifying confused and agitated patients' behavior because, as noted earlier, these patients may consider being ignored by the clinician a positive consequence rather than a negative one.

The response contingencies used and the schedule on which they are delivered change as the patient recovers. When patients are confused and agitated, only a few important behaviors are treated, response-contingent stimuli have incentive value, and consequences follow every occurrence of the targeted behavior. Negative reinforcement may be an important treatment procedure. As the patient recovers, the number and complexity of behaviors targeted for treatment increase, the emphasis shifts from negative reinforcement to positive reinforcement, and partial reinforcement schedules (in which not every occurrence of the target behavior receives consequences) replace continuous schedules of reinforcement.

Pharmacologic Management

Sedatives or antipsychotic drugs may be prescribed to reduce some traumatically-brain-injured patients' agitation and assaultiveness. The positive result of such medication is that the patient becomes calmer and less assaultive. The negative result is that many patients become lethargic and sleepy. Finding the dosage at which a patient's agitated behavior is controlled without making the patient too lethargic and sleepy to benefit from treatment requires careful tuning of the patient's dosage and medication schedule.

Stimulant drugs sometimes are prescribed to improve a traumatically-brain-injured patient's alertness and attention, thereby increasing the potential benefits of treatment. (Some stimulants also have antidepressive effects.) Although some studies have shown apparent acceleration of recovery by administration of stimulant drugs, others have shown no meaningful effects. At this time there is no conclusive evidence for their efficacy in facilitating traumatically-brain-injured adults' recovery of cognitive abilities.

Some traumatically-brain-injured patients become clinically depressed in the later stages of recovery, perhaps in part as a consequence of their experiences with social and vocational dislocation, compromised physical and mental abilities, financial hardship, isolation, and inactivity. Depression also may occur, in part, as a consequence of neurochemical imbalances. Antidepressant medications may be prescribed for these patients. However, some antidepressant medications have potential side effects that can compromise memory and motor performance. If possible, these antidepressants should be avoided, and antidepressants (or other medications) that are fatal in overdose should, of course, not be prescribed if a patient has suicidal tendencies.

A few traumatically-brain-injured patients eventually develop psychotic conditions (paranoia, delusional states, schizophrenic-like disorders). Antipsychotic medications may be prescribed for these patients. However, most of these medications may cause extrapyramidal side effects such as dyskinesia, suppressed volitional movement, tremor, and other such symptoms. Antipsychotic medications should be administered at minimum effective dosage, and patients must be monitored carefully for side effects.

Anticonvulsant medications are prescribed routinely for patients in the acute stages of recovery from traumatic brain injuries, whether or not the patient actually has had a seizure. These medications have several potential side effects, including sedation, depression, motor impairments, and memory impairments. Consequently, anticonvulsants should not be prescribed indiscriminately or continued unnecessarily.

Orientation Training

In some respects, procedures to enhance traumatically-brain-injured patients' orientation resemble procedures used in environmental control, and orientation training often is the next stage of treatment for patients who are becoming less confused and agitated. Orientation training typically relies on environmental prompts in the patient's living space, verbal orientation information delivered by caregivers, orientation drills, and behavior management.

Environmental prompts come in a variety of forms. Signs, notes, appointment calendars, and appointment books help the patient anticipate upcoming events and assume responsibility for daily routines. Prominently displayed calendars, clocks, and schedules help orient the patient to time. Signs, labels, and maps showing city, state, and facility names and locations and signs, posters, and pictures identifying significant locations within the treatment facility (e.g., the patient's room, lounges, and dining areas) help the patient orient to place. The patient's room may be identified by signs displaying the patient's name and photograph and by the presence of significant personal possessions. Orientation to person is facilitated by pictures of home and family members displayed in the patient's room and by name tags worn by staff.

These passive reminders of time, place, and person are augmented by overt reminders provided by patient-care staff and family members. Patient-care staff and family members include references to time, place, and person in routine interactions with the patient and may carry out orientation drills to stimulate the patient to acquire and retain a sense of time, place, and person.

Orientation drills come in two basic forms (Cherney, Halper, & Miller, 1991). *Passive orientation drills* are best suited for patients in the immediate post-coma phase of recovery, whose confusion, agitation, and profound attentional and memory impairments make their active participation in structured treatment activities unlikely. In passive orientation, the clinician provides didactic instruction, demonstration, prompts, and cues to help the patients understand who they are, what has happened to them, and where they are and to help the patients recall current hour, day, month, and year.

Passive orientation sometimes is carried out in group settings. Patients are asked to repeat orientation information after the clinician, but they are not expected to produce it without prompts or cues. When patients can repeat orientation information after the clinician, the clinician may train them to verbalize accurate information about person, place, and time in response to prompts or requests. However, the ability to verbalize this information does not mean that the patient has internalized the concepts well enough to incorporate the concepts into daily life activities. That often requires active orientation training.

Active orientation training helps patients incorporate their imperfectly developed sense of person, place, and time into daily life activities. In active orientation training the patient is given responsibility for carrying out daily life activities that depend on internalized concepts of person, place, and time. Passive orientation training usually precedes active orientation training. For example, patients are taught how to tell time (passive orientation) before they are expected to monitor the passage of time or follow appointment schedules (active orientation), and they are taught where they are (passive orientation) before they are expected to find their way around their environment (active orientation).

Component Training

As traumatically-brain-injured patients become less disoriented and their confusion dissipates, the focus of treatment shifts toward remediation of impaired cognitive and linguistic processes. Individual processes (e.g., *attention, memory, language and communication*) may be treated individually and in a sequence governed either by a theoretic rationale or the clinician's intuitions and preferences—an approach called *component training.*

The goal of component training is to facilitate cognitive and linguistic processes by means of drill activities. The drill activities often have little surface similarity to natural contexts. Specific cognitive or linguistic impairments are targeted sequentially for treatment, and treatment usually consists of repetitive drill, often with paper-and-pencil or computer-based materials, to facilitate and repair the targeted processes. The expectation is that as the cognitive and linguistic processes improve, general skills that depend on the processes also will improve. In this respect, component training has much in common with the *treat underlying processes* approach to aphasia treatment described previously. Component training is the mode of treatment for most confused but appropriate or automatic and appropriate patients (Rancho Los Amigos Scale levels 6 and 7), although some confused but nonagitated patients (Rancho Los Amigos level 5) may be ready for low-level component training.

Attention Treatment of attentional impairments occupies a prominent place in component training, in part because most traumatically-brain-injured adults have attentional impairments and in part because attention is so important for other cognitive processes.

Sohlberg and Mateer (1989) described an organized program of treatment for attentional impairments called *Attention Process Training*

(APT). APT is based on Sohlberg and Mateer's five-component model of attentional processes *(focused attention, sustained attention, selective attention, alternating attention, and divided attention)* and provides treatment activities to target each of the last four, in the belief that attentional impairments are best treated by targeting specific attentional processes. Sohlberg and Mateer recommend that training address *sustained attention, selective attention, alternating attention,* and *divided attention* in that order, apparently in the belief that the order represents a hierarchy and that focused, selective, and sustained attention are prerequisites for alternating and divided attention.

> According to Sohlberg and Mateer, focused attention usually is disrupted only in the early stages of emergence from coma. Consequently, it is not a concern for most patients who can participate in structured treatment activities.

Sustained attention is treated with a series of ATP tasks. In *visual cancellation tasks* the patient scans and crosses out specified targets in visual arrays. In *auditory vigilance tasks* the patient pushes a button to sound a buzzer whenever they hear specified targets. The auditory vigilance tasks range from simple ("Push the buzzer every time you hear the number 6.") to complex ("Push the buzzer every time you hear 2 months in a row, such that the second month comes just before the first one on the calendar."). In *serial numbers activities* patients perform tasks such as backward counting, adding 4 and subtracting 2 from successive numbers, and so on.

ATP treats *visual selective attention* with materials such as those used in visual sustained-attention activities but in which overlays with distracting designs are placed over the stimuli. *Auditory selective attention* is treated with audiotapes containing the same stimuli as the ATP auditory sustained-attention tasks but with targets presented against a background of distracting noise (e.g., conversations, news broadcasts).

ATP treats *alternating attention* with several response-switching activities. In *alternating cancellation tasks* the patient begins crossing out a specified target, such as all the even numbers in an array of numbers. Then, when the examiner says "change," the patient crosses out all the odd numbers. This continues for several changes in target. In *add-subtract alternation* the patient begins by adding numbers presented in pairs until the examiner says "change," at which time the patient begins subtracting, and so on, for several changes in direction. In *Stroop-like activities* the words *high, mid,* and *low* are printed in high, middle, and low positions on a line. The patient is directed to alternate between reading the words and saying their position on the line. They do the same when the words big and little are printed in large and small letters.

Divided attention is treated with tasks requiring simultaneous attention to two aspects of a single task or requiring simultaneous attention to two different tasks. An example of the former is the *card-sort task*, in which the patient sorts playing cards by suit, but cards whose name contains a designated target letter must be turned face-down. For example, if the target letter is *e*, all *1s, 3s, 5s, 7s, 8s, 9s, 10s,* and *queens* must be turned face down. An example of the latter is requiring the patient to do a letter-cancellation task while simultaneously saying "yes" each time the examiner says the number 5 in a string of randomly arranged spoken numbers.

Sohlberg and Mateer (1989) present some preliminary evidence supporting the efficacy of APT in improving four traumatically-brain-injured patients' attentional abilities, but conclusive evidence of APT's efficacy awaits additional empiric investigation. Nevertheless, APT represents an innovative, model-driven approach to attention training and provides a worthwhile source of procedures for systematic treatment of attentional processes. (Chapter 8 has more information on treating attentional impairments.)

Visual Processing Treatment of traumatically-brain-injured patients' visual perceptual impairments has received less attention than treatment of their attention, memory, and language impairments, and for speech-language pathologists, treatment of visual impairments may seem to lie somewhat outside their usual clinical territory. However, as Sohlberg and Mateer (1989) have noted, visual and visuospatial processing are crucial for carrying out activities of daily living, for adequate job performance, and for performing academic and clerical tasks. Consequently, speech-language pathologists may find that treatment of visual processing impairments is an important part of the overall plan of care for a traumatically-brain-injured patient, especially if the visual processing impairments compromise the adequacy or effectiveness of the patient's communication. Some treatment programs for visual processing impairments focus on *discrimination and recognition* of visual stimuli, and others focus on *visuospatial processes.* Work on discrimination and recognition usually precedes work on visuospatial processes, the rationale being that discrimination and recognition are prerequisites to more complex visuospatial processing.

> Treatment of attention often precedes treatment of visual perception and discrimination and sometimes accompanies it.

Visual discrimination and recognition treatment activities include visual scanning drills in which the patient scans an array of symbols, designs, or pictures to find those that match a target; visual closure tasks in which the patient must identify familiar objects or scenes based on partial information; and visual figure-ground discrimination tasks in which the patient must identify familiar objects or scenes presented on an interfering or distracting background. Sometimes these tasks are presented with a time limit to increase the speed and efficiency of the patient's visual processing. (Chapter 8 has examples of some of these tasks.)

Treatment of visuospatial processing impairments usually incorporates drills that emphasize analysis of spatial relationships. Tasks that require the patient to copy or draw simple or complex geometric figures from memory or to construct duplicates of a model constructed by the clinician with sticks or blocks commonly are used in treating visuospatial impairments. These tasks usually are arranged from simple to complex. For example, paper-and-pencil tasks might begin with copying two-dimensional figures, then progress to drawing two-dimensional figures from memory, copying three-dimensional figures, and drawing three-dimensional figures from memory.

Tasks that require the patient to mentally rotate printed visual stimuli (Figure 9-17) are sometimes used to treat visuospatial impairments. These tasks usually are presented in hierarchical fashion. For example, the patient may begin by arranging blocks in a row to replicate a model constructed by the clinician. Then the patient may be required to arrange blocks in several rows with different numbers in each row based on the clinician's model. Finally the patient may be required to reproduce complex three-dimensional constructions (Figure 9-18). More naturalistic tasks that require visuospatial processing such as interpreting maps, floor plans, and flowcharts also can be incorporated into treatment of visuospatial impairments.

Memory Impairments Memory impairments are a common and stubborn consequence of traumatic brain injury, often persisting for years despite intensive treatment. The pervasiveness of memory impairments following traumatic brain injury and their resistance to treatment have challenged patients, clinicians, and scientists for decades. In response to that challenge, clinicians and scientists have developed numerous programs for improving traumatically-brain-injured adults' memory.

Most of the early programs attempted to *restore* memory by means of what Sohlberg and

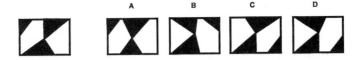

Figure 9-17 ■ A visual-rotation test item. The test-taker chooses from patterns *A* through *D* the one that represents a rotated version of the pattern on the left.

Mateer (1989) call the *muscle building* approach to memory rehabilitation. Memory restoration (muscle building) programs entail repetitive drills to strengthen and revitalize memory. These drills typically require patients to memorize and recall lists of numbers or words or to read printed texts or listen to spoken narratives and later retell them or answer questions about them.

As personal computers became more common and less expensive, computer-based memory retraining programs were marketed to clinics and individuals. These programs resembled their noncomputerized ancestors in that they focused on drills in which patients practiced remembering letters, numbers, words, pictures, shapes, and stories. They differed from their predecessors in that they controlled stimulus presentation rate and exposure time with great consistency and accuracy, they kept precise records of correct and error responses and of how long it took a patient to respond to each stimulus, and they did not require the presence of a clinician throughout the treatment session. These advantages contributed to a proliferation of computerized memory rehabilitation programs and their incorporation into the activities of clinics throughout the United States and in many other countries.

It gradually became apparent that the payoff of these computerized programs was considerably less than their promise. Articles began to appear in the literature asserting that stimulation approaches to memory rehabilitation in general, and computerized stimulation programs in particular, are of little value for creating meaningful changes in traumatically-brain-injured adults' daily life memory performance (Brooks, 1984; Gloag, 1985;

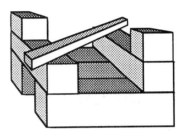

Figure 9-18 ■ A complex block-construction test item. The test-taker constructs from a set of blocks a duplicate of a model constructed by the examiner.

Godfrey & Knight, 1985; Hart & Hayden, 1986; Kreutzer & Wehman, 1991; Prigitano & associates, 1984; Robertson, 1990; Schacter, Rich, & Stampp, 1985; and others). As a consequence, stimulation treatment to restore traumatically-brain-injured adults' memory has been largely abandoned in favor of compensatory approaches. However, there are indications that treating attentional impairments may indirectly facilitate memory (Sohlberg & Mateer, 1989).

Reasoning and Problem-Solving Reasoning and problem-solving are involved in almost any treatment activity that a clinician might carry out with traumatically-brain-injured adults. Nevertheless, clinicians often focus treatment specifically on reasoning and problem-solving, either with paper-and-pencil workbook-like exercises or with on-line coaching and training in simulated or (less often) actual daily life problem-solving situations.

Many workbooks and paper-and-pencil programs for treating reasoning and problem-solving have been published. There is no strong evidence that doing such paper-and-pencil activities has any significant effects on patients' ability to reason and solve problems in daily life. Nevertheless, many clinicians incorporate them into their treatment, usually as homework. Because such exercises may do at least some patients some good and are unlikely to cause harm their use in treatment programs seems appropriate, provided clinicians ensure that improved performance on the paper-and-pencil exercises also leads to improved reasoning and problem-solving in daily life activities and provided that the paper-and-pencil exercises do not take the place of other activities with documented effectiveness.

Training in daily life problem-solving typically entails practice, coaching, and role-playing in simulated daily life situations. Patients with substantial impairments practice reasoning and problem-solving in simple, highly structured activities such as planning a meal, planning a trip to a shopping center on public transportation, or balancing a checking account. Patients with less severe impairments practice with less structured and more complex activities such as planning a vacation, role-playing the return of a defective item to a store for a refund, or role-playing an employment interview. (Chapter 8 has more information on treatment of reasoning and problem-solving.)

Language and Communication As noted earlier, except for dysarthria, most traumatically-brain-injured patients' language and communication impairments are attributable to underlying impairments in basic cognitive processes such as attention, memory, reasoning, abstract thinking, and problem-solving.

Attentional impairments can contribute to:
- Poor comprehension of spoken and written verbal materials, especially when they are long or complex
- Missing the details in spoken and written material
- Fragmented, disjointed, noncoherent spoken discourse
- Failure to observe turn-taking rules and conventions and weak or inappropriate topic maintenance

- Failure to appreciate and respond appropriately to social cues in conversational interactions
  Memory impairments can contribute to:
- Tangentiality, irrelevance, and failure to stay on topic in conversations and writing
- Excessive repetition and redundancy in spoken and written language
- Inability to keep goals, objectives, and strategies for improving communication in mind
  Impairments in reasoning and abstract thinking can contribute to:
- Concrete language and inability to appreciate inferences and indirectly stated material
- Inability to appreciate relationships in spoken or written discourse
- Egocentrism in social interactions and inability to appreciate others' points of view
  Impairments in problem-solving can contribute to:
- Failure to implement prescribed strategies to enhance communicative effectiveness
- Inappropriate conversational content and maladaptive interpersonal behaviors

These secondary effects of cognitive impairments on communication are most effectively and efficiently treated by treating the underlying cognitive impairments. However, many patients can benefit from direct treatment of communication impairments concurrently with work on the underlying impairments. Direct treatment of communication impairments for traumatically-brain-injured patients most often targets the social and interpersonal (pragmatic) aspects of communication. The general objective is to increase the appropriateness, relevance, and efficiency of the traumatically-brain-injured patient's participation in conversational interactions, to enhance the patient's ability to follow shifts in topic, and to improve the patient's appreciation of nonliteral aspects of communication.

Traumatically-brain-injured patients and patients with right-hemisphere brain damage often exhibit similar impairments in communicative interactions. Both tend to be impulsive and egocentric in interpersonal interactions; to miss nonliteral and implied meanings; to make faulty assumptions based on first impressions; and to be tangential, verbose, circumlocutory, and inappropriate in what they say. Consequently, treatment for traumatically-brain-injured patients' impairments in communicative interactions often resembles that for patients with right-hemisphere brain damage (discussed in Chapter 8).

Compensatory Training

When component treatment leaves a patient with residual impairments that interfere with daily life activities, the focus of treatment shifts to teaching the patient compensatory strategies by which the patient can circumvent the impairments. These compensatory strategies are deliberate, volitional (and sometimes unconventional) behaviors that allow a patient to carry on activities that would otherwise be impossible. For example, a traumatically-brain-injured college student who cannot take notes fast enough to keep up with lectures may be trained to record the lectures, write down only major points while the lecture is going on, and later use the tape recording to fill in the details.

Ylvisaker and Holland (1985) cite four principles of compensatory training:

1. Select strategies that fit the patient's strengths and weaknesses.
2. Train the patient in the use of efficient and effective strategies.
3. Help the patient control or eliminate inefficient, maladaptive, or escapist strategies.
4. Guide the patient through practice with the strategies until they become automatic, thereby limiting demands on attention, memory, and other cognitive processes.

Not every traumatically-brain-injured patient can learn compensatory strategies, and many who can learn them cannot apply them outside the environment in which they were learned. According to Ylvisaker and Holland, the success of compensatory strategy training depends partly on the patient and partly on the strategy. The patient must recognize the existence of impairments that cannot be alleviated by restitution of underlying processes; must be capable of recognizing problems as they occur or, better yet, anticipate problems before they occur; and must be capable of invoking a strategy based on recognition of a present or potential problem situation. The strategy must be fitted to the patient's needs, personality, and abilities. It must fulfill an obvious and apparent need that is personally felt by the patient. (Teaching a patient a strategy for remembering information from printed texts will be of little use for a patient who is uninterested in reading.) It must fit the personal inclinations and attitudes of the patient. (Teaching a shy and reclusive patient strategies that require assertiveness and social poise is unlikely to lead to the patient's use of the strategy in daily life.) It must be easy enough that the patient can eventually invoke it automatically and effortlessly. (Strategies that require substantial mental effort from the patient are unlikely to be used outside the environment in which they are learned.)

Barco and associates (1991) addressed the problem of matching compensatory strategies to the ability of the patient by dividing compensatory strategies into four categories, each of which is appropriate for patients at a given level of ability.

External compensations are appropriate for patients who are oriented and responsive but unaware of their impairments and do not recognize when their impairments cause problems. External compensations are changes in the environment initiated by an agent other than the patient. External compensation appears to be synonymous with *environmental control.*

Situational compensations are appropriate for patients who are aware of their impairments but do not recognize problems as they occur. These patients are taught compensatory strategies to be used habitually in all situations in which they might be appropriate. The patient routinely invokes the strategy whenever entering the situation and continues it throughout the situation whether or not problems targeted by the strategy occur. For example, a patient who occasionally misses some of the steps in a daily life procedure routinely may use a checklist whenever performing that procedure.

Recognition compensations are appropriate for patients who can recognize problems when they occur but do not anticipate them. These patients are trained to invoke a strategy when they perceive that a problem of a given nature is occurring. For example, a patient may be trained to begin writing down key points whenever they find themselves becoming confused when reading printed materials. Situational and recognition compensations may be identical in content. The difference is that situational compensations are invoked routinely within a specified context, whereas recognition compensations are invoked only when the patient gets into difficulty.

Anticipatory compensations are appropriate for patients who can anticipate problems before they occur. These patients are taught to invoke a strategy at the first signs of an impending problem, thereby avoiding the problem. Anticipatory compensations are flexible and effective but require relatively high levels of awareness and problem-solving ability. Consequently, they are beyond the reach of many traumatically-brain-injured patients.

The following short list gives examples of some compensatory strategies that may be useful for traumatically-brain-injured patients, if the strategies are appropriately matched to the patients.

- Keeping a daily log or journal in which the patient (or those around the patient) record daily life happenings, to help orientation
- Posting photographs of people who are significant participants in the patient's daily life activities, with printed names attached, to help the patient's orientation to person
- Using printed maps or diagrams showing routes to and from familiar destinations to help patients who get lost easily
- Using checklists that show the steps of commonly performed daily life activities and procedures
- Posting symbols or printed reminders in prominent places as cues to perform certain activities
- Writing down important information and covertly or overtly rehearsing it to facilitate memory
- Developing and using standard routines for organizing thinking and problem-solving

(e.g., ordering elements from first to last, most important to least important, or best known to least known)
- Mentally rehearsing problem situations and using visual imagery and written plans to organize responses to problem situations
- Organizing the workspace and materials, with tools and materials used together grouped together, and arranged in the order in which they are used
- Eliminating distractions from the workspace
- Asking for repetition or clarification when confused or uncertain about others' instructions, plans, or wishes
- Asking others to write down important information and instructions and asking others to speak slowly or to repeat key points
- Requesting extra time for performing tasks or taking tests

Helping traumatically-brain-injured patients compensate for memory impairments is a major focus of treatment for most patients. Compensatory strategies with which traumatically-brain-injured adults can circumvent problems generated by impaired memory can be divided into two general categories—those entailing the use of *internal strategies* and those entailing the use of *external aids* (Sohlberg & Mateer, 1989).

Approaches that teach patients to make use of *internal strategies* depend primarily on mnemonic devices or imagery and are best-suited for facilitating *retrospective memory*. Most mnemonic devices are verbal. In *verbal chaining strategies* patients are taught to arrange lists of to-be-remembered items into sentences or short stories to facilitate subsequent recall of the items. For example, a patient who has to remember the words *dog, book, rain,* and *bus* might mentally put them into a sentence such as "The dog chewed up the book and ran under the bus to get out of the rain." In *first-letter mnemonic strategies* patients are taught to associate the first letters of words to be remembered with words that can be arranged into easy-to-remember sayings, phrases, or rhymes. (The mnemonic for remembering the names of the cranial nerves is an example of a first-letter mnemonic strategy.)

Sometimes patients may be trained to create a mental image that organizes the words in a to-be-remembered list into a visual scene (e.g., a dog lying beside a bus in the rain and chewing on a book) or puts to-be-remembered items in a certain location within an imagined scene. When it comes time to retrieve the item from memory, the patient mentally "looks" for it in the imagined scene.

Giles and Clark-Wilson (1993) described a method for helping traumatically-brain-injured adults encode, store, and retrieve information from printed materials. They called the method the *PQRST* method (for *preview, question, read, state, test*). First the patient skims the material to learn its general content *(preview)*. Then the patient makes up questions about the central features of the material *(question)*. Then the patient actively reads the material with emphasis on answering the questions *(read)*. Then the patient repeats and rehearses the information from the printed material *(state)*. Finally, the patient evaluates the information to ensure that the questions were satisfactorily answered *(test)*.

Some studies have shown that training traumatically-brain-injured adults to use such internal strategies improves their performance on tests of recall (Cermak, 1975; Wilson, 1981; and others), but others have shown that the beneficial effects of training decay rapidly over time and do not generalize to natural situations (Glisky & Schacter, 1986; Lewinsohn, Danaher, & Kikel, 1977; Schacter & Glisky, 1986; and others). Sohlberg and Mateer (1989) point out that most traumatically-brain-injured patients do not have sufficient cognitive resources to carry out such internal strategies successfully:

> The utility of internal memory aids for this population should be suspect. These techniques place heavy demands on patients' already deficient cognitive systems; they are thus ineffectual for many persons with significantly compromised intellectual functions. (p. 153)

Parente and DiCesare (1991) also have pointed out that the practical application of internal mnemonic strategies is likely to be limited by traumatically-brain-injured patients' general impairments in attention, planning, and encoding, all of which are necessary for successful use of mnemonic strategies. However, step-by-step strategies such as *PQRST* may be used successfully by some higher-level traumatically-brain-injured adults provided that they write down the results of each step in the strategy before moving on to the next step.

External memory aids usually prove more practical for traumatically-brain-damaged adults than internal strategies. External memory aids provide cues and reminders that allow traumatically-brain-injured patients to compensate for their problems in remembering. External memory aids are well-suited for improving *prospective memory*—remembering to do things at some point in time. External memory aids span a range of sophistication from handwritten notes, calendars, and checklists to electronic organizers that permit the patient to organize, store, and retrieve complex information. External memory aids also include modifications to a patient's environment to facilitate prospective memory.

The simplest, cheapest, and easiest-to-use prospective memory aids are calendars, schedules, checklists, and memory notebooks. Carrying a pocket calendar or printed schedule in which appointments and important events are listed may be sufficient for some high-level traumatically-brain-injured patients who can remember to carry the calendar or schedule and look at it. However, many traumatically-brain-injured patients cannot remember to check the calendar or schedule often enough to prevent missing appointments or other important events. Checklists are helpful for patients who cannot keep track of which tasks they have accomplished and which remain undone, but checklists, like calendars, are of little value if the patient cannot remember to check the checklist. The solution for many of these patients is a signaling device (e.g., an alarm watch) that can be set to sound an alarm at preset times to remind them to check their calendar, schedule, or checklist.

Another solution for patients who cannot manage portable memory devices is *environ-*

mental modification, in which memory props are posted in conspicuous locations in the patient's living environment. For these patients, reminder notes may be posted on mirrors and in other conspicuous places, and large-print schedules of appointments and activities and check-off sheets to permit the patient to keep track of completed and pending tasks may be posted in strategic locations. Cupboards, shelves, and drawers may be labeled according to their contents, and closets and cupboards may be arranged systematically (e.g., items that are used together may be placed adjacent to each other, or items may be arranged alphabetically or by color).

Electronic memory devices may be appropriate for some higher-level traumatically-brain-injured adults. Electronic organizers (pocket-sized electronic devices for storing and retrieving information) and computer-based personal information managers are more expensive and not as easy to use as calendars, schedules, and checklists, but they provide more power and greater flexibility in storing names, addresses, phone numbers, appointments, and other personal information and are more versatile in sounding alarms and displaying reminders at times programmed into the device. Some of these devices also permit users to print a paper copy of appointment lists or calendars, which may be kept in a notebook. Programming these devices requires sustained attention, reasoning ability, and problem-solving skills, which means that programming will not be feasible for many traumatically-brain-injured patients. However, many who cannot program the devices can use them successfully in daily life, provided someone in the patient's life is available to do the programming.

Environmental Compensation

Another way to help traumatically-brain-injured adults compensate for residual impairments is to restructure the patient's daily life environment to minimize the effects of the impairments on the patient, family members, and associates. Such restructuring may require physical modifications to the patient's home, school, or work environment to facilitate access and ease of movement (e.g., installation of ramps and modifications of living spaces to accommodate a patient in a wheelchair). Such physical modifications usually are the province of physical and occupational therapists.

Environmental modifications may entail educating family members, teachers, supervisors, and others who associate with the patient to promote constructive attitudes and to minimize unrealistic expectations. Such education is especially important for families and associates of traumatically-brain-injured patients with residual cognitive impairments but few or no major physical impairments who talk and behave much as they did before their injury. Because these patients appear so normal, family members, friends, teachers, and supervisors often expect the patient to perform as they did before their injury. When the patient does not meet their expectations, these individuals may become irritated or angry and conclude that the patient is uncooperative, unmotivated, stubborn, or acting out hostility and anger. In such situations, environmental modification may entail education of family members about why the patient behaves as he or she does, teaching family members appropriate strategies for interacting with the patient, and helping the patient and family organize the patient's daily life environment to maximize successful interactions and minimize unsuccessful ones.

Environmental modifications might include:
- Establishing consistent routines and regular schedules for daily life activities.
- Instructing family members, friends, and associates in how best to facilitate the patient's success in daily life activities.
- Limiting or eliminating distractions by keeping radios and televisions turned down and closing doors and windows to reduce noise from outside or from other rooms.
- Keeping the patient's possessions in designated places and putting them away when they are not being used.

- Organizing the patient's workspace and scheduling work at difficult tasks for times at which the patient is rested and alert.
- Setting time limits (using alarms, timers) for working at difficult tasks to avoid fatigue and minimize mistakes.

Environmental compensation for higher-level traumatically-brain-injured patients resembles *environmental control* for confused and agitated patients. The primary difference is one of intent. The intent of environmental control, as the label implies, is to bring the patient's agitated, confused, and maladaptive behaviors under control. The patient does not plan, initiate, or use environmental control procedures in a purposeful way. The patient's behavior is controlled by the environment, rather than the other way around. The intent of environmental compensation is to provide strategies, prompts, or cues to enhance patients' performance in certain contexts or in certain cognitive or linguistic domains. The patient typically participates in planning the compensations, is actively trained in their use, and uses them in a purposeful and goal-directed way.

GENERAL CONCEPTS 9-5

- Most early treatment programs for adults with traumatic brain injuries relied on *drill activities* designed to stimulate and enhance mental processes. When it became obvious that stimulation programs were not effective, other approaches took center stage. Current treatment programs usually combine elements of *functionally oriented treatment, cognitive rehabilitation,* and *behavior therapy.*
- *Sensory stimulation* is a common form of treatment for comatose or semi-comatose patients, although there currently is no empiric verification of its effectiveness.
- *Environmental control* is an important part of treatment for confused and agitated patients, whose confusion and agitation may be reduced by making their environment stable, secure, and predictable.
- *Behavior management* techniques may control problem behaviors and enhance desired

behaviors by manipulating antecedent stimuli and response contingencies.
- *Medications* may be prescribed for traumatically-brain-injured patients to control agitation and restlessness, improve alertness and attention, manage depression, diminish psychotic symptoms, or control seizures. Dosages and effects must be monitored carefully to ensure that the medications do not adversely affect the patient.
- *Orientation training* may be appropriate for patients who are confused but who can attend to orientation training procedures and remember orientation information for more than a few minutes. Orientation training may include environmental prompts (e.g., signs, calendars), overt reminders by caregivers and patient-care personnel, passive orientation drills, or active orientation training.
- *Component training,* in which individual cognitive processes are treated with repetitive drill activities, may be appropriate for traumatically-brain-injured patients with reasonably good attention and memory. Treatment of attentional impairments occupies a prominent place in component training. Visual processing, reasoning, and problem-solving also may be addressed by component training.
- *Memory improvement programs* for adults with traumatic brain injury generally have failed to generate meaningful improvements in memory beyond the treatment programs themselves. Consequently, memory drills have largely been abandoned in favor of compensatory approaches to memory impairments.
- *Compensatory training* is appropriate when component treatment does not rectify impairments that interfere with a traumatically-brain-damaged individual's daily life competence.
- *External compensations* are changes in the environment initiated by an agent other than the patient. They are appropriate for patients who are oriented and responsive but unaware of their impairments.

- *Situational compensations* are appropriate for patients who are aware of their impairments but do not recognize problems as they occur. These patients are taught to use compensatory strategies habitually in certain situations.
- *Recognition compensations* are appropriate for patients who can recognize problems when they occur but do not anticipate them. These patients are trained to invoke a strategy when they perceive that a problem of a given nature is occurring.
- *Anticipatory compensations* are appropriate for patients who can anticipate problems before they occur. These patients are taught to invoke a strategy at the first signs of an impending problem.
- Compensatory techniques for memory impairment can be divided into *internal strategies* (e.g., mnemonic devices, imagery) or *external aids* (e.g., checklists, calendars, electronic organizers). Internal strategies best compensate for impaired retrospective memory. External aids are more practical for traumatically-brain-injured adults than internal strategies (which require substantial cognitive resources). External aids best compensate for impaired prospective memory.
- Modifying a traumatically-brain-injured individual's daily life environment may help to minimize the effects of the individual's impairments on their daily life competence.

Group Treatment

Group treatment usually is an integral part of the overall treatment plan for patients with traumatic brain injuries who can participate in group activities without disrupting them. (This usually means patients at *Rancho Los Amigos Scale* level 5 and above.) Group treatment provides a number of benefits, not all of which are related to improvements in cognitive and behavioral adequacy. Some of these auxiliary benefits include helping patients overcome feelings of isolation and loneliness, increasing patients' self-confidence and sense of self-esteem, and helping patients express and deal with negative feelings such as anger and hostility.

Groups for traumatically-brain-injured patients may serve several purposes, either separately or in combination. The most common purposes are *support, self-assessment, communication, cognitive rehabilitation, generalization,* and *education*. Less common purposes are *sensory stimulation* and *orientation*.

Sensory Stimulation Sensory stimulation of groups of patients with traumatic brain injuries is controversial, owing in large part to the questionable efficacy of sensory stimulation for individual patients. Sensory stimulation groups usually are made up of patients who are confused but not extremely agitated. Group sessions typically are short (30 minutes or less) and include a mix of orientation activities and sensory stimulation. Orientation activities may include activities in which the group leader and support staff:

- Greet each patient by name and announce to the group each patient's name and an item or two of interest about each patient.
- Announce the date, day of week, and time of day (often supported by visual aids such as a large clock and calendar).
- Give the name of the treatment facility, its location, and purpose.
- Describe the current weather and give the weather forecast.

Group stimulation may be provided with recorded music, recordings of radio or television programs or sporting events, movies, slide shows, or other auditory or visual materials. Group stimulation activities sometimes are supplemented with tactile, taste, or movement stimulation of individual patients.

Orientation Group orientation activities are most appropriate for patients at Rancho Los Amigos Scale levels 5 and 6. Group orientation activities are similar to those for patients in sensory stimulation groups, except that patients actively participate by acknowledging and repeating the information provided by the group leader and support staff. Some basic interactional skills, such as acknowledging and taking turns, also may receive attention.

Support Group support activities are most appropriate for patients at Rancho Los Amigos Scale level 6 and higher. Participation in support activities with other traumatically-brain-injured patients may help individual patients dispel feelings of isolation, loneliness, and having been unfairly singled out by fate. Observing other group members who are coping with their impairments and progressing may help motivate individual patients and provide them with hope for the future. Support from other group members may help individual patients deal with failure and overcome disappointments, and by providing a forum for expression of feelings, group activities may help individual patients express and deal with feelings of anger, rage, hostility, and frustration.

Self-Assessment Group self-assessment activities are most appropriate for patients at Rancho Los Amigos Scale levels 7 and 8, although some level 6 patients may profitably participate. Participation in self-assessment activities may help traumatically-brain-injured patients develop a more realistic sense of their abilities and disabilities. Group experiences may serve this function both for patients who minimize or deny their impairments and who have unrealistic expectations and for patients who exaggerate their impairments and minimize or ignore their remaining strengths. (One-on-one treatment, with its highly structured format and the presence of a supportive and helpful clinician, sometimes gives patients an unduly optimistic impression of their potential success in daily life interactions.) Group experiences also may provide opportunities for individual patients to observe and evaluate others' successful and unsuccessful performance as a prelude to evaluating their own performance. (Traumatically-brain-injured patients, like those with right-hemisphere brain injuries, usually are better at evaluating others' behavior than they are at evaluating their own behavior.)

Communication Group communication activities are most appropriate for patients at Rancho

Los Amigos Scale levels 6, 7, and 8. Group communication activities may provide traumatically-brain-injured patients with a sheltered but realistic context in which to work on interpersonal interactions. Group members may practice conversational and pragmatic skills such as turn-taking; topic maintenance; requesting, asserting, and clarifying; repairing conversational breakdowns; and monitoring and responding to others' verbal and nonverbal communication. Feedback concerning appropriate and inappropriate behavior may come from group leaders or, more importantly, from other group members. Videotaped role-playing activities in which participants act out and discuss daily life problem situations are a common vehicle for providing participants with practice to develop communication and interactional skills. Group review and discussion of the videotapes provides the opportunity for group members to exchange opinions and ideas regarding appropriate and inappropriate behavior in communicative interactions.

Erlich and Sipes (1985) described a communication group format for traumatically-brain-injured adults in which group activities center around videotaped role plays. Target behaviors are specified by group leaders in advance of each role play. Group leaders make the first videotape, in which they act out a common problem situation to illustrate appropriate and inappropriate behaviors. Then the interactions are replicated by group members in a second videotaped role play. The videotaped role plays are reviewed and commented on by the group, with emphasis on behaviors that contribute to or interfere with communicative success. Group members are assigned personal goals in each interaction, and members' successes and failures relative to their goals are discussed by the group. Erlich and Sipes's group format addresses *nonverbal communication* (voice inflection, facial expression, eye contact, posture, and gesture), *communication in context* (topic initiation, topic maintenance, and responsiveness to social context), *message repair* (awareness of communication failure, appreciation of listener needs, and clarification strategies), and *cohesive-ness* (organization and sequencing of information, temporal and spatial integrity).

Sohlberg and Mateer (1989) describe several group activities for working on traumatically-brain-injured patients' communication skills, including a collaborative drawing task in which group members are divided into pairs. One participant in each pair draws, out of sight of the other, three simple geometric shapes in two colors. Then the participant who drew the shapes tells the other how to reproduce the drawings without seeing them. When the second participant has finished, they compare drawings and discuss communication successes and failures. In another activity participants wear hats labeled with phrases such as "ignore me" or "talk down to me." (Group members cannot see what is printed on the hat they are wearing.) The group members discuss a topic and respond to each participant according to what is printed on their hat. After the discussion each member tries to guess what is printed on their hat, and the group talks about what happened and how they felt.

Cognitive Rehabilitation Group cognitive rehabilitation activities may address attention, memory, reasoning and problem-solving, and visual processing, either individually or in combination. Activities may resemble those used in one-to-one treatment activities, but group members may be divided into teams that compete with one another, collaborate on solving problems posed by the group leader, or take turns in game-like activities that call on the cognitive processes that are the focus of the day. Competition among teams to finish a task first or to finish a task with the highest accuracy often has a prominent place in cognitive rehabilitation group activities, both to motivate group members to participate and to keep levels of interest and attention high.

Generalization Generalization of skills, attitudes, strategies, and behaviors acquired in one-to-one treatment to less structured and more natural contexts is an objective of most group activities. Generalization is targeted by means of

group activities in which members may practice in controlled, structured, and supportive group situations strategies that they have learned in one-to-one treatment.

Education Instruction about the physical, cognitive, emotional, psychosocial, and vocational effects of brain injury sometimes is incorporated into group activities. Some instruction may be didactic, with group leaders providing group members with instruction and handouts. Videotapes or films about the effects of traumatic brain injury may be shown to and discussed by the group. Group exercises in which group members make lists of changes in their own lives caused by their brain injury, present the lists to the group, and discuss them with the group also may serve an educational purpose. Guest speakers, such as physicians, social workers, vocational counselors, or survivors of traumatic brain injury may talk to the group and lead subsequent group discussions.

Efficacy of Group Activities Just as there is no convincing empiric evidence for the efficacy of group treatment of aphasic or right-hemisphere damaged adults, there is no convincing empiric evidence for the efficacy of group treatment of adults with traumatic brain injuries, although numerous anecdotal reports have appeared in the literature. Deaton (1991) concludes her discussion of group interventions for traumatically-brain-injured adults as follows:

> At present, the most glaring gaps in the use of group interventions have to do not with the availability of various models and formats, but rather with the documentation of group effectiveness in improving cognitive skills in particular, as these skills generalize to other social environments. This remains the most significant issue needing to be addressed in future work in this area. (p. 199)

By far the most controversial purpose of group treatment is that of sensory stimulation. The appropriateness of sensory stimulation for groups of traumatically-brain-injured patients is questionable because, as noted earlier, there is no evidence that sensory stimulation of individual patients hastens their return to consciousness or accelerates their recovery of orientation to person, place, and time.

Group experiences for patients at Rancho Los Amigos Scale level 5 and below seem unlikely to provide unique benefits because these patients are at best only dimly aware of other group members and are unlikely to contribute to or benefit from a group experience. Proponents might argue that group stimulation, like individual patient stimulation, is unlikely to do harm and should be administered because it may do some good. Proponents also might argue that stimulation groups represent a cost savings over individual-patient stimulation. Whether the possible good merits the time and expense of professionals to provide the stimulation remains an important question, and one might argue that providing an ineffective treatment more cheaply is no bargain.

Although there is no convincing evidence for the efficacy of purely orientation groups, the fact that participants are actively responding to the group leaders and to other group members suggests that the group experience may enhance participants' orientation and help them get started on the road toward interpersonal adequacy. However, it is unlikely that patients who qualify for purely orientation groups receive much benefit from the group experience itself. Consequently, the primary advantage of putting them into a group for orientation may be cost savings. Whether orientation groups require professionals as leaders, however, seems questionable.

The widespread use of group activities to provide support, facilitate self-assessment, improve communication, enhance cognitive processing, promote generalization, and educate traumatically-brain-injured patients about the effects of brain injury—and the presence of numerous anecdotal reports of the positive effects of such group activities on traumatically-brain-injured patients' performance—provides some nonempiric support for their efficacy. At present, there is no compelling reason to reject group activities for traumatically-brain-injured adults, provided group members are appropriately selected (they must have adequate comprehension, expressive abilities, and intellectual function to participate, and they must be able to control disruptive behavior), there is at least some degree of homogeneity among group members, and activities and objectives are appropriately selected and matched to the group. However, as Deaton has noted, there is an immediate and pressing need for objective verification of the effectiveness of group treatment for traumatically-brain-injured adults.

COMMUNITY REENTRY

The final stage of rehabilitation for many traumatic-brain-injury patients is reentry into family, vocational, and community settings. Preparation for community reentry may take several months and usually takes place in residential facilities *(transitional living facilities),* where a group of traumatically-brain-injured patients lives around the clock. Patients in transitional living facilities spend their daytime hours in activities to prepare them for reentry into the community. Less often, preparation for community reentry is carried out in day treatment centers, where patients spend their daytime hours, returning home at the end of each workday.

Treatment objectives in reentry facilities differ across facilities and, of course, differ for different patients. However, most facilities offer programs directed toward the following objectives.

- Provide patients with a supportive context in which to practice and perfect strategies and procedures for increasing their daily life competence.
- Prepare patients for carrying out routine self-care activities (e.g., personal hygiene, eating, sleeping, grooming) in daily life.
- Develop patients' interest in domestic, vocational, leisure, and social activities, and develop the patient's ability to perform them.
- Establish routines for commonly occurring daily life domestic, vocational, leisure, and social activities, and train patients to perform them.

- Train patients to allocate appropriate amounts of time for daily activities and to use time constructively.
- Evaluate patients' competence for vocational, school, and leisure-time activities.
- Place patients in appropriate work, school, and leisure activities and work with employers, teachers, family, and others to ensure success.

These objectives are approached by means of one-to-one training sessions, group activities, and structured experiences in real-life situations. Patients typically spend part of the day working on specific behavioral strategies for increasing daily life competence and part of the day in group activities wherein they practice daily living skills, discuss problems and their potential solutions, and provide each other with social and emotional support. Sometimes patients spend time in real-life or simulated vocational, school, or social settings in which they may practice strategies that may be needed for success in work, school, or social endeavors. Family members, employers, and other individuals who may play important parts in a patient's daily life also may participate.

Treatment activities within reentry facilities are carried out by teams made up of occupational therapists, recreational therapists, speech-language pathologists, vocational counselors, neuropsychologists, social workers, and other professionals. As the patient progresses, the team gradually withdraws structured treatment, training, and support and expects increasing independence on the part of the patient. Discharge from the facility and return to home, family, work, or school mark the end of formal rehabilitation for most patients, although periodic counseling visits may continue for some.

WORKING WITH THE FAMILY

Providing support, reassurance, information, and direction to family members is an important part of the clinical management of patients with traumatic brain injuries. The family's need for support, reassurance, and information is greatest in the acute post-injury interval, and their need

for direction is greatest in the middle and later stages of recovery. Polinko (1985) has divided the time following traumatic brain injury into three stages: *injury to stabilization, return to consciousness,* and *rehabilitation.*

For the family the first stage *(injury to stabilization),* when the patient remains unconscious, is a period of apprehensive waiting. The patient is in the care of strangers and is surrounded by an alarming array of monitors and support systems. The family may have been told that the patient may not recover. They anxiously watch for the first signs of consciousness and often misinterpret the patient's purposeless activity as purposeful behavior. According to Polinko, this is a time of shock and denial, with occasional breakthroughs of panic, and family members need extensive support and reassurance. During this time, family members also need objective information about what has happened and what the outcome is likely to be, but they may have difficulty assimilating it because of their emotional upset. Consequently, information may have to be reiterated a number of times. As time goes on, denial may be replaced by bargaining, in which family members attempt to strike a deal with a deity or with fate by promising acceptance of the patient's condition, acts of contrition, changes in attitudes, or changes in behavior if only the patient survives.

The second stage *(return to consciousness)* usually brings feelings of relief that the patient will live, together with apprehension about the extent to which the patient will recover. Family members continue to watch anxiously for hopeful signs and may continue to interpret incidental patient behaviors as signs of recovery. Because the patient's emergence from coma often occurs rapidly, family members may be led into overly optimistic predictions about the patient's eventual recovery. Educating family members about the usual course of recovery from traumatic brain injury and helping them separate true prognostic indicators from fallacious ones is an important part of the clinician's responsibility during this stage.

By the time the third stage *(rehabilitation)* is reached, most families have accommodated to the accident and its aftermath and have moved past the stage of denial to reasonably realistic expectations about the future. The beginning of structured treatment activities usually is a time of increased hope and optimism for family members, often leading to optimistic expectations of what will be accomplished in treatment. This time of hope and optimism often gives way to anxiety, confusion, and eventually anger with the patient and with professional staff, as the patient's recovery fails to meet expectations. The unpredictable nature of recovery from traumatic brain injury adds to the family's confusion and sometimes to their anger. When periods of rapid recovery alternate with periods of little change, family members may accuse the patient of slacking off or accuse clinicians of not doing their job. When it becomes apparent that the patient will not recover to premorbid levels, the family will need help in planning how they will cope with a future that includes an impaired family member.

As time goes on, families usually return to a semblance of normal functioning. Family members who once stayed with the patient during major parts of the day return to work, and the patient no longer is the central focus of family life. Responsibility for the patient may be divided among family members. One family member may assume primary responsibility for visiting the patient and interacting with caregivers, and another may take responsibility for dealing with financial and logistic adjustments. During this time the family may need the help of psychologists, social workers, rehabilitation therapists, speech-language pathologists, and community service agencies in setting up a long-term plan for incorporating the brain-injured patient into family life in a way that is maximally beneficial for the patient and the family. Throughout the course of the patient's recovery the family will need continuing and conscientious assistance from all members of the patient-care team to survive the mental, emotional, and physical consequences of the patient's injury.

GENERAL CONCEPTS 9-6

- *Group treatment* may help patients overcome feelings of isolation and loneliness, increase patients' self-confidence and sense of self-esteem, and help patients express and deal with negative feelings such as anger and hostility, provided the patients can attend and participate in group activities without disrupting them.

- Group treatment may provide *sensory stimulation* and promote *orientation* of more severely impaired patients with traumatic brain injuries. For higher-level patients, group activities may provide *psychologic support, promote realistic self-assessment and personal goals, provide communication practice* in a controlled environment, *enhance cognitive abilities* in game-like activities, *provide for generalization* of skills to group settings, or *provide instruction* about aspects of brain injury and its effects on individuals and families.

- There is no empiric evidence for the efficacy of group treatment for adults with traumatic brain injuries. Many anecdotal reports suggest that some group treatment activities may be beneficial for some traumatically-brain-injured individuals, but specification of the what, when, and who remains to be accomplished.

- *Reentry into family, vocational, and community settings* is the final stage of rehabilitation for many traumatic-brain-injury patients. Preparation for community reentry usually takes place in residential transitional living facilities. Treatment activities in transitional living facilities are carried out by teams of professionals.

- Providing support, reassurance, information, and direction to family members is an important part of the clinical management of patients with traumatic brain injuries. The family's needs for support, reassurance, information, and direction change as the traumatically-brain-injured family member recovers. Support and reassurance are important in the early stages of the brain-injured family member's recovery. The family's need for information and direction becomes greater as the patient's survival is ensured and issues of coping and management become salient.

THOUGHT QUESTIONS

Question 9-1 Mary Jones slips on the ice at her front door and hits her head on the concrete step. She does not lose consciousness but immediately gets up, goes into the house, and tells her husband what happened. Except for some swelling and a small laceration at the back of her head, she appears to be fine. She complains of a severe headache 30 minutes later. She takes two aspirin. She complains that she feels nauseous and still has the headache 45 minutes after taking the aspirin. She vomits and complains of a stiff neck 15 minutes thereafter. Speculate about the neurologic events that might explain Mary's symptoms.

Question 9-2 Jerry Smith is a 25-year-old man who was riding his motorcycle along a rural road at approximately 50 mph. As he approached a farm driveway, a pickup truck pulled out into his path. He braked and swerved to avoid the truck but lost control and was thrown from the motorcycle, which was at that time traveling about 30 mph. He was thrown forward, flipped upside down, and struck the door of the pickup with his upper back and the back of his head. He was wearing a motorcycle helmet.

What would you expect the location and nature of his head injuries to be? How would your answer change if he were not wearing a helmet?

Question 9-3 You receive a referral for a 23-year-old male who is 9 days post-traumatic brain injury from a motor-vehicle accident. He emerged from coma 2 days ago and is now at Rancho Los Amigos level 4. The referring neurologist wishes you to evaluate the patient and make recommendations. You have a 1-hour time interval in your schedule in which you can see this patient.

Summarize what you would plan to do in your initial contact with the patient. What are your preliminary thoughts regarding prognosis? What information contributes to them?

Question 9-4 You have been asked to evaluate Ronald, a 20-year-old man who is now 6 months post-traumatic brain injury received in a motor-vehicle accident. At the time of his injury he was a sophomore at a state university where he majored in environmental studies and received mostly grades of B and some grades of A. He was injured in his college town, which is in another state, and received his post-accident medical care and 6 weeks of rehabilitation in that city. Since his discharge from the rehabilitation facility he has been living locally at home with his parents. He wishes to return to college at the beginning of the next term, 3 months from now, and resume his studies. He feels that he is ready to return to school, but his parents insist on a professional opinion regarding his potential for success at school before they agree to pay for his college expenses. You have a report from the rehabilitation institute, which contains standardized achievement test scores obtained at the time of Ron's discharge from that facility:

Mathematics: Grade 12+

Spelling: Grade 10

General knowledge: Grade 12+

Reading comprehension—sentences: Grade 12+

Reading comprehension—paragraphs: Grade 9

The report also states that at discharge Ron was capable of living independently—he competently performed activities of daily life without supervision, organized his daily schedule, remembered and kept appointments, and interacted appropriately with those around him.

What additional information would you need to offer an opinion about Ron's potential success at school? How would you get the information you need? (Assume that Ron's parents are willing and able to pay for extensive testing, if needed, and that Ron has agreed to participate.)

10

Dementia

DEFINING DEMENTIA

Dementia is a common consequence of several degenerative central nervous system diseases, especially those that affect older adults. Dementia is characterized by diffuse impairment of memory, intellect, and cognition. Alterations in behavior and personality are common, and physical impairments such as movement disorders or sensory disturbances often accompany dementia. The most widely used definition of dementia is that of the *Diagnostic and Statistical Manual of Mental Disorders-IV* (DSM-IV; American Psychiatric Association, 1994). Individuals diagnosed as having dementia according to the DSM-IV definition must exhibit the following:

- Impaired short-term memory
- Impaired long-term memory
- Impairment in at least one of the following
  —Abstract thinking
  —Personality
  —Judgment
  —Constructional abilities
  —Language
  —Praxis
  —Visual recognition

> Albert and associates (1974) and Cummings and Benson (1984) have commented that the DSM-IV criteria for diagnosing dementia are insensitive to the intellectual impairments of patients with dementia caused by subcortical brain damage.

The patient's impairments must meet the following requirements:

- They must be insidious in onset.
- They must be not accounted for by delirium, schizophrenia, or major depression.
- They must be acquired (which distinguishes dementia from congenital conditions such as mental retardation).
- They must be persistent (which distinguishes dementia from transitory states such as delirium or confusion).
- They must cross several areas of mental function (which distinguishes dementia from focal impairments such as aphasia or psychiatric disturbances).
- They must be severe enough to interfere with work, social activities, and relationships with others.

Many of the early signs of dementia are exaggerated forms of the minor day-to-day lapses of normal adults.

Memory failure. Normal adults occasionally forget an appointment, miss a deadline, forget a neighbor's name, or forget a birthday or anniversary. Adults with dementia may not remember making an appointment, may forget that they have a deadline, may not recognize a neighbor, or may not have any idea whose birthday is July 12.

Disorientation. Normal adults occasionally forget what day of the week it is and occasionally get lost in unfamiliar places. Adults with dementia routinely may not know what day it is; may not know if it is morning, afternoon, or evening; and may get lost in their own neighborhood or even in their own home.

Lapses in judgment. Normal adults occasionally run a red light, dress inappropriately for the weather, or unintentionally violate social conventions. Adults with dementia may fail to notice red lights, wear a wool overcoat on a hot day, or address strangers on the street as close friends or relatives.

Difficulty performing activities of daily life. Normal adults occasionally get distracted and leave the casserole in the oven too long or forget to provide towels for overnight guests. Adults with dementia may forget that they made the casserole and not only forget the towels but forget that they have overnight guests.

Difficulty performing mentally challenging tasks. Many normal adults are challenged by having to balance a checkbook, program a VCR, or double a recipe. Adults with dementia may be unable to perform simple calculations, remember what a VCR is used for, or keep the steps in a recipe in order.

Misplacing things. Normal adults occasionally misplace regularly used articles such as purses, keys, and cordless telephones. Adults with dementia may put regularly used items in odd places, such as a purse in the refrigerator or the car keys in the cookie jar and later have no idea how they got there.

Apathy and loss of initiative. Normal adults sometimes get mentally worn down by work, social obligations, housecleaning, and other activities of daily life, but most recover their initiative as time passes. Adults with dementia may abandon, avoid, and withdraw from previously enjoyed activities and never return to them.

Changes in mood. Normal adults typically experience a range of emotions in response to life events. Adults with dementia may exhibit rapid changes in mood that occur for no apparent reason or for trivial reasons.

Dementia usually begins late in life, and its incidence increases rapidly with age. Approximately 2% of 65-year-olds are likely to be affected by dementia, whereas approximately 20% of 80-year-olds are likely to be so affected (Evans & associates, 1989; Katzman, 1976; Kokmen & associates, 1989). Alzheimer's disease accounts for more new cases of dementia than any other single cause (Figure 10-1).

Dementia is the most common single diagnosis for nursing-home residents. Estimates of its prevalence differ greatly because of differences in where samples are obtained, variable definitions of dementia, and differences in the ages of the patients studied. In the year 2000 the U.S. population contained about 37 million adults older than age 65. Because of declining birth rates and longer life expectancy, the proportion of elderly persons in the world population is increasing, and with it the incidence of age-related illnesses, including dementia.

According to Jorm, Korten, and Henderson (1987), the presence of dementia in the U.S. population doubles with every 5-year increment in age after age 65. Gao and associates (1998) suggest, however, that the number of new cases of dementia is not consistent across age groups—it declines in the oldest age groups. According to Gao and associates, the number of new cases of dementia triples from age 55 to age 64, doubles from age 65 to age 74, and increases by 1.5 times from age 75 to age 95 (Figure 10-2). Gao and associates suggest that the slowing incidence rates for the oldest age groups may be because individuals with demen-

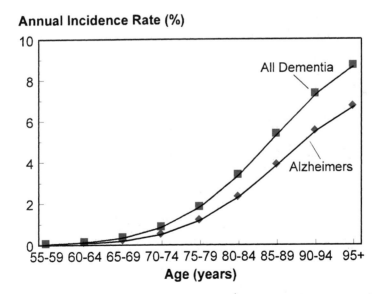

Figure 10-1 ■ **Yearly percentage incidence of dementia and Alzheimer's disease by 5-year age increments.** (Data from Gao, S., Hendrie, M. B., Hall, K. S., & Hui, S. (1998). The relationships between age, sex, and the incidence of dementia and Alzheimer disease. *Archives of General Psychiatry, 55,* 809-815.)

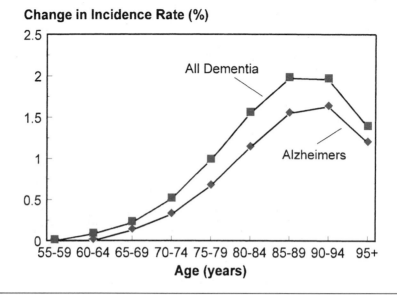

Figure 10-2 ■ **Change in yearly incidence of dementia and Alzheimer's disease as a function of age. (The slowing rate of incidence in the oldest age groups may represent the effects of attrition for patients who are susceptible to Alzheimer's disease, who may be less healthy and die earlier.)** (Data from Gao, S., Hendrie, M. B., Hall, K. S., & Hui, S. [1998]. The relationships between age, sex, and the incidence of dementia and Alzheimer disease. *Archives of General Psychiatry, 55,* 809-815.)

tia die earlier, leaving biologically stronger individuals (who presumably would be less likely to develop dementia) disproportionately well represented in the oldest age groups.

Dementia often occurs as the primary (or only) symptom of neurologic disease, as in *Alzheimer's disease* and *Pick's disease.* Vascular disease sometimes causes dementia, and dementia often appears in the late stages of extrapyramidal diseases such as *Huntington's disease* or *Parkinson's disease.* Depression, metabolic disorders, nutritional deficiencies, drug overdoses or drug side effects, infections (encephalitis, meningitis), and poisoning with toxic substances (mercury, lead, arsenic) also may lead to dementia. Some dementias (e.g., those caused by metabolic and nutritional disorders, drugs, infections, or toxins) are reversible, but most are irreversible and progressive.

Reversible dementia tends to occur in younger persons. Approximately 20% of dementias occurring in persons younger than age 65 are reversible, but only about 5% of dementias occurring in persons older than age 65 are reversible (Cummings & Benson, 1983).

Dementia syndromes can be divided into three major categories based on the location of pathologic changes in the central nervous system. *Cortical dementias* are caused by pathologic changes in the cerebral cortex. *Subcortical dementias* are caused by pathologic changes in the basal ganglia, thalamus, and brain stem. *Mixed dementias* are caused by pathologic changes in both cortical and subcortical struc-

Percent of Cases

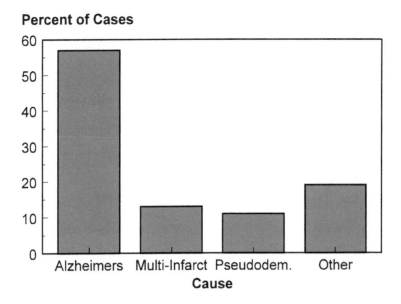

Figure 10-3 ■ Probable cause of dementia for patients referred for evaluation of dementia. Clarefield obtained these estimates by reviewing 32 published reports of diagnoses for patients referred for evaluation of dementia. *Pseudodem,* Pseudodementia (depression, reversible dementias); *Other,* Parkinson's disease, Huntington's disease, tumor, etc.). (Data from Clarefield, A. M. [1988]. The reversible dementia: do they reverse? *Annals of Internal Medicine, 109,* 472-478.)

tures. The most common causes of cortical dementia are *Alzheimer's disease* and *Pick's disease.* The most common causes of subcortical dementia are *Parkinson's disease* and *vascular disease.* The most frequent single cause of dementia is Alzheimer's disease (Figure 10-3).

SUBCORTICAL DEMENTIA

Impairments of cortical functions (memory, intellect, language) appear early in cortical dementia but not until the late stages of most subcortical degenerative diseases. Motor impairments typically are prominent in the early stages of subcortical dementia but are not common in early-stage cortical dementias. The first signs of dementia in patients with subcortical disease typically appear months to years after the appearance of the motor impairments symptomatic of the subcortical disease, presumably when pathologic changes have

progressed from subcortical structures to the brain cortex.

Parkinson's Disease

Parkinson's disease (also known as *paralysis agitans* or *primary parkinsonism*) is a degenerative disease affecting nuclei in the midbrain and brain stem. Parkinson's disease was first described in 1817 by James Parkinson, a British paleontologist and surgeon. Parkinson's disease sometimes is called *idiopathic parkinsonism* because the cause of the neural degeneration in Parkinson's disease is not known. Another variant, called *Parkinson-plus disease* or *multiple-system degeneration,* includes diseases in which the major symptoms of Parkinson's disease are accompanied by other symptoms of central nervous system pathology. Progressive supranuclear palsy, described later in this chapter, is an example of a Parkinson-plus disease.

> The term *idiopathic* means "of unknown cause." Diseases that resemble Parkinson's disease but whose causes are known are called secondary parkinsonism. Parkinsonism is a generic label for several diseases in which tremor, muscle rigidity, and slowness of movement are present.

The primary symptoms of Parkinson's disease are motoric and include muscle rigidity, tremor, slowness or abolition of movement, and loss of balance. Parkinson's disease affects about 1% of the U.S. adult population and is slightly more likely to affect men than women. Parkinson's disease usually becomes evident between the ages of 50 and 65 years.

Neuropathology Parkinson's disease is caused by deterioration of dopaminergic (dopamine-producing) neurons in the basal ganglia and the brain stem (especially a part of the basal ganglia called the *substantia nigra*). Dopamine is a neurotransmitter that inhibits neuronal activity and prevents unintended movements. When 60% or more of the dopamine-producing neurons in the brain are destroyed, the first symptoms of Parkinson's disease emerge. They include the following:

- Resting tremor ("pill rolling" tremor of the hands often is the first sign of tremor to appear)
- Muscle rigidity (patients may complain of unusual stiffness and difficulty moving)
- Slowness of movement and difficulty initiating movement *(bradykinesia)*
- Postural instability (impaired balance)

Although the causes of the neuronal degeneration in Parkinson's disease are not known, the causes of some kinds of secondary parkinsonism are known. An influenza epidemic in 1918 and 1919 was followed by development of parkinsonism in some survivors. Some cases of secondary parkinsonism have been attributed to poisoning with heavy metals (manganese, lead, mercury) or poisoning with aluminum, carbon monoxide, or cyanide. Recently a form of parkinsonism has developed in individuals who have used heroin contaminated with a neurotoxin called MPTP. Repeated minor head trauma such as that incurred by boxers can cause a Parkinson's-like condition called *pugilistic parkinsonism.*

Medical Management The primary treatment for Parkinson's disease is administration of *levodopa (L-dopa),* a chemical precursor to dopamine, which the body converts to dopamine. Treatment with levodopa or similar medications suppresses tremor and slows mental deterioration for about two thirds of patients with Parkinson's disease. Other medications, such as deprenyl (which slows the breakdown of dopamine in the body) and bromocriptine (which mimics the effects of dopamine) sometimes are used to control the symptoms of parkinsonism. Many patients eventually reach the point at which their disease progresses despite medications, at which time their mental functions also deteriorate.

Two relatively new surgical procedures sometimes may help patients whose symptoms cannot be controlled with medications. In *pallidotomy* tissue in the basal ganglia (the globus pallidus—hence the name pallidotomy) is surgically destroyed to relieve tremor and rigidity. *Fetal tissue transplant* is a controversial experimental technique in which dopamine-producing tissues from human fetuses are transplanted into the brains of patients with parkinsonism to replace lost dopaminergic neurons.

Evolution Parkinson's disease is characterized by slowly progressive deterioration of motor and mental functions. The usual first symptom of Parkinson's disease is tremor, but sometimes immobility and "poverty of movement" (Adams & Victor, 1981) appear before tremor develops. As Parkinson's disease progresses, memory, problem-solving, abstract reasoning, and other mental functions requiring sustained mental effort become increasingly compromised. Affect becomes progressively flattened, and many patients become depressed. Significant dementia develops in 15% to 20% of patients with Parkinson's disease (Levin, Tomer, & Rey, 1992), and up to 50% develop some signs of dementia (Duffy, 1995).

Speech and Language Patients with Parkinson's disease often first complain that their voice has become weak and that others cannot hear them in noisy environments. As Parkinson's disease progresses, patients' speech becomes rapid and phonetic distinctions diminish or disappear. Rapid, stuttering-like repetitions of syllables, words, and phrases may appear. Micrographia (extremely small writing) is common in the early stages of Parkinson's disease. Vocabulary, syntax, and grammar usually are preserved until the very late stages of the disease. Drooling and swallowing difficulties may appear in the middle stages of Parkinson's disease. In the late stages of Parkinson's disease comprehension of complex verbal materials may begin to deteriorate and the patient may have difficulty in tasks requiring sustained attention and mental effort. Although some patients with Parkinson's disease become profoundly demented by the very late stages of their disease, most retain sufficient intellect to function adequately in familiar environments with caregiver supervision. Most patients with Parkinson's disease die within 15 to 20 years of the onset of their disease.

Huntington's Disease

Huntington's disease is an inherited degenerative neurologic disorder first described in print (in 1872) by George Huntington, an American general practitioner. The disease soon became known as *Huntington's chorea* to highlight the movement disorder that is the primary sign of the disease. Because there are several other signs of the disease, and because chorea is not always present, the label *Huntington's disease* has become the preferred label for this disease. The genetic abnormality responsible for Huntington's disease apparently originated in Britain, and seventeenth-century British immigrants probably carried the abnormality to many parts of the world, including the United States and Canada. Diagnostic markers for Huntington's disease *(the HD triad)* include *chorea, cognitive decline,* and *neurobehavioral symptoms* (e.g., personality changes, agitation, depression, paranoia, delusions). In the United States, Huntington's disease affects about 1 person in 20,000.

> Huntington was never on a medical faculty and apparently never published another article, but his name is well known because of his accurate description of the disease that bears his name.

Neuropathology Huntington's disease is characterized neuropathologically by loss of neurons and shrinkage of the caudate nucleus and putamen in the basal ganglia together with patchy loss of neurons in the frontal and temporal regions of the brain cortex, with occasional extension of neuron loss to the cerebellum.

Medical Management There is no cure for Huntington's disease. Medical intervention for patients with Huntington's disease is most effective in treating the movement disorder and the emotional and psychologic consequences of the disease. Antidepressants may be prescribed for depression; antipsychotics for delusions, hallucinations, or paranoia; and anxiolytics for anxiety and agitation. Antipsychotic medications may diminish the severity of chorea, at least in the early stages of Huntington's disease, but they may exacerbate depression or agitation and may cause parkinsonian symptoms to appear.

Evolution Huntington's disease usually appears between age 40 and age 60, but the symptoms of about 10% of patients begin before 20 years of age. Huntington's disease progresses inexorably, and most patients die within 15 to 20 years after onset. The juvenile-onset form of the disease usually progresses more rapidly, with death occurring 5 to 10 years after onset.

The first symptoms usually are involuntary movements (chorea). The first choreic movements are undramatic and may be attributed to simple nervousness. The patient appears clumsy, restless, and fidgety. As time passes, the choreic movements become more obvious and personality changes develop.

> Patients begin to find fault and complain about everything and to nag other members of the family; they may be suspicious, irritable, impulsive, eccentric, or excessively religious, or may exhibit a false sense of superiority. (Adams & Victor, 1981, p. 804)

Irritability and emotional outbursts are common. Mental deterioration follows, often becoming salient several years after the first signs of chorea. When mental deterioration begins, memory typically is affected first, followed by slowing of intellectual functions and compromised attention. Progressive motor impairments, dementia, and incontinence eventually culminate in institutionalization, followed by death from infection or poor nutrition 15 to 20 years after onset.

Language and Communication Dysarthria caused by chorea is the most common communicative impairment in early-stage to middle-stage Huntington's disease. When chorea affects the muscles of articulation or respiration, irregular interruptions of speech and voice occur. As a patient's chorea increases, speech intelligibility declines and dysphagia (swallowing impairment) often develops. Language usually is preserved until the late stages of Huntington's disease, except for language tasks requiring sustained attention, memory, and judgment. In the final stages, patients with Huntington's disease become mute, incontinent, and profoundly demented.

Progressive Supranuclear Palsy

Progressive supranuclear palsy (PSP) was described as a clinical entity by Steele, Richardson, and Olszewski in 1964. Progressive supranuclear palsy is a rare disease (affecting about 1 in 20,000 adults in the United States). It usually begins between age 50 and age 80, with peak incidence in the early 60s. Progressive supranuclear palsy resembles Parkinson's disease in the presence of rigidity and slowness of movement, but it differs from Parkinson's disease in the absence of tremor and in the presence of rigidity affecting muscles of the neck and trunk, rather than the muscles of the limbs. Nevertheless, Lees (1990) claims that as many as 12% of patients with progressive supranuclear palsy are first diagnosed as having Parkinson's disease. Men develop progressive supranuclear palsy slightly more often than women do.

Neuropathology Progressive supranuclear palsy is caused by neuronal loss, neuronal abnormalities, and proliferation of glial cells throughout the brain stem and basal ganglia. Cortical neurons are largely spared. Early symptoms of progressive supranuclear palsy include paralysis of muscles responsible for downward gaze, rigidity of neck muscles, and facial muscle weakness. As progressive supranuclear palsy progresses the patient loses vertical movements of the eyes and then lateral movements of the eyes. Next the patient's limbs become stiff and rigid, dysarthria appears, and swallowing becomes difficult.

The combination of neck rigidity and paralysis of downward gaze produce early difficulties with walking for patients with progressive supranuclear palsy because they cannot see their feet. Patients report frequent falls, usually backward. Adams and Victor (1981) report the experience of a large man with progressive supranuclear palsy who fell repeatedly, wrecking furniture as he fell, but whose stance and gait appeared normal in the neurologic examination. Some neurology texts allude to the "dirty tie" sign caused by patients' inability to see food dropped as they eat.

The patient's personality typically changes as progressive supranuclear palsy progresses. Some patients become apathetic and seemingly euphoric. Others become restless and irritable. Depression is common. Dementia appears in the middle to late stages of progressive supranuclear palsy. The dementia is characterized by slowing of mental processes and increasing forgetfulness. In the final stages of progressive supranuclear palsy the patient becomes mute, immobile, and helpless.

Medical Management The cause of progressive supranuclear palsy is unknown, although viruses or slowly acting toxins are considered possible causes. Recent studies suggest that some forms of progressive supranuclear palsy may have a genetic origin. There is no effective medical treatment for progressive supranuclear palsy. Levodopa and similar medications sometimes provide temporary improvement, but no medical regimen provides long-term benefit. Medications to manage psychologic and neurobehavioral sequelae of progressive supranuclear palsy (e.g., depression, anxiety) may be appropriate.

Evolution The first symptoms of progressive supranuclear palsy are subtle. The patient reports frequent falls and complains of stiffness (rigidity) in neck and trunk muscles. As progressive supranuclear palsy advances the patient may complain of double vision (the first signs of ocular muscle weakness) and changes in mood. As the disease continues the patient loses up-and-down eye movements, muscle rigidity progresses to the patient's arms and legs, and pseudobulbar palsy (exaggerated palatal and laryngeal reflexes, drooling, swallowing disturbances, and heightened emotionality) appears. By this stage of progressive supranuclear palsy many patients become apathetic and some are clinically depressed. During the late stages of the disease the patient loses side-to-side eye movements, facial muscles become rigid, and walking becomes impossible because of frequent falls. Patients with very late-stage progressive supranuclear palsy usually are bedridden or confined to a wheelchair and require full-time care. Most patients with progressive supranuclear palsy die within 4 to 7 years after diagnosis, either from aspiration pneumonia or from respiratory failure as a result of central nervous system dysfunction.

Language and Communication Dysarthria appears early and can be severe even in the early stages of progressive supranuclear palsy. The patient's speech becomes slow and littered with stuttering-like repetitions, and the patient's voice intensity diminishes. Slowly progressive dementia often begins in the middle to late stages of progressive supranuclear palsy, but language usually remains well preserved until the very late stages. In the very late stages of this disease, the patient's speech becomes unintelligible and mutism is common.

Human Immunodeficiency Virus Encephalopathy

Acquired immunodeficiency syndrome (AIDS) is a complex of signs and symptoms caused by infection with the human immunodeficiency virus (HIV) transmitted by body fluids (primarily blood and semen). The virus weakens the immune system, leading to the appearance of various opportunistic diseases, including bacterial, parasitic, and fungal infections and several forms of cancer. According to the World Health Organization, about 22 million adults are living with HIV infections worldwide, most in developing countries. Most AIDS patients are younger than age 35. More than 90% of deaths from AIDS occur in individuals younger than 50.

> Opportunistic infections are infections made possible by a patient's lowered resistance. One of the hallmarks of AIDS is the occurrence of opportunistic infections.

Neuropathology HIV encephalopathy (also called AIDS dementia complex) is the most common neurologic consequence of AIDS, affecting up to 70% of patients with AIDS (Aminoff, Greenberg, & Simon, 1996). AIDS dementia complex is caused by infection of the brain with the human immunodeficiency virus. The infection causes pathologic changes in the subcortical white matter and basal ganglia, and these changes eventually progress to the cortex (Navia, Jordan, & Price, 1986). The HIV infection of the brain produces a pattern of impairment in which early symptoms (weakness, slowness, rigidity, dyskinesia) are characteristic of extrapyramidal pathology, and later-developing symptoms (impaired perception, memory, intellect, and language) signify cortical involvement. The exact cause of these pathologic changes is unknown, but neurotoxins triggered by the virus appear to be likely candidates. AIDS dementia complex usually develops late in the course of AIDS, but it sometimes occurs early and occasionally is the first sign of AIDS.

Medical Management There is no cure for AIDS or for AIDS dementia complex. However, a number of drugs have been shown to prolong AIDS patients' lives, and there are preliminary indications that these drugs also may lessen the severity of dementia in patients with AIDS dementia complex. Currently most practitioners believe that a combination of several powerful antiviral drugs provides the best treatment for AIDS, and the search continues for more effective drugs that may control or even cure the disease.

Evolution The onset of AIDS dementia complex is variable. Usually it begins insidiously and progresses slowly, but occasionally onset is abrupt and progression is rapid (Price & Perry, 1994). Initially the patient becomes forgetful and apathetic and has difficulty concentrating and carrying out complex mental tasks. As AIDS progresses, motor impairments representing combinations of subcortical pathology (weakness, rigidity, ataxia) and cortical pathology (spasticity, hyperreflexia, primitive reflexes) appear, followed by seizures and incontinence. Cognitive impairments prevent the patient from working and maintaining a household. Impairments in visuospatial abilities, abstract thinking, and reasoning appear. Patients in the final stages of AIDS are mute, disoriented, incontinent, immobile, and require around-the-clock nursing

care. Without aggressive medical treatment, death usually occurs within 6 months after the onset of central nervous system pathology, usually from aspiration pneumonia or opportunistic infection.

Language and Communication In the early stages of AIDS dementia complex, the patient's speech and language are generally within normal limits, although careful testing may reveal subtle impairments in word retrieval and comprehension of complex printed and spoken materials. As AIDS progresses and motor systems are affected, the patient's spontaneous speech becomes slow, labored, sparse, and dysarthric; the patient gets lost in conversations; and comprehension of printed and spoken materials declines. As the patient's dementia progresses into later stages, spontaneous speech is limited to single words and short phrases, and the patient comprehends only highly familiar spoken or printed material. In the final stages of AIDS dementia complex, the patient's speech is confined to a few overused words and phrases, comprehension of even simple printed materials is nonfunctional, and comprehension of speech is limited to short and simple utterances.

Identifying Subcortical Dementia

Most subcortical dementias are delayed consequences of extrapyramidal system disease and are preceded by characteristic impairments of volitional movements (e.g., the rigidity, tremor, and slowed movements of Parkinson's disease; the choreiform movements of Huntington's disease; the eye and trunk muscle paralysis of progressive supranuclear palsy).

Identifying subcortical dementia is somewhat less ambiguous than identifying cortical dementia because the clinician knows that several extrapyramidal diseases progress to dementia. When signs of mental decline appear in otherwise healthy patients with extrapyramidal disease, the signs may signal the onset of progressive dementia. Assessment of these patients' dementia usually is preceded by assessment and treatment of earlier-to-appear speech impairments (e.g., dysarthria). A few patients with extrapyramidal disease exhibit signs of intellectual deterioration before detectable motor impairments appear. For these patients no pre-existing disease points to a diagnosis of dementia, and the clinician must base the diagnosis on the pattern and progression of the patient's mental impairments. The diagnostic routine for these patients resembles the diagnostic routine for patients with cortical dementia, discussed later.

MIXED DEMENTIA

Vascular disease is an important cause of dementia in adults. It is second to Alzheimer's disease as a cause of dementia, accounting for 15% to 20% of all dementias (Cummings & Benson, 1992). The umbrella term for dementias caused by vascular disease is *multi-infarct dementia* (MID). As the label suggests, multi-infarct dementia is caused by repeated infarcts, usually at various locations in the brain. Three etiologic subgroups of vascular dementia have been described in the literature. They are *lacunar state, multiple cortical infarcts,* and *Binswanger's disease.* Lacunar state and Binswanger's disease represent primarily subcortical pathology, but multiple cortical infarcts (not surprisingly) represent primarily cortical pathology.

Most patients with vascular dementia have a history of hypertension, heart disease, or both, and patient histories of multiple strokes are common. The first symptoms of vascular dementia typically are abrupt in onset and generate focal neurologic signs (perceptual, motor, or sensory impairments), which represent the localized effects of the first incident. Subsequent incidents produce a stepwise progression of symptom development, as additional focal impairments are added with each new incident. The slow accumulation of neurologic events eventually produces diffuse cerebral involvement and dementia. The patient's personality and intellect usually are preserved until the late stages of vascular dementia, although depression, irritability, and emotional lability may appear early.

Lacunar state is caused by multiple small infarcts in the arteries supplying the basal ganglia, thalamus, midbrain, and brain stem. The first symptoms are subcortical in nature and include dysarthria, swallowing disturbances, pseudobulbar palsy, weakness, and sometimes tremor because of involvement of extrapyramidal and brain stem structures. Intellect and language are preserved until late in the course of the disease. Dementia eventually appears in 70% to 80% of patients with lacunar state (Celesia & Wanamaker, 1972).

Multiple cortical infarcts are caused by a series of thrombotic or embolic occlusions of cortical arteries. Each occlusion causes focal neurologic symptoms, and multiple occlusions yield an increasingly diffuse pattern of impairment, eventually culminating in cortical dementia. The patient's symptoms depend on the cortical areas involved in each incident and include those commonly associated with cortical damage (e.g., aphasia, apraxia, neglect). Hemiparesis and hemiplegia commonly are associated with cortical infarcts, but dysarthria and swallowing impairments, which typically are associated with subcortical pathology, are not.

Binswanger's disease is a rare disease caused by multiple infarcts in subcortical white matter, usually in patients with severe hypertension. The infarcts are a consequence of thrombotic or embolic occlusion of long penetrating arteries from the cortex that supply subcortical white matter tracts. The first symptoms of Binswanger's disease are focal, but repeated infarcts yield more pervasive mental and physical impairments, eventually culminating in dementia. Clinically, the symptoms of Binswanger's disease resemble lacunar state, but the onset of symptoms is slow, combinations of cortical and subcortical neurologic signs are common, and motor impairments appear somewhat later in Binswanger's disease than in lacunar state.

Vascular dementia occasionally occurs as a consequence of diseases such as autoimmune disease (lupus erythematosus) or infections such as Lyme disease if the disease causes pathologic changes in cerebral blood vessels. However, multiple strokes are by far the leading cause of vascular dementia in adults. The symptoms of vascular dementia occasionally mimic those of Alzheimer's disease, but the acute onset of symptoms, fluctuating severity of symptoms, and a history of hypertension and stroke usually lead to the appropriate diagnosis. Unlike patients with Alzheimer's disease, patients with vascular dementia tend to remain aware of their disabilities, even in advanced stages of dementia. Consequently, patients with vascular dementia tend to have a higher incidence of depression than patients with Alzheimer's disease.

The *Hachinski Ischemia Index* (Hachinski, Lassen, & Marshall, 1974) is a widely used set of criteria for identifying vascular dementia. It is quick and easy to complete and has been shown to reliably differentiate between vascular dementia and Alzheimer's disease (Table 10-1).

CORTICAL DEMENTIA
Alzheimer's Disease

Alzheimer's disease was first described by Alois Alzheimer, a German professor of neuropathology who reported autopsy findings from a 55-year-old patient who had died following several years of severe dementia. Alzheimer examined the patient's brain at autopsy and found several pathologic changes, which he described in a paper published in 1906. These pathologic changes came to define the disease.

Alzheimer's disease is the fastest-growing and most expensive clinical population in the United States (Bayles, Kaszniak, & Tomoeda, 1987). About 4 million adults in the United States have Alzheimer's disease. Alzheimer's disease affects 5% to 10% of the over-65 population and from 15% to 30% of the over-80 population in the United States (Clarke & Witter, 1990). Alzheimer's disease accounts for 50% to 70% of all progressive dementias (Cummings, 1990). Alzheimer's disease is two to three times more common in women than in men (Cummings & Benson, 1983).

TABLE 10-1
Hachinski Ischemia Index

Feature	Score*
Abrupt onset	2
Stepwise deterioration	1
Fluctuating course	2
Nocturnal confusion	1
Relative preservation of personality	1
Depression	1
Somatic complaints	1
Emotional lability	1
History of hypertension	1
History of stroke	2
Evidence of atherosclerosis	1
Focal neurologic symptoms	2
Focal neurologic signs	2
Total score	

Data from Hachinski, V. C., Lassen, N. A., & Marshall, J. (1974). Multi-infarct dementia: A cause of mental deterioration in the elderly. *Lancet, 2,* 207-210.
Symptom, reported by the patient; *sign,* observed by the examiner.
*Total score = 4 or less: likely Alzheimer's disease. Total score = 5 to 7: uncertain diagnosis. Total score = 8 or greater: likely vascular dementia.

Neuropathology Alzheimer's disease is characterized by three microscopic changes in brain neurons first described by Alzheimer: *neurofibrillary tangles, neuritic plaques,* and *granulovacuolar degeneration.* These changes are detectable only by direct examination of brain tissue; they are not visible on computerized tomography (CT) scans or magnetic resonance imaging (MRI) scans. It is not known whether the neuronal abnormalities are themselves the cause of dementia or are a consequence of other neurochemical processes that actually cause the dementia, although it generally is believed that the abnormalities interfere with normal neuronal functions and either directly or indirectly contribute to dementia.

In the late stages of Alzheimer's disease the brain shrinks, the ventricles become larger, and the sulci become wider (Hedera & Whitehouse, 1995). These changes are the result of neuron loss and are visible on CT or MRI scans.

Neurofibrillary Tangles Neurofibrils are threadlike structures normally found in the cell bodies, dendrites, axons, and sometimes in the synaptic endings of neurons in the brain. In Alzheimer's disease, the neurofibrils become twisted, tangled, contorted, and clumped together. These changes are easily seen in samples of brain tissue using a standard microscope. Neurofibrillary tangles are not unique to Alzheimer's disease. Neurofibrils may be present in the brains of patients with Parkinson's disease, in the brains of patients with progressive supranuclear palsy, and occasionally in the brains of elderly patients with no obvious neurologic disease. Neurofibrillary tangles may be a neuron's nonspecific reaction to central nervous system damage (Cummings & Benson, 1983; Bayles, Kaszniak, & Tomoeda, 1987).

Neuritic Plaques Neuritic plaques (sometimes called *senile plaques* or *dendritic plaques*) are "minute areas of tissue degeneration consisting of granular deposits and remnants of neuronal processes" (Cummings & Benson, 1992, p. 67). Neuritic plaques tend to concentrate in the cortex and subcortical regions of the brain. They cause marked reductions in neuronal synapses, thereby adversely affecting synaptic transmission. Neuritic plaques sometimes are found in the brains of patients with Down syndrome or Creutzfeldt-Jakob disease (a rare disease characterized by progressive degeneration of corticospinal nerve fibers) and in the brains of some normal elderly adults, but they are far more common in the brains of patients with Alzheimer's disease.

Granulovacuolar Degeneration Granulovacuolar degeneration is a pathologic process in which small fluid-filled cavities containing granular debris appear within nerve cells. The pyramidal neurons in the hippocampus (a deep brain structure that seems to be important in memory) most frequently are affected, accounting, at least in part, for the insidious deterioration of memory common in Alzheimer's disease. Granulovacuolar degeneration may be present in several neurologic diseases other than those causing dementia. Granulovacuolar degeneration occasionally appears in the brains of normal elderly persons, but Tomlinson and Henderson (1976) contend that if 10% or more of hippocampal neurons are affected, dementia always is present.

Other Abnormalities Lower-than-normal levels of acetylcholine (a neurotransmitter) have been noted in the brains of individuals with Alzheimer's disease—perhaps a significant difference because acetylcholine is believed to play an important part in memory. Abnormal levels of aluminum have been found in neurofibrillary tangles and neuritic plaques, but it is not known what potential role aluminum might play in causing or perpetuating Alzheimer's disease.

The neuropathologic changes in Alzheimer's disease are not diffuse and equally distributed throughout the brain but most frequently affect the temporoparietal-occipital junctions and the inferior temporal lobes (Figure 10-4). The frontal lobes, the motor and sensory cortex, and the occipital lobes usually are spared.

Medical Management The cause of Alzheimer's disease is unknown, although several causes have been proposed, including aluminum poisoning, disturbed immune function, infection with a slow virus, and genetically transmitted disturbance of neuronal functions.

Some cases of early onset Alzheimer's dementia have a familial pattern, apparently caused by a genetic abnormality transmitted from parents to children.

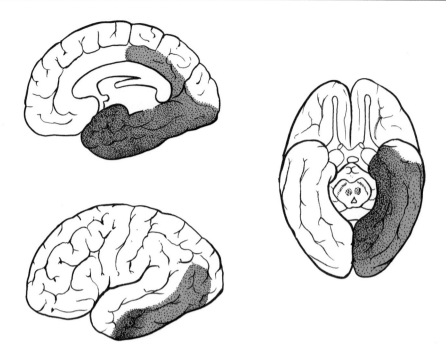

Figure 10-4 ■ Cortical brain regions most often affected by Alzheimer's disease. The darker shading represents the cortical regions most frequently affected.

The development of symptoms in Alzheimer's disease differs somewhat among individuals, suggesting that not all cases of Alzheimer's disease are caused by the same pathologic process. Although no medical treatment prevents or cures Alzheimer's disease, some symptoms of the disease may be amenable to treatment. Patients with Alzheimer's disease may be given tranquilizers to control combativeness and aggression or antidepressants to lessen depression. Diet and fluid intake may be monitored and managed to prevent dehydration and to maintain adequate nutrition. The environment of patients with Alzheimer's disease may be manipulated to stimulate the patient, to maintain orientation and cognitive abilities, and to prevent social isolation. Counseling and other support services may be provided to the patient and the patient's family.

During the past decade scientists have been searching for the causes of Alzheimer's disease and for effective medical treatments. Although a few medical treatments (neurotransmitter augmentation, nerve growth enhancement, antiinflammatory medications) have shown promise, no large-scale clinical trails have identified an effective treatment and the search for prevention, control, and cure continues. The drug tacrine *(Cognex)* reportedly improves cognition for some patients with Alzheimer's disease, but its toxic side effects (liver damage) preclude its long-term use for many patients. The drug donepezil *(Aricept)* has fewer side effects and may improve cognition and general functioning. Two drugs, rivastigmine and galantamine, are under U.S. Food and Drug Administration review. These drugs do not cure or slow the progression of Alzheimer's disease, but they provide some improvement in cognition and behavior for patients with mild to moderate Alzheimer's disease. They may not be effective for patients in the advanced stages of the disease.

> Some recent reports suggest that caffeine may slow or even prevent the appearance of Alzheimer's disease. Coffee growers and distributors eagerly await the results of additional research.

Evolution The development of Alzheimer's disease is characterized by progressive deterioration of intellect. The first symptoms are subtle and include lapses of memory (usually the first symptoms reported), faulty reasoning, poor judgment, disorientation except in highly familiar environments, and alterations of mood (depression, apathy, irritability, suspiciousness). The patient's personality and interpersonal behaviors remain relatively intact during the early stages of the disease, although the patient may withdraw from social contact. As Alzheimer's disease progresses the patient's mental impairments become more obvious. Intellect and cognition become increasingly impaired, and disturbances of language and communication appear. The patient becomes restless and agitated, gets lost even in familiar environments, and wanders off when not supervised. Episodes of incontinence appear. These symptoms gradually worsen, and the final stages leave the patient with profound motor deficits (rigidity or spasticity), complete incontinence, and loss of almost all intellectual and cognitive abilities. Motor abilities usually are spared until the very late stages of Alzheimer's disease, at which time signs of pyramidal system involvement (weakness, paralysis) may appear. Patients with Alzheimer's disease usually die of aspiration pneumonia or infection 5 to 10 years after their disease is diagnosed.

Language and Communication Language is less affected than cognition, memory, and intellect in the early stages of Alzheimer's disease. As Alzheimer's disease progresses, increasingly obvious impairments in language and communication appear. For most patients with Alzheimer's

disease the early language impairments reflect the effects of the disease on memory and intellect and do not represent specific language impairment (aphasia). There may be some similarities between the communicative abilities of early-stage Alzheimer's disease patients and patients with anomic aphasia and between later-stage Alzheimer's disease patients and patients with Wernicke's aphasia (Hier, Hagenlocher, & Shindler, 1985). However, patients with Alzheimer's disease always have conspicuous problems with memory and intellect that clearly separate them diagnostically from patients with aphasia.

As a general rule, the communicative performance of patients with Alzheimer's disease depends on the amount of mental effort required. Communicative activities that require greater mental effort are affected first and most dramatically by Alzheimer's disease, and communicative activities that require less mental effort are affected later and less dramatically. "Automatic" language processes, which require little mental effort *(grammar, syntax, social conventions),* usually are preserved until the very late stages of Alzheimer's disease.

> Although patients with Alzheimer's disease do not usually have significant problems with language, their impaired memory may compromise their retention of what they read or hear and what they have previously said. Patients with early-stage Alzheimer's disease often annoy caregivers by failing to remember what they have been told for more than an hour or so and by their propensity to tell the same story or ask the same question over and over.

Early Stages Phonology, syntax, articulation, and voice quality are well preserved in the speech of patients with early Alzheimer's disease, although mild word-retrieval problems, occasional verbal paraphasias, and subtle comprehension impairments may appear early. When word-retrieval failures occur these patients usually recognize and repair them, often by talking around the missing word (". . . and she was pushing the baby in a wagon . . . no, that's not it . . . in a cart . . . no . . . in a stroller, going down the street"). Patients with early-stage Alzheimer's disease may complain that they sometimes cannot think of the right word as they speak or write and that their spelling is not what it used to be. Patients with early-stage Alzheimer's disease make few grammatic errors in speaking or writing, and their production of syntactic structures in speech matches that of normal elderly speakers (Kempler, Curtiss, & Jackson, 1987; Figure 10-5).

Patients with early-stage Alzheimer's disease typically have functional reading comprehension for newspapers and magazines, although their reading rate is slow and they have difficulty comprehending and retaining long or complex materials. They may miss the meaning of complex syntactic structures (e.g., passive sentences, comparatives) and they may fail to recognize low-frequency words. Highly practiced speech responses (e.g., counting, reciting the alphabet, reciting the days of the week) are preserved, but responses calling for sustained attention and mental flexibility (e.g., explaining proverbs, comprehending abstract material) are compromised early.

Patients with early-stage Alzheimer's disease are adequate conversationalists. They usually observe conversational conventions (e.g., turn-taking, eye contact). As listeners they may have difficulty following conversations in which topics or speakers change and may fail to get the point of nonliteral material such as humor, irony, or sarcasm. As speakers, patients with early-stage Alzheimer's disease tend to talk too long, drift from the topic, unnecessarily repeat material, and make tangential and irrelevant comments.

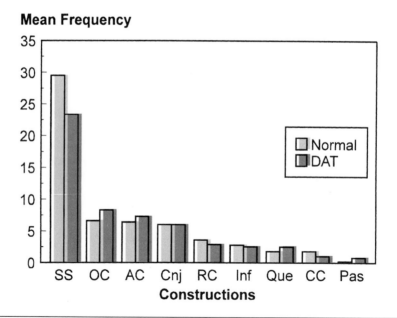

Figure 10-5 ■Mean frequency of syntactic structures in the speech of normal adults or adults with dementia. *DAT,* Dementia of Alzheimer's type; *SS,* simple sentences; *OC,* other complements; *AC,* adverbial clauses; *Cnj,* conjunctions; *RC,* relative clauses; *Inf,* infinitivals; *Que,* questions; *CC,* complex comparatives; *Pas,* passives. (Data from Kempler, D., Curtiss, S., & Jackson, C. [1987]. Syntactic preservation in Alzheimer's disease. *Journal of Speech and Hearing Research, 30,* 343-350.)

Middle Stages As patients progress into the middle stages of Alzheimer's disease communicative impairments become more obvious. Word-retrieval failures in spontaneous speech become more frequent and the patients' success in repairing them declines. Sentence fragments and ungrammatic sentences begin to appear in the patient's spontaneous speech. Reading rate continues to decline and eventually becomes nonfunctional for all but the most familiar material. Most patients in the middle stages of Alzheimer's disease abandon recreational reading.

Conversations with patients in the middle stages of Alzheimer's disease become more difficult. Some patients become apathetic and withdraw from conversational interactions. Most become passive conversational partners, allowing others to set the topic, tone, and content of conversations, and offer trivialities, automatisms, and irrelevant comments in place of substantive contributions. Unnecessary repetition of ideas increases. Patients get lost even in simple conversations on familiar topics. Conformity with conversational conventions deteriorates. Turn-taking violations become more frequent, although most patients retain a general sense of when to talk and when to listen. Comprehension of nonliteral material is grossly impaired.

Late Stages Communicative performance of patients in the late stages of Alzheimer's disease is severely compromised. Reading is nonfunctional, although patients may recognize some highly familiar words. Writing is nonfunctional, although some patients may be able to complete simple overlearned sequences (numbers, the alphabet) if given the first items in the sequence. Comprehension of spoken materials is limited to simple familiar phrases and words. Speech consists primarily of single words and sentence fragments, which are often bizarre, devoid of meaning, and repeated in robot-like fashion. Syntax begins to break down and stereotypic utterances ("great day in the morning . . . great day in the morning") and neologisms ("take it down the cranbibby") appear. Patients in the late stages of Alzheimer's disease generally are un-aware of errors and make no attempt to revise or correct them.

Patients in the late stages of Alzheimer's disease are nonfunctional conversationalists. They fail to observe social conventions (e.g., greetings, farewells) and are insensitive to conversational rules such as those governing turn-taking, topic maintenance, eye contact, and relevance. Patients tend to dwell on personal experiences (usually past events, and often misinterpreted) regardless of their conversational partner's intent. In the very late stages of Alzheimer's disease some patients become mute and others become echolalic (endlessly repeating what others say) or pallilalic (endlessly repeating a self-generated word or phrase). Those patients who still speak are limited to a few overused words produced indiscriminately and without regard to listeners. By the final stages of Alzheimer's disease the patient loses all orientation to self and surroundings and does not use language in any meaningful way. Table 10-2 summarizes the progression of communication impairment as Alzheimer's disease progresses.

Pick's Disease

Some patients become demented as a consequence of pathologic changes in the frontal lobes. The most common cause of dementia-causing frontal lobe pathology is Pick's disease, but cases of frontal lobe dementia have been reported in which the pathologic changes symptomatic of Pick's disease are not present. However, Neary and associates (1988) suggest that these anomalous cases actually may represent a form of Pick's disease.

Pick's disease was first described in 1892 by Arnold Pick, a professor of psychiatry at the University of Prague. Pick's disease is a progressive degenerative disease beginning in the cerebral cortex of the frontal lobes. It is a rare disease, affecting less than 1% of the United States population and accounting for only about 2% of dementia patients. Pick's disease usually begins between the ages of 40 and 60, although it appears sporadically in younger or older persons.

T A B L E   1 0 - 2
Effects of dementing illnesses on communication

Early stages

Sounds	Used correctly.
Words	May omit a meaningful word, usually a noun, when talking in sentences. May report trouble thinking of the right word. Vocabulary is shrinking.
Grammar	Generally correct.
Content	May drift from the topic. Reduced ability to generate series of meaningful sentences. Difficulty comprehending new information. Vague.
Use	Knows when to talk, although may talk too long on a subject. May be apathetic, failing to initiate a conversation when it would be appropriate to do so. May have difficulty understanding humor, verbal analogies, sarcasm, and indirect and nonliteral statements.

Middle stages

Sounds	Used correctly.
Words	Difficulty thinking of words in a category. Anomia in conversation. Difficulty naming objects. Reliance on automatisms. Vocabulary noticeably diminished.
Grammar	Sentence fragments and deviations common. May have difficulty understanding grammatically complex sentences.
Content	Frequently repeats ideas. Forgets topic. Talks about events of past or trivia. Fewer ideas.
Use	Knows when to talk. Recognizes questions. May fail to greet. Loss of sensitivity to conversational partners. Rarely corrects mistakes.

Late stages

Sounds	Generally used correctly, but errors are not uncommon.
Words	Marked anomia. Poor vocabulary. Lack of word comprehension. May make up words and produce jargon.
Grammar	Some grammar is preserved but sentence fragments and deviations common. Lack of comprehension of many grammatic forms.
Content	Generally unable to produce a sequence of related ideas. Content may be meaningless and bizarre. Subject of most meaningful utterances is the retelling of a past event. Marked repetition of words and phrases.
Use	Generally unaware of surroundings and context. Insensitive to others. Little meaningful use of language. Some patients are mute; some are echolalic.

From Bayles, K.A. (1994). Management of communication disorders associated with dementia (p. 542). In R. Chapey (Ed.). *Language intervention strategies in adult aphasia.* Baltimore: Williams & Wilkins.

Neuropathology Pick's disease is characterized by two neuronal abnormalities: proliferation of enlarged neurons *(Pick cells)* and the presence of *Pick bodies* within neurons. (Pick bodies are dense globular formations within the neuron cytoplasm. They are about the same size as the cell nucleus and contain numerous neurofibrils.) The progression of Pick's disease is marked by shrinkage of the brain (typically confined to the posterior inferior frontal lobes and the anterior superior temporal lobes) together with loss of neurons and proliferation of glial cells throughout the cortex. The cause of Pick's disease is unknown, although a genetic component (suggested by a pattern of familial inheritance) may be present in 20% to 50% of cases.

> In some contemporary technical literature, Pick's disease has been renamed frontotemporal dementia, but the label *Pick's disease* continues to be used by the general public, patients, caregivers, and many practitioners.

Medical Management At present there is no cure for Pick's disease, and its treatment, like that of Alzheimer's disease, is symptomatic, consisting of medications to control changes in mood and temperament and behavioral intervention to maintain the patient's orientation and to manage the patient's daily life behavior.

Evolution Pick's disease is commonly first diagnosed as stress, depression, or Alzheimer's disease, with the diagnosis changing as early subtle symptoms become more dramatic. The progression of symptoms in Pick's disease differs from that in Alzheimer's disease. In *Alzheimer's disease* intellect is compromised early and personality is spared until the late stages. In *Pick's disease* alterations in personality and emotion usually are the first symptoms to appear. Alterations in personality and emotion are closely followed by apathy and indifference toward the patient's usual interests and activities. The patient's ability to independently plan, initiate, and follow through on familiar activities declines, although the patient may be able to carry out the activities when prompted by others. The patient's social behavior deteriorates, and the patient becomes impulsive, disinhibited, and inappropriately jocular; makes inappropriate comments (often sexual in nature); talks indiscriminately with strangers; laughs inappropri-

ately; and generally behaves with "loss of personal propriety" (Cummings & Benson, 1992). Some patients with Pick's disease become hyperoral, making overeating and weight gain a problem.

As Pick's disease progresses the patient's judgment and insight become progressively more impaired, and obsessional, ritualistic behaviors appear (e.g., repeated hand washing, folding and refolding articles of clothing). Some patients become profoundly apathetic, sitting placidly for hours unless directed by a caregiver to perform an activity. Others become profoundly restless, fidgeting and pacing for hours unless a caregiver intervenes. In the late stages, patients with Pick's disease become mute and may exhibit motor rigidity. Patients with Pick's disease usually die from an infection, usually pneumonia.

Language and Communication Changes in language and communication in Pick's disease differ from those in Alzheimer's disease. In Alzheimer's disease memory and orientation are compromised early, but language remains relatively intact until the late stages. In Pick's disease memory and orientation usually are well preserved until the later stages of the disease, but language breakdown appears early and remains prominent in the middle and late stages of the disease. Word-retrieval failures, impaired confrontation naming, circumlocution, and use of generic words for specific words ("I got the thing and did that other, but it wasn't there.") are common expressive abnormalities. Echolalia and verbal stereotypies ("mama-mama-mama, me-me-me") may be present. The patient may tell the same story over and over, unaware of the repetition.

Comprehension impairments for both spoken and printed materials are prominent in the middle stages of Pick's disease and become progressively more profound as Pick's disease progresses. By the final stages, patients with Pick's disease are mute and profoundly demented, with severely impaired memory, orientation, and cognition. Patients with Pick's disease usually die from aspiration pneumonia or infection 6 to 12 years after their disease is diagnosed.

Differentiating Pick's Disease from Alzheimer's Disease Mendez and associates (1993) suggested that Pick's disease can be differentiated from Alzheimer's disease by the following characteristics:

- Onset of symptoms in Pick's disease begins before age 65.
- Personality change is among the first symptoms observed in Pick's disease.
- Patients with Pick's disease are hyperoral (eat excessively, indiscriminately put things in mouth).
- Patients with Pick's disease are impulsive and lack social inhibitions.
- Patients with Pick's disease roam or wander when left unsupervised. (Author's note: Patients with Alzheimer's disease also roam and wander but not until later in the disease.)

Mendez and associates assert that if three of the foregoing characteristics are present, Pick's disease is the most likely cause.

Kertesz and Munoz (2000) identified the following differences between early Pick's disease and early Alzheimer's disease:

- Personality and language changes are much more common in early Pick's disease.
- Memory impairments are much more prevalent in early Alzheimer's disease.
- Patients with early Pick's disease have significantly greater impairment in activities of daily living (e.g., *grooming, bathing, managing personal affairs*).

Other Causes of Dementia

Normal-Pressure Hydrocephalus Normal-pressure hydrocephalus (sometimes called *nonobstructive* or *communicating* hydrocephalus) usually is caused by physiologic conditions that interfere with resorption of cerebrospinal fluid from the brain ventricles and the spinal cord. The compromised resorption causes accumulation of excess cerebrospinal fluid in the ventricles and spinal cord, increases intracranial pressure, and causes the ventricles to enlarge. In-creased intracranial pressure eventually inhibits production of cerebrospinal fluid by the choroid plexus and forces cerebrospinal fluid into brain tissue, at which time intracranial pressure gradually decreases, often to normal levels. The ventricles, however, remain enlarged.

The preferred medical treatment of patients with normal-pressure hydrocephalus is *shunting,* in which a hollow needle connected to a flexible tube is inserted into a ventricle and excess cerebrospinal fluid is siphoned off, usually into the thorax, where it is eventually resorbed. About two thirds of patients so treated improve and about one third show no change in symptoms or worsen, usually as a result of complications (hematoma, infection).

Patients with normal-pressure hydrocephalus typically exhibit dementia, gait disturbance, and urinary incontinence. The gait disturbance exhibited by patients with normal-pressure hydrocephalus is unusual. The patient is unsteady while standing and has difficulty initiating walking, appearing as if "glued to the floor" (Aminoff, Greenberg, & Simon, 1996, p. 55). Once initiated, walking is slow and shuffling. The patient easily performs leg movements (kicking, bicycling, walking) to command while lying down or sitting but is unable to do so when standing and bearing weight on the legs (a condition called *apraxia of gait*).

The dementia exhibited by patients with normal-pressure hydrocephalus is first characterized by slowing of mental functions, impaired memory, emotional dullness, and mild attentional impairments. Focal impairments (e.g., aphasia, agnosia) are uncommon. Most patients recover spontaneously following placement of a ventricular shunt; some stabilize at levels of mild to moderate dementia; and a few progress to global cognitive dysfunction, muteness, and total obliviousness to surroundings, followed by death from infection or respiratory failure.

Creutzfeldt-Jakob Disease Creutzfeldt-Jakob disease is a rare, invariably fatal disease that causes rapidly progressing dementia and neuro-muscular disorders. It is caused by invasion of the central nervous system by protein particles called *prions* (for *proteinaceous infectious particle*). Prions are thought to transform normal and benign brain proteins into an infectious and deadly form by altering the shape of molecules in healthy proteins. Most cases of Creutzfeldt-Jakob disease are sporadic—there is no known source of infection and no pattern of familial infections, although in about 10% of cases there seems to be a familial pattern of infection. At this time the only documented mode of transmission from person to person is by unintended consequences of medical procedures using prion-tainted human tissues (grafts, transplants) or contaminated surgical instruments. However, there is widespread belief in the scientific community that ingestion of prion-infected animal tissue (primarily from beef cattle) is responsible for many cases of Creutzfeldt-Jakob disease.

A prion-caused disease called *kuru* was common in the Fore tribe in Papua, New Guinea during the 1950s and early 1960s. Kuru was essentially eliminated when the tribe stopped the ritual handling and eating of deceased relatives' brains and internal organs.

Infection with the prion causing Creutzfeldt-Jakob disease causes widespread neuronal loss and proliferation of glial cells throughout the brain, together with the appearance of numerous microscopic cavities throughout the brain substance. These cavities cause the brain to become soft and spongy. For this reason Creutzfeldt-Jakob disease sometimes is called *subacute spongiform encephalopathy*. Creutzfeldt-Jakob disease resembles several diseases of animals, including *scrapie* in sheep and goats, *chronic wasting disease* in deer and elk, and bovine spongiform encephalopathy in cattle (popularly known as *mad cow disease*). All are thought to be caused by prions. Although at this time there is no direct evidence of transmission of prion-caused diseases from animals to humans, many scientists believe that consumption of beef from infected cattle was responsible for an increase in Creutzfeldt-Jakob disease in England in the early 1990s.

Creutzfeldt-Jakob disease is rare in the United States, affecting about 1 in 1 million inhabitants. It can occur at any age, although most cases are adults in their 50s and 60s. There is no effective treatment for Creutzfeldt-Jakob disease; once contracted, the disease is rapidly progressive and invariably fatal, with death occurring within 1 year of the first symptoms.

Patients in the early stages of Creutzfeldt-Jakob disease exhibit a variety of signs and symptoms, but dementia is almost always present. Memory impairments, slowing of mental processes, impaired reasoning and problem-solving, insomnia, and flattened affect are prominent early in the disease. Neuromuscular abnormalities (extrapyramidal signs, cerebellar ataxia, myoclonus) quickly develop as Creutzfeldt-Jakob disease progresses. Hallucinations, confusion, and delusions often follow. The patient's condition rapidly deteriorates. Changes in the patient's intellect, behavior, and affect are rapid, often being obvious from week to week and sometimes from day to day. Patients with Creutzfeldt-Jakob disease eventually become completely unresponsive to stimulation, with death, usually from an infection (most often pneumonia), following.

Occasional Causes of Dementia Other progressive neurologic diseases sometimes lead to dementia, although often it is not clear if the disease causes dementia or if the dementia is the result of a different pathologic process. Patients in the late stages of amyotrophic lateral sclerosis and multiple sclerosis sometimes develop mild to moderate dementia. Brain tumors and chronic subdural hematomas may lead to dementia if they cause chronic elevation of intracranial pressure. Bacterial or viral infections of the brain (meningitis, encephalitis) may cause dementia. Dementia from tumors, hematomas, or infections often are reversible with appropriate medical or surgical intervention.

Prolonged (3 years or more) hemodialysis (usually for kidney failure) occasionally is associated with slowly progressive dementia (called *dialysis dementia*). The earliest neurologic signs typically are dysarthria, myoclonus of muscles, and seizures, with dementia developing later. At first the symptoms of dialysis dementia are confined to times immediately following dialysis sessions, but as time goes on the symptoms persist and eventually become continuous.

GENERAL CONCEPTS 10-1

* Dementia is characterized by diffuse impairment of *memory, intellect,* and *cognition,* which usually appears late in life, develops gradually, and worsens over time.

* Dementia syndromes can be divided into three major categories: *cortical dementia, subcortical dementia,* and *mixed dementia.* Impairments of *memory, intellect,* and *language* appear early in cortical dementia. *Motor impairments* appear early in subcortical dementia.

* *Parkinson's disease, Huntington's disease, progressive supranuclear palsy,* and *AIDS* are the most common causes of subcortical dementia. *Alzheimer's disease* is the most common cause of cortical dementia. *Vascular disease* sometimes causes a combination of subcortical and cortical dementia. *Pick's disease* also causes cortical dementia.

* *Pick's disease* sometimes is misdiagnosed as *Alzheimer's disease.* However, changes in personality (impulsivity, diminished social inhibitions) and deterioration of language are more common in early Pick's disease, whereas memory impairment is more common in early Alzheimer's disease.

* *Alzheimer's disease* is the single most common cause of dementia, accounting for up to 70% of all cases of dementia. *Vascular disease* is the second most common cause of dementia, accounting for 15% to 20% of all dementia.

* Alzheimer's disease is characterized by three microscopic changes in the brain: *neurofibrillary tangles, neuritic plaques,* and *granulovacuolar degeneration.* There is no effective medical treatment for Alzheimer's disease.

* The speech and language of patients in the early stages of Alzheimer's disease resembles that of patients with *anomic aphasia* (impaired word retrieval; subtle comprehension problems; fluent, syntactically correct speech). The speech and language of patients in the middle stages of Alzheimer's disease resembles that of patients with moderate *Wernicke's aphasia* (semantic paraphasias, empty and excessive speech, moderate-to-severe comprehension problems). The speech and language of patients in the late stages of Alzheimer's disease is generally nonfunctional. Comprehension of all but the simplest and most familiar material is grossly impaired, and speech consists mostly of single words and automatisms, usually devoid of meaning.

* Patients with *hydrocephalus, Creutzfeldt-Jakob disease, amyotrophic lateral sclerosis,* or *multiple sclerosis* or patients who experience prolonged *kidney dialysis* sometimes develop dementia, although these conditions account for a very small proportion of all cases of dementia.

Pseudodementia Many nondemented elderly adults become clinically depressed because of illness, physical limitations, changes in lifestyle, or social and financial difficulties. The symptoms of depression (cognitive impairments, loss of appetite, difficulty sleeping, social withdrawal, apathy) may mimic those of dementia (a condition called *pseudodementia*). Elderly depressed adults may experience memory disturbance, confusion, and attentional impairments, which may mimic signs of true dementia. Accurate and timely diagnosis of depression in elderly adults is crucial because medications and psychotherapeutic intervention often lessen or eliminate the depressive symptoms. Ripich and Ziol (1998) offered the following diagnostic guidelines for discriminating pseudodementia from true dementia:

- Pseudodementia has an identifiable onset, with rapid symptom development. Dementia has insidious and gradual onset with slow symptom development.
- Patients with pseudodementia make little effort to perform clinical tests. Patients with true dementia (in early stages) try hard to prove themselves adequate on tests.
- The test performance of patients with pseudodementia is highly variable from test to test and day to day, even on tests of equivalent difficulty. The test performance of patients with true dementia is consistent across tasks and test occasions.

Several rating scales and questionnaires have been developed to assess the presence and severity of depression in elderly adults. The *Geriatric Depression Scale* (Brink & associates, 1982; Sheikh & Yesavage, 1986) may be useful for estimating the severity of depression in normal elderly adults or adults with mild dementia. The long form consists of 30 questions related to feelings and mood ("Are you basically satisfied with your life?" "Do you often feel helpless?" "Do you frequently worry about the future?"). The short form consists of 15 questions taken from the long form. The long form permits users to categorize respondents as *normal, mildly depressed,* or *severely depressed* based on the number of answers suggesting depression. The short form permits users to categorize respondents as *normal* or *suggestive of depression.* Because the *Geriatric Depression Scale* requires the potentially depressed person to reliably answer questions it is not suitable for persons with moderate or severe dementia and it may not be suitable for persons with mild dementia who deny feelings of depression.

The *Cornell Scale for Depression in Dementia* (Tueth, 1995; Table 10-3) is better suited for documenting depressive signs in patients with dementia because it uses family member or caregiver ratings. The ratings are based on the family member's or caregiver's observations during the week prior to the rating.

The 19 signs of the Cornell Scale (Table 10-3) provide a useful list of signs likely to be associated with depression in older adults.

Delirium and Dementia Delirium (sometimes called *confusional state*) is a (usually transient) condition in which a person experiences confusion, disordered thinking, disorientation, agitation, hyperactivity, distractibility, and sometimes delusions and hallucinations—symptoms that cannot be accounted for by a pre-existing dementia. The onset of delirium usually is rapid, taking place within hours to a few days. Delirium can be caused by the following:

- Medications (especially antidepressants, antipsychotics, anxiolytics)
- Infections
- Metabolic disorders
- Surgery, anesthesia
- Substance withdrawal (e.g., alcohol, cocaine, barbiturates)
- Kidney or liver disease
- Toxins (e.g., heavy metals, food poisoning)

Delirium in elderly adults sometimes follows sudden environmental changes (changes in surroundings, location, activities, caregivers), but by far the most common cause of delirium in elderly adults is medications. Delirium should be suspected whenever elderly adults who are taking medications suddenly become confused, especially if the patient's medication regimen has changed recently.

Although the behavioral manifestations of delirium may resemble those of dementia, rapid onset and rapid progression of symptoms, the presence of delusions or hallucinations, and the presence of identifiable precipitants should point to a diagnosis of delirium. Delirium may, however, appear in adults with pre-existing dementia. Whenever an adult with confirmed dementia suddenly exhibits rapid worsening of intellect, behavior, and personality, the patient's history should be examined to rule out delirium

T A B L E   1 0 - 3

Cornell Scale for Depression in Dementia

Mood-Related Signs	Score*			
Anxiety (anxious expression, ruminations, worrying)	a	0	1	2
Sadness (sad expression, sad voice, tearfulness)	a	0	1	2
Lack of reactivity to pleasant events	a	0	1	2
Irritable, easily annoyed, short-tempered	a	0	1	2
Behavioral Disturbance				
Agitation (restlessness, hand wringing, hair pulling)	a	0	1	2
Retardation (slow movements, slow speech, slow reactions)	a	0	1	2
Loss of interest (less involved in activities in past 1 month)	a	0	1	2
Multiple physical complaints	a	0	1	2
Physical Signs				
Loss of appetite (eats less than usual)	a	0	1	2
Weight loss (score 2 if greater than 5 pounds in 1 month)	a	0	1	2
Lack of energy (fatigues easily, does not sustain activities—acute change in less than 1 month)	a	0	1	2
Cyclic Functions				
Diurnal mood variation (symptoms worse in morning)	a	0	1	2
Difficulty falling asleep (later than usual)	a	0	1	2
Multiple awakenings from sleep	a	0	1	2
Awakens earlier than usual	a	0	1	2
Ideational Disturbance				
Suicidal thoughts (life not worth living, suicidal wishes, suicide attempts)	a	0	1	2
Self-deprecation (self-blame, poor self-esteem, feelings of failure)	a	0	1	2
Pessimism (anticipates the worst)	a	0	1	2
Mood congruent delusions (delusions of poverty, illness, or loss)	a	0	1	2

Total Score (>7 = Probable Depression)

Data from Tueth, M. J. (1995). How to manage depression and psychosis in Alzheimer's disease. *Geriatrics, 50,* 43-49.
*a, unable to evaluate; 0, absent; 1, mild or intermittent; 2, severe.

or the occurrence of another pathologic event such as stroke.

IDENTIFYING CORTICAL DEMENTIA

Identifying the subtle signs of early-stage cortical dementia is a challenge. Patients in the early stages of cortical dementia rarely have motor impairments, and they do not exhibit overt signs of mental decline that point unequivocally to a diagnosis of dementia. They usually arrive at the medical facility with vague complaints of forgetfulness, mental slowing, apathy, depression, fatigue, and similar nonspecific symptoms. The reports of family members often are not helpful in diagnosing dementia because family members tend to focus on the most disruptive alterations in the patient's behavior and overlook the subtle signs of cognitive decline that signal the beginning of dementia.

Identifying cortical dementia in its beginning stages requires comprehensive testing to detect subtle disturbances of intellect and cognition. The most sensitive tests for detecting early cortical dementia are mentally challenging tests that require *abstraction, analysis, integration of information, reasoning,* and *problem-solving.* Highly practiced and automatic activities (counting, reciting the days of the week, reciting the alphabet) or structured tasks with highly constrained responses (confrontation naming, phrase and sentence repetition, copying) are too easy to be of much use in detecting early dementia. The most sensitive tests of language and communication are likely to be those requiring mental flexibility and creativity, such as generative naming ("Tell me all the words you can that start with the letter __."), story telling or story retelling, or comprehension of abstract or implied spoken or printed material.

Identification of middle-stage and late-stage cortical dementia usually poses no great clinical challenge to experienced practitioners. Patients in the middle and late stages of cortical dementia exhibit such striking impairments of intellect, orientation, and behavior that a careful review of the patient's history; an interview with the patient; an interview with family members and caregivers; and brief assessment of orientation, memory, and intellect usually are sufficient to confirm the presence of dementia.

One diagnostic question that occasionally confronts speech-language pathologists is whether a patient has dementia or is aphasic. Patients with early-stage cortical dementia are most likely to be confused with patients who have *anomic aphasia* because of their word-retrieval problems and their subtle comprehension impairments. Patients with middle-stage cortical dementia are most likely to be confused with patients with *Wernicke's aphasia* because of their vague, empty, paraphasic and circumlocutory speech and their significant comprehension impairments.

> Physicians and other health care personnel sometimes use the label *aphasia* in a broad sense to refer to any language impairment caused by brain damage, whether or not it is the patient's primary impairment. Speech-language pathologists use the label in a narrow sense to refer to specific patterns of language impairment disproportionate to any other cognitive or behavioral impairments the patient may have.

The key to differential diagnosis of dementia versus aphasia is administering nonverbal tests of intelligence and problem-solving. Patients with aphasia do better on nonverbal tests than on verbal ones, whereas patients with dementia perform poorly on both. Additional diagnostic help may come from knowledge of the onset and progression of symptoms. Dementia usually is insidious in onset and develops slowly, with gradual worsening from subtle impairments of memory, reasoning, and problem-solving to gross impairments of intellect, personality, and behavior. Aphasia usually is abrupt in onset and symptoms develop rapidly, peaking within a few minutes to a few hours, followed by slow improvement over weeks to years.

There are several reports in the literature of patients whose aphasia was mild at onset but slowly increased in severity with no apparent general mental decline (Duffy, 1987; Heath, Kennedy, & Kapur, 1983; Kirshner & associates, 1987; Mesulam, 1982). The label *slowly progressive aphasia* has been assigned to these patients. Slowly progressive aphasia is a poorly understood phenomenon, and apparently some patients who initially exhibit slowly progressive aphasia eventually become demented. Nevertheless, the potential existence of slowly progressive aphasia slightly diminishes the utility of rate of symptom development for differentiating dementia from aphasia.

GENERAL CONCEPTS 10-2

- The symptoms of *depression* (cognitive impairment, loss of appetite, difficulty sleeping, social withdrawal, apathy) sometimes are mistaken for symptoms of dementia. However, depression, unlike dementia, usually has an identifiable onset with rapid symptom development, patients with depression make little effort to perform on clinical tests, and the performance of patients with depression is highly variable from test to test.

- The symptoms of *delirium* (a transient confusional state) sometimes resemble symptoms of dementia. However, delirium, unlike dementia, usually has an identifiable precipitant (e.g., changes in medications, infections, metabolic disorders), symptoms appear abruptly and progress rapidly, and delusions and hallucinations are common.

- Although some of the symptoms of dementia may resemble some symptoms of *aphasia,* patients with dementia do poorly on verbal and nonverbal tests, whereas patients with aphasia do better on verbal tests than on nonverbal tests. Dementia has insidious onset and symptoms slowly worsen, whereas symptoms of aphasia appear abruptly and gradually improve.

ASSESSMENT OF PATIENTS WITH CONFIRMED DEMENTIA

Rating scales occupy a prominent place in the assessment of patients with confirmed dementia. Rating scales provide a quick but not very sensitive estimate of a patient's intellectual abilities, competence in activities of daily living, or both. Most rating scales permit the user to identify the presence of moderate to severe dementia but are insensitive to subtle intellectual decline; consequently, most are not suitable for evaluating patients with suspected early-stage dementia. Detecting the subtle signs of early dementia requires standardized, sensitive, and reliable tests of cognitive and linguistic performance administered by a specialist trained in their administration and interpretation.

Most rating scales require little or no specialized training to complete and can be completed after observing the patient and interviewing family members and caregivers. More than a dozen scales for rating dementia severity have been published, of which six or eight are in fairly general use. Two popular rating scales are the *Blessed Dementia Scale* (BDS; Blessed, Tomlinson, & Roth, 1968) and the *Global Deterioration Scale* (GDS; Reisberg & associates, 1982).

The *Blessed Dementia Scale* uses information obtained from family members, caregivers, and the patient's medical record to estimate the patient's ability to get along in daily life activities. The BDS has two sections (Table 10-4). In one section the patient's performance of eight daily life activities is rated. In the other section 14 aspects of the patient's behavior and personality are rated. For some items (eating, dressing, sphincter control) the severity of the patient's impairments, as well as their presence, is rated. Increasing scores on the BDS represent increasing severity of impairment. The maximum possible score is 28. Patients scoring below 4 are considered unimpaired; scores of 4 to 9 represent mild impairment; and scores of 10 or higher represent moderate to severe impairment (Eastwood, Lautenschlaeger, & Corbin, 1983).

The *Global Deterioration Scale* permits users to assign patients to one of seven levels representing increasing severity of intellectual impairment (Table 10-5). The GDS is completed by a clinician after interviewing the patient, family members, and caregivers. Ratings are based on general descriptions of behavior provided in the GDS, and, because few patients are likely to match precisely the descriptions provided, raters must use subjective judgment and intuition to arrive at a rating. The GDS provides for relatively coarse estimates of intellectual level. However, it covers a wide range of levels of impairment and ratings are easy to make and fairly reliable. Consequently, it occupies a place in rating dementia similar to the place occupied by the *Rancho Los Amigos Scale of Cognitive Levels* (Hagen & Malkamus, 1979) for rating cognitive functioning following traumatic brain injury.

T A B L E 1 0 - 4	
Blessed Dementia Scale	
Feature	**Score**
Changes in Performance of Everyday Activities	
1. Unable to perform household tasks	1
2. Unable to cope with small sums of money	1
3. Unable to remember short lists of items (e.g., in shopping)	1
4. Unable to find way about indoors	1
5. Unable to find way about familiar streets	1
6. Unable to interpret surroundings	1
7. Unable to recall recent events	1
8. Tends to dwell in the past	1
Changes in Habits	
9. Eating	
Messily with spoon only	1
Simple solids (e.g., biscuits)	2
Has to be fed	3
10. Dressing	
Occasionally misplaced buttons, etc.	1
Wrong sequence, commonly forgetting items	2
Unable to dress	3
11. Sphincter control	
Occasional wet beds	2
Frequent wet beds	2
Doubly incontinent	3
12. Increased rigidity	1
13. Increased egocentricity	1
14. Impairment of regard for feelings of others	1
15. Coarsening of affect	1
16. Impairment of emotional control	1
17. Hilarity in inappropriate situations	1
18. Diminished emotional responsiveness	1
19. Sexual misdemeanor (appearing first in old age)	1
20. Relinquished hobbies	1
21. Diminished initiative or growing apathy	1
22. Purposeless hyperactivity	1

From Blessed, G., Tomlinson, B. E., & Roth, M. (1968). The association between quantitative measures of dementia and senile change in the cerebral gray matter of elderly subjects. *British Journal of Psychiatry, 114,* 791-811.
The presence of a characteristic receives the indicated score. The total score is used to judge the severity of depression.

T A B L E 1 0 - 5

Stages of the *Global Deterioration Scale* and clinical characteristics of patients at each stage

GDS stage	Clinical phase	Clinical characteristics
1. No cognitive decline	Normal	No complaints of memory impairment. No evidence of memory impairments in the clinical interview.
2. Very mild cognitive decline	Forgetfulness	Subjective complaints of memory impairment, such as forgetting where one has placed familiar objects or forgetting formerly well-known names. No objective evidence of memory impairment in the clinical interview. No objective impairment in work or social situations. Patient is appropriately concerned with regard to symptoms.
3. Mild cognitive decline	Early confusional	The patient exhibits the first obvious impairments. Exhibits more than one of the following: (1) The patient gets lost when traveling to an unfamiliar location. (2) Co-workers are aware of patient's impairments. (3) Family or caregivers note word-retrieval and naming impairments. (4) The patient does not remember information from recently read printed material. (5) The patient has unusual difficulty in remembering names on introduction to new people. (6) The patient loses or misplaces items of value. (7) Attentional impairments are obvious in clinical testing. Objective evidence of the patient's memory impairment is observable only with an intensive interview conducted by a trained professional. The patient exhibits impaired performance in demanding work and social situations. The patient begins to deny impairments and exhibits mild to moderate anxiety.
4. Moderate cognitive decline	Late confusional	The patient exhibits obvious impairments in a careful clinical interview. Impairments consist of: (1) diminished knowledge of current and recent events, (2) mild impairment in giving personal history, (3) attentional impairments on difficult tasks, and (4) impaired ability to travel, handle personal finances, and so on. The patient usually has minimal or no impairments in: (1) orientation to time and person, (2) recognition of familiar persons and faces, and (3) ability to travel to familiar locations.
5. Moderately severe cognitive decline	Early dementia	The patient can no longer survive without assistance from others. In a clinical interview the patient cannot provide major, relevant, current information (such as their address or telephone number, the names of close members of their family, the name of the high school or college from which they graduated). The patient frequently exhibits some disorientation to time (date, day, season) or place. The patient knows his or her own name and usually knows the names of spouse and children. They eat and toilet themselves unassisted but may need assistance in choosing what to wear.
6. Severe cognitive decline	Middle dementia	These patients occasionally may forget the name of their spouse or primary caregiver. The patient is largely unaware of recent events and experiences, but retains sketchy knowledge of his or her past life. The patient generally is disoriented to time and place. The patient usually requires assistance with activities of daily living and may be incontinent. The patient may retain the ability to travel to familiar locations but cannot travel to unfamiliar locations without assistance. The patient remembers his or her own name and recognizes familiar persons. Personality and emotional changes become obvious, and may include: (1) Delusional behavior. They may accuse their spouse of being an imposter, talk to imaginary persons, or talk to their own image in the mirror. (2) Obsessive behavior, such as continual repetition of a simple cleaning activity. (3) Anxiety, agitation, and occasional violent behavior. (4) Loss of willpower because the patient cannot maintain thought long enough to determine a purposeful course of action.
7. Very severe cognitive decline	Late dementia	The patient loses all verbal ability. Speech may consist only of grunting. The patient is incontinent of urine and requires assistance with eating and toileting. The patient loses the ability to walk. Generalized neurologic signs and symptoms are obvious.

Modified from Reisberg, B., Ferris, S. H., DeLeon, M. J., & associates. (1982). The global deterioration scale for assessment of primary degenerative dementia. *American Journal of Psychiatry, 139,* 1136-1139.

ASSESSING LANGUAGE AND COMMUNICATION IN PATIENTS WITH DEMENTIA
Comprehensive Test Batteries

Speech-language pathologists make perhaps their most important contribution to management of dementia by administering standardized and reliable tests to identify the patient's communicative strengths and weaknesses and to provide dependable baseline measures against which the time-course of dementia and the effects of interventions can be assessed. Tests of language and communication supplement tests of verbal and nonverbal intelligence, tests of immediate and remote memory, and tests of attention and perception to provide a comprehensive description of the patient's impairments.

The *Arizona Battery for Communication Disorders of Dementia* (ABCD; Bayles & Tomoeda, 1991) is a clinical assessment instrument for identifying and quantifying communicative deficits of persons with dementia (specifically those caused by Alzheimer's disease). The ABCD contains four screening subtests to evaluate *speech discrimination, visual perception and literacy, visual fields,* and *visual agnosia,* plus 14 subtests to evaluate *mental status, linguistic expression, verbal memory, linguistic comprehension,* and *visuospatial construction.* The subtests in the ABCD are based on the authors' research on the language performance of 175 normal older adults and 300 adults with dementia-producing illnesses. The ABCD is standardized on 50 adults with Alzheimer's disease and 50 age-matched normal adults. Reliability and validity information and cut-off scores for normal performance are provided in the test manual. The ABCD appears to be an efficient and informative instrument for assessing communicative disabilities of persons with either suspected or confirmed dementia, and the authors report that the ABCD correlates with several other measures of dementia severity.

In-depth evaluation of the patient's *speech, language,* and *communicative abilities* may include a comprehensive aphasia test such as the *Boston Diagnostic Aphasia Examination* (Goodglass, Kaplan, & Barresi, 2001) or the *Western Aphasia Battery* (Kertesz, 1982) to measure the patient's general language abilities and to track change in language abilities over time. A test of functional communication such as *Communicative Activities in Daily Living* (Holland, Frattali, & Fromm, 1999) may be administered to estimate the patient's daily life communicative ability and to provide a baseline measure against which future changes in functional communication may be compared.

The *Western Aphasia Battery* and *Communicative Abilities in Daily Living* (Holland, 1980) have been used to evaluate communicative abilities of persons with dementia, and some normative information has been published (Appell, Kertesz, & Fishman, 1982; Fromm & Holland, 1989; Murray & associates, 1984).

Comprehension and Retention of Spoken Language

Information from a comprehensive test battery may be supplemented by the results of additional tests that sample specific speech, language, and communicative abilities. A receptive vocabulary test such as the *Peabody Picture Vocabulary Test* (Dunn & Dunn, 1981) may be administered to detect subtle changes in receptive vocabulary. Bayles & associates (1989) reported that performance on the *Peabody Picture Vocabulary Test* dependably discriminated adults with mild Alzheimer's disease from normal elderly adults.

A *delayed story retelling task,* in which the examiner tells the patient a short story then later asks the patient to retell it, may be administered to evaluate the patient's encoding, retention, and recall of verbal material. Bayles and associates (1989) reported that delayed story recall was the single most useful test for discriminating patients with mild Alzheimer's disease from normal elderly adults. On the average, normal elderly adults recalled about 96% of the information from the stories, whereas adults with mild Alzheimer's disease recalled only about 2% of the information, and adults with moderate Alzheimer's disease recalled none of the information.

A spoken-sentence comprehension test such as the *Test of Auditory Comprehension of Language* (Carrow-Woodfolk, 1999) or a sentence-comprehension subtest from an aphasia test battery may help detect sentence-level comprehension impairments, although most early-stage dementia patients are likely to have difficulty only on syntactically complex items. A test of discourse comprehension such as the *Discourse Comprehension Test* (Brookshire & Nicholas, 1993) may estimate the patient's comprehension and short-term retention of directly and indirectly stated main ideas and details from spoken stories. Patients with mild dementia are likely to have difficulty with implied details, are likely to have minor difficulty with stated details, and have little difficulty with main ideas either stated or implied. As a patient's dementia progresses, deficient performance is likely to extend to main ideas, with implied main ideas affected first.

Speech Production

A generative naming test may be administered to evaluate the patient's mental flexibility and attention. The most sensitive generative naming tests for patients in the early stages of dementia are those in which the patient is asked to provide examples of a given semantic category (e.g., animals, fruits) in a fixed time interval (usually 1 minute). Patients in the early stages of dementia usually do better on generative naming tests in which they provide words beginning with a given letter than on category-membership tests, although performance on beginning-letter tests declines as patients' dementia progresses (Butters & associates, 1987).

The *Boston Naming Test* (Kaplan, Goodglass, & Weintraub, 2001) may be administered to evaluate the patient's confrontation naming. The *Boston Naming Test* is sensitive to early-stage dementia patients' word-retrieval impairments and disturbed visual recognition. Performance on the *Boston Naming Test* usually is superior to performance on generative naming tests for patients at early and middle stages of dementia. (Most patients with late-stage dementia are unable to perform either test.)

A sample of connected speech elicited by asking the patient to describe a pictured scene such as the "cookie theft" picture from the *Boston Diagnostic Aphasia Examination* (Goodglass, Kaplan, & Barresi, 2001) provides information about the patient's ability to make sense of a pictured situation and to formulate and produce a cohesive and topically relevant narrative. Patients who are in the early stages of dementia may exhibit word-retrieval failures, insert tangential comments, and have difficulty staying on topic. As patients progress into the middle stages, word-retrieval failures become more common, neologisms appear, and gross failures to maintain a coherent topic and to convey a central theme become evident. By the late stages of dementia, patients' responses contain little more than automatisms, stereotypic words and phrases, and tangential and irrelevant comments. The following transcripts trace the decline in a dementia patient's connected speech as Alzheimer's dementia progresses.

At diagnosis:

C: Now, Mrs. ___, I'd like you to tell me what's going on in this picture.

P: Well, there's a woman . . . a mother . . . she's managing the . . .she's drying the dishes, but she isn't . . . she doesn't know that the sink is too full and it's flouting . . . no . . . it's drailing or going onto the floor. She'll notice it when her feet get wet, I guess. And behind her there there's two kids, a boy and a girl. The boy is up on a bench . . . a chair . . . that's not it but you know what I mean. And the one there is going to tip over and the girl is laughing about it and it looks like the top one there was stealing cookies while the mother is off lost in space. The mother. She's dishing the dishes. Is that what you mean?

C: That's it. Thank you very much.

Early stage, approximately 3 years post-diagnosis:

C: Now, Mrs. ___, I'd like you to tell me what's going on in this picture.

P: I don't care for this one. Can we do a different one?

C: Let's do this one. It's one of my favorites. I hope you don't mind.

P: Well, all right. If you like it. What was it again?

C: Tell me what's going on in this picture.

P: Well, there's a woman there and she's up to something. She's not looking at that other there, and I don't know why it's going and going and going and she's never mind and they must have had a meal or a dinner or something, and she's up to. . . dishes. Dishes and dishes. I wouldn't know. . . Is that it?

C: Can you tell me anything more?

P: Well there's these here little ones. A boy and a sister. Little urchins, or scapegoats. He's up to it and she's laughing and laughing and all that and I guess they must be playing some sort of game or contest or something but it's not clear to me why and their mama doesn't look like she's in the game or anything and that's about all I have to say about that.

C: Thank you. That was perfect.

Middle stage, approximately 5 years post-diagnosis:

C: Now, Mrs. ___, I'd like you to tell me what's going on in this picture.

P: This looks like an indeling one. A real American art machine.

C: Can you tell me what's happening there?

P: Yes I can. They're so scabble-de-goo that I wonder what all will come of it. They don't have the sense that God gave a goose if you ask me and I don't know why that other one there is not in the measure of this one but it doesn't matter because this one here is laughing and playing and I don't know why you never know about them these days. But anyway, if they were for me, I'd have to squelge and anoint that one there because I can't stand it when there's such chess and mirvir. Is that what you mean?

C: Thank you. That's exactly what I mean.

Late stage, approximately 9 years post-diagnosis:

C: Now, Mrs. ___, here's a picture that tells a story. Look at it and tell me what's happening in this picture.

P: Never mind.

C: Can you tell me what's happening here?

P: I said never mind.

C: Mrs. ____, can you do me a big favor? Tell me what's happening here.

P: Oh, all right. It looks like somebody lost the way and was the other way. Not under and over, but imbulation.

C: Can you tell me anything more?

P: That's the usual something for under and over. And that's all.

C: Thank you very much. You did fine.

According to Bayles and associates (1989) the best combination of tests for discriminating adults with mild dementia from normal elderly adults are the following:

- Delayed story retelling
- Mental status (orientation to time, place, person, and general knowledge)
- Pantomime expression
- The *Peabody Picture Vocabulary Test*

All of these are included in the *Arizona Battery for Communication Disorders of Dementia.*

GENERAL CONCEPTS 10-3

- *Rating scales* provide a quick but not very sensitive way to identify the presence of moderate-to-severe dementia. Detecting mild dementia requires sensitive and reliable tests of cognitive and linguistic performance administered by a qualified professional.

- The *Arizona Battery for Communication Disorders of Dementia* is a standardized assessment battery for identifying and quantifying the communicative impairments of adults with dementia. Aphasia test batteries and standardized tests of speech, language, and comprehension may be administered to obtain detailed information about the language and communicative abilities of adults with dementia.

• The most sensitive tests for detecting early dementia are tests that require *effortful mental processing.* Bayles and associates reported that the best combination of tests for detecting mild dementia is *delayed story retelling, mental status, pantomime expression,* and the *Peabody Picture Vocabulary Test.*

HELPING PATIENTS AND FAMILIES COPE WITH DEMENTIA

The progressive nature of irreversible dementia rules out restoration of lost abilities as a practical clinical objective for most patients with dementia. As the dementia patient's neurologic condition deteriorates, mental functions inevitably decline. Efforts at restoring a dementia patient's declining intellectual capacities are no match for the implacable loss of neuronal function taking place within the patient's brain. The clinical effort becomes a tenacious holding action in which the advancing effects of the patient's neurologic disease are lessened by helping the patient, caregivers, and family members counteract the effects of the disease. The clinical objectives of intervention are to *minimize the disruptive effects of the dementia* on the patient, caregivers, and family members; to *ensure the patient's safety;* to *keep the patient healthy;* and to *provide support and direction* for the patient, caregivers, and family members. Reaching these objectives requires the coordinated efforts of professionals in several disciplines, including medicine, nursing, speech-language pathology, occupational therapy, recreational therapy, physical therapy, neuropsychology, clinical psychology, social work, and dietetics, plus the patient, family members, and caregivers.

Experiencing Dementia: The Patient and the Family

The magnitude and the nature of the problems, stresses, and issues faced by the family inexorably increase as the patient's intellectual and behavioral dysfunction progress from annoying to enervating. Clinicians who intend to provide appropriate and effective care for dementia patients and their families must understand what the patient and the family experience as the patient's dementia progresses. Only by matching clinical efforts with the needs of the patient, family members, and caregivers can clinicians provide the best and most effective care for patients who struggle with dementia and for those who share that struggle with the patient.

The first symptoms of dementia usually are subtle and may be overlooked by the family. The patient becomes forgetful, irritable, and inattentive but remains oriented and socially appropriate. The first symptoms of dementia may be interpreted by family members as depression, stubbornness, or normal aging. As the patient's gradual decline continues, family members may remain unaware that something ominous is happening until the patient's deteriorating intellect and changing behavior begin to interfere seriously with family life.

As the family's concern deepens, they seek professional help in finding out what is wrong. The diagnosis of dementia almost always begins a time of intense stress for the patient and family members, during which counseling and support for the patient and family is crucial. The patient often goes through a time of frustration and anger about what has been lost, combined with worry and anxiety about the future. As time goes on, the patient may become depressed and apathetic and withdraw from family and friends, with intervals of self-imposed social isolation punctuated by angry outbursts over trivial incidents. The patient needs help in dealing with feelings of grief and anger about what is happening, help with diffuse anxiety about the future, and a plan for coping with the future. The family needs information about what is happening to the patient and about the probable course of the patient's illness. The family, like the patient, needs help in dealing with the grief, anger, and anxiety that almost invariably follow the diagnosis.

During the very early stages of dementia, most of the patient's symptoms are inconveniences, and families often spontaneously adapt to them. They no longer permit the patient to

---

Interview with the wife of a patient with early Alzheimer's dementia

It took us a while to realize what was happening. George was always real easygoing, you know. Nothing got under his skin. Then—it must have been a year or so ago—little things started to set him off. Like—this is the first one I remember— one morning when George got up we were out of coffee. He had gone to the store the day before and forgot to get coffee, though he knew we were out. Well, anyway—when things like that happened he usually would just shrug it off, you know—like ordinarily he would have just gone to the store to get more coffee. But this time he got really ticked off. He was slamming cupboard doors and swearing—which was really strange, because George never used profanity—and he started yelling at me and telling me I was no good. Finally I just left him there in the kitchen and walked over to the neighbors and when I came back about an hour later, George was all settled down and he had gone out and got the coffee.

That's the first real incident I recall, but as I think back there were other times before that. Little things—nothing dramatic. Like he'd always been a real reader. A book a week. And he stopped doing that. And he'd forget things. Like the grandkids coming over for the day. And he seemed to have lost interest in socializing with our friends. But what really got me to thinking something was really wrong was when he started thinking the neighbors were spying on him. He'd close all the blinds so they couldn't see in and I'd come by and open them up again. But next time I'd come by the blinds would be closed again. Then he started threatening to confront the neighbors about their spying. And so I took him to see Dr. Wells and he did some tests and suggested we make an appointment at the university. And so we went there, and that's when we found out that George probably had Alzheimer's.

---

run errands unaccompanied because they discover that the patient tends to get lost. They take away the patient's car keys because they sense that impaired judgment and slow reactions place the patient and other drivers in danger. They gradually assume the patient's responsibilities for shopping, paying bills, and housecleaning and take over the patient's legal and financial affairs. They shape family routines around the patient's eccentricities. If the patient lives alone, the family keeps track of the patient with frequent telephone calls and visits, but gradually the family is forced to assume more and more responsibility for the patient, until they decide that the patient must move in with a family member. This decision often is precipitated by a dramatic incident (the patient may start a fire by leaving a stove or iron unattended, may get lost and be picked up by the police, or may enter neighbors' houses uninvited).

As the patient's dementia progresses the patient's lapses of memory increase in frequency and duration until they constitute a profound impairment in storing and retrieving new information. The patient begins to neglect self-care and has to be reminded, cajoled, or nagged to bathe, keep clothing clean, and maintain oral hygiene. Progressive impairments in judgment, attention, and memory put the patient and others at risk when the patient uses gas stoves, ovens, power tools, ladders, or machinery. The patient becomes progressively more anxious, depressed, and irritable and withdraws from interactions with family members and others. Periodic violent emotional outbursts may occur. The patient takes frequent naps during the day and wakes up and wanders about during the night. For some patients the wake-sleep cycle is reversed, and the patient sleeps all day and is awake all night. Some patients become indifferent to food and fail to maintain adequate caloric and fluid intake without supervision. Others become gluttonous, eating continuously and indiscriminately unless they are supervised.

> ## Interview with the wife of a patient with middle-stage Alzheimer's disease
>
> Well, it's pretty much like living with a stranger. Actually a child who's also a stranger. But a child remembers things, and you can reason with a child. That's not true with Harry any more. He doesn't remember and when you remind him he blows his top. He blames me for all the problems and that hurts. And Jim and Nancy [son and daughter] think I'm exaggerating because when they come over, Harry gets on his best behavior and he's very good at covering up when he wants to. Then as soon as they leave he's back to his old self again. They notice that Harry forgets things and that a lot of times what he says doesn't make sense, but they say that's just normal aging. So I'm not getting much support from them. Sometimes I just think, "Oh what's the use!"

During the middle stages of dementia the patient and family members must cope with the patient's increasingly severe mental impairments and the disruptive effects of the impairments on family relationships and routines. Family members are distressed by the patient's increasing mental impairments and unpredictable changes in mood. Family members may be angry and resentful about the burden that has been imposed on them, although they are unlikely to openly express or acknowledge their anger and resentment and may feel guilty about their feelings. Family relationships and routines are disrupted as caregivers become increasingly responsible for the patient and are forced to neglect other activities and responsibilities.

As the patient's deterioration progresses and the patient's appreciation of reality declines, the patient's depression and apathy may give way to hyperactivity, wandering, and stereotypic repetitive behaviors. The patient can no longer be left alone and requires continuous supervision. Family members take responsibility for bathing the patient and supervising the patient's oral hygiene. When incontinence develops, the burden of caring for the patient escalates. Additional deterioration often brings verbal abusiveness, aggressiveness, and episodes of threatened or actual physical violence, further disrupting family relationships and increasing family members' anger, resentment, and guilt.

This phase of the patient's illness requires continuing education, support, and therapy for the family. Family members need education about why the patient behaves disruptively and about how disruptive behaviors can be controlled or eliminated. Family members need help in setting up a safe, predictable, and stable environment for the patient. They may need help in dividing caregiving responsibilities among family members, and they may need encouragement and direction in taking advantage of respite-care and day-care services and support groups. As the burden of caring for the patient escalates, family members need help in planning for and accomplishing placement in an extended-care facility (nursing home). Throughout this phase of the patient's illness family members need help in dealing with their feelings of resentment, anger, apprehension, and guilt; guilt becomes especially prominent as the family begins to contemplate the patient's placement in an extended-care facility.

Most dementia patients are cared for at home until the burden becomes intolerable, at which time the patient is placed in a nursing home. The period of at-home care may range from 1 or 2 to 10 or 15 years, depending on how rapidly the patient's dementia progresses and on the family's tolerance for the disruptions caused by the patient's dementia.

Most demented patients spend their last years in an extended-care facility. Although the physical burden of caring for the patient has been alleviated by extended-care placement, the emotional burden carried by family mem-

---

Interview with the husband of a patient with late-stage Alzheimer's disease

(Interviewer: What led you to place Mrs. Baxter in a nursing home?)

Well, it was probably several things. Things were just gradually getting worse and I was getting near the end of my rope. She'd get up in the middle of the night and roam around. We had to put key locks—the ones you can lock from inside with a key—on all the doors going outside to keep her from getting out of the house in the middle of the night. And she was having accidents—wetting herself and now and then messing herself. But I could handle that. Then one day I came home and she was asleep on the couch and the house was full of smoke. She had put a loaf of bread in a plastic bag in the oven and set the oven as high as it would go. Then she must have forgot about it and took a nap. The oven was a terrible mess—we were lucky it didn't start a fire. So the kids and I sat down and talked things over and we decided that she should go to a home where she could be supervised 24 hours a day. She had become a danger to herself and to others. It was the hardest thing I've ever done in my life but it had to be done. It's the best thing for her and for me and for the family. I still feel guilty about it though.

---

bers continues, often augmented by feelings of guilt over abandoning the patient to the care of strangers and by feelings of loss that accompany the patient's departure from home. As the patient's physical condition becomes more fragile, family members are faced with decisions about whether heroic measures should be used to sustain the patient's life. During this time family members need continuing help in resolving their often conflicting feelings about their own needs and their obligations to the patient and in making decisions about when and how to end procedures for prolonging the patient's life.

The patient's death does not end the family's need for advice, support, and reassurance. The period of mourning following the death of the demented family member may be brief, perhaps because the family has been mentally preparing for the patient's demise for months or years. Although the mourning period may be short, the grief felt by family members may be intense, owing perhaps to the release of emotional tensions that have built up over years of the patient's illness. Professional counseling and support during this period may help family members acquire knowledge and understand their feelings and their reactions to what they have been through and may help them reconstruct and repair family relationships that have been damaged or distorted by the pressures of caring for the demented patient.

MANAGEMENT ISSUES
Early Stages

Memory Impairments Memory impairments characteristically are the first and most troublesome of the patient's early symptoms. These early memory impairments typically affect *declarative memory* (memory for the past, such as the names of children or yesterday's visit by a family member) and *prospective memory* (remembering to do things at specific times, such as keeping an appointment or bringing in the mail). Early-stage dementia usually does not affect *procedural memory* (how to do things, such as how to make coffee with a drip coffee maker), at least for procedures that are well practiced and not too complex. Impaired declarative memory is most annoying to early-stage dementia patients; impaired prospective memory is most annoying to their caregivers.

> Attentional impairments may interfere with early-stage dementia patients' completion of well-remembered procedures. Patients who are interrupted or distracted while performing a remembered procedure may forget where they were in the procedure and may either start again from the beginning or abandon the procedure in confusion.

> I'll tell her something and she's saying "yes-yes" and then 10 minutes later she's acting like I never said it. I don't think she pays enough attention. I tell her to listen and even have her say it back to me. She'll do it but then later on it's like it never happened. Sometimes I think she's just trying to get my goat.

A patient with early-stage dementia may forget to bring the groceries in from the car on returning from a shopping trip, but if reminded, the patient has little difficulty carrying out the procedures involved in bringing the groceries in and putting them away. However, the early-stage dementia patient may do the following:

- Forget the grocery list, forget to consult the shopping list when at the store, or misplace the list while shopping.
- Forget the names of brands customarily purchased and return home with other brands.
- Retrace a route down aisles previously taken and place items in the shopping cart that duplicate items previously placed there. (But the patient is unlikely to forget the shopping procedure—such as pushing the cart down the aisles and placing items in the cart, taking the items to the checkout counter.)
- At home the next day, forget having purchased the groceries and may return to the store and purchase the same list of groceries.

It is not unusual for caregivers to feel that a patient's memory lapses can be resolved if the patient would just try harder. They may badger the patient with well-intentioned but inappropriate admonitions to remember important items and may drill the patient on the information, not understanding that neither admonitions nor drills are solutions. Caregivers can help the patient cope with memory impairments by maximizing the orderliness and predictability of the patient's living environment (more on this later).

GENERAL CONCEPTS 10-4

- In the early stages of dementia, the patient's memory lapses, personality changes, and behavioral changes are primarily inconveniences, and caregivers usually find ways to adapt to them or to work around them, often with professional guidance. As the patient's dementia progresses, caregiver burden increases as troublesome behaviors become more frequent, the patient begins to neglect self-care, and the patient's impaired judgment place the patient and others at risk. Eventually caregiver burden becomes intolerable, at which time the patient is likely to be transferred to an extended-care facility.
- *Memory impairments* usually are the first symptoms of Alzheimer's dementia. The impairments typically affect *declarative memory* and *prospective memory* but largely spare *procedural memory.* As dementia progresses, memory impairments become more profound until all aspects of memory are grossly impaired in the very late stages of dementia.

Impaired Language and Communication
Patients in the early stages of dementia usually have sufficient language comprehension and speech to manage routine daily-life situations. However, subtle attention and memory impairments compromise the patient's retention of spoken or printed materials. The patient's comprehension deteriorates in noisy and distracting environments or when several people are talking, and intermittent word-retrieval failures create annoying gaps in the patient's output, although they

do not seriously interfere with communication. Patients in the early stages of dementia (and their families and caregivers) need help in identifying how communication is affected by the patient's impairments, assistance in identifying the most important targets for management, help with devising strategies for working around the patient's communication impairments, and direction in putting the strategies into practice.

> The main thing I notice is how he's gotten sort of vague. Like his thinking is fuzzy or something. He's always been a very precise speaker but now he hesitates and fumbles and stumbles around. And he misses words. Like this morning when he was talking about getting the car serviced and he called the car the bathtub. . . . I think he mostly understands what people say, but sometimes he misses things. Especially if you tell him several things in a row, like what we're having for dinner or what we need from the store. I think maybe he's not paying enough attention.

Anxiety and Depression Anxiety and depression are common in patients with early-stage dementia. Anxiety typically begins as the patient senses loss of control and independence in daily life activities. The patient's anxiety is perpetuated by fear of what the future may bring, uncertainty about coping with upcoming difficult or stressful events, perception of unwanted changes in social status and interpersonal relationships, and a variety of other concerns about an uncertain future or an unsatisfactory present.

> You know, she's always been an upbeat kind of person but now it's like she's drawing into a shell. It's like she's pulled down some sort of inner curtain between herself and the world outside. Disconnected herself. She doesn't fuss or cry or things like that. Disconnected— emotionally disconnected. That's how it seems.

Behavior Change The onset of dementia typically brings with it alterations in the patient's behavior. Some become apathetic and lose interest in activities that formerly were an important part of his or her life. Others become hyperactive and seemingly unable to sit still, ceaselessly pacing about the house and engaging in ritualistic, obsessive activity (e.g., repeatedly asking the same questions, raising and lowering window shades, opening and closing drawers and cupboards).

Many patients in the early stages of dementia become irritable and easily frustrated. Minor annoyances and petty inconveniences precipitate angry outbursts and sometimes threatened or real physical aggression. Some experience exaggerated mood swings, laughing excessively at minimally amusing or neutral material or propelled into tears by innocuous events.

> She's always been pretty calm and collected. I was the one who would fly off the handle and she was the one to tell me to take it easy and calm down. But that's changed. Now it seems like she's just generally harder to get along with. Seems like she's never satisfied. She complains a lot, even about trivial things, which she never used to do. And that irritates me and we usually end up arguing, but we never seem to get things straightened out.

Denial Patients in the early stages of dementia often deny or minimize their impairments. Memory lapses are explained away, blamed on others, or denied. Impairments in reasoning, problem-solving, and sustained attention are dismissed. Denial usually arises from the patient's need to appear normal, but it annoys caregivers and complicates the patient's daily life. These patients need coaching in constructive alternatives to denial. Sometimes what seems to be denial arises from the patient's genuine confusion about the specifics of an event or a situation or by the patient's faulty memory. These patients need help with interpreting and remembering events and situations, not advice about denial.

> I think he's gotten more defensive lately. When he slips up he usually finds a way to pass it off or shift the blame. Like last week he forgot to take our bill payments to the post office. When I asked him about it he said I was the one who was supposed to take them even though I clearly remember him agreeing to do it. And just now, when we were talking to the other doctor he said he wasn't having any problems with his urine, but we both know that he's had several accidents in the last few months. I'm having to just bite my tongue and not argue with him because it doesn't do any good. But I think it's unhealthy for him to be so defensive.

Excess Disability Sometimes the functional impairments exhibited by early-stage dementia patients exceed the limitations attributable to the patient's cognitive impairments (a phenomenon called *excess disability*). Excess disability may be caused by coexisting illness, by coexisting emotional and psychologic states (e.g., anxiety or depression), by medication, or by environmental influences including how the patient is treated by caregivers. Removing or abating the causes of excess disability (treating coexisting illness or coexisting emotional and psychologic states, modifying medications, and changing the patient's environment) may have remarkable positive effects on the early-stage dementia patient's performance in activities of daily life.

Caregivers sometimes unintentionally contribute to a patient's excess disability by rewarding dependent behavior and ignoring or discouraging independent behavior. This often happens when a caregiver, frustrated by how long a patient takes to perform an activity or by how imperfectly the patient performs it, takes over an activity the patient is capable of performing. For example, a caregiver may dress the patient, take over meal planning and preparation, or arrange

vacations and outings without the patient's participation, thereby increasing the patient's dependence and contributing to the patient's sense of helplessness and incompetence.

Excess disability can be reduced by adapting daily life activities and responsibilities to the patient's ability level. The patient who can no longer independently plan meals may help caregivers plan menus. The patient who can no longer arrange a vacation may help caregivers choose where to go, how long to stay, and what to do. Including the patient with dementia in such activities helps the patient to feel competent, respected, and needed.

Sleep Disturbances Most people sleep less as they get older, and disrupted sleep patterns are particularly common in dementia. Sleep medications commonly are prescribed to normalize dementia patients' disrupted sleep-wake cycles, probably more often than necessary. Adjusting the patient's daily schedule and sleep environment may normalize the patient's sleep pattern and should be tried before medications are prescribed. Even when medications are prescribed, changes in daily schedules and in the patient's sleep environment can lower the dosage needed. Patients' sleep schedules often can be normalized by cutting back on the number of naps the patient takes during the day, ensuring that the patient goes to bed at the same time every night, ensuring that the patient gets mild exercise early in the evening, and keeping doors and windows in the patient's bedroom closed while the patient is sleeping.

> I feel tired all the time. I hardly ever get a good night's sleep because she's constantly getting up in the middle of the night and rummaging around. That wakes me up, and I have to get up and talk her back to bed. But I'm never sure she'll stay there so I lay there awake until I hear her snoring. Then it takes me a while to get back to sleep. This usually happens once or twice every night. If I could get some help with that it would really help me.

Health The mental impairments associated with dementia often disrupt the patient's normal eating and drinking habits and compromise the patient's judgment about nutrition and fluid intake. Consequently, maintaining adequate nutrition and fluid intake is an important part of the patient's general health care. Ensuring that the patient has properly fitting dentures and maintaining oral hygiene are additional important, but sometimes overlooked, aspects of patient care.

Other illnesses often accompany dementia. Diabetes, heart disease, pulmonary disease, kidney failure, and metabolic or chemical imbalances are common in both the normal and demented elderly. Patients with dementia are particularly susceptible to bacterial and viral infections; therefore, prevention and treatment of infections is an important part of a general program of healthcare. Providing hearing aids for the hard-of-hearing patient and properly fitting eyeglasses for those with impaired vision prevent sensory deprivation and contribute to the patient's constructive interaction with the environment. Providing canes, walkers, crutches, or wheelchairs provides physically impaired patients with the mobility needed to get around.

Middle Stages

When the patient enters the middle stages of dementia, impairments of memory and attention increase in severity and affect more dimensions of the patient's daily life. Ironically, the patient's awareness of the severity and extent of the impairments diminishes as the impairments become more pronounced. Caregivers are likely to be experiencing heightened feelings of loss, anxiety, anger, and hostility as the patient's impairments become more profound and the burden of management shifts increasingly to caregivers. Physical care problems now become more salient, as the patient becomes more confused, neglects self-care, sleeps less, wanders more, and perhaps experiences bowel and bladder incontinence. Incidents of hostility, verbal abuse, and actual or threatened physical violence from the patient increase in frequency. Caregivers become resigned,

despondent, and tired of coping with the patient's ever-increasing impairments and with increasingly frequent troublesome behaviors.

Troublesome Behaviors Rabins, Mace, & Lucas (1982) surveyed the families of 55 patients with irreversible dementia to find out what families considered the major problems in caring for their demented family member. The results of their survey are summarized in Figure 10-6. The five most frequently reported *trouble-*

Behavior	Mention Behavior (%)	Considered Problem (%)
Memory disturbance	100	93
Catastrophic reactions	87	89
Demanding, critical behavior	71	73
Night waking	69	59
Hiding things	69	71
Communication difficulties	68	74
Suspiciousness	63	79
Making accusations	60	82
Uncooperative at meals	60	55
Daytime wandering	59	70
Uncooperative at bathing	53	74
Hallucinations	49	42
Delusions	47	83
Physical violence	47	94
Incontinence	40	86
Unsafe cooking	33	44
Hitting	32	81
Unsafe driving	20	73
Unsafe or excessive smoking	11	67
Inappropriate sexual behavior	2	0

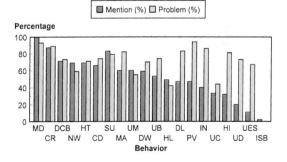

Figure 10-6 ■ **Percentage of families reporting the occurrence of problem behaviors and the percentage considering a behavior to be a problem.** (Data from Rabins, P. V., Mace, N. L., & Lucas, M. J. [1982]. The impact of dementia on the family. *Journal of the American Medical Association, 248,* 333-336.)

some behaviors were *memory disturbance, catastrophic reactions, demanding and critical behavior, night waking,* and *hiding things.* The five behaviors most frequently reported as *major problems* were *physical violence, memory disturbance, catastrophic reactions, incontinence,* and *delusions.* Every respondent reported the presence of memory failure and almost all (88%) considered it a major problem. However, fewer than half of the respondents (47%) reported the presence of physical violence, but almost all (94%) who reported it considered it a major problem. Only 11% reported unsafe or excessive smoking, but two thirds of those reporting it considered it a major problem. Clearly, the perceived importance of a troublesome behavior is not determined by its frequency of occurrence alone, but it reflects the amount of emotional stress or inconvenience the behavior causes for family members.

As the patient progresses into the middle and late stages of dementia, the patient's behavior becomes less predictable. Emotional outbursts are triggered by trifling events. The patient becomes sullen, hostile, and uncooperative for no apparent reason. The patient resists the caregiver's help with self-care, then complains that the caregiver neglects them. The patient's volatility in mood and behavior heighten caregiver stress.

> It used to be that he gave some sign that he was about to blow his top. I could see it coming, so usually I could distract him and he'd calm down. Now it seems like I never know what's going to set him off. We'll be going along okay, then, bam! He's hollering and shaking his fist at me and telling me I'm no good. I'm always walking on pins and needles. There's nothing I can do to keep the explosions from happening, and that's hard to take.

Insight, Judgment, and Orientation As patients pass into the middle stages of dementia,

problems with insight, judgment, and orientation become salient. The patient needs continual supervision. The patient's independent access to appliances, tools, the telephone, and the outdoors must be increasingly restricted. The restrictions irritate and anger the patient, who by now lacks insight into the reasons for the restrictions.

> He's always liked puttering around the house, but he got so that we couldn't trust him not to get hurt or do something that might flood or burn down the house. For example, one day he was building something out of copper pipe and he was using one of those propane torches to solder with, and he went off and got the mail and was sitting in the house looking through a magazine and the torch was sitting in the garage blazing away. Fortunately I went out in the garage and saw it, but he could have burned the house down. So now we don't let him use the torch or any of his power tools unless there's someone there to watch him. He's not at all pleased about it, but that's the way it's got to be.

> It's like a 24-hour-a-day-job. There's just no letup. It's up to me to get everything done. Get her up. Get her dressed. Make her meals. It just goes on and on. Sometimes Martha [a daughter] or Fran Elliott [a neighbor] come in and take over to give me a break. That helps. But it really wears on a person. To have total responsibility for someone else—it's like carrying this 500-pound weight around on your back, day after day. I don't resent it, and I'm not feeling sorry for myself. But sometimes I wonder if I'm strong enough. Mentally, I mean.

Physical Dependence The patient's physical dependence on caregivers steadily increases as the patient's dementia progresses. The patient no longer carries out personal care activities without assistance and must be helped with bathing, dressing, toileting, and grooming. The patient's medication regimen must be supervised carefully. Diet and fluid intake must be monitored and adjusted to ensure adequate nutrition and hydration. The patient's interest in leisure activities declines, and the caregiver becomes the patient's primary source of stimulation.

Language and Communication Communication with the patient becomes increasingly one-sided as the patient progresses into the middle stages of dementia. The patient no longer initiates conversations but becomes a passive conversational partner. The patient's responses consist primarily of trivialities and automatisms ("you don't say," "gracious sakes") or tangential comments, but the patient makes no substantive contribution to either the content or the continuity of the conversation.

> We have what you might call conversations, but there's no real connection. You know what I mean? She says things, but it's like there's nothing behind what she says. Thought-wise, I mean. She's pleasant enough, and I'm sure she's trying, but there's nothing there. No matter what we talk about, she says pretty much the same things. Empty. And like I said, no real connection.

Late Stages

Patients in the late stages of dementia are no longer capable of collaborating in programs to enhance their quality of life and maximize their participation in daily life activities. Helping patients at this stage of dementia means helping their caregivers manage troublesome behaviors, ensuring the patient's health and security, and maintaining the patient's participation in daily life activities so far as the patient's intellectual and psychologic attributes permit.

GENERAL CONCEPTS 10-5

- Patients in the early stages of Alzheimer's dementia retain sufficient language and communicative abilities to get along in daily life, although subtle problems in comprehension and word retrieval may prove annoying. As dementia progresses, comprehension impairments become more obvious, word-retrieval failures in speech become more obvious, the patient's contributions become less relevant and less efficient, and violations of communicative rules and conventions become more frequent. By the very late stages of dementia the patient has lost essentially all volitional communication.

- Many patients with dementia become anxious and depressed, first in response to the diagnosis of dementia and later in response to changes in abilities, social status, and personal relationships. Anxiety and depression often diminish as the patient's dementia progresses and the patient becomes less attuned to the environment and to personal relationships.

- Patients in the early stages of dementia often deny or minimize impairments of which they are aware. As the dementia progresses, the patient becomes less aware of impairments and consequently neither denies nor acknowledges them.

- *Troublesome behaviors* (e.g., wandering, hiding things, aggression) and *sleep disturbances* begin to appear in the early stages of dementia and increase in frequency and magnitude as the patient's dementia progresses. Troublesome behaviors add to caregiver stress in proportion to the amount of inconvenience or disruption the behaviors create. Helping caregivers manage troublesome behaviors is an important objective of intervention.

- Sometimes patients who have dementia exhibit functional impairments that exceed the limitations imposed by the patient's dementia *(excess disability)*. Excess disability can be caused by coexisting illness, emotional states, medications, and the patient's environment, including how they are treated by caregivers. Caregivers may contribute to excess disability by encouraging dependent behavior and discouraging independent behavior (usually unintentionally).

INTERVENTION

Early Stages

Intervention programs for patients in the early stages of dementia represent a three-way collaboration among the patient, the caregiver, and the clinician. Early-stage dementia patients are intensely aware of their impairments and willingly participate in programs to help them compensate for or work around their impairments. Most can identify problems they would like addressed in the intervention program and can help the clinician select intervention strategies. Caregivers participate in planning the intervention program, practice compensatory strategies with the patient, help to modify the patient's daily life environment to facilitate the patient's performance, monitor the patient's performance, and help with modifications to the intervention program as the patient's needs change. The clinician instructs the patient and caregivers about the nature of the patient's problems, helps the patient and caregivers select targets for intervention, directs the design and implementation of the intervention program, and supervises changes in the intervention program as the need arises.

Memory Impairments The problem for early-stage dementia patients is with recalling the past *(declarative memory)* and remembering to do things in the present *(prospective memory)* but not with remembering how to do familiar procedures *(procedural memory).* Their problem is *remembering that* versus *remembering how.* There are no effective procedures for directly improving dementia patients' memory, so intervention focuses on developing compensatory memory strategies, providing the patient with portable memory aids, and modifying the patient's environment to minimize the effects of the patient's memory impairments on the patient's daily life competence.

Compensatory memory strategies may be useful for some patients in the very early stages of dementia, who retain sufficient cognitive resources to remember, organize, and execute the strategies. Mental imagery or the PQRST (for *preview, question, read, state, test*) method (see Chapter 9) may help some patients whose dementia is very mild. Mnemonic strategies require too much mental effort to be useful to patients with dementia, even those whose dementia is very mild. Compensatory memory strategies may provide short-term help for mildly impaired patients but will not be retained as the patient's dementia progresses. Consequently, they are less commonly used than portable memory aids and environmental modification in managing the memory impairments of patients with dementia.

Some portable memory aids help dementia patients' prospective memory. *Electronic organizers* (personal information managers) with built-in alarms help with prospective memory by signaling the patient and displaying textual reminders of appointments and other time-based responsibilities. *Pocket-sized checklists* remind the patient of scheduled obligations, which the patient can check off when the obligations are satisfied.

Some portable memory aids help with declarative memory—usually with memory for personal information (e.g., addresses, phone numbers, names, dates). *Memory wallets* are pocket-sized booklets that may contain printed personal information, photographs of family members or familiar locations, printed sentences relating to the patient's daily life, or other personal material. Bourgeois (1990, 1992) reported that memory wallets, when combined with patient and caregiver training, improved the factual content of dementia patients' conversation and that the improvements were maintained across time. The scope and complexity of the information included in memory wallets and other portable aids can be matched to the patient's needs and abilities and can be adjusted as the patient's ability to use them changes.

Modifying the patient's daily life environment can help most patients in the early to middle stages of dementia cope with declining memory. Some environmental modifications target prospective memory:

- A schedule of activities that remains constant from day to day

- An alarm clock or an alarm watch worn by the patient set to sound when it is time to perform given activities (often accompanied by a checklist to permit the patient to keep track of which activities have been attended to)
- Checklists posted in strategic locations to remind patients to accomplish scheduled activities and to permit them to check off completed activities (e.g., checklists next to exit doors listing things the patient is to do when leaving—turn off lights, close windows, get keys)

Some environmental modifications help the patient with procedural memory:

- Items used in an activity are kept together (coffee pot, filters, and coffee are kept on the same shelf). Arranging the items in the order they are used helps some patients keep procedural steps in order.
- Checklists for complex procedures are posted where the procedure is to be accomplished. Steps in the procedure are listed in chronologic order (e.g., the steps in sorting laundry, washing, and drying are posted next to the washer).

Bourgeois (1991) identified several advantages of external memory aids for patients with dementia:

- External memory aids are useful in daily life, and their use by the patient elicits natural positive reinforcement.
- External memory aids enhance the patient's interaction with the environment by providing many opportunities for daily use.
- External memory aids can be modified to meet the changing needs of the patient or caregivers or to accommodate changes in the patient's ability to use them.
- External memory aids are tangible, permanent prompting mechanisms that are immediately accessible to the patient.

Bourgeois also commented that the best self-prompting memory aids are likely to be those the patient used before developing dementia because using the old memory aid may be in the patient's repertoire of automatic skills. Portable memory aids are useful, however, only if the patient remembers to use the aid. Consequently, their usefulness typically disappears by the time the patient is in the middle stages of dementia.

Confusion Intermittent episodes of confusion often occur during the early stages of dementia. The first episodes are frightening to the patient and worrisome to family members, although they do not seriously compromise the patient's safety or well-being. As the patient's dementia progresses and episodes of confusion increase in frequency and magnitude the episodes may threaten the patient's safety (e.g., the patient gets lost and ends up in an unsafe neighborhood, drives the wrong way down a one-way street, takes medications intended for another family member). Managing confusion is an important aspect of intervention for patients in the early stages of dementia. When confusion can no longer be managed adequately, restrictions on the patient's independence and freedom of movement become necessary. Many of the procedures for managing memory impairments also make patients less vulnerable to confusion, but strategies that focus more directly on confusion may be useful.

- A large calendar is posted in a highly visible location. The patient circles the correct day on arising in the morning. If the patient cannot remember to do this, caregivers may do it.
- The patient wears a watch that shows the date and time with AM and PM indicated.
- Doors and drawers in cabinets, dressers, and bureaus are labeled with their contents.
- The patient's personal possessions are kept in a consistent location and put back when not in use.
- Maps and printed instructions depicting familiar routes are prepared and given to the patient before the patient sets out.
- The patient carries a card on which are printed constructive responses to disorientation. *(Stop. Stay calm. Think about where you came from and where you are going. Look around for helpful cues, such as street signs and house numbers. Try retracing your path*

until you see something familiar. If you are still confused, ask someone for help.)

Every adult should carry an identification card showing the person's name, address, home telephone number, and the name of someone to notify in case of emergency. Adults with dementia should carry a card with that information, plus the names and telephone numbers of several close relatives or caregivers.

Impaired Communication Patients who are in the early stages of dementia remain functional communicators in most everyday situations, although subtle problems with word retrieval and impaired comprehension of spoken and printed materials may prove annoying to patients and caregivers. Patients in the early stages of dementia typically are acutely aware of their communicative miscues and readily cooperate with remedial programs. Patients in the early stages of dementia can learn strategies to prevent, work around, or repair communicative mishaps, provided that the strategies do not demand greater mental flexibility, creativity, attention, and memory than the patient has available.

Some communicative strategies can be characterized as *adaptive* (Clark & Witte, 1991). Adaptive strategies are used by the patient to regain control when communication failure occurs. The patient who fails to understand a spoken message might ask the speaker to repeat the message, speak more slowly, or write it. The patient who has word-finding difficulty or problems organizing speech output might ask the listener for help ("Bear with me and give me a little more time. I'm having difficulty organizing my thoughts."). The patient who loses track of the topic of a conversation might ask the conversational partner to remind them of the topic ("I seem to have lost my train of thought. What was it we were talking about?").

An appealing characteristic of adaptive behaviors such as these is that they do not strike conversational partners as abnormal because they resemble what normal adults do when they stumble in a conversation. The major hindrance to their use by early-stage dementia patients is the patient's reluctance to engage in behaviors that might mark them as impaired. Persuasion may be needed to get the patient to try the strategies, but once the patient discovers how much easier it is to use the strategies than to expend energy on concealment and to bear the consequences of communication failure, persuasion usually is no longer necessary.

Other communication strategies are *facilitative* (Clark & Witte, 1991). Facilitative strategies are used by the patient to prevent or repair communication failure. Facilitative strategies allow patients to circumvent communication breakdown caused by word-retrieval failure, comprehension impairments, and compromised ability to organize and communicate thoughts coherently. A patient who experiences word-retrieval failure might circumlocute ("I had the letter all ready to go, but I didn't have a . . . with flaps . . . you lick it and seal it . . . an envelope."), use semantic self-cueing ("My wife doesn't want me to drive so she hides the lock . . . ring . . . lock . . . keys."), or use phonemic self-cueing ("They played hard, but they lost the team . . . tame . . . game.").

Clark and Witte recommend what they call *script strategies* to help early-stage dementia patients maintain topic and cohesion within spoken discourse. The patient who uses a script strategy is trained to organize spoken discourse according to the parts of a story (theme, setting, characters, events, actions, consequences, outcomes). However, many patients with mild dementia may be overwhelmed by the terminology and the memory demands of the script strategy. Giving them a set of questions makes it easier: *What is it about? Where did it happen? Who was there? What happened? What is the point?* The questions can be printed on a card if the patient has difficulty remembering them or keeping them in order.

Clark and Witte recommend what they call *life-experience strategies* to help patients who have difficulty expressing abstract ideas. By illustrating abstract ideas with life experiences patients may convey the abstract character of their ideas without explicitly conveying the abstraction. For example, a patient who wishes to communicate the concept of trust might say, "When I was young I knew I could always depend on Mom and Dad. Even when I didn't agree with them I knew that they wanted what was best for me and would never mean to do anything to hurt me. That's an important thing to have between people."

Group Treatment Group treatment may be a useful addition to intervention programs for patients in the early stages of dementia. Rationales and procedures differ across programs but all share similar goals:

- Stimulate self-expression.
- Stimulate cognitive processes.
- Promote social interaction.
- Enhance feelings of self-worth.

Structured group activities may provide patients with a comfortable environment in which they can try out newly acquired communicative strategies. Group activities may provide patients with a supportive climate in which to talk about problems, feelings, and emotions. Group activities may provide a venue in which patients can share stories of success and failure. Group activities may enhance patients' feelings of self-esteem and self-worth by helping them feel that they are actively helping themselves and other group participants. Group activities may stimulate patients' remaining intellect by involving them in activities such as planning trips or outings, discussing problems, role-playing daily life situations, and playing games such as *password* or *twenty questions.*

GENERAL CONCEPTS 10-6

- The effects of the early-stage dementia patient's memory impairments may be lessened by teaching *compensatory memory strategies,* by providing *portable memory aids,* and by *modifying the environment* to provide prompts and cues that lessen the effects of the patient's memory impairments on the patient's daily life.

- The dementia patient's confusion can be lessened by *controlling the patient's environment* and *providing prompts and cues* to enhance orientation.
- *Adaptive* and *facilitative* communicative strategies may help early-stage dementia patients maintain communicative abilities. *Script* strategies may help early-stage dementia patients maintain topic and cohesion in discourse. *Life-experience* strategies may help early-stage dementia patients express abstract ideas.
- *Group treatment* is a common component of intervention programs for early-stage dementia patients. The goals of group treatment usually include stimulating self-expression and cognitive processes, promoting social interaction, and enhancing patient feelings of self-worth.

Middle Stages

As the patient progresses into the middle stages of dementia, caregiver burden increases. The patient becomes less able to monitor behavior and to adjust it to the needs of others. Behavioral conflicts between the patient and the caregiver increase in frequency and magnitude. The patient's ability to remember and use previously acquired compensatory strategies declines. Environmental modifications that once helped the patient compensate for impaired attention and memory lose their power. The patient's awareness of impairments declines, and the patient no longer is capable of active participation in intervention programs. Intervention goals change from helping the patient find ways to compensate for impairments to helping caregivers find ways to keep the patient physically and mentally active and oriented, to promote the patient's psychologic well-being, and to facilitate patient–caregiver communication.

Intervention now requires collaboration between the clinician and the caregiver. Caregiver and clinician work together to identify targets for intervention and to rank them in order of importance. Targets for intervention include patient behaviors that the caregiver wishes to modify or control and patient skills that the caregiver wishes to maintain or enhance.

When targets for intervention have been selected, the clinician and the caregiver work together to devise procedures to accomplish the objectives of intervention. Then the caregiver practices the procedures, and the clinician monitors and gives feedback and advice. The intervention procedures are modified and adjusted based on the caregiver's experience and are organized into a comprehensive intervention program. The caregiver puts the program into operation, and the clinician monitors the results and suggests alterations and adjustments as needed.

Environmental control becomes increasingly important as the patient is governed less and less by internal reasoning and judgment and more and more by the characteristics of the external environment. Environmental prompts and cues that previously helped the patient compensate for impairments lose their power as the patient becomes increasingly inattentive to the prompts and cues and becomes increasingly distracted by incidental stimuli. Maintaining environmental control requires intensification of stimuli that govern the patient's behavior. Environmental cues are made more striking. Color and attention-getting graphics are added to checklists, posters, signs, and calendars. Caregivers increasingly direct the patient's attention toward environmental prompts and cues.

As the patient's ability to remember and use adaptive and compensatory strategies declines, intervention focuses on preserving the patient's use of the most effective strategies. The remaining strategies may be simplified and more powerful external cues may be incorporated to keep them within the patient's repertoire.

As the patient's impairments become more pronounced, supervision increases and the patient's independence in risky activities is curtailed. Control of major financial decisions may be assumed by caregivers, but the patient may be permitted freedom to make routine and innocuous financial decisions (e.g., spending on incidental self-care items, personal clothing) in consultation with caregivers.

Managing Troublesome Behaviors
Caregivers for patients in the middle and late stages of dementia face numerous problems related to the patient's declining intellect, exaggerated mood swings, and changes in behavior. Although the decline in the patient's abilities cannot be arrested or reversed, the effects of the patient's intellectual impairments can be minimized, the patient's mood swings can be diminished, and distressing behaviors often can be controlled or eliminated by environmental manipulation and behavior management techniques similar to those used with traumatically-brain-injured adults.

Combative, aggressive, and accusatory behaviors rank high on caregivers' lists of problems as the patient reaches the middle stages of dementia. Caregivers are better equipped to manage the patient's problem behaviors if they understand that emotional outbursts, combativeness, and physical attacks often are predictable based on previous incidents, that they frequently are preceded by warning signs, and that they often represent the patient's response to being pushed beyond their ability to deal with a situation or event. Many times such outbursts can be eliminated by removing their precipitating stimuli.

A man with dementia became violently angry when he saw his wife paying the monthly bills, perhaps because he felt that she was usurping his role as head of the household. The wife realized what precipitated her husband's outbursts and began paying the bills while her husband took his usual morning nap. This change in routine eliminated the outbursts.

Warning signs can be diverse and tend to be idiosyncratic. They range from subtle signs such as increased body rigidity, aversion of gaze, or increased respiration rate to more obvious behaviors such as crying and arguing. Teaching caregivers to recognize such warning signs and to respond to them by slowing the pace of the activity, doing something else, or diverting the patient's attention can reduce the frequency of such outbursts.

If caregivers understand that the demented patient's outbursts may be an involuntary response to demanding or too-difficult situations, their responses to the outbursts are likely to change in constructive ways. They are less likely to regard the patient as stubborn and uncooperative and less likely to see the patient's emotional outbursts as a personal affront. They are more likely to look for what pushed the patient out of control and to eliminate or control the precipitating stimuli. Understanding that accusations and suspicion may be the patient's attempts to account for misplaced possessions, forgotten appointments, and unexpected changes in routine may lead caregivers to increase the predictability and orderliness of the patient's environment, rather than argue with the patient about the accuracy of the patient's suspicions.

Finally, caregivers should know that hostile and aggressive behavior can be caused by physical pain or illness and that patients who exhibit sudden increases in aggressive behavior may need medical evaluation. Because some medications may cause increased aggressiveness, changes in mood or diminished tolerance for frustration that occur when medications are begun or dosages changed should be evaluated by a physician. Sometimes medication may be prescribed to control a patient's violent behavior, but because of their depressive effects on alertness and general mental functioning, they should be prescribed only when behavioral methods fail to provide sufficient control.

Mace and Rabins (1991) described six ways in which caregivers may manage disruptive behaviors and maintain appropriate behavior for patients who are in the middle to late stages of dementia. They call their suggestions *The Six Rs of Behavior Management.*

- *Restrict.* If the person is doing something undesirable, try to get them to stop, especially if the person might harm self or others. Do not be confrontational or argumentative. Be calm and reasonable.
- *Reassess.* Ask yourself: Might a physical illness or drug reaction be causing the problem? Is the person having difficulty seeing or hearing? Is something upsetting the person? Can the annoying situation or person be removed? Would a different approach upset the person less?
- *Reconsider.* Imagine how things seem from the person's point of view. It is understandable that a person becomes upset when things happen that do not make sense.
- *Rechannel.* Look for a way that the behavior can continue in a safe and nondestructive way. The behavior may be important to the person in a way that we do not understand.
- *Reassure.* Take time to reassure the person that things are all right and that you still care for them. Take time to reassure yourself that you are doing the best you can in a difficult and demanding situation.
- *Review.* Afterward, think about what happened and how you managed it. What can you learn from this experience that will help you next time? What led up to the behavior? How did you respond to it? What did you do right? What might you try next time?

Communication As the patient progresses into the middle stages of dementia, communication strategies previously used by the patient to compensate for impaired word finding and comprehension are neglected or forgotten, and the patient becomes less and less capable of managing communicative interactions. Automatisms and stereotypic utterances become more frequent, the informational content of the patient's speech declines, and the patient has difficulty following the gist of everyday conversations. The patient rattles on about trivial past events and neglects conversational behaviors such as turn-taking and eye contact. Reminding the patient to use previously learned communicative strategies may have transitory effects on the patient's communicative behavior, but the effects soon evaporate, leaving the patient rattling on and the caregiver frustrated.

Because patients in the middle stages of dementia cannot acquire new communicative strategies and because they cannot dependably use previously learned strategies, intervention concentrates on preserving the patient's residual communicative abilities to the extent permitted by the patient's declining intellect.

The focus of intervention now shifts away from training the patient to use communicative strategies and toward stimulating the patient, maintaining the patient's remaining communicative abilities, and preserving the patient's interest in communicating. Intervention is now caregiver-centered. The caregiver carries out the day-to-day requirements of the intervention program. The clinician trains the caregiver, monitors progress, gives encouragement and advice, and helps the caregiver modify the intervention program as the patient's communicative abilities change.

The clinician helps the caregiver make the transition from communicative partner to facilitator and supporter of the patient's communicative behavior. The traditional concept of communication as a two-way exchange of information is revised to emphasize the role of communication in maintaining the caregiver–patient interpersonal relationship, maintaining the patient's ability to communicate, and preserving the patient's willingness to participate in communicative interactions. The caregiver no longer arranges conversations to orient the patient or to train the patient to use compensatory strategies, although if the patient uses previously learned strategies the caregiver reinforces their use. Instead of instructing, training, and correcting, the caregiver does the following:

- Accepts the patient's contributions at face value. The caregiver treats the patient as a conversational partner whose ideas and opinions are important, although what the patient says may not make complete sense to the caregiver. The caregiver does not correct the patient, argue with the patient, or test the patient by asking the patient to repeat what the

caregiver has said. The caregiver may restate, repeat, or paraphrase *some* of the patient's contributions to verify the patient's communicative intent.

- Adapts his or her contributions to the patient's comprehension impairments. The caregiver keeps sentences short, uses simple and concrete vocabulary, and puts only one idea in each sentence. The caregiver speaks slowly and distinctly (but not artificially so) and adds redundancy to utterances by repeating key elements and paraphrasing information. The caregiver clearly establishes the topic at the beginning of conversations and repeats or paraphrases the topic periodically thereafter or whenever the patient seems to be losing the topic. The caregiver clearly signals topic changes ("Now let's talk about something different. Let me tell you about . . .").

- Encourages the patient's participation by periodically asking for the patient's opinion and by asking questions that can be answered in a few words and that limit the number of alternative responses from which the patient must choose. Two-choice questions (yes-no, either-or) are useful, but caregivers must use them sparingly because overuse may turn the conversation into a drill.

- Communicates respect for the patient and interest in what the patient contributes. Demonstrating respect and interest often proves a more powerful incentive for the patient's participation in conversations than positive comments following individual patient contributions.

- Sets aside consistent times every day for structured conversation with the patient. The caregiver chooses topics that are relevant and interesting to the patient and to which the patient is likely to have something to contribute. If the patient reads and gets some information from newspaper or magazine articles, the caregiver may select an article the patient has read, adding props such as photographs or illustrations to increase the patient's interest and enhance the patient's participation. The caregiver may use photographs or personal memorabilia relating to significant patient life experiences to stimulate the patient's desire to communicate. The caregiver guides these conversations but does not overtly attempt to control the relevance or accuracy of what the patient says, although the caregiver may guide the patient in less obvious ways, such as by repeating main ideas in a conversational manner.

- Ensures that incidental communicative interchanges (e.g., *comments, rhetorical questions, exclamations*) are not neglected. Offhand comments ("I'm so tired today."), rhetorical questions ("Is it going to rain, I wonder?"), exclamations ("What a miserably hot day!"), and the like are a common part of the everyday life of adults who live together. When the dementia patient neither initiates such incidental interchanges nor overtly responds to them, caregivers are likely to forego them, thereby further isolating the patient from the daily give-and-take that is an important part of normal adult-to-adult relationships.

Group Activities Group activities may provide structured stimulation and structured interactions for patients in the middle stages of dementia. Group activities for middle-stage dementia patients who live at home typically are offered at day treatment centers, rehabilitation centers, university clinics, and the outpatient departments of some medical facilities. The goals of group activities for middle-stage dementia patients usually include the following:
- Maintaining orientation
- Stimulating cognitive processes
- Maintaining communicative abilities
- Reinforcing appropriate interpersonal behavior

GENERAL CONCEPTS 10-7

- As a patient moves into the middle stages of dementia, reliance on compensatory strategies declines and *environmental control* becomes increasingly important.
- *Aggressive and accusatory behaviors* usually become important concerns as the patient

progresses into the middle stages of dementia. Helping caregivers understand why these behaviors occur and providing them with the means to control the behaviors is an important part of intervention for patients in the middle stages of dementia.

- In the middle and late stages of the patient's dementia, the purposes of communication between the caregiver and the patient become to *stimulate the patient,* to *maintain the patient's remaining communicative abilities,* and to *preserve the patient's interest in communicating.* Caregiver–patient communication no longer serves the traditional purpose of exchange of information, and the caregiver no longer uses communication to orient the patient or to teach the patient new strategies. The caregiver treats the patient as a conversational partner whose contributions are important, regardless of their accuracy or relevance.

Late Stages

Helping Caregivers of Late-Stage Dementia Patients at Home The focus of intervention for caregivers of late-stage dementia patients who still live at home is on environmental control and management of behavioral contingencies. (Most late-stage dementia patients are cared for in nursing homes or other extended-care facilities. Clinical management for these patients is discussed in the following section.) The objective of at-home care for late-stage dementia patients is to maintain the patient's ability to carry out familiar and well-learned daily-life routines and to help the patient participate in life experiences to the extent permitted by the patient's cognitive and physical abilities.

A structured approach to at-home care is important. The caregiver and the clinician make a list of behavioral routines that caregivers would like to see the patient maintain, then rank the list in order of importance to the patient and caregiver. The list is limited to simple and highly familiar everyday routines the patient has practiced repeatedly throughout adulthood (e.g., *bathing, brushing teeth, hanging up clothes*). A small set of target routines is selected from the highest-ranked items and an intervention program is formulated. The intervention program focuses on *eliciting* the routines by means of environmental stimuli and *maintaining* the behaviors in the routines by applying contingencies to the behaviors.

Environmental cues are used to elicit the routines. The patient's daily life environment may be modified to make naturally occurring cues more prominent (e.g., placing the patient's toothbrush and toothpaste on the bathroom counter where the patient will see them on arising), or new and salient cues may be invoked to elicit the desired routine (e.g., taping a colored picture of a person brushing their teeth to the bathroom mirror). The patient's completion of behavioral routines may be reinforced by natural consequences (the toothpaste tastes good and the patient's mouth feels clean) but may require additional contingencies provided by caregivers ("I see you brushed your teeth. That's great! Because you did such a good job, I have a special treat for you at breakfast.").

Intervention and Management for Institutionalized Patients with Dementia Numerous programs for maintaining and enhancing institutionalized dementia patients' cognitive, communicative, and social functioning have been described in the literature. Although the specifics differ, most fall into one of two general categories. One category *(environmental manipulation)* consists of programs that manipulate the characteristics of patients' living environments to maintain and enhance their cognitive status, communicative competence, and social participation. The other category *(behavior management)* consists of programs that manipulate specific response-eliciting stimuli and response contingencies to increase the frequency of desired behaviors and diminish the frequency of undesired behaviors. Although designed primarily for institutionalized patients in the middle to late stages of dementia, most of the principles and procedures of these programs

should be useful for middle-stage to late-stage dementia patients who are cared for in the home.

Environmental Manipulation Perhaps the oldest and most common approach to management of institutionalized dementia patients is called *reality orientation*. Reality orientation seeks to preserve and enhance patients' cognitive functioning and social adequacy by repeatedly exposing them to information about the daily life environment (e.g., *what day it is, what the weather is like, activities for the day*). The information is provided orally by staff during their interactions with patients and is posted in printed and/or pictorial form at strategic locations. Reality orientation is designed to help patients attend to and remember environmental information by repeatedly stimulating them with the information, usually in both spoken and printed form and often enhanced by bright colors, attention-getting graphics, and so forth.

Numerous anecdotal reports suggest that reality orientation enhances dementia patients' orientation and promotes appropriate social interactions, provided that several criteria are met:

- The orientation information is not too complex. Few patients with significant dementia attend to or understand complex printed lists, schedules, and instructions.
- Each posted informational item presents a single piece of information in an attention-getting format. Patients will be more likely to attend to the information if it is enhanced with vivid color and illustrated with appealing drawings.
- Caregivers ensure that patients attend to the information. Training caregivers to routinely call patients' attention to orientation information is crucial.
- The information is accessible to the patient when the patient needs it. A poster in the patient lounge that gives the schedule of activities for the day will not help the patient who is elsewhere in the facility and needs to know what is on the schedule.
- The information is actually relevant to the patient. It may be less important that the patient

know that the date is March 21 than to know that a party is scheduled for 2 PM that day.

Milieu therapy sometimes is combined with reality orientation. Milieu therapy endeavors to enhance patients' alertness and increase appropriate social behavior by making the patient's environment more interesting and more conducive to social interactions. Environmental changes in milieu therapy range from simple adjustments such as providing refreshments during activity periods to more complex changes such as rearranging furniture; adding plants, pictures, and other decorative items; introducing pets; and providing conversational partners.

A few controlled studies have shown that milieu therapy can increase the frequency of socially appropriate behaviors (Blackman, Hoover, & Pinkston, 1976; Quatrocchi-Tubin & Jason, 1980). However, Cartensen and Erickson (1986) report that although milieu therapy may increase the frequency of appropriate behaviors (sitting quietly, speaking, listening, touching), it also may increase the frequency of inappropriate behavior (bizarre, nonsensical utterances; verbal harassment and threats; physical violence). It may be necessary to combine milieu therapy with behavior management procedures to ensure that desired behaviors are enhanced and undesired behaviors are minimized.

Behavior Modification Whereas environmental manipulation seeks to affect patients' overall level of orientation, cognitive status, communication, and social participation, behavior modification focuses on specific categories of behavior to diminish undesirable behaviors (e.g., *shouting, hitting, wandering*) and to augment desirable behaviors (e.g., *bathing, grooming, participating in activities*). Behavior modification relies heavily on the consequences for responses. Positive consequences may be delivered contingent on instances of desirable behaviors *(positive reinforcement),* and negative consequences may be delivered contingent on instance of undesirable behaviors *(punishment).* Positive reinforcement may use intangible consequences such as caregiver praise or attention or coupons that the patient may exchange for desired items or tangible consequences such as sweets, cigarettes, or trinkets. Punishment may use removal of positive consequences contingent on specified behaviors, intervals of "time out" in which the patient is ignored or isolated, verbal reproof, or a combination of several negative consequences.

Sometimes undesirable behaviors may be controlled or eliminated by providing positive consequences for behaviors that are incompatible with the undesirable behaviors. For example, a patient who wanders might receive positive consequences for sitting quietly and participating in games, hobbies, or group activities. Positively reinforcing a desired behavior that is incompatible with an undesirable behavior and punishing the undesirable behavior may have stronger effects on behavior than either positive reinforcement or punishment alone.

No large-scale, well-controlled studies confirm the effectiveness of behavior modification for adults in the middle to late stages of dementia, although several small-group and single-case studies suggest that behavior modification procedures are effective in diminishing the frequency of specific undesired behaviors and increasing the frequency of specific desired behaviors (Allen-Burge, Stevens, & Burgio, 1999; Coyne & Hoskins, 1997; Heard & Watson, 1999; Hussian, 1988; Stokes, 1990; Vaccaro, 1988; and others). However, the durability of changes in behavior achieved by means of behavior modification is not well established. Few published reports address the issue of maintenance—that is, whether the behavior changes achieved by means of behavior modification persist when response contingencies are discontinued. The maintenance issue is important because some published studies report that modified behaviors revert to pretreatment levels when response contingencies are no longer in force (Allen-Burge, Stevens, & Burgio, 1999; Spector & associates, 2000).

The literature suggests that environmental manipulation has somewhat more dependable and more powerful effects than behavior modification on the behavior of adults with dementia. However, those who write about environmental manipulation generally agree that it, like behavior modification, generally is effective only while the manipulations are in place. If the environmental manipulations are discontinued, the behaviors affected by the manipulations usually return to pretreatment levels. At this time, a combination of environmental manipulation and behavior modification appears to provide the best means of modifying and maintaining behavior change for adults in the late stages of dementia. Additional research clearly is needed to clarify the effectiveness and efficiency of existing behavior modification procedures and to propose new procedures or combinations of procedures to create and maintain behavioral changes in adults who are in the late stages of dementia.

GENERAL CONCEPTS 10-8

- In the very late stages of dementia, intervention focuses almost exclusively on *environmental control* to stimulate the patient and preserve the patient's remaining cognitive and communicative abilities, using enhanced environmental prompts and cues.
- Intervention programs for institutionalized dementia patients typically depend on *environmental control, behavior management,* or a combination of the two. *Reality orientation* and *milieu therapy* are forms of environmental control. *Behavior modification* manipulates antecedent stimuli and response consequences to influence the frequency and form of specific patient behaviors.
- The evidence suggests that environmental control and behavior management can be effective in modifying and controlling dementia patients' behavior, but the durability of the changes achieved has not been clearly established.
- Controlled investigations are needed to evaluate the effectiveness of existing procedures and to devise new procedures for managing patients who are in the late stages of dementia.

THOUGHT QUESTIONS

Question 10-1 You are preparing for a first interview with the spouse of a man with suspected early-stage Alzheimer's dementia. You may ask 10 questions during the interview. List the questions you would choose to ask and tell why you would ask each question.

Question 10-2 The following items resemble items that might be found in a screening test of mental status. Arrange them in what you think would be increasing order of difficulty for persons with moderate Alzheimer's dementia. Briefly describe the rationale for your ordering of items.

    Count backward from 20 to 1.

    How old are you?

    What does "a stitch in time saves nine" mean?

    What is your name?

    Who is the current U.S. President?

    Point to the ceiling, then point to the floor, and blink three times.

    What day of the week is it?

    Who was the first U.S. President?

    What is your phone number?

    Say "please put the groceries in the refrigerator."

    Tell me the days of the week, beginning with Sunday.

    How would your uncle's daughter be related to you?

Question 10-3 The following utterances were produced as patients described the Boston Diagnostic Aphasia Examination "cookie theft" picture (Figure 5-22). The patients had the diagnoses listed here. Match the utterances with the diagnoses. (Some utterances may fit more than one diagnosis.)

Broca's aphasia

Wernicke's aphasia

Conduction aphasia

Right-hemisphere syndrome

Alzheimer's dementia

1. The mother is drinking . . . no . . . the mother is drying the cups and the plates . . . or the dishes.
2. If you don't know what's going on there I'm not going to be the one to tell you.

3. The wasker ... waster ... walter ... water is running on the floor.
4. There's a window with some curtains and a woman looking out.
5. I can't tell you what it is. My eyes aren't what they used to be.
6. Cookies and ... and ... swipe ... kids ... and mother ... and ... and ... dishes and water ... and floor ...
7. There's a major biskelorum happening there in that frenellation ...
8. ...And the ... what do you call it ... the dripper ... or the spigot ... or the hydrant ... it's flushing ... or rushing on the floor ...

11

Motor Speech Disorders

APRAXIA OF SPEECH

The label *apraxia of speech* first appeared in the literature in the late 1800s and early 1900s as part of a syndrome called *oral apraxia.* During the first half of the twentieth century, writers began separating apraxic speech movements from apraxic non-speech movements, and labels such as *apraxic dysarthria, peripheral motor aphasia, articulatory dysarthria,* and *apraxia of vocal expression* were applied to the speech syndrome, and labels such as *buccofacial apraxia, facial apraxia,* and *oral nonverbal apraxia* were applied to the non-speech syndrome. Darley (1969) settled on the label *apraxia of speech* for the speech syndrome, and since then most speech-language pathologists and many others have used this label for the collection of articulatory impairments described by Darley, Aronson, and Brown (1975):

> Apraxia of speech is a distinct motor speech disorder distinguishable from the dysarthrias (speech disorders due to impaired innervation of speech musculature) and aphasia (a language disorder due to impairment of the brain mechanism for decoding and encoding the symbol system used in spoken and written communication). Apraxia of speech is a disorder of motor speech programming manifested primarily by errors in articulation and secondarily by compensatory alterations of prosody. The speaker shows reduced efficiency in accomplishing the oral postures necessary for phoneme production and the sequences of those

postures for production of words. The disorder is frequently associated with aphasia but may also occur in isolation. Oral (non-speech) apraxia may co-occur. (p. 267)

Neuropathology

The presence of apraxia of speech almost always signifies pathology affecting the frontal lobe in the language-dominant hemisphere—usually in the posterior inferior region (in, around, or under Broca's area). Stroke is the leading cause of apraxia of speech in adults, but apraxia of speech also may appear as a consequence of degenerative nervous system diseases such as multiple sclerosis, traumatic brain injury, or brain tumor (Figure 11-1).

Related Findings

Most patients with apraxia of speech also exhibit hemiparesis or hemiplegia, spasticity, exaggerated reflexes, and somesthetic sensory impairments contralateral to the side of brain injury (the right side for right-handed individuals). Many patients with apraxia of speech also exhibit buccofacial apraxia, although either may occur independent of the other. Some patients with apraxia of speech exhibit limb apraxia. (See Chapter 4 for descriptions of buccofacial apraxia and limb apraxia and their neurophysiologic bases.)

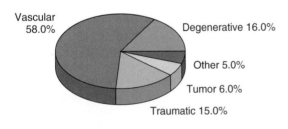

Figure 11-1 ■ **Causes of dysarthria for 107 Mayo Clinic patients with a primary diagnosis of apraxia of speech.** (Data from Duffy, J. R. [1995]. *Motor speech disorders: Substrates, differential diagnosis, and management.* St Louis, MO: Mosby.)

Apraxia of speech usually occurs in association with nonfluent (Broca's) aphasia. In fact, descriptions of the speech output of patients with Broca's aphasia usually resemble those for apraxia of speech (Benson, 1979; Goodglass & Kaplan, 1983; Wertz, LaPointe, & Rosenbek, 1984).

> The verbal output in Broca aphasia . . . is sparse, poorly articulated, consists of very short phrases (characteristically one word in length, or, following improvement, telegraphic), is produced with considerable effort, particularly on initiation of speech, and is strikingly dysprosodic. The output consists almost exclusively of substantives such as nouns, action verbs, significant modifiers or stock phrases (cliches). (Benson, 1979a, p. 65)

When apraxia of speech accompanies Broca's aphasia the patient's speech may be *agrammatic* and *telegraphic,* as Benson notes. Most patients with Broca's aphasia plus apraxia of speech also exhibit word-retrieval impairments and subtle to moderate comprehension impairments, which are not characteristics of apraxia of speech in isolation.

Duffy (1995) reported that 78% of a sample of 107 Mayo Clinic patients with a primary diagnosis of apraxia of speech also had evidence of aphasia. Duffy also commented that if patients with apraxia of speech as a secondary diagnosis were included in the Mayo Clinic sample, the percentage of patients exhibiting both apraxia of speech and aphasia would be much greater than 78%. In most clinics the percentage probably exceeds 90%.

Dysarthria sometimes appears in combination with apraxia of speech. Duffy (1995) reported that 29% of the 107-patient Mayo Clinic sample of patients with a primary diagnosis of apraxia of speech also exhibited dysarthria—usually appearing as unilateral upper motor neuron dysarthria or spastic dysarthria.

Speech Characteristics

Apraxia of speech is characterized by highly variable articulation errors embedded in a pattern of speech made slow and effortful by trial-and-error gropings for the desired articulatory postures. The off-target productions are usually complications of articulatory performance, that is, substitutions (many of them unrelated to the target phoneme), additions, repetitions, and prolongations. Less frequently the errors are simplifications, that is, distortions and omissions. Errors are most often on consonants occurring initially in words, predominantly on those phonemes and clusters of phonemes requiring more complex muscular adjustment. Errors are exacerbated by increase in length of words and the linguistic and psychologic "weight" of a word in a sentence. They are not significantly influenced by auditory, visual, or instructional set variables. Islands of fluent, error-free speech highlight the marked discrepancy between efficient automatic-reactive productions and inefficient volitional-purposive productions. (Darley, Aronson, & Brown, 1975, p. 267)

Apraxia of speech (sometimes called *verbal apraxia*) resembles other forms of ideomotor apraxia in several ways. It is not caused by weakness, paralysis, or sensory loss in the speech muscles. Unplanned, automatic speech is less clumsy and effortful than speech requested by the examiner. Speech elicited in natural contexts is less effortful and sounds more nearly normal than speech elicited in artificial contexts (such as a typical speech evaluation).

Several characteristics of apraxia of speech differentiate it from neurogenic communication impairments that otherwise resemble it (particularly dysarthria and aphasia). Two important identifying characteristics are *articulatory error patterns* and *consistency of errors.*

Articulatory Error Patterns Darley, Aronson, and Brown (1975) and Wertz, LaPointe, and Rosenbek (1984), among others, have described characteristic articulatory error patterns of patients with apraxia of speech. These error patterns define relationships between articulatory or linguistic variables and error probabilities. Wertz, LaPointe, and Rosenbek (1984) describe the following error patterns:

- Substitution errors are more frequent than distortion, omission, or addition errors. Many substitution errors replace an easy-to-articulate sound with a more difficult one. Kearns and Simmons (1988) suggest, however, that what listeners perceive as substitutions actually may be extreme phonetic distortion errors.
- Errors are more likely to be errors in placement of the articulators than errors of voicing, manner, or resonance.
- Most errors resemble the target sound.
- Consonant clusters are more likely to be in error than single consonants.
- Front-of-the-mouth sounds are more likely to be correct than back-of-the-mouth sounds.

Wertz, LaPointe, and Rosenbek (1984) suggest that the following characteristics are true for apraxic speakers as a group but may not always be true for an individual apraxic speaker:

- Voiceless sounds are more frequently substituted for voiced sounds than vice versa.
- Anticipatory errors (producing a sound before it occurs in a word or phrase, as in *thoothbrush* for *toothbrush*) are more frequent than either perseverative errors (inappropriately repeating a sound in a word or phrase, as in *manina* for *manila*) or metathetic errors (transposing adjacent sounds, as in *tevelision* for *television*).
- Consonant errors are more frequent than vowel errors.

Consistency of Errors Darley, Aronson, and Brown (1975), Wertz, LaPointe, and Rosenbek (1984), Kearns and Simmons (1988), and others have identified articulatory inconsistency as an important feature of apraxia of speech. Articulatory inconsistency is manifested as correct articulation of phonemes at one time and incorrect articulation of the same phonemes at another time. Inconsistency in articulation often is related to variations in the context in which the phonemes are produced. A phoneme may be articulated correctly in one phonemic context (e.g., when the same phoneme is repeated in words or phrases, as in *Don did the dishes*) and misarticulated in another (e.g., when contrasting phonemes occur in words or phrases, as in *Don bought a car*).

Apraxic speakers' articulation usually is better in natural situations than in artificial ones. An apraxic patient's production of "see you later" is likely to be better when the patient is actually leaving than when the patient is asked by a clinician to say it in the middle of a treatment session. This phenomenon is related to what Darley, Aronson, and Brown (1975) referred to as *islands of fluent, error-free speech,* in which an apraxic speaker produces occasional fluent words, phrases, or sentences in the midst of effortful, struggling speech. Such periods of fluent speech in an overall context of nonfluency help to differentiate apraxia of speech from the dysarthrias, in which such intermittent periods of correct articulation rarely occur. The primary exceptions are dysarthrias accompanying cerebellar ataxia and some dysarthrias caused by extrapyramidal disease, wherein speech may be intermittently dysarthric and normal. These variations in fluency and articulatory accuracy usually are unpredictable and are not strongly related to situational variables, as is true for apraxia of speech.

Posterior Apraxia of Speech

Several writers (Buckingham, 1979; Deutsch, 1984; Square, Darley, & Sommers, 1982; and others) have described a *posterior apraxia of speech* syndrome caused by damage in the anterior parietal lobe or the anterior parietal-temporal region. Patients exhibiting this syndrome are less likely to be weak or paralyzed on one side but are more likely to exhibit contralateral somesthetic sensory impairments than patients with apraxia of speech following frontal-lobe injury.

The speech characteristics of patients with posterior apraxia of speech differ in several respects from the speech of patients with apraxia of speech caused by frontal-lobe damage. Square, Darley, and Sommers (1982) reported that the speech errors of patients with posterior apraxia of speech include more substitutions and fewer distortions than the speech of patients with apraxia of speech caused by frontal-lobe damage. Deutsch (1984) reported that the speech errors of patients with posterior apraxia of speech include more transpositions of sounds and syllables (e.g., *tevelision* for *television*) than the speech of patients with apraxia of speech caused by frontal-lobe damage. The speech of patients with posterior apraxia of speech often is described as less effortful, more fluent, and having more nearly normal prosody than the speech of patients with apraxia of speech caused by frontal-lobe damage.

The concept of posterior apraxia of speech has come under fire from some writers who assert that the syndrome does not represent an apraxia but is part of the symptom-complex of *conduction aphasia* (Buckingham, 1979, 1992; Canter, 1973). According to these writers, patients who speak effortlessly and with normal prosody between instances of breakdown are more properly described as exhibiting *conduction aphasia* than posterior apraxia of speech, and their speech errors are more properly described as *literal paraphasias* than apraxic errors. Regardless of the labels one chooses, it seems clear that there are differences in speech output between patients with damage in the posterior frontal lobe and patients with damage in the anterior parietal or temporal lobes of the language-dominant hemisphere (McNeil, Robin, & Schmidt, 1997).

- Patients with frontal-lobe damage speak slowly and with great effort, distorted consonants and vowels are prominent, and runs of normal speech are rare.
- Patients with parietal-temporal lobe damage speak fluently and with little effort, and runs of normal speech are common.
- Patients with frontal-lobe damage exhibit consistent prosodic disturbances—prolonged interword intervals, prolonged vowels, prolonged articulatory movement durations.
- The prosodic characteristics of patients with parietal-temporal lobe damage are variable but usually are within a normal range.
- Patients with frontal-lobe damage tend to make the same kinds of errors in the same locations from trial to trial.

- Patients with parietal-temporal lobe damage tend to make different kinds of errors and make them at different locations from trial to trial.
- Patients with frontal-lobe damage tend not to move toward correct productions on repeated attempts.
- Patients with parietal-temporal lobe damage tend to move toward correct productions on repeated attempts.

> Although arguments about what constitutes apraxia of speech and what constitutes conduction aphasia are not settled, almost all of the literature on treatment for apraxia of speech is based on patients with frontal-lobe damage, Broca's aphasia, and apraxia of speech. In what follows, the reader may assume that the label *apraxia of speech* refers to that group of patients.

Testing for the Presence of Apraxia of Speech

Tests to detect apraxia of speech typically include the following:

- Producing non-speech oral movements, in isolation and in sequence. These tests are sensitive to the presence of *buccofacial apraxia*
- Producing speech movements, in isolation and in sequence
- Producing words with increasing phonologic complexity
- Producing phonologically complex phrases and sentences

Tests for limb apraxia usually complement tests for buccofacial apraxia and apraxia of speech. Tests for limb apraxia typically require sequential movements of hand and arm, such as waving goodbye or flipping a coin. As noted in Chapter 4, limb apraxia is more severe distally than proximally. Consequently, test items requiring wrist and finger movements are more sensitive to limb apraxia than test items requiring

only shoulder and arm movements, such as saluting or thumbing a ride. Because many patients with limb apraxia are paralyzed on one side, tests for limb apraxia should include movements that can be demonstrated with one arm and hand. Box 11-1 lists tasks for identifying buccofacial apraxia, apraxia of speech, and limb apraxia.

Treating Apraxia of Speech

According to Rosenbek and Wertz (1972), treatment for patients with apraxia of speech should:

> . . . concentrate on the disordered articulation and, therefore, be different from the language stimulation and auditory and visual processing therapies appropriate to the aphasias.

> . . . emphasize the relearning of adequate points of articulation and the sequencing of articulatory gestures.

> . . . provide conditions such that the apraxic patient can advance from limited, automatic-reactive speech to appropriate, volitional purposive communication. (p. 192)

> Rosenbek and Wertz were addressing treatment of apraxia per se. This does not imply that "therapies appropriate to the aphasias" are not appropriate for patients who are both apraxic and aphasic.

Most apraxic speakers can produce individual sounds and one-syllable words correctly and with little effort, but problems arise when they are called on to produce multisyllabic utterances and phonologically complex words. Speech that is smooth and effortless when the apraxic patient produces short and phonologically simple utterances becomes slow, halting, and riddled with articulatory missteps when utterances are long and phonologically complex.

Apraxic speakers' problems do not arise because they cannot hear or discriminate the

---

Box 11-1 Screening Tasks for Identifying Apraxia of Speech and Related Conditions

Nonverbal Oral Movements (Examiner may demonstrate, if necessary.)

Cough.
Stick out your tongue.
Puff out your cheeks.
Pucker your lips.
Smile.
Click your teeth.

Nonverbal Oral Movement Sequences (Examiner may demonstrate, if necessary.)

Lick your lips all the way around.
Show me how you would blow out a candle.
Pucker your lips, then smile.
—One time.
—Three times in succession.
Click your teeth, pucker your lips, then smile.
—One time.
—Three times in succession.

Repetition—Syllables

Say *puh-puh-puh-puh* as long as you can and as fast as you can.
Say *tuh-tuh-tuh-tuh* as long as you can and as fast as you can.

Say *kuh-kuh-kuh-kuh* as long as you can and as fast as you can.
Say *puh-tuh-kuh—puh-tuh-kuh* as long as you can and as fast as you can.

Repetition—Words

Say: *bob dad pop kick gag lap mat rap*
Say: *gingerbread snowman artillery impossibility*
Say three times in succession: *gingerbread artillery impossibility*

Repetition—Phrases

Say: *Please put the groceries in the refrigerator.*
Say: *The shipwreck washed up on the shore.*
Say: *Nelson Rockefeller drives a Lincoln Continental.*

Limb Movements

Show me how you would comb your hair.
Show me how you would salute.
Show me how you would wave good-bye.
Show me how you would play a piano.
Show me how you would wind a watch.

See also Dabul, 2000; Darley, Aronson, and Brown, 1975; Disimoni, 1989; Duffy, 1995; Wertz, LaPointe, and Rosenbek, 1984.

---

sounds of speech—apraxic speakers do not need auditory discrimination training. Some early studies of apraxic speakers suggested that many were deficient in oral sensation and oral form identification (Guilford & Hawk, 1968; Larimore, 1970; Rosenbek, Wertz, & Darley, 1973), but subsequent studies have failed to replicate these findings (Deutsch, 1981; Square & Weidner, 1976). Sensory abnormalities sometimes coexist with apraxia of speech, but the abnormalities appear not to be strongly related to its severity, making work on oral sensation a questionable treatment option for most apraxic patients.

Patients with Severe Apraxia of Speech

Characteristics at Intake Patients with severe apraxia of speech usually have no volitional speech. Many emit stereotypic speech responses during the first month or two post-onset. These stereotypic responses usually disappear by 2 months post-onset, unless the patient also is severely aphasic. Most patients with severe apraxia of speech have moderate to severe buccofacial and limb apraxia. They are almost always hemiparetic or hemiplegic and most are at least moderately aphasic.

Progression of Treatment Treatment of severely apraxic patients begins at elemental levels. Many cannot phonate voluntarily. Most who can phonate cannot modify their phonation to produce vowels, and few can produce consonant–vowel syllables. Consequently, early stages of treatment usually are concerned with developing volitional vocalization and a small repertoire of vowels and consonant–vowel syllables. Treatment procedures make use of *phonetic placement* (use of drawings, models, descriptions, or mechanical positioning of the patient's articulators), *phonetic derivation* (deriving a new speech sound from a non-speech movement or position—for example, deriving a *buh* sound by having the patient close the lips, puff air, and vocalize), and *progressive approximation* (deriving a new speech sound from one the patient can make—for example moving from *mah* to *bah*).

Phonetic contrasts (training a series of syllables or words in which elements in the series differ by a single feature—for example, *pan - tan - fan - van*) may help expand the patient's repertoire. Severely apraxic speakers usually are poor imitators. Consequently, imitation drills may not be appropriate, although *integral stimulation (watch me and do what I do)* may be useful for some patients.

Some severely apraxic speakers occasionally utter single words, but the words are likely to have little or no communicative value and are likely not to be under the speaker's volitional control. Helm and Barresi (1980) have suggested that such words can be brought under the patient's control and have described a program for incorporating such involuntary utterances into treatment.

Alternative communication devices such as communication boards and communication books may be used to provide a means of communication for patients with severe apraxia of speech, at least on a temporary basis. Severely apraxic patients' use of gestural communication also may be emphasized and trained. Education and counseling of those who care for the patient are crucial aspects of treatment for severely apraxic patients.

Outcome As noted earlier, apraxia of speech usually accompanies Broca's aphasia, although occasionally a patient appears with mild to moderate apraxia of speech and no detectable aphasia. Whether an apraxic and aphasic patient will benefit from treatment depends both on the severity of the patient's apraxia and the severity of the patient's aphasia. The more severe the patient's impairments (after the first 3 or 4 weeks post-onset), the poorer the prognosis for recovery. As noted earlier, patients who, a month or more post-onset, have no volitional speech, emit stereotypic speech responses, and are severely aphasic are unlikely to recover functional speaking abilities, even with intensive treatment.

Only a small proportion of patients who remain severely apraxic at 3 or more months post-onset develop more than rudimentary functional speech. Some patients with severe apraxia of speech who are also severely aphasic (and usually hemiplegic) end up in nursing homes. For these patients, it may be particularly important to develop a means of rudimentary communication between the patient and caregivers.

Patients with Moderate Apraxia of Speech

Characteristics at Intake Patients with moderate apraxia of speech usually have some volitional speech at 1 to 2 months post-onset. Stereotypic utterances may be present immediately after onset but disappear as the patient recovers. Many patients with moderate apraxia of speech exhibit mild to moderate buccofacial and limb apraxia. Almost all are hemiparetic or hemiplegic. Mild to moderate aphasia often accompanies the patient's apraxia of speech.

Progression of Treatment Because patients with moderate apraxia of speech usually have some volitional speech, treatment usually begins at the syllable, word, or phrase level. Patients with moderate apraxia of speech actively participate in treatment. They are motivated to recover. They work independently. They learn and can generalize what they learn to new situations. They collaborate with the clinician in setting goals and in designing and carrying out treatment procedures, and they take responsibility for independent practice. Patients with moderate apraxia of speech usually move quickly from single-syllable to multiple-syllable speech production. Consequently, treatment activities can emphasize volitional control of sequenced articulatory movements, together with manipulations of rate, pauses, and intonation.

Wertz, LaPointe, and Rosenbek (1984) recommend *contrastive stress drill* for the early phases of treatment for patients with moderate apraxia of speech and suggest that oral reading may be suitable in later phases of treatment. In contrastive stress drill the clinician says a sentence such as "Bake a pie" then asks the patient questions such as "DO WHAT to a pie?," "Bake a WHAT?," and so on. The patient answers each question, putting emphatic stress on words that answer the question ("BAKE a pie.").

Relaxation training in conjunction with speech retraining may help moderately apraxic patients speak better and with less effort. Many patients with moderate apraxia of speech can learn a problem-solving approach to communication, in which they learn to anticipate difficult words and difficult speaking situations, recognize communication failure when it occurs, and respond to communication failure in a planned and systematic way.

Outcome Most patients with moderate apraxia of speech regain functional speech, although speech tends to be slow and agrammatic. Many continue slow improvement in speech over many years—even after formal treatment has ended. Most return to their homes following discharge from the hospital, and most function independently in common daily life activities. A few whose work does not depend heavily on speech may return to work, but most do not.

Patients with Mild Apraxia of Speech

Characteristics at Intake Many patients with mild apraxia of speech at the end of the first month or so post-onset spontaneously recover enough speech to be functional talkers in daily life. Most patients with mild apraxia of speech are mildly aphasic, but a few show no signs of measurable aphasia.

Progression of Treatment Patients with mild apraxia of speech usually profit from articulation drills, instruction in strategic approaches to communication, and instruction on how to cope with the communicative disruptions created by their slow speech rate and their articulatory miscues. Treatment usually consists of repetition drills coupled with exercises in which the patient formulates and produces phrases, sentences, and multiple-sentence utterances. The emphasis of treatment is on increased articulatory agility, improved articulatory accuracy, and closer-to-normal prosody and rate.

Outcome Patients with mild apraxia of speech almost always return home. Some may return to work. Almost all communicate independently in most daily life situations, but they speak slowly with exaggerated effort and often miss articulatory targets.

General Principles of Treatment for Apraxia of Speech McNeil, Robin, and Schmidt (1997) offer several principles for treating apraxia of speech:

- Intensive treatment is required. Treatment should consist of massed practice over a long interval (weeks, months, or years).
- Many repetitions are needed to stabilize newly acquired responses and make them automatic.
- The patient should revert to a neutral position between trials. A brief rest interval should occur before the patient begins a new series of trials.
- Treatment should progress systematically through a hierarchy of task difficulty (e.g., from non-speech movements to syllables, to sequences of syllables, to words, to sequences of words).
- Treatment of prosody (rhythm, stress, intonation) should accompany articulation treatment.
- Treatment should provide successful experiences for the patient. Successful communication, not perfection, is the goal.

Several of McNeil and associates' principles for treatment of apraxia of speech apply equally to treatment of other communication disorders and have been discussed elsewhere in this book.

Stimulus Manipulations and Response Accuracy in Apraxia of Speech

Automacity Overlearned sequences (counting, reciting the alphabet, reciting the days of the week) may be surprisingly easy for some patients who are severely apraxic and can produce little or no volitional speech. For these patients, drill with overlearned sequences may increase oral agility and oral motor control in preparation for work on volitional production of less automatic words and phrases.

Many apraxic patients do well as they count from 1 to 10 but are tied in knots by the multisyllabic numbers above 10. An apraxic patient asked to count to 20 gave the following response: "One ... two ... thee ... four ... five ... six ... seven ... eight ... nine ... ten ... neeleven ... telve ... thriteen ... tritheen ... thirty-teen ... forty-teen ... five-tithy-teen ..."

Visibility, Length, and Articulatory Complexity Visible and motorically simple movements are the easiest articulatory movements for apraxic speakers. Visibility and complexity interact to some extent because visible movements tend to be motorically simpler than non-visible movements. As word length increases, the probability of apraxic speech errors increases (Johns & Darley, 1970; Shankweiler & Harris, 1966), although short words with complex articulation may be more difficult than long words without complex articulation. Apraxic errors tend to increase as the distance between successive points of articulation increases (Wertz, LaPointe, & Rosenbek, 1984).

Rate Apraxic speakers' articulatory selection and sequencing impairments make it impossible for them to speak at their old normal rate, but many try to push their articulators beyond their capacity. An important early goal of treatment for such impatient apraxic speakers is to convince them that by speaking slower they will speak better. Helping the patient understand that a few well-chosen and carefully articulated words yield better communicative success than a flood of poorly articulated words helps. Showing the patient that slow, well-controlled speech is less effortful than fast, poorly controlled speech also helps. Providing experiences in which slow, controlled speech leads to successful communication in daily life usually puts the patient's doubts to rest. Most apraxic patients eventually adopt a slow, highly controlled, and carefully monitored speaking style. Getting the patient to this stage is an important early clinical responsibility.

Delay Many apraxic patients have difficulty keeping mental articulatory plans in place over time. This phenomenon often becomes apparent in articulation drills in which the clinician says a word, phrase, or sentence that the patient then repeats. Apraxic patients who do well when permitted immediately to reproduce the clinician's model often break down if they must delay their responses for 10 to 30 seconds. Clinicians sometimes build greater reserve capacity into apraxic patients' speech production by gradually increasing the time the patient must wait between the clinician's model and the patient's response.

Context The phonologic characteristics of the word or phrase in which a particular sound is located may affect the likelihood that it will be produced correctly by an apraxic speaker. There is some evidence suggesting that the first sound in a word is more likely to be produced correctly than subsequent sounds (Shankweiler & Harris, 1966; Trost & Canter, 1974). However, others have failed to confirm this effect (Dunlop

& Marquardt, 1977; Johns & Darley, 1970; LaPointe & Johns, 1975).

The linguistic context in which a word is produced usually affects how difficult it is for an apraxic patient to say. Placing a word in a frequently occurring phrase usually makes it easier. For example, the word *coffee* is likely to be easier if it is elicited by a phrase such as *I want a cup of . . .* than if it is elicited by a picture. Situational context also may affect apraxic speakers' success. Most speak better to friends and relatives (and clinicians) than they do to strangers. Most speak better face-to-face than on the telephone. Most speak better when they express their own knowledge, opinions, and wishes than they do when they must speak about topics prescribed by others.

Cues The nature of cues provided to apraxic patients has strong effects on their success in producing speech. In general, the probability of successful responses increases as more information about target responses is provided by the cues. Love and Webb (1977) studied the effects of three cues on picture naming by patients with Broca's aphasia and apraxia of speech. The cues were *a sentence with the target word missing, the first sound of the target word,* and *the printed target word.* They found that, on the average, providing the first sound of the target word was most successful in eliciting the target word (60% success). Sentence completion was the next most effective cue (34% success), followed by the printed word (28% success). The differences were statistically significant except the difference between sentence completion and printed word cues.

Love and Webb do not report whether individual subjects all generated the same hierarchy as the group. It is unlikely that they did. Furthermore, it seems likely that many of Love and Webb's subjects' were both apraxic and aphasic, with word-retrieval impairments complicating their attempts to produce spoken words (a probability to which Love and Webb allude). Love and Webb's results do, however, show that cues may have strong effects on the

accuracy of apraxic speakers' retrieval and production of single words. Love and Webb's hierarchy also may provide a starting point for clinicians who wish to construct a cueing hierarchy for an individual patient.

Rosenbek and associates (1973) proposed an eight-step continuum of cues for treatment of patients with apraxia of speech. The continuum gradually reduces the salience of cues while gradually increasing response requirements.

1. The clinician and patient produce the target utterance in unison.
2. The clinician produces the target utterance. The patient produces the utterance while the clinician silently mouths the utterance with the patient.
3. The clinician produces the utterance. The patient says the utterance.
4. The clinician produces the utterance. The patient says the utterance several times in succession.
5. The patient reads the target utterance aloud from a printed card.
6. The patient studies the utterance printed on a card. The card is taken away. The patient says the utterance.
7. The clinician asks a question that is answerable with the target utterance. The patient says the target utterance.
8. The clinician and patient interact in a role-playing situation in which previously practiced utterances are appropriate. The patient produces the utterances when appropriate.

Clinicians can add additional levels to Rosenbek and associates' continuum by imposing delayed-response requirements at some or all of the stages in the continuum.

Stimulus Modality Most treatment programs for apraxic patients manipulate the modalities in which stimuli are delivered, although not all do so systematically. Despite the frequently encountered assertion that multimodality stimulation is better than unimodality stimulation, no experimental evidence supports the claim, and the assertion almost certainly does not apply to every apraxic patient. Some patients are confused rather than helped by the additional information provided by multimodality stimulation.

Visual stimulation in apraxia treatment consists primarily of two procedures. The most common is *watch me and do what I do (integral stimulation)*. If integral stimulation fails, the clinician may add mirror work to increase visual input. In mirror work, the clinician and patient sit side-by-side in front of a mirror and watch as the patient repeats the clinician's models. The clinician directs the patient's attention toward visual aspects of speech production, such as lip and jaw position, rounding, and so forth. Sometimes videotapes of the patient may take the place of the mirror, but the clinician–patient visual monitoring procedure resembles that for mirror work. Some apraxic patients' performance improves when visual input is embellished with mirrors or videotapes. Mirror and videotape work sometimes helps patients with impaired oral tactile sensation or position sense by allowing them to see the position of their articulators as they speak. Others seem confused by the additional information and do worse when they watch themselves talk than when they do not.

Emphasizing the patient's attention to *tactile and kinesthetic stimuli* during speech sometimes improves the accuracy of apraxic patients' speech. (This does not imply that tactile stimulation by itself, outside of speech activity, is likely to be beneficial; usually it is not.) Clinicians sometimes enhance kinesthetic stimulation by manually touching, positioning, or moving the patient's jaw, tongue, and lips. Clinicians typically use manual manipulations to help the patient position the articulators for specific sounds and gradually eliminate the manipulations as the patient becomes proficient at volitionally producing the targeted sounds.

Clinicians usually resort to manual manipulation when integral stimulation and mirror work fail to produce the intended performance (although they often combine mirror work and manual manipulation).

Although the *auditory modality* is not usually written about in treatment of apraxia of speech (Wertz, LaPointe, & Rosenbek, 1984, is an exception), most treatment programs depend strongly on the patient's auditory self-monitoring as the patient talks. Most clinicians encourage apraxic patients to concentrate on listening as they speak, believing that the additional information coming into the patient's ears will improve what comes out of the patient's mouth. Clinicians also typically teach patients to evaluate each utterance to tell if it is adequate (not necessarily *correct*). Few clinicians spend time training auditory discrimination (teaching the patient to identify phonemic differences in words spoken by the clinician), but many spend time training the patient to tell how their own productions differ from targets. Pointing out consistent mismatches (e.g., syllable transpositions, articulatory substitutions) often accelerates progress.

Meaningfulness In general, the more meaningful a speech response is, the easier it is for an apraxic speaker. Consequently, most clinicians structure treatment around meaningful words, phrases, and sentences. Dabul and Bollier (1976), however, recommend that treatment for patients with apraxia of speech should begin by concentrating on production of *nonmeaningful* articulatory sequences to teach the patient volitional control of speech production prior to attempts at meaningful words. There is no conclusive evidence for either position. Majority opinion at this time seems to favor using real words as soon as possible. However, if an apraxic patient is having trouble moving from isolated sounds to sound sequences in real words, the clinician might consider using Dabul and Boller's strategy to see if it might help the patient bridge the gap.

Neurobehavioral Reorganization Approaches to Treatment Rosenbek, Collins, and Wertz (1976) and Rosenbek (1978) have described two innovative procedures for enhancing apraxic patients' speech production—*intersystemic reorganization* and *intrasystemic reorganization.*

Intersystemic Reorganization Intersystemic reorganization adds non-speech behaviors (tapping, gesturing, pantomiming) to speech, thereby facilitating speech production for apraxic individuals. (For example, a patient might pantomime the act of raising a glass and drinking from it while saying, "A drink of water.") Intersystemic reorganization takes apraxic patients through a predetermined sequence of activities (Rosenbek & LaPointe, 1978):

- The clinician and the patient compile a set of simple, meaningful, and easily recognizable gestures.
- The patient learns to recognize each gesture and its associated word or phrase when the gesture and the word or phrase are produced by the clinician.
- The patient learns to imitate the gesture. (Rosenbek and associates stress the importance of feedback from the clinician at this stage because they have observed that many apraxic patients have difficulty judging the adequacy of their own gestures.) The clinician may manipulate the patient's hand and arm to bring about the gesture, or the patient may be given real objects to use in the movement.
- When the patient can produce each gesture without effort, the patient learns to combine each gesture with a word or phrase.
- When the patient can reliably and appropriately produce speech and gesture combinations inside and outside the clinic, the gestures may be deemphasized gradually. Rosenbek and associates recommend that even at the last stage of treatment patients should be encouraged to continue using gestures for self-cueing and self-correction of errors.

According to Rosenbek and associates, patients who cannot learn gestures, who cannot learn to pair gestural and speech responses, and who are severely aphasic are not candidates for intersystemic reorganization. According to Rosenbek and

associates, patients who are severely aphasic usually do no better when treated using intersystemic reorganization than when they are treated using other procedures.

Intrasystemic Reorganization Intrasystemic reorganization elicits and enhances movements by shifting the locus of control from one level of the motor system to another. The shift usually is from automatic action to volitional action. The typist who slows down and types words syllable by syllable when typing unfamiliar or complicated words uses intrasystemic reorganization. (The typist who subvocally spells words while typing uses intersystemic reorganization.) Many treatment activities for apraxic patients qualify as intrasystemic reorganization, although they are not so labeled. Teaching patients to speak slowly and with consciously controlled articulatory movements is one example of intrasystemic reorganization. Teaching them to speak with exaggerated prosody and teaching them to concentrate on kinesthetic feedback during speech are other examples.

Wertz, LaPointe, and Rosenbek, (1984) described an intersystemic reorganization treatment program for moderate apraxia of speech in which speech is combined with tapping gestures. They call this program *gestural reorganization.* In gestural reorganization the patient is trained to emphasize the rhythm or pacing of speech by pairing tapping movements with speech. Gestural reorganization typically proceeds through an eight-step continuum.

- *Step 1: Explaining the program's purpose.* This step is necessary for patients who may be reluctant to add gestures to speech because they do not wish to appear abnormal. A patient may be told that the gestures are to help them get started and that the gestures may be phased out eventually. The clinician may compare gestures to other prosthetic devices such as eyeglasses and hearing aids.
- *Step 2: Diagnostic treatment.* The clinician and the patient identify one or more simple, repetitive gestures that the patient can do reliably (e.g., tapping one finger, tapping with all

the fingers on one hand, tapping one foot, tapping one hand against a thigh). The patient is trained to do the gesture in isolation. Then the patient is trained to use the gesture while producing a simple nonsense syllable or word.

- *Step 3: Stabilizing the gesture.* The clinician and the patient increase the patient's volitional control of the gesture by manipulating the rate, complexity, and length of tapping and by inserting delays between the clinician's model and the patient's response.

- *Step 4: Pairing gesture and speech.* The patient is trained to pair speech and gesture for simple speech responses. The clinician taps and says words or phrases. The patient and the clinician tap and say the words or phrases together.

- *Step 5: Fading cues.* The clinician gradually fades out cues. The clinician may tap only at the beginning of utterances, tap only for the most important words, or tap only for difficult words. The clinician may speak more softly or may speak only for some words in each utterance.

- *Step 6: Gesture and contrastive stress.* The clinician asks questions to which the patient responds by tapping simultaneously with speech. (Contrastive stress drill is described earlier in this chapter.)

- *Step 7: Greater volitional-purposive control.* The patient answers questions and produces phrases and sentences in response to a variety of clinician prompts, some of which may resemble conversational behaviors.

- *Step 8: Fading the gesture.* For patients who do not spontaneously stop using gestures while they speak but could do so, the clinician may help the patient move away from gesture with drills containing successively larger proportions of utterances unaccompanied by gestures. Patients may, however, be advised to resort to gesture when they encounter difficulty getting words out.

Helm (1979) described a simple apparatus for gestural reorganization, called a *pacing board*. Helm's pacing board is about 14 inches long and 2 inches wide. It is divided by ridges into eight

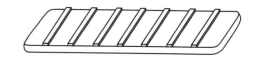

Figure 11-2 ■ **A pacing board similar to the one described by Helm (1979).**

sections (Figure 11-2). Patients are trained to tap out rhythm and stress patterns from left to right on the pacing board. Then speech and tapping are combined, and the length and complexity of tapped speech responses gradually increase. As a patient becomes proficient at speaking with the full-size pacing board, a pocket-size pacing board may be substituted, and more natural tapping or gestures gradually may replace tapping on the pacing board.

There are no reliable data to support the efficacy of reorganization in eliciting speech from apraxic patients or in reinstating speech that apraxic patients are likely to use in daily life communication, and there are no data comparing reorganization with other treatments. Anecdotal reports suggest that reorganization is effective in eliciting speech from many apraxic patients and that it makes meaningful changes in the daily life communicative ability of some of them. Intersystemic reorganization provides a way to elicit volitional speech; intrasystemic reorganization provides a way to polish it.

Melodic Intonation Therapy Melodic intonation therapy (MIT; Sparks, Helm, & Albert, 1974; Sparks & Holland, 1976) was designed to elicit speech from severely aphasic (and apraxic) patients who have little or no volitional speech by increasing the participation of the nondominant hemisphere in speech activities. (The nondominant hemisphere is thought to be important for perception and production of musical and rhythmic material.) MIT places the patient in structured drills in which phrases are produced with exaggerated stress, rhythm, and pitch, and the patient taps out the rhythm of each phrase while producing the phrase (e.g., *cup . . . of . . . CO . . . fee,* spoken with rising intonation and emphatic stress on *CO*).

In MIT the patient is trained to utter propositional phrases and sentences, using sung intonation patterns that are similar to the natural intonation patterns of the spoken phrases or sentences. First the clinician intones sentences and helps the patient tap the stress patterns of the sentences in unison with the clinician's utterances. Then the patient and clinician intone the sentences and tap their stress patterns together. Then the clinician gradually fades her or his participation in production and tapping, until the patient is intoning and tapping phrases without assistance in response to the clinician's intoned model. If a patient cannot tap and say the phrase, some clinicians substitute gesture for tapping.

When the patient's simultaneous intonation and tapping have stabilized, speech production moves away from melody toward natural prosody. First there is a transition from melodic intonation to *sprechgesang* (speech song), in which words are no longer sung but are spoken with exaggerated inflection. The next transition is from *sprechgesang* to natural prosody.

> Having a patient tap or gesture while speaking is a form of intersystemic reorganization; having a patient speak rhythmically and with exaggerated intonation is a form of intrasystemic reorganization.

According to Sparks, Helm, and Albert (1974), MIT is appropriate for patients with the following characteristics:

- Auditory comprehension is better than verbal expression. (Spontaneous recognition and self-correction of errors by the patient is considered a favorable sign.)
- The patient is emotionally stable and has good attention span.
- The patient has severely impaired verbal output and has little or no ability to name, repeat, or complete sentences.

- The patient makes vigorous attempts at self-correction.
- The patient emits clearly articulated, stereotyped utterances.

There are no controlled evaluations of the efficacy of MIT, either by itself or relative to other treatment approaches, although in 1994 a committee of the American Academy of Neurology described MIT as "promising." Anecdotal reports suggest that MIT is effective in eliciting speech from patients who otherwise cannot produce volitional speech. The most significant problem with MIT appears to be generalization of speech learned in the clinic to daily life. Little generalization of what patients learn in MIT to other activities usually occurs until the patient is in the final stages of MIT, and many patients do not make it to the final stages. A particularly difficult transition seems to be the transition from sung phrases to *sprechgesang*.

Non-Speech Communication Systems

Some severely apraxic patients never regain enough volitional speech to permit them to communicate even simple messages by talking. Non-speech communication systems may help some of them communicate. However, many severely apraxic patients also have significant aphasia, which may compromise their ability to use alternative communication systems that depend on verbal skills. Some patients with apraxia of speech may learn gesture and pantomime as part of reorganization. The gestures and pantomime may function both as a substitute for speech and as a facilitator for the patient's production of speech. Some patients with apraxia of speech may learn to use sign languages, either temporarily as they are reacquiring speech or as a permanent substitute. Producing such signs also may facilitate speech through intersystemic reorganization.

GENERAL CONCEPTS 11-1

- *Apraxia of speech* (verbal apraxia) is characterized by variable articulatory errors and trial-and-error articulatory groping in a context of slow and effortful speech.

- Apraxia of speech is caused by damage in posterior regions of the *frontal lobe* in the language-dominant brain hemisphere.
- Patients with apraxia of speech usually also exhibit *Broca's aphasia,* which adds *agrammatism* and *telegraphic speech* to the signs of apraxia of speech.
- *Limb apraxia* and *buccofacial apraxia* often accompany apraxia of speech.
- Patients with apraxia of speech often have *contralateral motor and sensory impairments* (weakness, paralysis, spasticity, exaggerated reflexes, diminished somesthetic sensation).
- Apraxia of speech is characterized by *slow, effortful speech; articulatory inconsistency; substitution articulation errors;* and *strong effects of context* on articulatory accuracy.
- *Posterior apraxia of speech* is said to be caused by *parietal-temporal lobe damage.* Many practitioners consider the speech errors of patients with so-called posterior apraxia of speech to be the *literal paraphasias* of individuals with *conduction aphasia.*
- Treatment of patients with severe apraxia of speech typically begins with sound or syllable production and may require use of *phonetic placement, phonetic contrasts,* or *integral stimulation* to facilitate speech.
- Treatment of patients with moderate apraxia of speech usually begins at the *word or phrase level,* and may involve *contrastive stress drill* in early phases. *Relaxation training* may help some speak with less effort.
- Treatment of patients with mild apraxia of speech usually consists of *speech production drills* with *phrases, sentences,* and *multiple-sentence utterances* plus training in *coping* and *compensatory* strategies.
- Emphasizing attention to *tactile and kinesthetic feedback* helps many apraxic speakers talk better.
- *Visible, short,* and *motorically* simple speech materials are easiest for apraxic speakers.
- Slowing an apraxic speaker's *rate of speech* usually improves the quality of the speech and lessens the speaker's effort in producing speech.
- *Delay* imposed between a stimulus and an apraxic speaker's responses usually compromises response accuracy. Delay may be used in treatment to increase an apraxic speaker's reserve capacity.
- *Familiar* and *natural* linguistic and situational contexts and *meaningful* content usually facilitate speech for apraxic speakers.
- Many treatment programs for apraxia of speech use *cueing hierarchies* in which cues of gradually decreasing power are systematically provided.
- *Intersystemic reorganization* enhances apraxic speakers' speech by incorporating non-speech behaviors into speech production. *Intrasystemic reorganization* enhances apraxic speakers' speech by moving control from one level of the motor system to another.
- Some severely apraxic speakers may need *augmentative or alternative communication systems* for functional communication.

DYSARTHRIA

Dysarthria is a generic label for a group of speech disorders caused by impaired control of the muscles responsible for speech. Darley, Aronson, and Brown (1975) define dysarthria as follows:

> Dysarthria is a collective name for a group of speech disorders resulting from disturbances in muscular control over the speech mechanism due to damage of the central or peripheral nervous system. It designates problems in oral communication due to paralysis, weakness, or incoordination of the speech musculature. It differentiates such problems from disorders of higher centers related to the faulty programming of movements and sequences of movements (apraxia of speech) and to the inefficient processing of linguistic units (aphasia). (p. 246)

Neuropathology

As Darley, Aronson, and Brown assert, dysarthria is caused by weakness, paralysis, or incoordination of the muscles required for speech. Weakness or paralysis of speech muscles most often is caused by damage in the pons and medulla, which affects lower motor neurons serving the speech muscles, or by damage in tracts connecting motor neurons to the speech muscles. Dysarthria may be caused by diseases of nerve-muscle junctions (e.g., myasthenia gravis), diseases of muscles (i.e., myopathy), or psychosomatic conditions (wherein the physiologic mechanisms responsible for speech are unimpaired). Dysarthria often accompanies progressive neurologic diseases (e.g., Parkinson's disease) in which the dysarthria and the disease progressively worsen. Dysarthria caused by destruction of motor neurons or nerve fiber tracts is irreversible, as are most dysarthrias caused by diseases affecting nerve-muscle junctions and diseases of muscles. Patients may, however, compensate for impaired control of the speech muscles by various strategies, such as slowing the rate at which they speak or by exaggerating articulatory movements.

Darley, Aronson, and Brown (1975) divided dysarthrias among seven types, which reflect the nature of the underlying neuropathology and the nature of the motoric disturbances caused by the neuropathology (Table 11-1).

Dysarthria and Upper Motor Neuron Pathology Unilateral damage to upper motor neurons (neurons in the motor cortex, projecting to the motor nuclei in the brain stem) or to corticobulbar tracts usually does not cause persisting dysarthria because most of the speech muscles receive input from the motor cortex in both brain hemispheres. The muscles of the pharynx, larynx, tongue, and jaw are bilaterally innervated so that pathology affecting upper motor neurons in one brain hemisphere usually causes only transitory weakness of those muscles. The external muscles of the lower face receive most of their input from the motor cortex in the contralateral hemisphere so that pathology affecting the motor cortex or corticobulbar tracts usually causes weakness or paralysis of the lower facial muscles, including the lip muscles. Patients with unilateral upper motor neuron pathology typically exhibit mild dysarthria, but speech intelligibility is well preserved. Weak lip muscles may, however, create mild articulatory imprecision of sounds that depend on lip position or lip movements. The patient's tongue rests on the midline but deviates to the weaker side when protruded.

T A B L E   1 1 - 1
Types of dysarthria described by Darley, Aronson, and Brown

Type	Neuropathology
Spastic	Upper motor neurons (usually bilateral)
Flaccid	Lower motor neurons
Ataxic	Cerebellar system
Hypokinetic	Extrapyramidal (usually Parkinson's disease)
Hyperkinetic	Extrapyramidal (chorea, dystonia, etc.)
Mixed	Multiple motor systems

From Darley, F. L., Aronson, A. E., & Brown, J. R. (1975). *Motor speech disorders.* Philadelphia, W.B. Saunders.

> The muscles of the tongue receive most of their input from the contralateral hemisphere but have sufficient ipsilateral input that unilateral upper motor neuron damage causes only mild weakness on the side contralateral to the damage (Duffy, 1995).

Now and then a patient with what seems to be unilateral upper motor neuron damage experiences persisting dysarthria, a condition Duffy (1995) calls *unilateral upper motor neuron dysarthria.* According to Duffy, unilateral upper motor neuron dysarthria has received little attention in the literature, perhaps because most writers consider it a temporary phenomenon. Darley, Aronson, and Brown (1975) declare that unilateral pathology in upper motor neurons produces only transitory speech disturbance that resolves within the first month post-onset. Duffy (1995), however, comments that unilateral upper motor neuron pathology may lead to persisting mild dysarthria.

According to Duffy, patients with unilateral upper motor neuron dysarthria are hemiplegic on the side contralateral to the brain injury, have weakness in the lower face contralateral to the brain injury, and sometimes have weakness in the tongue muscles contralateral to the brain injury. Patients with unilateral upper motor dysarthria speak slowly and with reduced loudness. Their voice quality tends to be harsh and occasionally hypernasal because of spasticity in the vocal cords and the muscles that close the velopharyngeal opening (Duffy, 1995). Box 11-2 lists characteristics of unilateral upper motor neuron dysarthria.

In contrast to the sporadic appearance of dysarthria following unilateral upper motor neuron pathology, bilateral upper motor neuron

---

> ### Box 11-2 Characteristics of Unilateral Upper Motor Neuron Dysarthria
>
> "Unilateral UMN dysarthria may be distinguished from other dysarthria types more by its mildness and somewhat nebulous speech characteristics than by any distinctive characteristics of its own." (Duffy, 1995, p. 352)
>
> **Distinguishing Speech Characteristics**
>
> Mild articulatory imprecision
> Slow/normal speech rate
> Normal voice quality
> Normal resonance
>
> **Related Signs**
>
> Hypertonus
> Hemiparesis, hemiplegia
> Exaggerated reflexes
> Pseudobulbar state

From Duffy, J. R. (1995). *Motor speech disorders: Substrates, differential diagnosis, and management.* St Louis, MO: Mosby.

---

pathology usually creates persisting dysarthria. The muscles responsible for articulation, velopharyngeal movements, and laryngeal movements become hypertonic and hyperreflexive and exhibit reduced strength and range of movement. Patients with bilateral upper motor neuron pathology typically experience bilateral facial weakness or paralysis, drooling, bilateral hemiparesis and slowness of movement, and dysarthria. Dysarthria from bilateral upper motor neuron pathology often appears as part of a syndrome called *pseudobulbar state,* in which the patient is dysarthric, has impaired swallowing (dysphagia), and has poor control of laughing or crying. The most common cause of bilateral upper motor neuron dysarthria is multiple strokes. Traumatic brain injuries, tumors, and demyelinating diseases such as multiple sclerosis are less common causes of bilateral upper motor neuron dysarthria.

Darley, Aronson, and Brown (1975) call dysarthria caused by bilateral upper motor neuron pathology *spastic dysarthria.* According to Darley, Aronson, and Brown, spastic dysarthria affects *phonation, articulation, resonation,* and *prosody.* Spastic laryngeal muscles create *strained-strangled-harsh* voice quality. Spastic articulatory muscles lose their agility, leading to imprecise consonant articulation, especially for consonants requiring rapid or complex articulatory movements. Spastic velopharyngeal muscles stiffen the velum and prevent it from occluding the velopharyngeal opening, creating hypernasality. Spastic laryngeal muscles vibrate at a slower-than-normal rate, reducing vocal pitch. Hypertonic laryngeal muscles impair vocal flexibility, diminish variability in pitch and loudness, and create strained, strangled, harsh voice quality. Reduced movement of muscles in the chest wall and abdomen compromise respiratory support for speech and contribute to weak voice and short utterances. Box 11-3 lists distinguishing features of spastic dysarthria.

Strokes and degenerative diseases are the most common causes of spastic dysarthria. Traumatic brain injury and demyelinating disease are less common causes (Figure 11-3).

Box 11-3 Characteristics of Spastic Dysarthria

Distinguishing Speech Characteristics

Imprecise consonants
Strained-strangled-harsh voice
Slow rate

Other Speech Characteristics

Hypernasality
Monopitch, low pitch
Monoloudness
Reduced stress
Distorted vowels
Short phrases
Pitch breaks
Continuous breathy voice
Excess, equal stress

Related Signs

Hypertonus (spasticity)
Hemiparesis, hemiplegia
Exaggerated reflexes
Psuedobulbar state

From Darley, F. L., Aronson, A. E., & Brown, J. R. (1975). *Motor speech disorders.* Philadelphia, W.B. Saunders; Duffy, J. R. (1995). *Motor speech disorders: Substrates, differential diagnosis, and management.* St Louis, MO: Mosby; and Rosenbek, J. C. & LaPointe, L. L. (1985). The dysarthrias: Description, diagnosis, and treatment. In D. F. Johns (Ed.), *Clinical management of neurogenic communication disorders* (2nd ed., pp. 97-152). Boston: Little-Brown and Company, 1985.

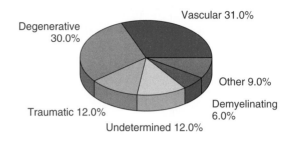

Figure 11-3 ▪ Causes of dysarthria for 107 Mayo Clinic patients with a primary diagnosis of spastic dysarthria. (Data from Duffy, J. R. [1995]. *Motor speech disorders: Substrates, differential diagnosis, and management.* St Louis, MO: Mosby.)

Dysarthria and Extrapyramidal System Pathology Darley, Aronson, and Brown (1975) divided dysarthrias caused by extrapyramidal system pathology into two categories—*hypokinetic dysarthria* and *hyperkinetic dysarthria*. Both are caused by damage in the basal ganglia, but they are differentiated by the nature of the movement abnormalities caused by the damage.

Hypokinetic dysarthria is characterized by slowness of volitional movement and difficulty initiating volitional movements (a phenomenon called *bradykinesia*), muscle rigidity, and tremor. Parkinson's disease is the most common cause of hypokinetic dysarthria. Hypokinetic dysarthria sometimes appears in other nervous system diseases, such as progressive supranuclear palsy and Wilson's disease, and occasionally appears following anoxia, overuse of some medications, or repeated blows to the head. (See Chapter 10 for more on Parkinson's disease and related conditions.)

Muscle rigidity is a prominent symptom of Parkinson's disease, affecting muscles of ambulation, respiration, speech, and facial expression. Rigid respiratory muscles compromise respiration, making the patient's utterances short and separated by long pauses. Rigid laryngeal muscles resist vibration and fail to fully adduct the vocal folds, making the patient's voice strained and breathy. Respiratory insufficiency, rigid laryngeal muscles, and incomplete adduction of the vocal folds combine to compromise vocal intensity. Patients with Parkinson's disease speak softly—sometimes inaudibly. Rigid articulatory muscles have restricted range of movement. Articulation of patients with Parkinson's disease is imprecise and indistinct, with grossly diminished range of articulatory movements. The pathology causing Parkinson's disease disrupts initiation and timing of movements. The speech rate of patients with Parkinson's disease typically is highly variable, with periods of slow or normal rate interspersed with rushes of rapid and indistinct speech, punctuated by inappropriately

Box 11-4 Characteristics of Hypokinetic Dysarthria

Distinguishing Speech Characteristics

Blurring of consonant distinctions
Rapid rate, inability to modify rate
Short rushes of speech
Monopitch
Monoloudness
Reduced stress

Other Speech Characteristics

Harsh voice
Low pitch
Inappropriate silent intervals

Related Signs

Muscle rigidity
Slowness of movement
Tremor
Masked facies
Festinating gait*
Stooped posture

From Darley, F. L., Aronson, A. E., & Brown, J. R. (1975). *Motor speech disorders.* Philadelphia, W.B. Saunders; Duffy, J. R. (1995). *Motor speech disorders: Substrates, differential diagnosis, and management.* St Louis, MO: Mosby; and Rosenbek, J. C. & LaPointe, L. L. (1985). The dysarthrias: Description, diagnosis, and treatment. In D. F. Johns (Ed.), *Clinical management of neurogenic communication disorders* (2nd ed., pp. 97-152). Boston: Little-Brown and Company, 1985.

Festinating gait, Walking begins with slow steps. Steps increase in rate and become smaller, until the patient shuffles with short, rapid steps.

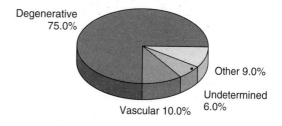

Figure 11-4 ■ **Causes of dysarthria for 107 Mayo Clinic patients with a primary diagnosis of hypokinetic dysarthria.** (Data from Duffy, J. R. [1995]. *Motor speech disorders: Substrates, differential diagnosis, and management.* St Louis, MO: Mosby.)

Patients with Parkinson's disease often have great difficulty taking the first steps when attempting to walk, but once they get going, they walk faster and faster with smaller and smaller steps until they are shuffling rapidly along on tiny steps. Parkinson's disease patients' speech disturbances and their gait disturbances may reflect the same underlying problems with initiating and controlling the rate of volitional movements.

placed pauses. Box 11-4 lists distinguishing features of hypokinetic dysarthria.

Hypokinetic dysarthria most often is associated with degenerative neurologic disease—usually Parkinson's disease. About three fourths of all cases of hypokinetic dysarthria are related to degenerative disease (Duffy, 1995). Multiple strokes in the basal ganglia account for about 10% of cases (Figure 11-4).

Hyperkinetic dysarthria is a consequence of basal ganglia pathology that causes involuntary, uncontrollable movements to appear. Darley, Aronson, and Brown (1975) divided hyperkinesia into two categories—*quick hyperkinesia* and *slow hyperkinesia.* In quick hyperkinesias (myoclonus, tics, chorea, ballism) involuntary movements are rapid, unpatterned, and unsustained or briefly sustained, and they do not occur repetitively in the same muscles. In slow hyperkinesias (athetosis, dystonia) involuntary movements build slowly to a peak, which may be maintained for intervals ranging from a few seconds to a few minutes before gradually subsiding. Muscle tone waxes and wanes, producing distorted postures of the head, trunk, and limbs.

The involuntary movements associated with hyperkinetic syndromes affect speech when they distort movements involved in respiration, phonation, or articulation. Respiration is disrupted when involuntary movements cause uncontrollable changes in breath pressure at the

Box 11-5 Characteristics of Hyperkinetic Dysarthria*

Quick Hyperkinetic (Chorea)

"...a highly variable pattern of interference with articulation; episodes of hypernasality; harshness and breathiness; and unplanned variations in loudness." (Darley, Aronson, & Brown, 1975, p. 210)

Distinguishing Speech Characteristics

Prolonged intervals between phonemes
Abnormal silent intervals
Variable rate
Distorted vowels, prolonged phonemes
Excess loudness variation

Other Speech Characteristics

Imprecise consonants
Monopitch
Harsh voice
Monoloudness
Short phrases
Irregular articulatory breakdown
Excess and equal stress, or reduced stress
Hypernasality
Strained-strangled-hoarse voice

Related Signs

Quick, unsustained involuntary movements

Slow Hyperkinetic (Dystonia)

"...the hyperkinetic dysarthria of dystonia shares with ataxic dysarthria and the hyperkinetic dysarthria of chorea characteristic and marked irregularities in precision of articulation, control of loudness, maintenance of steady rate, and efficiency of phonation..." (Darley, Aronson, & Brown, 1975, p. 222)

Distinguishing Speech Characteristics

Prolonged intervals between phonemes
Abnormal silent intervals, voice arrest
Irregular articulatory breakdown
Prolonged phonemes
Excess loudness variation

Other Speech Characteristics

Short phrases
Reduced stress
Voice stoppages
Slow rate
Imprecise consonants
Distorted vowels
Harsh voice
Strained-strangled-hoarse voice
Monopitch, monoloudness

Related Signs

Slow, sustained, unpredictable involuntary movements

From Darley, F. L., Aronson, A. E., & Brown, J. R. (1975). *Motor speech disorders.* Philadelphia, W.B. Saunders; Duffy, J. R. (1995). *Motor speech disorders: Substrates, differential diagnosis, and management.* St Louis, MO: Mosby; and Rosenbek, J. C., & LaPointe, L. L. (1985). The dysarthrias: Description, diagnosis, and treatment. In D. F. Johns (Ed.), *Clinical management of neurogenic communication disorders* (2nd ed., pp. 97-152). Boston: Little, Brown and Company.
*The visual characteristics of hyperkinetic movement disorders (jerks, tics, spasms, distorted postures) are diagnostically confirmatory of the disease syndrome. Speech abnormalities occur in conjunction with the movement disorders and are physiologically compatible with the movement disorders but usually are not the primary means of diagnosing the underlying disease.

vocal folds, leading to fluctuating vocal intensity. Articulation breaks down when involuntary movements disrupt the timing, force, and amplitude of speech movements. Patients with hyperkinetic dysarthria typically speak slowly and pause often. Their speech may have an uneven, jerky quality because normal variations in loudness and pitch are exaggerated by involuntary movements of respiratory muscles. The articulation of patients with hyperkinetic dysarthria may have an intermittently explosive quality when involuntary movements of the speech muscles exaggerate articulatory movements and interrupt the smooth flow of speech.

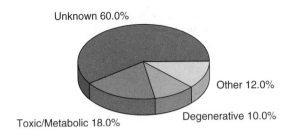

Figure 11-5 ■ **Causes of dysarthria for 86 Mayo Clinic patients with a primary diagnosis of hyperkinetic dysarthria.** (Data from Duffy, J. R. [1995]. *Motor speech disorders: Substrates, differential diagnosis, and management.* St Louis, MO: Mosby.)

Of all the types of dysarthrias, it [hyperkinetic dysarthria] is probably the one in which visual observation during speech helps to define the disorder because involuntary movements of the jaw, face, and tongue so obviously explain so many of its deviant perceptual characteristics. (Duffy, 1995, p. 351)

Box 11-5 lists distinguishing features of hyperkinetic dysarthria.

Hyperkinetic dysarthria is the most mysterious form of dysarthria when cause is considered. Duffy (1995) reported that the cause of dysarthria for approximately 60% of a sample of 86 patients with a primary diagnosis of hyperkinetic dysarthria was unknown. Toxic-metabolic conditions and degenerative disease accounted for the largest percentages of known causes (Figure 11-5).

Dysarthria and Cerebellar Pathology
Cerebellar pathology causes disruption of motor coordination and rhythm, usually with loss of muscle tone. Volitional movements are slow and awkward *(ataxia).* The range and force of movements are distorted *(dysmetria),* and movements become jerky and segmented *(decomposition of movement).* Intentional movements are accompanied by tremor that disappears when the muscles are at rest. Darley, Aronson, and Brown (1975) call the dysarthria associated with cerebellar pathology *ataxic dysarthria.*

The speech of patients with ataxic dysarthria is characterized by anomalies of force, timing,

---

Box 11-6 Characteristics of Ataxic Dysarthria

Distinguishing Speech Characteristics

Inconsistent consonant misarticulation
Excess, equal stress (scanning speech)
Irregular articulatory breakdown
Irregular, excessive loudness variability
Excessive rate variability

Other Speech Characteristics

Harsh voice
Prolonged phonemes
Prolonged interphonemic intervals
Falling intonation on vowels

Related Signs

Hypotonus
Diminished reflexes
Intention tremor
Dysmetria*

From Darley, F. L., Aronson, A. E., & Brown, J. R. (1975). *Motor speech disorders.* Philadelphia, W.B. Saunders; Duffy, J. R. (1995). *Motor speech disorders: Substrates, differential diagnosis, and management.* St Louis, MO: Mosby; and Rosenbek, J. C. & LaPointe, L. L. (1985). The dysarthrias: Description, diagnosis, and treatment. In D. F. Johns (Ed.), *Clinical management of neurogenic communication disorders* (2nd ed., pp. 97-152). Boston: Little-Brown and Company, 1985.
*Dysmetria, Inaccurate trajectory of goal-directed movements, causing overshoot or undershoot of targets.

---

and amplitude of movements. Uncontrollable changes in breath pressure at the vocal folds produce irregular, sometimes explosive, changes in pitch and loudness. Ataxic articulatory muscles create similar irregular disruptions of articulation. The patient's speech may be alternately normal in nasality and hypernasal as ataxic velopharyngeal muscles fluctuate in the force and amplitude of their movements. Box 11-6 lists distinguishing features of ataxic dysarthria.

Ataxic dysarthria may be caused by several conditions leading to cerebellar pathology. Cerebellar degeneration and demyelinating diseases account for about half the cases of ataxic

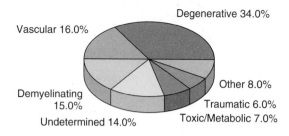

Figure 11-6 ■ **Causes of dysarthria for 107 Mayo Clinic patients with a primary diagnosis of ataxic dysarthria.** (Data from Duffy, J. R. [1995]. *Motor speech disorders: Substrates, differential diagnosis, and management.* St Louis, MO: Mosby.)

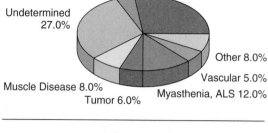

Figure 11-7 ■ **Causes of dysarthria for 107 Mayo Clinic patients with a primary diagnosis of flaccid dysarthria.** (Data from Duffy, J. R. [1995]. *Motor speech disorders: Substrates, differential diagnosis, and management.* St Louis, MO: Mosby.)

dysarthria, and vascular disease affecting the cerebellum accounts for about 15% (Figure 11-6).

Dysarthria and Cranial Nerve Pathology
Neuropathology in the pons and medulla often causes dysarthria by damaging corticobulbar tracts and the cranial nerve nuclei for nerves supplying the facial, oropharyngeal, and laryngeal muscles. If cranial nerves for the speech muscles are affected, *flaccid dysarthria* invariably follows. Pathology affecting cranial nerves can arise from several sources. Surgery involving the cervical spine, carotid endarterectomy (surgery to remove plaque from a carotid artery), or traumatic injuries to the head and neck may injure cranial nerves and create flaccid dysarthria. Strokes or tumors in the brain stem may cause flaccid dysarthria if cranial nerve nuclei are affected. Muscle diseases such as muscular dystrophy and degenerative diseases such as amyotrophic lateral sclerosis are less common causes of flaccid dysarthria (Figure 11-7).

Damage to cranial nerves or their nuclei causes flaccid paralysis of muscles on the side of the lesion, often accompanied by fasciculations (twitching) in the affected muscles followed by gradual muscle atrophy. The signs of cranial nerve damage depend on whether the pathology affects cranial nerve fiber tracts or the cranial nerve nucleus. Pathology affecting cranial nerve

fiber tracts causes paralysis of the muscles served by the nerve. Pathology affecting the cranial nerve nucleus causes paralysis of the muscles served by the nerve, often accompanied by spastic hemiparesis or hemiplegia of the contralateral arm and leg. This combination of signs happens because the corticospinal fiber tracts to muscles in the contralateral arm and leg pass through the brain stem next to the cranial nerve nuclei so that pathology affecting cranial nerve nuclei often impinges on corticospinal fibers serving the contralateral arm and leg (Figure 11-8).

> Corticospinal fibers decussate (cross) below the cranial nerve nuclei. Therefore pathology affecting cranial nerve nuclei on the left side of the brain stem creates right-sided hemiplegia and vice versa.

Pathology affecting the motor branch of the *facial nerve (CN 7)* causes weakness or flaccid paralysis of the ipsilateral eyelid muscles and the muscles of facial expression in the lower face. Pathology affecting the sensory branch of the facial nerve causes loss of taste in the anterior two thirds of the tongue.

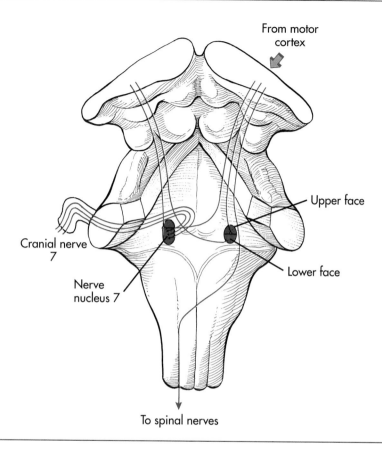

Figure 11-8 ■ Diagram of cranial nerves and their nuclei. A lesion that destroys a cranial nerve nucleus often destroys corticospinal tract fibers that descend alongside the nucleus. Muscles that depend on the destroyed cranial nerve nucleus are paralyzed on the side of the lesion. Because the corticospinal tract decussates below the level of the cranial nerve nuclei, a lesion that destroys a cranial nerve nucleus and adjacent corticospinal fibers causes contralateral paralysis of arm and leg muscles.

Pathology affecting the facial nerve often leads to a syndrome called *Bell's palsy*. Bell's palsy is a facial nerve syndrome in which the eyelid muscles and the muscles of facial expression on the side of the affected facial nerve are paralyzed. Bell's palsy is caused by inflammation of the facial nerve within the narrow bony channel through which it exits from the skull. Inflammation causes the facial nerve to swell. Swelling compresses the nerve within its channel, and paralysis and sensory loss in the ipsilat-

eral face follow. Bell's palsy usually resolves spontaneously within a few days or weeks. Sometimes the palsy does not resolve, the patient's facial muscles atrophy and droop, and the patient loses automatic eye blinks on the affected side. Loss of automatic eye blinks causes irritation of the eye because the eye no longer is moistened by tears. The patient may have to wear a bandage over the affected eye to control the irritation.

Unilateral facial nerve pathology usually has only minor effects on speech. Weakness, slowness, and restricted movement of the muscles that purse and retract the lips may cause imprecise articulation of sounds requiring lip movements *(p, b, m, f, v, w, wh)*. Weakness of muscles that tighten the cheeks may make sounds requiring oral breath pressure *(p, b, t, k)* weak and indistinct. These articulatory imperfections usually have only minor effects on intelligibility. The speech of patients with unilateral facial nerve pathology typically is intelligible and their speech deviations are annoying, rather than handicapping.

Bilateral facial nerve pathology has more significant effects on speech. Paralysis of lip muscles produces severe distortions of sounds requiring lip closure or lip rounding. Vowels requiring lip rounding are distorted. Sounds requiring oral breath pressure are weak and indistinct, and the patient's cheeks may flutter during conversations or spoken discourse.

> Some patients with bilateral facial paralysis use a finger to prop up the sagging weak side at rest or during speech or may use a finger to push up the lower lip to make sounds that require lip closure (Duffy, 1995).

Pathology affecting the *glossopharyngeal nerve (CN 9)* reduces or abolishes the gag reflex and weakens or paralyzes the (ipsilateral) muscles that elevate the palate and larynx plus the muscles that constrict the pharynx. Tactile sensation to the posterior wall of the pharynx and the back of the tongue on the side of the pathology may be reduced or abolished. Hypernasality and swallowing problems (dysphagia) are common consequences of glossopharyngeal nerve pathology. Pathology affecting the glossopharyngeal nerve may have minor effects on resonance because of compromised velopharyngeal elevation and constriction. These minor effects often are overshadowed by the effects of pathology affecting the vagus nerve (CN 10), which has more dramatic effects on speech.

> Because the glossopharyngeal nerve (CN 9), the vagus nerve (CN 10), and the spinal accessory nerve (CN 11) travel side by side as they leave the medulla and exit the skull, pathology affecting CN 9 usually also affects CN 10 and CN 11.

Pathology affecting the *vagus nerve (CN 10)* causes paralysis of the muscles of the soft palate on the side of the pathology, creating mild to moderate hypernasality of sounds requiring oral breath pressure. Pathology affecting the recurrent laryngeal branch of the vagus nerve causes unilateral vocal-fold paralysis and produces weak and breathy or hoarse voice, reduced vocal pitch, pitch breaks, and diplophonia (the presence of two pitches or tones in the voice). If the sensory branch of the vagus nerve is damaged, pharyngeal sensation is impaired and the mechanics of swallowing may be compromised.

Pathology affecting the *spinal accessory nerve (CN 11)* usually has no direct effects on speech because the spinal accessory nerve innervates external muscles in the neck and shoulders rather than muscles directly involved in speech. Bilateral accessory nerve pathology may have indirect effects on speech if muscle weakness causes shoulder and head droop, which in turn compromise respiration and phonation.

Pathology affecting the *hypoglossal nerve (CN 12)* causes (usually mild) ipsilateral weakness of the tongue. Patients with hypoglossal nerve damage have difficulty protruding the tongue, and the tongue deviates to the weak side because the muscles on the strong side pull the tongue out while the weak side lags behind. The patient also has difficulty moving the tongue laterally toward the side of the pathology because the weakened muscles on that side cannot move the tongue against the resistance created by the resting tone of the contralateral muscles.

Hypoglossal nerve pathology typically causes imprecise articulation of sounds that depend on tongue movements. The effects of unilateral hy-

Box 11-7 Characteristics of Flaccid Dysarthria

Distinguishing Speech Characteristics

Hypernasality
Continuous breathy voice
Nasal emission
Audible inspirations
Imprecise consonants

Other Speech Characteristics

Monopitch
Monoloudness
Harsh voice
Short phrases

Related Signs

Hypotonus (flaccidity)
Diminished reflexes
Fasciculations
Atrophy

From Darley, F. L., Aronson, A. E., & Brown, J. R. (1975). *Motor speech disorders.* Philadelphia, W.B. Saunders; Duffy, J. R. (1995). *Motor speech disorders: Substrates, differential diagnosis, and management.* St Louis, MO: Mosby; and Rosenbek, J. C. & LaPointe, L. L. (1985). The dysarthrias: Description, diagnosis, and treatment. In D. F. Johns (Ed.), *Clinical management of neurogenic communication disorders* (2nd ed., pp. 97-152). Boston: Little, Brown and Company.

poglossal nerve pathology typically are mild and do not seriously compromise intelligibility. Bilateral hypoglossal nerve pathology has more serious consequences, with sounds that require elevation of the tongue *(k, g, s, sh, tch, r, l)* particularly affected. If tongue weakness is severe, vocal resonance may be affected because of alterations in the shape of the oropharyngeal cavity. Hypoglossal nerve damage may affect swallowing if the patient cannot control the movement of food during chewing and cannot position the food preparatory to swallowing it.

Box 11-7 lists distinguishing features of flaccid dysarthria.

Dysarthria and Anterior Horn Cell Disease Several neurologic diseases are characterized by degeneration of anterior horn cells in the spinal cord. Most also cause degeneration of motor neurons serving cranial nerves, and some extend to the corticospinal and corticobulbar tracts. Degeneration of anterior horn cells causes symptoms typical of lower motor neuron disease, namely flaccid paralysis, fasciculations of muscles served by the damaged nerves, and eventual muscle atrophy. Anterior horn cell disease, by itself, has only indirect effects on speech. Weakness of respiratory muscles or muscles of the shoulders and rib cage may compromise breath support for speech, leading to diminished vocal intensity and short breath groups. When the disease also affects cranial nerves or corticospinal or corticobulbar tracts, speech movements may be compromised, affecting articulation, speech rate, speech prosody, and vocal quality, depending on which nerves are affected. Anterior horn cell diseases are almost always progressive (except for poliomyelitis). Consequently, many patients require augmentative or alternative communication systems during the final stages of their disease.

Dysarthria and Spinal Nerve Disease Spinal nerves sometimes are the focus of inflammatory or destructive disease. Inflammatory spinal nerve diseases (such as Guillain-Barré syndrome) usually are general rather than focal. Inflammatory spinal nerve diseases typically affect the longest nerve fibers first—muscles in the limbs are affected before the muscles in the torso, and distal muscles of the limbs are affected before proximal limb muscles. Motor fibers usually are affected before sensory fibers. Spinal nerve diseases produce symptoms typical of lower motor neuron disease—weakness, hypotonia, fasciculations, and diminished reflexes, together with variable sensory impairment. As is true for anterior horn cell disease, spinal nerve disease usually affects speech indirectly by compromising respiration. However, if the disease extends into the brain stem, corticobulbar tracts, or corticospinal tracts, speech movements may be directly affected, with changes typical of lower motor neuron pathology.

> Guillian-Barré syndrome is a progressive but self-limiting neurologic condition caused by axonal demyelination and characterized by progressive muscle weakness. Recovery usually begins spontaneously within 4 weeks of onset. Its cause is unknown, but it sometimes develops following inoculations or surgical procedures.

Diseases affecting cervical and thoracic spinal nerves may compromise respiratory support for speech by weakening or paralyzing respiratory muscles. Spinal nerve pathology affecting spinal nerves C3, C4, and C5, which innervate the muscles of the diaphragm, is especially likely to compromise respiratory support. Pathology affecting spinal nerves T2 through T12, which innervate muscles of the thoracic and abdominal wall, usually has less striking effects on respiratory support, unless it occurs in combination with pathology of cervical spinal nerves.

Respiratory muscles weakened by spinal cord pathology do not draw enough air into the lungs and fail to provide adequate breath pressure at the vocal folds. The effects of respiratory insufficiency may be exacerbated by weak and flaccid laryngeal muscles, which fail to fully adduct the vocal folds, leading to inefficient use of the patient's limited air supply. Patients with compromised respiratory support speak in short utterances, with frequent pauses for breath. Vocal intensity is weak and voice quality may be breathy, particularly at the end of utterances. Vocal pitch tends to be low and monotonous.

Dysarthria and Diseases of the Neuromuscular Junction Diseases of the neuromuscular junction are characterized by abnormalities in the neurotransmitters responsible for transmission of nerve impulses across synapses. The abnormalities are related to deficiency or excess of the neurotransmitters themselves or to alter-

ations in the sensitivity of receptor cells to neurotransmitters. *Myasthenia gravis* is the most common of the neuromuscular junction diseases. Myasthenia gravis is caused by autoimmune-mediated damage to the acetylcholine receptors on muscle cells, which interferes with neuromuscular transmission. Symptoms of myasthenia gravis include generalized and fluctuating muscle weakness (with a predilection for the extraocular, pharyngeal, oral, and proximal limb muscles), rapid muscle fatigue, and quick recovery of strength when the muscles are rested. Myasthenia gravis often causes a unique flaccid dysarthria syndrome, in which the patient's speech intelligibility deteriorates as the patient talks and recovers with rest.

> Injection of drugs that enhance acetylcholine uptake (Tensilon, neostigmine) causes dramatic improvement in the speech of patients with myasthenia gravis. The patient's dysarthria improves or disappears within 30 to 60 seconds after Tensilon injection or within 10 to 15 minutes after neostigmine injection. The effects of Tensilon last 4 to 5 minutes, and the effects of neostigmine last for 2 or 3 hours. (The differences in rate and duration of symptom remission exist because Tensilon is injected into a vein and neostigmine is injected into a muscle.)

Dysarthria and Primary Diseases of Muscle Some diseases affect muscle fibers, eventually producing atrophy of muscle tissue and flaccid dysarthria. Myotonic dystrophy is a relatively common inherited muscle disease (myopathy) that may affect muscles responsible for speech. Myositis, an acquired inflammatory muscle disease, usually does not affect speech but may affect respiratory muscles and sometimes produces swallowing problems. When myopathy affects muscles serving respiration and speech, characteristic signs of muscle weakness appear. If the patient's respiratory muscles are affected, the patient's utterances are short, long pauses occur between utterances, and vocal intensity is diminished because the patient does not possess the respiratory drive needed for normal utterance length and vocal intensity. If the patient's laryngeal muscles are affected, the patient's voice is weak and breathy because weakened laryngeal muscles cannot fully adduct the vocal folds and maintain the muscle tension needed for normal voice. If the patient's velopharyngeal muscles are affected the patient becomes hypernasal, and if the patient's articulatory muscles are affected the patient's articulation slows and becomes indistinct.

Dysarthria and Sensory Loss Damage to sensory branches of the cranial nerves or to the sensory cortex may impair sensation in the face, mouth, and neck and may cause transient speech disturbances, usually lasting no more than a few weeks. Persisting dysarthria from sensory disturbance alone is rare. However, when sensory disturbances are superimposed on coexisting motor impairments, the resulting dysarthria may be more severe than if the sensory disturbance were not present. A normal motor system usually has enough resilience to compensate for sensory disturbances, but an impaired motor system often does not.

Dysarthria and Disorders of Multiple Motor Systems What Darley, Aronson, and Brown called *mixed dysarthria* is common in clinical practice. According to Duffy (1995), slightly more than one third of patients with a primary diagnosis of dysarthria seen at Mayo Clinic over a 4-year interval exhibited mixed dysarthria. Mixed dysarthrias often are caused by combinations of neurologic events (e.g., multiple strokes, stroke plus demyelinating disease) and by diseases that affect more than one component of the motor system (e.g., amyotrophic lateral sclerosis).

> Mixed dysarthrias represent a heterogeneous group of speech disorders and neurologic diseases. Virtually any combination of two or more of the pure dysarthria types is possible, and in any particular mix any one of the components may

predominate. In spite of its heterogeneity, and the fact that sorting out the various components of mixed dysarthrias can be quite difficult, many mixed dysarthrias are perceptually distinguishable. And, like the pure forms, they may be the first, or among the first signs of neurologic disease. (Duffy, 1995, p. 234)

Spastic dysarthria plus flaccid dysarthria are common participants in mixed dysarthria types. According to Duffy (1995), spastic dysarthria was present in more than 90% of 300 Mayo Clinic cases with a primary diagnosis of mixed dysarthria. Flaccid dysarthria and ataxic dysarthria were present in 54% and 43% of the sample, respectively. Hypokinetic dysarthria and hyperkinetic dysarthria were less common, accounting for 21% and 13% of the sample, respectively. The combination flaccid–spastic was most common (42% of cases), followed by ataxic–spastic (23% of cases). Ataxic-flaccid-spastic and hyperkinetic-hypokinetic combinations were relatively uncommon.

Degenerative disease (especially amyotrophic lateral sclerosis) was the most common cause of mixed dysarthria in the Mayo Clinic sample, accounting for about two thirds of cases. Stroke was the second most common cause of mixed dysarthria, accounting for slightly more than 10% of cases. Demyelinating disease, traumatic brain injury, and tumor were occasional causes of mixed dysarthria (Figure 11-9).

Dysarthria Versus Apraxia of Speech Determining if a patient's speech abnormalities represent dysarthria or apraxia of speech usually is not difficult for experienced practitioners. Information from the neurologic examination may lead the way toward an appropriate diagnosis. The presence of cortical or near-cortical pathology in the language-dominant hemisphere points toward a diagnosis of *apraxia of speech*. The presence of pathology affecting the basal ganglia, brain stem, or peripheral nerves points toward a diagnosis of *dysarthria*.

Normal oral and velopharyngeal muscle strength and range of movement for simple nonspeech movements suggest *apraxia of speech;*

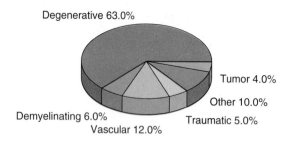

Degenerative 63.0%

Tumor 4.0%

Other 10.0%

Demyelinating 6.0%

Traumatic 5.0%

Vascular 12.0%

Figure 11-9 ■ Causes of dysarthria for 300 Mayo Clinic patients with a primary diagnosis of mixed dysarthria. (Data from Duffy, J. R. [1995]. *Motor speech disorders: Substrates, differential diagnosis, and management.* St Louis, MO: Mosby.)

impaired muscle strength and range of movement for simple non-speech movements suggest *dysarthria.* Hemiparesis, spasticity, and exaggerated limb reflexes are signs of upper motor neuron pathology, and their presence suggests that associated speech abnormalities are a manifestation of *apraxia of speech,* rather than dysarthria. The presence of aphasic symptoms (e.g., agrammatism, impaired comprehension, word-retrieval failure) points strongly toward a diagnosis of *apraxia of speech.*

Apraxia of speech and dysarthria usually affect speech processes in different ways. Because apraxia of speech is primarily a motor planning problem and not a problem with the muscles themselves, apraxic speakers' articulation and prosody are abnormal, but phonation and resonation usually are within a normal range. Because dysarthria is a product of weak or uncoordinated muscles, articulation, phonation, resonation, prosody, and sometimes respiration are abnormal.

The speech errors made by apraxic speakers differ from those made by dysarthric speakers. Most apraxic speech errors are *sound substitutions;* dysarthric speech errors tend to be *distortions* and *omissions.* Apraxic speakers often substitute a complex sound for a simple sound (e.g., substituting *ch* for *k*). Apraxic speakers of-

ten produce simple sounds and sound sequences without error but have trouble with complex sounds or with phonologically complex sound sequences. Dysarthric speakers usually have equivalent difficulty and make errors on the same sounds regardless of the length and phonologic complexity of the utterances.

Apraxic speakers typically produce what Darley, Aronson, and Brown (1975) called *islands of error-free speech,* in which automatic, unplanned utterances such as verbal asides and editorial comments ("wait a minute," "well whaddya know") are produced without error. Dysarthric speakers do not experience such interludes of error-free speech. (The speech of patients with ataxic dysarthria or hyperkinetic dysarthria may vary in accuracy across time, but the variability is related to physiologic changes in neuromotor control and not to the automaticity or phonologic complexity of what is said.) Table 11-2 summarizes the major differences between apraxia of speech and the dysarthrias.

Apraxia of speech and dysarthria sometimes co-occur. Most often the combination is one of apraxia of speech and unilateral upper motor neuron dysarthria. The combination produces the speech characteristics of apraxia of speech, plus those of unilateral upper motor neuron dysarthria—mild but consistent articulatory imprecision and (sometimes) mild strained-strangled-harsh voice quality. Bilateral hemispheric damage may produce apraxia of speech plus spastic dysarthria, in which slow speech rate, moderate to severe articulatory imprecision, and strained-strangled-harsh voice quality are superimposed on the signs of apraxia of speech. Apraxia of speech in combination with other varieties of dysarthria is less common and may prove more puzzling, but the presence of intervals of error-free speech and the positive effects of automaticity on apraxic speakers may help to identify apraxia that coexists with other varieties of dysarthria.

GENERAL CONCEPTS 11-2

• Dysarthria is a generic label for a group of speech impairments caused by *weakness,*

	T A B L E 1 1 - 2	
	Major differences between apraxia of speech and the dysarthrias. These differences are true for dysarthria in general. Specific dysarthria types may differ in some features.	
Feature	**Apraxia of speech**	**Dysarthria**
Neuropathology	Cortical, language-dominant hemisphere	Subcortical, peripheral
Neurologic signs	Aphasia, hemiparesis, hemiplegia, spasticity, exaggerated reflexes	Rigidity, dyskinesia, flaccid paralysis, diminished reflexes, fasciculations, atrophy*
Motor signs	Strength, range of movement, coordination intact in nonverbal oral movements	Strength, range of movement, coordination impaired in nonverbal oral movements
Related conditions	Aphasia, buccofacial apraxia, limb apraxia	Dysphagia, dyskinesia, rigidity, hypotonus*
Speech processes affected	Articulation, prosody	Articulation, phonation, resonation, prosody
Primary speech error type	Substitutions, transpositions	Distortions, omissions
Speech error pattern	Variable, unpredictable, intervals of error-free speech, automatic speech better than highly planned speech	Consistent, predictable; no intervals of error-free speech; no effect of automaticity†
Speech sounds in error	Consonants, primarily in phonologically complex utterances; vowels usually unaffected	Most consonants, vowels often distorted‡
Effects of length, complexity	Longer, phonologically complex utterances more likely to elicit errors	Short, phonologically simple utterances and long, phonologically complex utterances equally affected

*Depending on the type of dysarthria.
†Some patients with hyperkinetic dysarthrias may have intervals of relatively good speech, but these intervals are not predictable based on automaticity, phonologic complexity, etc.
‡However, more complex consonants are harder for most dysarthric speakers.

paralysis, incoordination, or *sensory loss* in muscle groups responsible for speech.

- The most common cause of dysarthria is *weakness or paralysis* of muscles needed for speech.
- Unilateral damage to upper motor neurons usually does not cause persisting dysarthria because most of the muscles responsible for speech are bilaterally innervated.

- A few patients may develop mild but persisting *unilateral upper motor neuron dysarthria* following apparent unilateral upper motor neuron pathology.
- Bilateral damage in upper motor neurons usually causes persisting *spastic dysarthria.*
- Pathology in the *pons* and *medulla* almost invariably causes *flaccid dysarthria* because of damaged nuclei for cranial nerves serving

speech muscles. Pathology affecting *cranial nerve fibers* causes *flaccid paralysis* of muscles served by the nerves.

- *Flaccid dysarthria* often follows damage to the *glossopharyngeal nerve* (CN 9), the *vagus nerve* (CN 10), and the *hypoglossal nerve* (CN 12) because these cranial nerves supply muscles that are important for speech. Damage to the *facial nerve* (CN 7) or the *spinal accessory nerve* (CN 11) usually do not cause significant dysarthria because the muscles they innervate do not have major responsibilities for speech production.
- Pathology affecting the *extrapyramidal system* often causes *hypokinetic* or *hyperkinetic dysarthria* plus associated motor abnormalities (impaired volitional movements, muscle rigidity, uncontrollable involuntary movements).
- *Parkinson's disease* is a common disease of the extrapyramidal system that causes *hypokinetic dysarthria* characterized by weak, strained, and breathy voice; rushes of rapid speech; and indistinct articulation.
- Pathology affecting the *basal ganglia* often causes *hyperkinetic dysarthria,* in which speech and respiration are compromised by sporadic, involuntary movements of muscle groups.
- *Cerebellar pathology* often causes *ataxic dysarthria,* in which relatively well-controlled speech is punctuated by intervals of dysarthria caused by aberrations in the force and amplitude of respiratory and articulatory movements.
- *Degenerative neurologic diseases* often cause *mixed dysarthria.* Mixed dysarthria usually represents a combination of *spastic* and *flaccid* signs.
- Diseases affecting *anterior horn cells* or *spinal nerves* sometimes affect speech by compromising muscles of respiration. Patients with anterior horn cell or spinal nerve pathology speak softly, in short utterances, and with abnormally long pauses between utterances because of respiratory insufficiency.
- Diseases of the *neuromuscular junction* often cause dysarthria. The most common of

these diseases is *myasthenia gravis.* The speech of patients with myasthenia gravis becomes increasingly dysarthric the longer they speak. The dysarthria diminishes or disappears with rest.
- *Sensory loss* in structures involved in speech may produce transient mild speech impairments but rarely causes significant dysarthria. However, sensory loss superimposed on coexisting motor speech impairments usually increases the severity of dysarthria.
- Dysarthria may be differentiated from apraxia of speech by the *types of speech errors,* the *consistency of speech errors,* the presence of *intervals of error-free speech,* and the *effects of context* on articulatory accuracy. *Phonation* and *resonation* usually are normal in apraxia of speech, but they are abnormal in dysarthria.

Evaluation

Dysarthric patients are referred to speech-language pathologists because their speech sounds abnormal to physicians, nurses, or family members or to the patients themselves. The speech-language pathologist's assessment of a dysarthric patient usually has five purposes:

1. To determine if the patient's speech is abnormal
2. To evaluate the nature and severity of speech abnormalities
3. To determine the cause(s) of speech abnormalities
4. To determine if treatment is appropriate
5. To identify potential directions for treatment

Because dysarthria is a problem with speaking, it seems logical that one should look to the mouth for its source. The mouth is the appropriate place to start, but the search also must extend down into the throat, chest, and abdomen and up into the pharynx and nasal cavities. To speak we must breathe, so assessment of dysarthria includes assessment of respiration. To speak we must produce voice, so assessment of dysarthria includes assessment of vocal-fold function. To speak normally we must nasalize and denasalize sounds, so assessment of dysarthria includes assessment of the muscles of the posterior pharynx and the soft palate. To speak intelligibly we must shape the breath stream into consonants and vowels, so assessment of dysarthria includes assessment of how well the tongue, lips, and jaw move and how accurately they reach their targets.

Structured assessment of dysarthria usually begins with administration of a *motor speech examination* in which the patient's respiration, phonation, resonance, prosody, and articulation are systematically evaluated. Phonation and resonance usually are estimated with a rating scale with which the examiner judges characteristics such as *pitch, loudness, voice quality,* and *nasality.* Prosody usually is estimated with a rating scale with which the examiner judges characteristics such as *rate, phrase length, stress,* and *intonation.* Respiration may be measured indirectly with measures such as *forced expiration time, sustained phonation time,* or *maximum utterance length,* although phonation time and utterance length are affected by the efficiency of glottal closure. Articulation usually is measured with a combination of rating scales and scoring of articulation in speech production tasks *(syllable repetition, word repetition, phrase repetition, and spontaneous speech).* Figure 11-10 shows a form for rating speech produced by dysarthric individuals.

Assessment of the processes involved in dysarthria entails assessment of *respiration, phonation, resonation,* and *articulation.* However, one cannot consider these processes piece by piece because they interact. Assessment of dysarthria is as much a search for interactions among processes underlying speech as it is a diagnosis of abnormalities within speech itself.

Evaluating Respiratory Support

Characteristics of Normal Respiration

In neurologically normal adults, respiration for biologic purposes and respiration for speech differ in subtle but important ways. In normal passive breathing, the diaphragm provides most of the respiratory drive by contracting during inhalation. This muscle contraction compresses the abdominal contents downward, increases the volume of the chest cavity, and generates negative

pressure within the lungs. Muscles in the chest wall and shoulder girdle contribute by elevating the shoulders and rib cage, further increasing the volume of the chest cavity and adding to the negative pressure within the lungs. Outside atmospheric pressure then forces air into the lungs.

Expiratory force for exhalation during normal passive breathing is generated by the torque of the expanded rib cage as it returns to its resting position and by upward pressure on the bottom of the diaphragm as the compressed abdominal contents regain their normal volume. When a person speaks, the elasticity of the rib cage and the pressure exerted by compressed abdominal contents do not generate enough breath pressure for speech (Hixon, 1987). The speaker provides the necessary respiratory boost by actively contracting the abdominal muscles to increase upward pressure on the diaphragm.

During passive breathing, normal adults inflate their lungs to about 20% of total capacity, but when they speak they inflate their lungs to from 35% to 60% of total capacity (Hixon, 1987). The usual respiratory pattern during speech consists of quick inhalation to about 60% of lung capacity, followed by slow exhalation until the lungs reach about 30% of total capacity, at which time the speaker takes another breath. The normal ratio of inhalation to exhalation is about 1:6—that is, the expiratory phase lasts about six times as long as the inspiratory phase (Yorkston, Beukelman, & Bell, 1988).

Passive Respiration A patient's posture and general appearance may suggest potential respiratory insufficiency. Patients who slouch and bend forward at the waist when standing or sitting or who sit or stand with dropped chin and drooping head may compress the chest cavity and lungs, compromising respiration for speech. (Slouched, drooping posture often is a sign of general muscle weakness, which in itself may compromise respiration.)

Abnormality in the rate and depth of a patient's resting respiration also may suggest respiratory insufficiency for speech. Normal resting respiration rates range from 12 to 20 cycles per minute, although there is substantial variability

Rating Scale for Motor Speech Disorders

Phonation

Overall pitch: Very low ☐   Somewhat low ☐   Normal ☐   Somewhat high ☐
Pitch breaks: Often ☐   Sometimes ☐   Never ☐
Monotone, monopitch: Severe ☐   Moderate ☐   Normal ☐
Tremor: Severe ☐   Moderate ☐   Normal ☐
Loudness: Very loud ☐   Somewhat loud ☐   Normal ☐   Somewhat soft ☐   Very soft ☐
Uncontrolled changes in loudness: Often ☐   Sometimes ☐   Never ☐
Diminishing loudness with sustained phonation: Severe ☐   Moderate ☐   Normal ☐
Harsh voice (rough, raspy): Severe ☐   Moderate ☐   Normal ☐
Hoarse voice (wet, gurgly): Severe ☐   Moderate ☐   Normal ☐
Breathy voice: Severe ☐   Moderate ☐   Normal ☐

Respiration

Forced inspiration, expiration: Often ☐   Sometimes ☐   Never ☐
Audible inhalation: Often ☐   Sometimes ☐   Never ☐
Audible exhalation: Often ☐   Sometimes ☐   Never ☐
Utterance length: Very short ☐   Somewhat short ☐   Normal ☐

Resonance

Very hyponasal ☐   Somewhat hyponasal ☐   Normal ☐   Somewhat hypernasal ☐   Very hypernasal ☐
Nasal emission: Severe ☐   Moderate ☐   Mild ☐   None ☐

Prosody

Rate: Very slow ☐   Somewhat slow ☐   Normal ☐   Somewhat fast ☐   Very fast ☐
Rate: Very variable ☐   Somewhat more variable than normal ☐   Normal variability ☐
Intermittent fast rate: Often ☐   Sometimes ☐   Never ☐
Stress: Reduced ☐   Excessive ☐   Uncontrolled changes ☐   Normal ☐
Excessive pauses: Between phrases ☐   Between words ☐   Within words ☐
Short rushes of speech: Often ☐   Sometimes ☐   Never ☐

Articulation

Imprecise consonants: Often ☐   Sometimes ☐   Never ☐
Weak plosive consonants: Severe ☐   Moderate ☐   Mild ☐   None ☐
Distorted vowels: Often ☐   Sometimes ☐   Never ☐
Prolonged phonemes: Often ☐   Sometimes ☐   Never ☐
Repeated phonemes: Often ☐   Sometimes ☐   Never ☐
Irregular articulatory imprecision: Often ☐   Sometimes ☐   Never ☐

Consistency of Errors

Phoneme errors: Consistent ☐   Inconsistent ☐
Syllable/word errors: Consistent ☐   Inconsistent ☐
Intervals of fluent, error-free speech: Many ☐   Some ☐   None ☐

Error Correction

Attempts to correct errors: Often ☐   Sometimes ☐   Never ☐
Successful error correction: Often ☐   Sometimes ☐   Never ☐

Spontaneous Speech versus Repetition

Spontaneous speech better ☐   Repetition better ☐   No difference ☐

Intelligibility

10% or less ☐   11% - 25% ☐   26% - 50% ☐   51% - 75% ☐   76% or above ☐

Overall Effect on Listener

Very distracting ☐   Somewhat distracting ☐   Minimally distracting ☐   Within normal range ☐

Figure 11-10 ■ **A rating form for rating various aspects of motor speech disorders.**

in the normal adult population. Overt movement of the shoulders or head does not occur during normal respiration. When it does, it suggests that the patient is compensating for weak respiratory muscles. Fast, shallow breathing (in the absence of exertion or heightened emotions) may be a sign of weakness in the muscles of respiration, and patients with weak respiratory muscles may have difficulty speaking with normal loudness and phrase length. Fluctuating breathing rate during passive breathing may be a manifestation of involuntary movements associated with cerebellar or extrapyramidal system pathology. The movement abnormalities creating the patient's fluctuating breathing pattern also may cause irregular disruption of the patient's phonation and articulation.

Evaluating Respiration for Speech The clinician's first objective in evaluating respiration for speech is to determine if comprehensive evaluation of respiratory function is necessary. The clinician asks the patient to produce sustained phonation and to repeat syllables. Most normal adults can sustain phonation of an open vowel for 7 to 8 seconds. However, if a patient can sustain effortless phonation of an open vowel *(ah)* with normal loudness for 4 to 5 seconds and can say at least three consonant-vowel syllables on a single breath with normal loudness, respiration is likely to be at least minimally adequate for speech, and direct work on respiration may not be needed.

Patients with 4- to 5-second maximum phonation times will be able to say only short phrases (one to three words) on a single breath. For these patients, respiration may be worked on indirectly by increasing the number of words the patient can say on a single breath.

If the patient fails to meet sustained-phonation criteria, the clinician cannot immediately conclude that the problem is with respiratory support because sustained phonation requires not only that the patient impound an adequate supply of air but that the patient has strong enough respiratory muscles to generate functional subglottic air pressure and enough laryngeal muscle movement and strength to keep the vocal folds adducted against the pressure of the breath stream. Problems with vocal-fold adduction usually are obvious during phonation. If the vocal folds are not closing, the patient's voice sounds weak and breathy. If the vocal folds are hypertonic, the patient's voice sounds harsh and strangled.

Measuring Respiratory Pressure and Flow Sophisticated instruments are available for measuring respiratory pressure and flow. They are not commonly available clinically. However, two inexpensive and relatively simple instruments for measuring breath pressure and flow can be constructed.

Netsell and Hixon (1978) described a U-tube manometer suitable for measuring breath pressure (Figure 11-11). The manometer is a U-shaped glass tube fastened to a board. The U-tube is half-filled with colored water and calibrated in centimeters (see Netsell and Hixon for specifications). A flexible tube is attached to one end of the U-tube. A rigid T-shaped tube serves as a mouthpiece and bleed tube. The patient blows into the mouthpiece and breath pressure displaces the column of water. The leak tube provides a constant escape for the air stream so that the person being tested must maintain continuous air flow to sustain displacement of the water. According to Netsell and Hixon, an individual who can maintain a 5 cm displacement of the water column for 5 seconds has sufficient breath pressure for basic speech requirements *(the 5 for 5 rule)*.

Hixon, Hawley, and Wilson (1982) suggested a similar but simpler and easier-to-use device. A tall drinking glass (12 cm or more) is filled with water. The glass is calibrated in centimeters (Figure 11-12). A drinking straw is affixed to the glass so that it reaches a prescribed depth (e.g., 5 cm). An individual blowing into the straw

Manometer

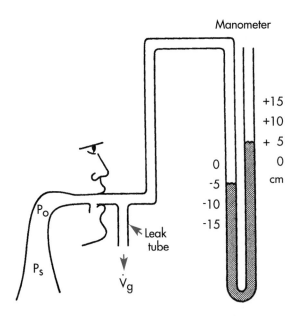

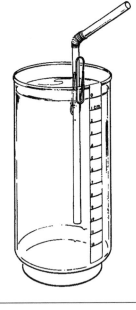

Figure 11-11 ■ A U-tube manometer. The patient blows into the mouthpiece. A leak tube permits a constant amount of air to escape. The height of the liquid in the U-tube is determined by the amount of breath pressure the patient can sustain. (From Netsell, R., & Hixon, T. J. [1978]. A noninvasive method for clinically estimating subglottal air pressure. *J Speech Hear Disord, 43,* 326-330.)

Figure 11-12 ■ A water glass manometer. The deeper the straw is in the water, the more breath pressure is needed to sustain a string of bubbles at the deep end of the straw. (From Hixon, T. J., Hawley, J. T., & Wilson, K. J. [1982]. An around-the-house device for the clinical determination of respiratory driving pressure. *J Speech Hear Disord, 47,* 413-415.)

must maintain breath pressure equal to the depth to which the straw is inserted in the water to generate a stream of bubbles at the end of the straw. By inserting the straw to 5 cm, one can evaluate whether a patient meets the *5 for 5 rule.*

Evaluating Phonation

Laryngeal Mechanics Assessment of laryngeal muscle function often precedes assessment of phonation. To determine the functional integrity of muscles that adduct the vocal cords, the examiner may ask the patient to *cough, grunt,* and *produce glottal stops* (voiceless grunts) individually and several times in succession. Weak, breathy, or indistinct coughs, grunts, and glottal stops suggest weakness of vocal cord adductor

muscles, impaired respiratory drive, or both. Patients with compromised respiratory support often produce sharper glottal stops and grunts than coughs because grunts and glottal stops require less respiratory drive than coughs. Patients with compromised vocal-fold adduction produce weak and indistinct coughs, grunts, and glottal stops (Duffy, 1995). The presence of audible inspiration (*inhalation stridor*—a rasping sound during inhalation) suggests weakness in the muscles that separate (*abduct*) the vocal cords.

Phonation Time and Voice Quality The typical first step in evaluating phonation is to ask the patient to sustain an open vowel (*ah*) until the patient runs out of breath while the clinician times the duration of the patient's phonation. As the patient phonates, the clinician also evaluates the loudness, pitch, and quality of the patient's voice. Phonation times below 12 to 15 seconds are considered abnormally low and suggest problems either with glottal valving or with breath support for speech.

Damage to cranial nerves, especially the laryngeal branches of the vagus nerve, may cause weakness or paralysis of laryngeal muscles. The weakened muscles cannot fully adduct the vocal folds, leading to air wastage and to diminished phonation time plus breathy and weak voice quality and abnormally low pitch.

Bilateral damage to upper motor neurons causes strained, strangled, harsh voice quality. Spastic laryngeal muscles constrict the glottal opening, increase glottal resistance to airflow, and reduce maximum phonation time. Most patients with bilateral upper motor neuron pathology should, however, have sufficient respiratory drive to produce 5 to 10 seconds of sustained phonation, although with strained, strangled, and harsh quality.

Most patients with cerebellar pathology can produce 5 to 10 seconds of sustained phonation, although voice quality is likely to be abnormal and both loudness and quality may fluctuate. Abnormalities in coordination of respiration and vocal-fold adduction may cause aspiration of voiced sounds or strained, strangled voice quality at the onset of phonation.

Extrapyramidal diseases may affect vocal-fold adduction, shortening phonation time and affecting voice quality. Maximum phonation times for patients with extrapyramidal disease range from substantially reduced (3 to 4 seconds) to normal, depending on the efficiency of glottal valving and the degree to which respiratory muscles are affected.

Patients with *Parkinson's disease* typically have breathy, hoarse voices, with maximum phonation time reduced by laryngeal-muscle rigidity. Patients with Parkinson's disease often begin phonation normally but sound progressively more strangled as phonation continues, often culminating in a whisper or squeak. Patients

with movement disorders caused by extrapyramidal disease typically experience altered vocal pitch, loudness, and quality during episodes of involuntary movements. The alterations may be slow or rapid, continuous or intermittent, depending on the nature of the patient's movement disorder. Patients with *tremor* usually produce regular, cyclic perturbations of pitch and loudness. Patients with *chorea* produce irregular prolonged distortions of vocal pitch and loudness during episodes of choreiform movement.

Vocal Flexibility and Coordination Assessing phonation time and voice quality provides important information about the efficiency of laryngeal valving and respiratory support for speech. Continuous phonation requires that the vocal folds be adducted and maintained in a constant state of tension, but continuous phonation does not provide much information about how well the laryngeal muscles accomplish the intricate movements required by connected speech. That information is obtained by asking the patient to change vocal pitch and loudness in prescribed ways. The patient may be asked to do the following:

- Count aloud from 1 to 10, beginning with a whisper and ending with a shout.
- Count from 10 to 1, beginning with a shout and ending in a whisper.
- Sing up and down a musical scale.
- Count aloud, beginning with the lowest pitch that the patient can produce and gradually increasing pitch until the patient can go no higher.
- Say short sequences of numbers aloud, alternating loud and soft voice or high and low pitch.
- Repeat sentences at a whisper, normal loudness, and a shout.
- Read a paragraph or story aloud with exaggerated emphatic stress.

The changes in pitch and loudness achieved by the patient in these tasks may be compared with what the patient does in less structured speech tasks, such as conversational speech. Many dysarthric patients sound better in structured tasks when their attention is focused on controlling the pitch and loudness of their speech than in unstructured tasks in which they must attend to other tasks, such as formulating ideas and taking turns in addition to controlling pitch and loudness.

The patient's ability to coordinate respiration and speech may be evaluated by asking the patient to do the following:

- Produce a series of short vowels *(uh-uh-uh—, ee-ee-ee—)*.
- Alternate aspirate-vowel and voiced continuant-consonant pairs *(huh-muh—huh-muh)*.
- Alternate voiced and voiceless consonant-vowel pairs *(puh-buh—puh-buh)*.

If nervous system pathology is sufficient to produce significant dysarthria, vocal flexibility almost always is reduced. Constricted range of pitch and loudness may be caused by upper motor neuron pathology, lower motor neuron pathology, extrapyramidal pathology, or cerebellar pathology. Incoordination between respiration and voice onset most often are related to extrapyramidal system pathology or cerebellar pathology.

Evaluating Velopharyngeal Function and Resonation Velopharyngeal structures serve to isolate the pharyngeal and oral cavities from the nasal cavity during swallowing and production of denasalized speech sounds. Although the exact means by which velopharyngeal closure is achieved differs somewhat across individuals (Yorkston, Beukelman, & Bell, 1988), closure is achieved primarily by movement of the velum (soft palate) up and back to meet the posterior pharyngeal wall and by movement of the lateral pharyngeal walls toward the midline to meet the sides of the velum. Occasionally the posterior pharyngeal wall may move forward toward the velum (Croft, Shprintzen, & Rakoff, 1981). When normal speakers produce denasalized sounds, velopharyngeal muscles contract to close the nasopharyngeal opening and prevent the passage of air from the oral cavity through the nasal cavity. When the speaker produces nasal sounds, the velopharyngeal muscles relax, opening the na-

sopharyngeal port and allowing part of the air stream to pass through the nasal cavity, adding nasal resonance to the sounds.

Velopharyngeal Mechanics Evaluation of the mechanics of velopharyngeal functions begins with visual assessment of the resting palate and pharynx through the patient's open mouth. Bilateral droop of the palate at rest suggests bilateral weakness of muscles that elevate the palate (served by CN 9 and 10); unilateral droop suggests weakness of palatal muscles on the drooping side. Spontaneous rippling or dimpling of palatal muscles suggests loss of input from CN 9 and 10. Sporadic or rhythmic movements or pulsations of the resting palate suggest pathology affecting the basal ganglia or cerebellum.

Indirect assessment of velopharyngeal mechanics may be accomplished by having the patient puff out the cheeks with air. Failure, especially when accompanied by nasal escape of air, suggests poor velopharyngeal closure. Success, however, does not ensure velopharyngeal closure because a patient may compensate for weak velopharyngeal muscles by pushing the velum up with the back of the tongue. A *tongue-anchor test* (Dalston, Warren, & Dalston, 1990; Fox & Johns, 1970), in which the patient protrudes the tongue between closed lips while puffing out the cheeks, prevents the patient from using the tongue to help occlude the velopharynx.

Evaluation of velopharyngeal mechanics continues with the patient producing an open-mouth sustained *ah* several times in succession while the examiner watches for movement of the palate and oropharynx as phonation begins and ends. Failure to elevate the palate during phonation suggests bilateral weakness in palatal muscles. Asymmetric elevation of the palate during phonation suggests unilateral weakness of palatal muscles on the non-elevating side.

Evaluating Resonance To evaluate velopharyngeal function in speech the clinician listens for *hypernasality, nasal escape of air,* and *distorted consonants* while the patient produces sustained phonation and repeats syllables. Judging hypernasality is one of the clinician's most difficult tasks. Such judgments often are unreliable, in part because they are affected by other speech characteristics (Moll, 1968). The more severe a patient's articulatory deviations, the more likely the patient will be judged hypernasal. Patients who speak loudly tend to be judged more hypernasal than those who speak softly (Yorkston, Beukelman, & Bell, 1988). However, no satisfactory substitute for subjective judgments of hypernasality exists.

One of the easiest tests for hypernasality is to alternately pinch and release the nostrils as the patient produces a sustained vowel. If the patient is hypernasal, the sound of the vowel changes as the nostrils are occluded and opened. However, this test does not always predict hypernasality in connected speech. Some patients can successfully occlude the velopharyngeal port during sustained phonation but cannot do so during the more complex movement patterns of connected speech. One can, of course, pinch and release the patient's nostrils as the patient produces connected speech. If the hypernasality is dramatic, changes in vocal resonance will be apparent, although moderate hypernasality may not be apparent and mild hypernasality will not be apparent. Fortunately, moderate hypernasality, either by itself or in combination with mild articulatory imprecision, usually does not make speech grossly unintelligible. Hypernasality usually is a primary focus of treatment for those patients in whom velopharyngeal incompetence is so severe that it significantly compromises speech intelligibility.

The primary means of assessing nasal escape of air also is perceptual. The clinician listens for sounds of air escaping through the nose as the patient sustains phonation or repeats syllables, phrases, or sentences containing stop consonants. Other techniques have been used (feathers or small pieces of tissue on a card held under the nose, a cold mirror held under the nose), but they usually yield positive results only when a patient has severe velopharyngeal incompetence. Instrumentation to measure nasal emission is available, but it is expensive and not available in most clinics. Consequently, the clinician's ears (and sometimes, eyes) remain the most common instrument for measuring nasal escape.

Velopharyngeal incompetence often causes distortion of consonants; especially consonants that require interruption or constriction of the air stream (stop consonants such as *p* and *b* and continuants such as *s* and *sh*). When velopharyngeal incompetence is present, stop consonants and continuants are weak and may be accompanied by nasal emission of air, and voiced consonants (such as *b* or *d*) are weak and hypernasal. When articulation of consonants requiring increased oral breath pressure (stops and continuants) seems markedly poorer than articulation of other sounds, velopharyngeal incompetence is the likely reason.

Evaluating Articulation

Articulatory Mechanics Assessment of articulatory mechanics typically precedes assessment of speech-sound production. The examiner observes the patient's face at rest, looking for drooping, atrophy, or involuntary movements of muscles. Then the examiner asks the patient to open his or her mouth and observes the tongue at rest, noting whether it is on the midline and looking for dimpling, rippling, or involuntary movements. Off-midline resting tongue position and dimpling or rippling may suggest pathology affecting the hypoglossal nerve (CN 12). Involuntary movements may suggest extrapyramidal or cerebellar pathology.

Next the examiner tests the strength, agility, and range of movement of muscles in the jaw, lips, and tongue. The patient is asked to open and close the jaw several times while the examiner watches for slowness, restricted movement, or deviation from the midline. If the masseter muscles on one side are weak, the jaw deviates toward the unaffected side. Then the patient is asked to open and close the jaw and move it from side to side while the examiner grasps the patient's chin and resists the movements. Weakness and restricted range of movement suggest weakness of the masseter muscles (served by CN 5).

Next the patient is asked to open and close the jaw several times ("click your teeth together") while the examiner notes the speed and timing of the movements. Irregular rate and timing of jaw movements may suggest problems in the extrapyramidal system.

Lip movements and strength are evaluated by asking the patient to purse, protrude, and retract the lips ("show me your teeth," "smile"), first unopposed and then while the examiner resists the movements. Asymmetry of lip retraction and protrusion and one-sided weakness of lip muscles suggests unilateral pathology affecting the facial nerve (CN 7) on the side of the weakness.

> Some patients who smile asymmetrically when asked to smile volitionally produce symmetric smiles when spontaneously smiling. This phenomenon suggests that different motor systems perform volitional smiles (sometimes called *pyramidal smiles*) than perform spontaneous smiles.

Tongue movements and strength are assessed by asking the patient to protrude the tongue and move it from side to side. Tongue deviation away from the midline suggests weakness of tongue muscles on the side toward which the tongue deviates. Restricted range of movement on one side suggests weakness of tongue muscles on the side of restricted range of movement. Tongue strength may be assessed by asking the patient to push out each cheek with her or his tongue. If the patient is successful, the examiner may push against the cheek to assess the strength of the tongue muscles on each side. Tongue strength also may be assessed by asking the patient to protrude the tongue while the examiner resists the movement with a tongue depressor.

Speech Movements Syllable and phrase repetition are the primary vehicles for assessing dysarthric patients' articulatory accuracy. The syllables and phrases are chosen to highlight the contribution of the various articulatory structures to the overall speech product. Lip closure is evaluated by asking the patient to repeat bilabial consonant-vowel combinations *(puh-puh-puh—, buh-buh-buh—)*. Tongue-tip elevation is evaluated by asking the patient to repeat tongue-tip alveolar-ridge combinations *(tuh-tuh-tuh—, duh-duh-duh—)*. Elevation of the back of the tongue is evaluated by asking the patient to repeat high-back consonant combinations *(kuh-kuh-kuh—, guh-guh-guh—)*. Articulatory flexibility and coordination are evaluated by asking the patient to repeat strings of syllables in which articulation points change *(puh-tuh-kuh, duh-buh-guh)*. Articulatory accuracy in longer segments of speech is estimated by asking the patient to repeat multisyllabic words *(gingerbread-gingerbread-gingerbread, artillery-artillery-artillery)*, phrases *(the national Republican convention)*, and sentences *(Nelson Rockefeller drives a Lincoln Continental)*.

Articulation Versus Intelligibility Standard articulation inventories such as those used to evaluate children rarely are administered to dysarthric patients. Articulatory problems in dysarthria usually are part of a constellation of respiratory, phonatory, and resonance disturbances. Consequently, clinicians are more interested in which impaired speech processes account for a patient's pattern of articulatory impairment than in which sounds are in error. The goal of most treatment for dysarthric patients is intelligibility, rather than articulatory accuracy. Because articulatory accuracy has only a general relationship to intelligibility, measuring intelligibility usually provides more therapeutically valuable information than measuring articulatory accuracy.

Yorkston, Beukelman, and Bell (1988) offer three objections to the use of traditional articulation inventories with dysarthric speakers:

1. A judge's perceptions of articulatory accuracy may not reflect the adequacy of the patient's articulatory movements.
2. Articulation inventories fail to discriminate between sounds that are accurate and sounds

that are distorted but still within phoneme boundaries.

3. When judges know the target words, as in traditional articulation inventories, they are likely to overestimate a patient's articulatory accuracy.

Yorkston and associates (1986) advocate use of the *phoneme identification task* as a substitute for traditional articulation inventories. In the phoneme identification task, the speaker is recorded while reading aloud a list of single words and sentences. The list is designed to elicit 57 target phonemes. A judge (not the examiner) then listens to the recording and identifies the target phonemes, using the following procedure:

- A word or sentence is played.
- The judge is given a card showing a word with the target phoneme missing (e.g., *ma_* for *mat*) and is asked to identify the missing phoneme.
- The judge rates the patient's production of the perceived phoneme using a four-point scale, ranging from *no basis for a guess* to *correct, undistorted.*

Evaluating Intelligibility Yorkston and Beukelman (1981) published an assessment tool called *Assessment of Intelligibility of Dysarthric Speech.* The test has two sections. One measures single-word intelligibility; the other assesses sentence intelligibility and speaking rate. In the *single word task* a patient's oral reading of 50 single words is recorded. Each word is selected by the examiner (before the test) from a corpus of similar-sounding words. One or more judges (not the examiner) then listen to the recording and either write down each spoken word or choose each spoken word from a set of 12 words that are similar in sound to the target word.

In the *sentence task* the patient reads aloud 22 sentences, ranging in length from 5 to 15 words (2 sentences at each length). One or more judges (not the examiner) then listen to the recording and write down the sentences. Judges' transcriptions are scored by the examiner to yield several measures:

- Percent intelligibility
- Speech rate for sentences (words per minute)
- Intelligible words per minute
- Unintelligible words per minute
- Communicative efficiency ratio (intelligible words per minute divided by normal speech rate—190 words per minute)

Assessment of Intelligibility of Dysarthric Speech appears to be a sensitive and reliable estimator of speech intelligibility if administered and scored according to instructions. The measures obtained are useful for predicting a speaker's intelligibility in daily life, for measuring changes in intelligibility over time, and for planning treatment to improve a speaker's intelligibility. Patients who are both aphasic and dysarthric may have difficulty with the sentence production part of the test because of reading problems, problems in auditory comprehension and retention, or paraphasic errors in oral reading. Consequently, the test may not be practical for patients who are both dysarthric and more than mildly aphasic.

GENERAL CONCEPTS 11-3

- Comprehensive assessment of dysarthria requires assessment of *respiration, phonation, resonation,* and *articulation* and their interactions.
- Respiration for speech requires that normal passive exhalation be assisted by active contraction of the muscles of the diaphragm to produce sufficient breath pressure for speech.
- Comprehensive assessment of respiration for speech entails measurement of *respiratory pressure and flow* in non-speech activities; assessment of *sustained phonation;* and assessment of *breath support* for speech as the patient produces words, phrases, and connected speech.
- *Coughs, grunts,* and *glottal stops* provide indications of the adequacy of glottal valving in non-speech activities.
- *Abbreviated sustained phonation times* (less than 12 to 15 seconds) suggest a problem either with respiratory support or with

glottal valving for speech. Several neurologic conditions may affect glottal valving for speech, including *spastic vocal folds* caused by bilateral upper motor neuron pathology, *flaccid vocal folds* caused by lower motor neuron pathology, *rigid vocal folds* caused by Parkinson's disease, and *intermittent contractions of vocal folds* caused by extrapyramidal system or cerebellar pathology.

- Dysarthric patients' control of voice and articulation often is better in highly structured tasks such as *continuous phonation* and *production of single syllables and short phrases* than in less structured tasks such as *story telling* or *conversation*. Assessment of patients with dysarthria should include assessment of their performance in both structured tasks and unstructured tasks.

- Visual examination of the palate at rest and during vowel production provides information about the integrity of velopharyngeal muscle functions. Asking the patient to puff out his or her cheeks provides an indirect indication of velopharyngeal competence in non-speech activities.

- *Hypernasality, nasal escape of air,* and *distorted consonants* during production of denasalized speech sounds are signs of impaired velopharyngeal closure. One of the easiest tests for hypernasality is alternately to pinch and release the patient's nostrils as the patient speaks, listening for changes in the quality of the patient's speech as the nostrils alternately are occluded and opened.

- Poor articulation of consonants requiring oral breath pressure and good articulation of other consonants is a sign of inadequate velopharyngeal closure.

- Drooping, atrophy, or involuntary movements of facial muscles; off-midline resting tongue position; and dimpling or rippling of the tongue suggest compromised innervation of the affected muscles.

- The examiner evaluates the strength, timing, and range of movement of the jaw, lips, and tongue by asking the patient to move them both freely and against resistance applied by the examiner.

- Standard articulation inventories are not commonly used in assessing the speech of dysarthric patients. *Syllable and phrase repetition* is the most commonly used way to assess these patients' articulatory accuracy.

- Intelligibility, rather than articulatory accuracy, is the primary concern for most patients with significant dysarthria.

- *Assessment of Intelligibility of Dysarthric Speech* (Yorkston & Beukelman, 1981) provides a consistent procedure for assessing the intelligibility of single words and sentences produced by dysarthric speakers.

Treatment

Dysarthria is one consequence of neurologic disorders that causes weakness, slowness, incoordination, diminished range of movement, or sensory loss in speech structures. Some patients do not have the muscle strength or range of movement needed for normal speech. Others may have the muscle strength but not the coordination. Still others may lack the respiratory support necessary for normal speech. Consequently, there is no single treatment for dysarthria.

Treatment of dysarthria must take into account both the causes of a patient's dysarthria and the nature of the speech disturbances. Some treatment procedures may be concerned with causative mechanisms, whereas others may focus on the speech disturbances themselves. The goal of dysarthria treatment is to maximize the dysarthric patient's communicative effectiveness and efficiency. This goal can be achieved in various ways—for example, by improving the physiologic support for speech; by direct work on speech; by environmental control, education, and counseling; by providing compensatory techniques or alternatives to speech for communication; by providing prosthetic facilitation of speech; or occasionally, by medical or surgical intervention.

Treatment of dysarthric patients may rely on indirect approaches, whereby speech is improved by improving sensory and motor functions involved in speech, rather than directly, by working on speech itself. Indirect treatment procedures include *sensory stimulation, muscle strengthening, modifying muscle tone,* and *modifying respiration.* Direct procedures include *modifying phonation, modifying resonation, modifying articulation,* and *modifying prosody.* For most dysarthric patients, treatment is a combination of direct and indirect procedures. If a patient is severely dysarthric and can produce little or no volitional speech, treatment is likely to focus on physiologic support for speech. If a patient can produce some voice, approximate a few vowel sounds, and produce a few articulatory movements, treatment is likely to focus on production of speech. Non-speech exercises to strengthen muscles and increase their agility and range of movement may be appropriate for these latter patients but primarily as an adjunct to direct work on speech.

The more severe a patient's dysarthria, the more likely it is that the clinician will work to strengthen muscles and improve sensory function outside the context of speech. Patients with mild or moderate dysarthria may get stronger muscles and improved sensory function from treatment, but almost always this is better accomplished by controlled speaking practice, rather than by stimulation of oral structures or by movement exercises in isolation.

Indirect Treatment Procedures

Sensory Stimulation Sensory stimulation procedures seek to increase the dysarthric patient's motor control by increasing the amount and fidelity of sensory feedback from oral structures. Stimulation may include brushing, stroking, vibrating, or applying ice to the patient's lips, tongue, pharyngeal walls, or soft palate. There is little empiric evidence that sensory stimulation improves motor performance in dysarthria, and its use remains controversial, except, perhaps, for stimulation of the soft palate.

Rosenbek and LaPointe (1985) suggest that massaging and lifting the soft palate concurrent with the patient's attempts to raise it may improve velopharyngeal competence. Johns (1985) reports that movement of the lateral pharyngeal walls toward the midline sometimes increases following installation of palatal prostheses. He attributes this movement to increased sensory feedback generated by contact of the pharyngeal walls with the prosthesis. However, Dworkin and Johns (1980), after reviewing various approaches to managing velopharyngeal insufficiency, assert that neither stimulation nor muscle strengthening are likely to be effective if the insufficiency is caused by neurologic impairment.

It may be that clinicians' willingness to use stimulation to remediate velopharyngeal incompetence comes as much from the lack of other methods for remediation as from the clinician's belief that stimulation actually works. Nevertheless, stimulation of the soft palates and pharyngeal walls of dysarthric patients with gross velopharyngeal incompetence is likely to continue, at least until something better comes along.

Muscle Strengthening Muscle-strengthening exercises seek to improve the dysarthric patient's respiration, phonation, articulation, and resonance by enhancing movement of weakened muscles. There is no conclusive evidence confirming the efficacy of muscle strengthening in treating dysarthria, but it appears to have positive effects for at least some patients (Liss, Kuehn, & Hinkel, 1994; Massengill & associates, 1968; Powers & Starr, 1974; Yules & Chase, 1969). Rosenbek and LaPointe (1978) suggest that muscle strengthening is most appropriate for patients with severe flaccid dysarthria whose physiologic support for speech is substantially compromised. They recommend muscle strengthening when adjustment of posture, muscle tone, and respiration are ineffective and when direct treatment of articulation, phonation, and prosody leave the patient unintelligible, but only if the patient will remain in treatment for several weeks and can carry out assignments outside the clinic. In practice, muscle strengthening usually is reserved for patients with weak muscles and severe flaccid dysarthria who can produce little intelligible speech or can produce speech only in fragments and under ideal conditions.

It is important that clinicians not exaggerate the importance of muscle strength for adequate speech intelligibility. Intelligible speech rarely requires forceful muscle activity. In fact, forceful articulatory movements, such as those seen in ataxia, dystonia, and chorea, actually may diminish intelligibility. Agility and range of movement are more important contributors to intelligible speech than strength. Consequently, muscle-strengthening exercises that include movement (*isotonic* exercise) are likely to be more effective than those requiring exertion against stationary resistance (*isometric* exercise). As a general rule, clinicians should move from isometric to isotonic movements as soon as the patient can accomplish short sequences of simple movements. Muscle-strengthening activities should lead into agility and range of motion exercises as soon as the muscles have enough strength to carry out the exercises at low levels of speed and efficiency.

Liss, Keuhn, and Hinkel (1994) have suggested that changes in muscle strength seen in the early stages of strength training are a result of neural adaptation (increased rate of firing of motor neurons, participation of previously non-participating motor neurons) rather than increased muscle mass. These neural adaptations apparently are movement-specific—strength training movements must closely match the target movements in direction, force, range, and velocity. These findings suggest that strength-training exercises such as those in which a patient pushes against a tongue depressor with tongue or lips are unlikely to produce beneficial changes in speech precision, agility, or endurance but that training exercises that mimic speech movements may produce beneficial neural adaptations (Hageman, 1997; Liss, Kuehn, & Hinkel, 1994).

If a dysarthric patient with weak speech muscles can produce a vowel or two and approximate a few consonants, muscle strengthening may be supplemented by direct work on speech production. Patients whose muscles do not have the strength, agility, or range of movement to talk but who can produce a few speech sounds usually will develop increased strength, agility, and range of movement in the muscle groups needed for speech as quickly (and more efficiently) if they are talking than if they are moving speech structures against resistance or in non-speech movement drills.

Modification of Muscle Tone Some dysarthric patients exhibit abnormalities in muscle tone that interfere with speech intelligibility. Some are *hypertonic*. Hypertonicity appears as *spasticity* when patients have upper motor neuron pathology and as *rigidity* in Parkinson's disease. Both kinds of hypertonicity are constant over time and uniform across affected muscle groups. Hypertonicity also appears as a consequence of extrapyramidal diseases such as dystonia and chorea. In dystonia and chorea muscle tone tends to wax and wane and may move from muscle group to muscle group. Abnormally diminished muscle tone (hypotonicity) usually follows lower motor neuron or peripheral nervous system pathology. Hypotonicity is almost always constant over time and does not move from one muscle group to another.

A variety of procedures for relaxing hypertonic muscles have been reported in the literature. *Progressive relaxation* reduces the hypertonic patient's overall level of muscle tension. *Shaking* and *chewing* exercises (Froeschels, 1943, 1952) may help the patient relax muscle groups involved in speaking. Lying down while speaking may help some hypertonic patients by lowering their overall level of muscle tension. *Biofeedback,* in which the electrical activity in selected muscle groups is amplified and converted to auditory or visual signals monitored by the patient, may help patients selectively relax muscles (Hand, Burns, & Ireland, 1979; Netsell & Cleeland, 1973; Rubow & associates, 1984). When hypertonicity is caused by extrapyramidal pathology (such as Parkinson's disease), medications to reduce muscle tone may be more effective than behavioral treatment. In fact, hypertonicity caused by extrapyramidal disease usually is not responsive to behavioral treatment.

Hypotonicity (as in flaccid dysarthria) typically is treated by raising the patient's overall level of muscle tension. Simply asking the patient to increase the overall level of effort sometimes improves the intelligibility of patients with flaccid dysarthria (Rosenbek & LaPointe, 1985). If this approach is not effective, the patient's general level of muscle tension may be increased by asking him or her to push or pull against a stationary resistance while speaking. Pushing down on a table or on the arms of a chair or wheelchair or clasping the hands together and pulling may increase overall muscle tone and improve the speech of hypotonic patients.

Posture and Speaking Position Modifying a dysarthric patient's posture and speaking position may improve the patient's speech, especially when general muscle weakness is present, as in myopathies and diseases affecting neuromuscular transmission. Straightening a slouching patient's spine and neck and bringing the patient's head to an upright position with a brace or a support may improve the mechanical relationships among the structures involved in speech and improve the quality of the patient's speech. Postural adjustments may help the patient compensate for weak muscles and stabilize the structures with which speech movements are carried out. Cervical collars, body braces, slings, and restraints, singly or in combination, may be used to get a weak patient into a more efficient position for speech and help the patient maintain that position. (Posture and positioning most often are useful for patients with weak neck and trunk muscles who have difficulty sitting up and keeping their head erect.)

When the patient has been positioned in a better speaking posture, stabilization and support of selected muscle groups may enhance the intelligibility of the patient's speech. If a patient's neck muscles are weak, a cervical collar or neck brace may stabilize the patient's head. Girdles, stomach bands, or stomach boards (Rosenbek & LaPointe, 1985) may be used to stabilize and support weak abdominal muscles.

(Stomach boards are boards, usually fastened across the arms of a wheelchair, against which the patient can compress the abdomen and generate greater expiratory pressure for speech.) Girdles and stomach bands compress the abdomen, compensate for weak abdominal muscles, and provide a firm base for exhalation during speech. Patients with movement disorders may wear cervical collars, neck braces, or body braces to limit involuntary movements.

Postural adjustment, positioning, stabilization, and support should be carried out in collaboration with a physician because changes in posture or bracing, banding, and belting may contribute to medical complications. For example, abdominal banding or girdling may restrict breathing and predispose patients to pneumonia. Cervical collars and neck braces may compress muscles and nerves in the patient's neck and shoulders.

Respiratory Capacity and Efficiency Respiratory capacity is most likely to be a problem for patients with generalized weakness, as in demyelinating disease, spinal nerve pathology, and diseases of the neuromuscular junction. Increasing respiratory capacity may improve these patients' speech, but only if they can use the breath stream efficiently. Respiratory capacity often is less important to speech than efficient use of the air stream. If a patient's glottal valving, velopharyngeal porting, and articulation are poor, increasing respiratory capacity will do little for the intelligibility of speech, except, perhaps, for boosting its loudness.

Treatment procedures for enhancing respiratory support take several forms. Postural adjustments, positioning, and stabilization may improve the mechanical background for respiration. Muscle-strengthening activities may be directed toward the muscles of respiration. Sometimes techniques for increasing muscle tone (e.g., pushing and bearing down) are used to increase respiratory drive. Training in more efficient glottal valving and increasing articulatory precision may have indirect positive effects on respiratory support.

Exercises that deal directly with respiration also may be appropriate. Controlled exhalation, in which the patient slowly exhales a uniform stream of air over a certain period, may improve respiratory capacity and enhance control of exhalation. In most cases, direct treatment of respiration is an early phase of treatment, and the focus of treatment usually moves to speech production as soon as the patient achieves basic respiratory support for speech.

Direct Treatment Procedures

In direct treatment procedures, dysarthric patients produce speech under controlled conditions. Treatment of dysarthric patients usually includes both indirect and direct procedures, and indirect procedures tend to fade into direct procedures, as when controlled exhalation leads into controlled phonation. Direct treatment procedures tend to overlap and merge one into another, as when controlled phonation progresses into articulation drills. Direct treatment procedures may address *phonation, resonation, articulation,* or *prosody,* either singly or in combination.

> Technically, one cannot treat speech—one treats speech by changing the amplitude, speed, or accuracy of movements that generate speech or by improving the laryngeal mechanics necessary for phonation. Consequently, even "direct" treatment procedures are indirect, in this sense.

Phonation Speech activities to enhance phonation emphasize *efficient laryngeal valving* of the air stream and *adjusting utterance length* to the patient's respiratory capacity. Controlled phonation is the primary vehicle for increasing dysarthric patients' laryngeal efficiency. In the early stages of treatment, the patient may be asked to produce prolonged vowels with gradually increasing vowel duration. When the patient's vowel production has stabilized, the patient may be trained to produce

strings of vowels or consonant-vowel syllables, with the length of the strings gradually increasing as the patient masters shorter strings. Gradual changes in intensity then may be superimposed on the strings to further enhance respiratory control.

When the patient can say short phrases, treatment may incorporate the concept of *optimal breath group* (Linebaugh, 1983). The optimal breath group for a patient is the number of syllables the patient can produce comfortably on one breath. The optimal breath group approach entails determining the patient's optimal breath group, teaching the patient to keep the number of syllables per breath within the optimal breath group, then gradually increasing the length of the patient's optimal breath group by means of drills to enhance respiratory control and glottal valving.

When glottal valving is compromised by spastic laryngeal muscles, procedures for reducing laryngeal tension, including relaxation, massage of the larynx, or providing postural support, may be combined with work on voice production. When laryngeal muscles are flaccid, pushing and bearing down during phonation may be incorporated into voice drills, and in some cases visual feedback, such as that provided by a VU (loudness) meter or an oscilloscope tracing, may be used to help the patient control (and increase) loudness.

When loudness is a problem in dysarthria, it usually is a case of too little, rather than too much. Dysarthric patients' speech may be made louder by improving respiratory support (teaching appropriate breath groups, positioning, bracing, banding, bearing down), by increasing the efficiency of phonation, or by speech exercises that directly target vocal intensity.

Contrastive stress drill (Rosenbek & LaPointe, 1985) is one way of giving dysarthric patients concentrated vocal intensity training. In contrastive stress drill, the clinician says a sentence, such as "Bob hit Bill," and then asks the patient questions such as "WHO hit Bill?", "WHAT did Bill do?", and so on. The patient answers each question, putting emphatic stress on elements that answer the questions ("Bob hit BILL.").

If adequate vocal intensity cannot be obtained by means of behavioral treatment, a portable voice amplification system may be necessary. Portable amplification systems include either a throat-mounted or headset-mounted microphone connected to a small amplifier and speaker that can be worn in a pocket or on a strap or belt. However, as Rosenbek and LaPointe (1985) caution, amplification is appropriate for patients with intelligible speech. Amplifying unintelligible speech only produces louder unintelligible speech.

Increasing *vocal pitch range* may be appropriate for some patients, particularly those with flaccid dysarthria. Techniques for increasing pitch range include the following:

- Phonation with gradually rising and falling pitch
- Counting aloud with rising or falling pitch
- Reciting the alphabet or the days of the week with rising or falling pitch
- Producing sequences of syllables or words with gradually rising or falling pitch
- Contrastive stress drill
- Asking questions (for rising pitch) and making assertions (for falling pitch) with exaggerated intonation

Maintaining *constant pitch* may be important for patients with ataxic dysarthria, whose pitch fluctuates because of abrupt changes in the force, timing, and amplitude of movements. Techniques for controlling unintentional pitch changes include continuous phonation while keeping pitch constant and continuous phonation with slowly rising or falling pitch.

Resonance Speech resonance is affected by the size and configuration of the oral cavity and by the size of the opening between the oral and nasal cavities. Although aberrations in the shape of the oral cavity may change the resonance characteristics of speech, such changes are primarily cosmetic, affecting speech quality rather than speech intelligibility. (However, aberrations in the shape of the oral cavity usually are produced by abnormal positions of the articulators, so that articulatory errors are superimposed on the resonance abnormalities. The combination can de-

stroy intelligibility.) By far the most important resonance aberration in dysarthria is hypernasality, caused by failure to close the velopharyngeal opening during denasalized speech segments. Failure to close the velopharyngeal opening has two effects. It produces excessive nasal resonance. More importantly, it distorts or destroys sounds that require oral breath pressure because the air required to produce them escapes through the nose.

Increasing velopharyngeal competence can create dramatic improvements in intelligibility for many hypernasal patients. Several behavioral techniques for controlling hypernasality have been described in the literature. The techniques rely on *ear training* to teach the patient to recognize hypernasality plus *pushing and bearing-down exercises* to increase the patient's overall level of muscle tension and facilitate the movement of velopharyngeal muscles. Behavioral remediation of hypernasality usually is practical only when hypernasality is mild to moderate. If hypernasality is severe, prosthetic or surgical management may be necessary.

Moderate to severe hypernasality caused by palatal insufficiency sometimes can be reduced by a palatal lift prosthesis. A palatal lift prosthesis is constructed by a prosthodontist, usually in collaboration with a speech pathologist. The body of the prosthesis consists of a plate that covers the hard palate. The plate is attached to the teeth by wires. The palatal lift, which is made of acrylic and shaped to fit the patient's oropharynx, is attached to the rear of the plate and is adjusted to fit the configuration of the patient's oropharynx. The lift mechanically pushes the patient's palate up and back to help close the velopharyngeal port.

> *Prosthesis:* A fabricated device that substitutes for a missing body part or physically compensates for deficient physical function. From a Greek word meaning "an addition."

The literature (Netsell & Rosenbek, 1985; Rosenbek & LaPointe, 1985; Yorkston, Beukelman, & Bell, 1988) suggests that patients with the following characteristics are the best candidates for palatal lift prostheses:

- Patients who are extremely hypernasal, who cannot achieve velopharyngeal closure, and for whom behavioral intervention has been unsuccessful.
- Patients whose soft palates and pharyngeal muscles are not spastic. (Spastic muscles resist displacement and may dislodge the prosthesis.)
- Patients who have teeth to which the prosthesis can be anchored. Prostheses have been fitted to dentures, but the results may be unsatisfactory if the lift dislodges the dentures.
- Patients who have reasonably good articulation and phonation. Hypernasal patients with severe articulatory or phonatory deficits generally will remain as unintelligible after the prosthesis is fitted as they were before.
- Patients who are likely to cooperate by wearing the lift and caring for it. Some patients may not tolerate the discomfort associated with wearing the prosthesis or put up with the inconvenience of wearing the prosthesis and caring for it.
- Patients who do not have swallowing difficulties. Palatal prostheses sometimes interfere with swallowing.
- Patients without degenerative disease. Although fitting a prosthesis to such patients may provide temporarily increased intelligibility, the effects are likely to be transitory and eventually will be negated by the progression of the disease.

Articulation Improving dysarthric patients' articulation was for many years the core of treatment for dysarthria because dysarthria was considered to be little more than defective articulation. However, as Rosenbek and LaPointe (1985) assert, "Articulation is being forced to share its popularity with other speech processes . . . and dysarthria is coming to mean speech—not articulation—deficit" (p. 294). Most dysarthric patients receive articulation treatment. However, few receive *only* articulation treatment.

Treatment procedures for improving articulation include *imitation; phonetic derivation*

(deriving sounds that the patient cannot say from those that the patient can say); *phonetic placement* (physically adjusting or positioning the patient's articulators); and *sequential repetition* of sounds, syllables, and words. Articulation exercises usually focus on *speech movements* (production of syllables or words), rather than on *fixed positions* (individual sounds), although severely dysarthric patients may work on producing fixed articulatory positions. When a patient's articulatory movements are imprecise, the patient may be taught to exaggerate them, which helps make the movements more precise. When a patient cannot produce an articulatory movement or position, a compensatory movement or substitute position may be taught. Work on articulatory precision often is combined with slowing the patient's speech rate. Slower speech rate allows the patient more time to make articulatory adjustments, and it allows the patient's listeners more time to decode what the patient is saying.

Prosody Activities for changing the prosodic characteristics of dysarthric patients' speech may focus on rate, loudness, or pitch (intonation). Changes in patients' *speech rate* can be produced by changes in articulation rate (the rate at which individual speech sounds are produced) or by increasing the number or duration of pauses in the patient's speech. Most dysarthric speakers have great difficulty changing articulation rate, making rate manipulations by means of pauses the procedure of choice. If a patient is trained to produce optimal breath groups, pauses may occur automatically, but the pauses may not be at syntactic or semantic boundaries. These patients sound more natural and are easier to understand if they are trained to pause at phrase, clause, or sentence boundaries.

Several techniques are available for controlling dysarthric patients' speech rate. Most require the patient to speak in unison with an external timing stimulus. The clinician may tap, gesture, or speak along with the patient. The patient may speak to the beat of a metronome or a flashing light. The patient may tap, use a pacing board, drop beads in a cup, gesture, or produce other non-speech movements in unison with speaking. Teaching the patient to speak with exaggerated articulation and to exaggerate emphatic stress (contrastive stress drill) also may slow the patient's speech rate.

Beukelman and Yorkston (1977) provided two severely dysarthric speakers with a communication board on which were printed the alphabet, numerals from 0 to 9, and several phrases (e.g., *end of sentence, end of word*). The dysarthric speakers were trained to point to the first letter of each word as they said it. Both dysarthric speakers spoke more slowly and with greater intelligibility when using the first-letter procedure than when speaking without it. Beukelman and Yorkston attributed the effects of the procedure to (1) increased information provided to listeners by the first letter of each word and (2) the dysarthric speaker's slower speech rate.

GENERAL CONCEPTS 11-4

- Treatment of dysarthria may entail modification of underlying processes *(indirect procedures)* or modification of speech *(direct procedures)*. Indirect procedures include *sensory stimulation, muscle strengthening, modifying muscle tone,* and *modifying respiration.* Direct procedures include *modifying phonation, modifying resonation, modifying articulation,* and *modifying prosody.*
- There is no convincing evidence for the effectiveness of *sensory stimulation* in treatment of dysarthria, although sensory stimulation remains a common practice of many who treat dysarthric patients.
- *Muscle-strengthening* exercises may be appropriate for patients with severe dysarthria. Patients who can produce syllables or short phrases with reasonable intelligibility probably will benefit more from speech production exercises than from muscle strengthening per se.
- *Relaxation exercises,* shaking, chewing, and biofeedback may help dysarthric speakers with *hypertonic* speech muscles. Asking the patient to *increase overall muscle effort* or

pushing and bearing-down exercises may help dysarthric speakers with *hypotonic* speech muscles.

- *Improved respiratory capacity and efficiency* for speech for dysarthric patients may be obtained by *adjusting the dysarthric patient's posture and position, supporting weak muscles,* or having the patient do *exhalation and blowing exercises.*
- Dysarthric patients' *phonation* may be treated by *improving glottal valving, teaching optimal breath groups,* or doing *contrastive stress drills* or *vocal pitch change drills.*
- Dysarthric patients' *hypernasality* may be treated by combining *ear training* and *pushing or bearing-down exercises.* Severe hypernasality may be treated by providing the patient with a *palatal life prosthesis.*
- Dysarthric patients' impaired *articulation* may be treated by drills involving *imitation, phonetic derivation, phonetic placement,* or *sequential repetition.* Slowing dysarthric patients' rate of speech and teaching them to exaggerate articulatory movements also may improve their intelligibility.

Environmental Control and Education

Most dysarthric speakers eventually discover that intelligibility in the speech clinic, where rooms are quiet and well lit and where the dysarthric speaker is face-to-face with the clinician, is no guarantee of intelligibility in daily life, where rooms may be poorly lit and noisy and where listeners may not always be nearby or looking at the speaker. Skilled clinicians know this and teach dysarthric speakers how to compensate for less-than-ideal speaking conditions. When a dysarthric speaker reaches reasonable levels of intelligibility in the controlled environment of the clinic, the clinician may broaden the treatment program to maximize communication in less-than-ideal speaking situations. This usually requires both *environmental control* and *behavioral compensation.*

The patient and caregivers may be trained to use environmental controls to minimize adverse effects of environmental variables on speech intelligibility. The most effective controls relate to ambient noise, lighting, and the spatial relationships between dysarthric speakers and their listeners. Controlling ambient noise is a simple, but often overlooked, way to improve dysarthric speakers' communicative success. Turning the television set and radio down or off and closing windows or doors to shut out outside noise are simple ways to diminish ambient noise. Families may install draperies or other acoustic treatments to control ambient noise levels in dysarthric speakers' homes.

Controlling lighting and the position of dysarthric speakers relative to their listeners also may enhance dysarthric speakers' communicative effectiveness. Lighting may be adjusted to illuminate the dysarthric speaker's face, and dysarthric speakers routinely may position themselves so that listeners can see their face.

Dysarthric speakers may be trained to monitor their listeners' comprehension by maintaining eye contact and, if necessary, asking listeners whether they understand. They also may be trained when (and how) to repeat, simplify, paraphrase, or exaggerate articulatory movements (especially when the dysarthric speaker perceives communication breakdown). Those around the dysarthric speaker may be taught to control the situational variables described above, to indicate (either gesturally or verbally) to the speaker when they do not understand, and to ask the dysarthric speaker to slow down, exaggerate articulatory movements, repeat, paraphrase, or simplify when the dysarthric speaker fails to communicate.

Medical and Surgical Treatment

Medical Treatment Some conditions causing dysarthria are medically treatable. When they are, medical treatment precedes behavioral intervention, and when medical treatment is successful, behavioral intervention may not be needed. Medically treatable conditions causing dysarthria include extrapyramidal diseases such as Parkinson's disease, irritative and inflamma-

tory processes causing peripheral nerve dysfunction, and some metabolic and nutritional disturbances.

Parkinson's disease is caused by deficiencies in certain neurotransmitters (dopamines) and often responds well to medications such as levodopa (L-dopa) that replenish the missing neurotransmitters. These medications often diminish or eliminate the motor symptoms of the disease, including dysarthria. Movement disorders (such as chorea and dystonia) sometimes respond favorably to tranquilizers and related medications, although complete remission of symptoms with medication is unusual. Some facial paralyses are treatable with steroids. Neurologic diseases caused by abnormalities in central nervous system metabolism, such as Wilson's disease, may be medically treatable. When medical treatment of a dysarthric patient's neurologic disease is effective, the patient's dysarthria often improves enough to make direct treatment of dysarthria unnecessary. However, medical treatment often decreases, but does not eliminate, dysarthria, making behavioral treatment, in conjunction with or following medical treatment, necessary.

Wilson's disease: An inherited disease in which copper accumulates in body tissues, especially the brain, kidneys, liver, and eyes. Wilson's disease is treated with penicillamine, which removes the copper deposits.

Teflon Injections and Surgical Treatment When structural abnormalities produce severe hypernasality, physical modification of velopharyngeal structures may be appropriate. Teflon may be injected into the posterior pharyngeal wall to reduce velopharyngeal insufficiency (Lewy, Cole, & Wepman, 1965; Bluestone & associates, 1968). Teflon injections are most useful for mild to moderate hypernasality when behavioral modification of hypernasality has not been successful. When dysphonia is caused by inability to adduct the vocal folds, injection of Teflon into the vocal folds may improve voice quality. These procedures often do not eliminate the patient's speech abnormalities, so that behavioral treatment of the patient's residual speech abnormalities may be needed.

Surgical treatment of velopharyngeal insufficiency may help severe velopharyngeal incompetence, although the general opinion seems to be that surgery is a last resort to be tried only after less drastic approaches have failed. The most frequent surgical procedure for remediating velopharyngeal insufficiency is the *posterior pharyngeal flap*. In this procedure, bands of muscle tissue are surgically lifted from the posterior pharyngeal walls and attached to the soft palate. When the pharyngeal wall muscles contract, the bands shorten, pulling the soft palate toward the pharyngeal walls.

Pharyngeal flap procedures are most common in management of palatal insufficiency for children with cleft palates. Their use to treat hypernasality in dysarthria is controversial. Gonzalez and Aronson (1970) assert that prosthetic management of velopharyngeal insufficiency usually produces better results than surgery. Hardy and associates (1961) make a similar assertion regarding management of velopharyngeal insufficiency in children. Miniami and associates (1975) did pharyngeal flaps on five dysarthric patients with "palatal paresis" and reported disappointing results. However, after reviewing the literature and summarizing his own experience with surgical remediation of velopharyngeal insufficiency, Johns (1985) concluded that surgical management "holds great promise for a large number of dysarthric patients" (p. 175).

Augmentative and Alternative Communication

Many severely dysarthric patients do not regain enough intelligible speech to communicate even simple messages by talking. Non-speech communication systems enable many of these patients to communicate. Non-speech communication systems may be either *augmentative* or *alternative*. *Augmentative systems* supplement what the patient can say and permit the patient to communicate more elaborate messages or to communicate simple messages with greater intelligibility. Amplifiers are the most common augmentative systems for dysarthric speakers. *Alternative systems* replace speech as a means of communication. Alternative (non-speech) communication systems fall into four general categories: *communication boards and communication books, mechanical and electronic devices, gesture and pantomime,* and *sign language.*

Selection of a non-speech communication system for a dysarthric speaker requires consideration of the dysarthric speaker's perceptual, motor, and linguistic abilities because different non-speech communication systems require different user abilities and different levels of user skill. Some systems require that the user point to symbols or operate a keyboard. Patients with poor manual dexterity may not be able to use such systems. Some systems require that the user spell, read, or arrange words into phrases or sentences. Patients with linguistic impairments may not be able to use them.

Communication Boards and Communication Books Communication boards and communication books are similar in content but differ in form. A communication board is an array of symbols on a durable surface. A communication book is a collection of symbols arranged in book form. The symbols in either can be pictures, letters, words, phrases, or some combination of the four. To communicate, the patient points to the symbols, either singly or in sequence. Figure 11-13 shows examples of two kinds of communication boards. At the top is a simple board containing pictorial symbols and printed words. At the bottom is a more complex board containing letters, numerals, and words.

In general, communication boards and books containing letters, words, and phrases are best suited for patients without substantial linguistic impairments. The board shown at the top of Figure 11-13 would be usable by many

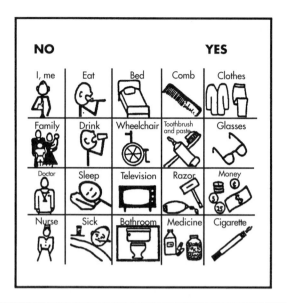

I CAN HEAR PERFECTLY	PLEASE REPEAT AS I TALK (THIS IS HOW I TALK BY SPELLING OUT THE WORDS)		WOULD YOU PLEASE CALL
A AN HE	AM ARE ASK BE BEEN BRING CAN		ABOUT ALL
HER I IT ME	COME COULD DID DO DOES DON'T		AND ALWAYS
MY HIM SHE	DRINK GET GIVE GO HAD HAS HAVE		ALMOST AS
THAT THE THESE	IS KEEP KNOW LET LIKE MAKE MAY		AT BECAUSE
THEY THIS WHOSE	PUT SAY SAID SEE SEEN SEND SHOULD		BUT FOR FROM
WHAT WHEN WHERE	TAKE TELL THINK THOUGHT WANT		HOW IF IN
WHICH WHO WHY	WAS WERE WILL WISH WON'T WOULD -ED		OF ON OR
YOU WE YOUR	-ER -EST -ING -LY -N'T -'S -TION		TO UP WITH

A	B	C	D	E	F	G	AFTER AGAIN
H		I	J	K	L	M	ANY EVEN / EVERY HERE
N	O	P	Qu	R	S	T	JUST MORE
U	V	W	X	Y	Z		ONLY SO
1	2	3	4	5	6	7	SOME SOON
8	9	10	11	12	30		THERE VERY

SUN. MON. TUES. WED. THUR. FRI. SAT. BATHROOM	PLEASE THANK YOU GOING OUT	$¢ ½(SHHH!!)?
	MR. MRS. MISS START OVER	_____
	MOTHER DAD DOCTOR END OF WORD	_____

Figure 11-13 ■ **Communication boards. The upper one is a picture communication board suitable for a patient with moderate-to-severe language impairment. The lower one is a more complex board containing words and phrases that would be appropriate for a patient with good language abilities and sufficient finger and arm dexterity to point to letters and words at a reasonably fast rate.**

linguistically impaired patients because its symbols are nonverbal. The board shown at the bottom of Figure 11-13 would be inappropriate for most linguistically impaired patients but would be appropriate for dysarthric patients without major linguistic impairment, provided they have the motor ability to point to the symbols on the board.

Versions of communication boards that do not require the user to directly select symbols have been developed. The simplest is the *eye gaze board.* Eye gaze boards are used when speechless patients have good language abilities but cannot move their limbs to directly select symbols from a board (e.g., patients who are quadriplegic following cervical spinal cord injuries). Eye gaze boards allow such patients to indicate letters, words, phrases, or symbols by looking at them. Message recipients watch the patient's eye movements and say what they believe the patient is looking at. The patient signals correct choices, usually by blinking. Because it is difficult for message recipients to tell exactly where a patient is looking, eye gaze boards have to be large, with large spaces between symbols. For this reason eye gaze boards cannot contain very many items. Most eye gaze boards contain an alphabet, numbers, and perhaps a few key words or phrases. Many are printed on transparent plastic sheets or have cutouts through which message recipients can monitor the patient's eye movements.

Mechanical and Electronic Devices Mechanical and electronic devices for augmenting or replacing speech differ in cost, complexity, portability, and output. They range in cost from less than a hundred dollars to several thousand dollars. They range in portability from small handheld devices to large units that cannot be carried. The most common units are portable electronic devices that translate keyboard input into messages that are displayed on electronic readouts, printed on paper tape, or translated into speech-like output. Some generate literal representations of what is entered on the keyboard, and what the auditor sees is what

the user has entered. Other units translate codes entered by the user into programmed output messages (e.g. a three-digit code entered by the user might generate a five- or six-word phrase). Many (especially the handheld devices) require finger dexterity and coordination to operate keyboards, and most require that the user read, spell, or remember codes, making them unsuitable for use with most aphasic patients, patients with moderate to severe cognitive impairments, or patients with poor motor control.

Gesture and Pantomime Some dysarthric patients may be taught gesture or pantomime to augment speech. Pairing gesture or pantomime with speech often improves intelligibility for patients whose speech is at least moderately intelligible without gestural augmentation. Gesture or pantomime may not help patients with severe intelligibility problems who usually do better with communication boards, communication books, or electronic devices.

Sign Languages Sign languages are practical for some dysarthric patients who have the cognitive ability and the motivation to learn and use them. *Amerind* (American Indian Sign; Skelly, 1979) contains signs that do not depend heavily on verbal skills and can be learned by some patients with linguistic impairments. Most Amerind signs are comprehensible to message recipients without extensive training. A major problem with most other sign languages is that the signs are not comprehensible to message recipients without training, so that patients who use them cannot communicate with untrained persons.

Considerations in Selecting Augmentative or Alternative Communication Silverman (1983) described several variables that should be considered when a clinician chooses an alternative or augmentative system for a patient.

- The *cost* of the system is important when resources for purchasing it are limited.
- The amount of *training* needed for the patient to learn to use the system is important. If the system is to be a permanent one, extensive training can be justified. If the system

is for temporary use, or if an alternative means of communication is needed immediately, systems requiring extensive training are not appropriate.

- *Interference,* or the extent to which using the system interferes with other activities, is important. A system that requires the patient to sit at a fixed terminal and use both hands to operate it is more disruptive than a portable system that can be operated with one hand.

- The *intelligibility* of the output of the augmentatative or alternative system affects both the time required to make it functional and the generality with which it can be used by the patient. Systems that generate output that is intelligible to untrained message recipients require less time to become operational and will be useful in more different places than systems producing symbols whose meanings message recipients must be taught. Systems that print messages on paper tape or in liquid crystal displays cannot be used in the dark, over the telephone, or when patient and auditor are more than a few feet apart. Systems that generate messages on illuminated displays can be used in the dark but not over the telephone or at a distance. Systems that generate speech-like output may be unintelligible in noisy environments and may not be intelligible over the telephone, depending on the fidelity of the augmentative or alternative system's output and the fidelity of the telephone system.

- The *acceptability* of the system to user and message recipients usually determines the extent to which it will be used in daily life. If the device or system is costly, cumbersome, complicated, or unnatural, it may be discarded in favor of less costly, less cumbersome, and less effective ways to communicate.

GENERAL CONCEPTS 11-5

- *Control of the dysarthric patient's everyday speaking environment* is an important, but sometimes overlooked, component of treatment. Keeping ambient noise levels low and en-

suring that the dysarthric speaker's face is visible to listeners may significantly enhance listeners' comprehension of the dysarthric patient.

- Some diseases causing dysarthria (e.g., Parkinson's disease) are treatable with *medications.* The medications usually have beneficial effects on associated dysarthria, but behavioral treatment of dysarthria may be needed when medication does not completely resolve a patient's dysarthria.

- *Teflon injections, palatal lifts,* and *pharyngeal flaps* may be appropriate for treating patients with *severe hypernasality.* These procedures usually are used only when hypernasality is severe and when behavioral treatment fails to make the patient's speech sufficiently intelligible for daily life communication.

- Some patients with severe dysarthria may need *augmentative or alternative communication systems* to permit them to communicate in daily life. Speech amplifiers, gesture, and pantomime may *augment* a patient's limited speech. Communication boards, communication books, and electronic devices may *replace* speech for severely impaired dysarthric speakers who have the manual dexterity needed to use them.

THOUGHT QUESTIONS

Question 11-1 Speculate as to the potential motor speech disorder likely to be exhibited by:

- A patient with a history of atrial fibrillations.
- A patient with 10 years of participation in professional boxing.
- A patient with a family history of Huntington's chorea.
- A patient with a traumatic brain injury incurred in a motor-vehicle accident.
- A patient with a 10-year history of transient ischemic attacks.

Question 11-2 A 57-year-old woman comes to a neurology clinic with the following complaints.

"I've been having increasing trouble getting up out of a chair and now I'm having trouble turning over in bed."

"Sometimes I have trouble walking. It's like I'm glued to the floor. It takes me three or four tries to get going."

"It seems like my voice has gotten fainter and I'm hoarse most of the time. At first I thought it was allergies or a cold or something, but it hasn't gone away. People complain that they can't hear me when there's noise in the background. And it seems like I'm beginning to stutter or something. I'll repeat things over and over—sounds and words."

The neurologist conjectured that the patient's complaints suggested neurologic disease and dysarthria—a conjecture borne out by a subsequent neurologic examination. What was the disease? What was the dysarthria type? Explain your reasoning.

Question 11-3 How might the focus of treatment differ for patients with apraxia of speech caused by damage in or near Broca's area *(frontal apraxia of speech)* versus patients with "apraxia of speech" caused by damage in parietal-temporal regions *(posterior apraxia of speech)?*

Question 11-4 What do you think Darley, Aronson, and Brown (1975) meant by "islands of error-free speech" in the speech of patients with apraxia of speech? Which characteristics of speech do you think they were thinking of? Write your own definition—try to make it specific to apraxia of speech and exclude the dysarthrias.

Question 11-5 A 56-year-old man is referred to you by a neurologist who asks you for help in diagnosing the nature of the man's speech impairment. The man's neurologic examination is within normal limits, except for questionable bilateral slowness of arm and hand movements. Your examination yields the following results:

- Normal strength and range of movement of tongue, lips, and jaw.
- Normal movement of palate and pharynx at beginning of phonation. Visible tensing of palatal, pharyngeal muscles on sustained phonation.
- Normal cough, grunt, glottal stop.
- Normal articulation for syllables, words, sentences, paragraphs.
- Normal voice quality, intonation, and loudness for single syllables and words.
- Unable to control voice loudness in longer speech segments. Initial words in phrases, sentences, and connected speech are produced at normal loudness, but loudness quickly increases as speech continues until the patient is shouting loudly. Spontaneous speech, repetition, and series speech (e.g., counting) are affected. Articulation and resonance are not affected by changes in loudness.
- No evidence of aphasia or cognitive impairment.

The patient reports that the changes in his speech occurred gradually over several months. He says that he knows that he shouts but cannot help it and is embarrassed by it. He reports no history of head injury, significant medical problems, or diagnosed neurologic problems. He works for a railway company as a laborer. His duties include repairing and maintaining the rail line, spraying weeds and grasses along the right-of-way with herbicides, and periodically checking switches and signal systems to ensure reliable operation.

Standard Medical Abbreviations

The following list contains some frequently encountered medical abbreviations. Most medical establishments have a list of standard abbreviations for use in their facilities, but the lists differ to some extent across establishments, and individual physicians often use idiosyncratic abbreviations that may force the reader to engage in reasoning, detective work, or both to deduce what the abbreviations mean.

~	approximately
△	change
≃	consistent with
†	death
↘	decrease
°	degree
≤	equal to or less than
>	greater than
<	less than
♀	female
♂	male
—	negative
#	number
%	percent
%ile	percentile
+	positive
1°	primary
2°	secondary
∴	therefore
c̄	with
Ø	without
AAROM	active assisted range of motion
abn	abnormal

a.c.	before meals
ACA	anterior communicating artery, anterior cerebral artery
ADL	activities of daily living
ad lib	as desired
AIDS	acquired immunodeficiency syndrome
AK, AKA	above the knee, above-knee amputation
alc, ETOH	alcohol
ALS	amyotrophic lateral sclerosis
AMA	against medical advice, American Medical Association
amb	ambulatory
AMI	acute myocardial infarction
angio	angiogram
ant	anterior
ante	before
AODM	adult onset diabetes mellitus
AP	anteroposterior
ARD	acute respiratory disease
ARF	acute renal failure
ASA	aspirin
ASAP	as soon as possible
ASCVD	arteriosclerotic cardiovascular disease
ASHD	arteriosclerotic heart disease
ASVD	arteriosclerotic vascular disease
AV	arteriovenous, atrioventricular
AVM	arteriovenous malformation
b.i.d.	twice a day
bil	bilateral
BK	below the knee
bm	bowel movement
BM	bone marrow
BMR	basal metabolism rate
BP	blood pressure

BRP	bathroom privileges	ECT	electroconvulsive therapy
bs	bowel sounds	EEG	electroencephalogram
BS	breath sounds	EENT	eye, ear, nose, throat
BUN	blood urea nitrogen	EMG	electromyogram
bx	biopsy	ENT	ear, nose, throat
C	celsius, centigrade	EOM	extraocular movements
CA	cardiac arrest	ER	emergency room
CA, ca	carcinoma	ETOH	ethanol (alcohol)
Ca⁺	calcium	exam	examination
CABG	coronary artery bypass graft	ext	external, exterior
CAD	coronary artery disease	F	Fahrenheit
cal	calorie	FB	foreign body
CAT	computerized axial tomography	FBS	fasting blood sugar
cath	catheter	FH	family history
CBC	complete blood count	fib	fibrillation
CBS	chronic brain syndrome	fl, fld	fluid
cc	cubic centimeter	FU	follow-up
CC	chief complaint	FUO	fever of unknown origin
CHF	congestive heart failure, chronic heart failure	fx	fracture
		GB	gall bladder
CHI	closed head injury	gen	general
cm	centimeter	GI	gastrointestinal
CMT	continuing medication and treatment	gm	gram
CN	cranial nerve	gr	grain
CNS	central nervous system	GSW	gunshot wound
c/o	complains of	GTT	glucose tolerance test
COLD	chronic obstructive lung disease	GU	genito-urinary
cont	continue(d)	GYN	gynecology
COPD	chronic obstructive pulmonary disease	h, hr	hour
CPR	cardiopulmonary resuscitation	HA	headache
CRF	chronic renal failure	Hb	hemoglobin
CSF	cerebrospinal fluid	HB	heart block
CT	computerized tomography	HBP	high blood pressure
cu	cubic	HCM	health care maintenance
CV	cardiovascular	HCVD	hypertensive cardiovascular disease
CVA	cerebrovascular accident	HEENT	head, eyes, ears, nose, throat
CXR	chest X-ray	Hg	mercury
d	day	Hg, Hgb	hemoglobin
DNR	do not resuscitate	HH	homonymous hemianopsia
DNT	did not test	H/O	history of
DOA	dead on arrival	H&P	history and physical
DOE	dyspnea (shortness of breath) on exertion	HPI	history of present illness
		HR	heart rate
d/t	due to	hs	bedtime
DT	delirium tremens	HTN	hypertension
DTR	deep tendon reflex	hx	history
DU	diabetic urine	H₂O	water
Dx	diagnosis	ICA	internal carotid artery
ECA	external carotid artery	ICP	intracranial pressure
ECG, EKG	electrocardiogram	ICU	intensive care unit

IM	intramuscular	OPD	outpatient department
imp	impression	OPT	outpatient treatment
inc	increase	OR	operating room
inf	inferior	OT	occupational therapy
I&O	intake and output	oz.	ounce
IU	international unit	p̱	pulse
IV	intravenous	p	after
kg	kilogram	PA	posteroanterior
KJ	knee jerk	PAR	postanesthesia recovery room
L, l	left	path	pathology
lab	laboratory	PC	presenting complaint
lat	lateral	p.c.	after meals
LCA	left coronary artery	PCA	posterior cerebral artery
LE	lower extremity	PCN	penicillin
liq	liquid	PE	physical examination
LMD	local medical doctor	PEG	percutaneous endoscopic gastrostomy
LOC	loss of consciousness	per	by
LOM	limitation of motion	PERRLA	pupils equal, round, reactive to light and accomodation
LOS	length of stay		
LP	lumbar puncture (spinal tap)	PET	positron emission tomography
LPN	licensed practical nurse	PH	past history
L&W	living and well	PI	present illness
MCA	middle cerebral artery	PMD	personal medical doctor
MH	marital history	PMH	past medical history
MI	myocardial infarction	PMR	physical medicine and rehabilitation
ml	milliliter	p.o.	by mouth
mm	millimeter	POD	postoperative day
mHg	millimeters of mercury	pos.	positive
MRI	magnetic resonance image	post.	posterior
MS	multiple sclerosis	PR	pulse rate
MVA	motor vehicle accident	preop	preoperative
NA	not applicable	prep	preparation
NAD	no acute distress	prn, p.r.n.	as needed
neg	negative	PROM	passive range of motion
neuro	neurologic, neurology	Psych	psychiatry
NG	nasogastric	Psychol	psychology
NKA	no known allergies	pt	patient
no.	number	PT	physical therapy
noc.	night	PTA	prior to admission
NP	neuropsychiatric	PX	physical
NPO, npo	nothing by mouth	q.a.m.	every morning
N/S	neurosurgery	q.d.	every day
NSC	not service connected	q.h.	every hour
N&V	nausea and vomiting	q.i.d.	four times per day
OBS	organic brain syndrome	q.o.d.	every other day
OD	officer of the day	R, r	right
OD	overdose	RBC	red blood cell
OM	otitis media	RIND	reversible ischemic neurologic deficit
OOB, oob	out of bed	RMS	rehabilitation medicine service
OP	outpatient	RN	registered nurse

RND	radical neck dissection	TB,TBC	tuberculosis
r/o	rule out	TBI	traumatic brain injury
ROM	range of motion	temp	temperature
RR	respiration rate	TIA	transient ischemic attack
Rt	right	t.i.d.	three times per day
RT	radiation therapy	TPR	temperature, pulse, respiration
RT	recreational therapy	tx	transplant
RTC	return to clinic	Tx	treatment
Rx	therapy	UA	urinalysis
s, sec	second	UCHD	usual childhood diseases
s	without	VD	venereal disease
SAB	subarachnoid bleed	VDRL	Venereal Disease Research Laboratory Test (for VD)
SAH	subarachnoid hemorrhage		
SC	service connected	VF	visual field
SCI	spinal cord injury	v fib	ventricular fibrillations
SH	social history	VHD	valvular heart disease
SI	seriously ill	VS	vital signs
SOB	shortness of breath	W	white
s/p	status post	w, wk	week
spec	specimen	WBC	white blood cells
ss	one-half	WD	well developed
SSN	Social Security number	WDWN	well developed, well nourished
stat	immediately	WNL	within normal limits
surg	surgery	wt	weight
Sx	symptoms	w/u	workup
Sz	seizure	Y/O	year old
T	temperature	yrs	years

Glossary

Acceleration injury: Brain injury caused when the moving head strikes a stationary surface or the stationary head is struck by a moving object in a way that causes the head to move quickly from its resting position. *Linear acceleration injury* is caused by forces that propel the head on a linear path. *Angular acceleration injury* is caused by forces that propel the head at an angle from the path of the impact and cause it to rotate. (See also *coup injury, contrecoup injury, diffuse axonal injury, translational trauma.*)

Afferent: Sensory.

Agnosia: Inability to recognize stimuli in a sensory modality despite intact sensation in the modality. Several varieties of agnosia have been described in the literature, including *auditory agnosia, visual agnosia, tactile agnosia,* and combinations such as *auditory-verbal agnosia* and *visual-verbal agnosia.*

Agrammatism: Speech in which content words (mainly nouns, verbs, adjectives) are present, but most function words (articles, prepositions, conjunctions) are missing. A common characteristic of the speech of adults with Broca's aphasia.

Agraphia (dysgraphia): Impaired writing.

Alertness, phasic: Rapidly occurring changes in receptivity to stimulation.

Alertness, tonic: Ongoing receptivity to stimulation.

Alexia (dyslexia): Impaired reading.

Alexia without agraphia: A rare syndrome in which the patient cannot read but can write. Usually caused by isolation of the visual cortex from Wernicke's area.

Alzheimer's disease: A progressive neurologic disease characterized by increasing dementia.

Amnesia: Loss of memory, inability to remember.

Anesthesia: Complete loss of sensation.

Aneurysm: Balloon-like bulges in an artery caused by weakness in the arterial wall. Aneurysms are susceptible to hemorrhage.

Angiography (arteriography): A laboratory procedure by which blood vessels can be visualized. A contrast medium is injected into the bloodstream and a series of X-ray exposures is made to determine the condition of the patient's blood vessels.

Angular gyrus: A prominent gyrus near the temporo-parietal-occipital junction, at the posterior end of the Sylvian (lateral) fissure. Damage in the region of the angular gyrus often causes problems with reading and arithmetic abilities.

Anomia: Inability or impaired ability to retrieve and produce words.

Anosagnosia: Denial of illness. Often a symptom of right-hemisphere brain pathology.

Anterior horn cells: Spinal motor neurons, located in the anterolateral part of the spinal cord.

Anton's syndrome (visual anosognosia): A condition in which a person is blind because of bilateral destruction of the visual cortex *(cortical blindness)* but denies being blind.

Aorta: The main artery from the heart.

Aphasia: A language impairment that crosses all input and output modalities. Can be divided into various syndromes.

Apraxia: Disruption of volitional movement sequences in the absence of sensory loss, weakness, paralysis, or incoordination of the muscles involved in the movements. Usually a consequence of damage in the premotor cortex. (See also *ideational*

569

apraxia, ideomotor apraxia, buccofacial apraxia, limb apraxia, verbal apraxia, dressing apraxia, and constructional apraxia.)

Aqueduct: A channel or opening.

Arachnoid villi: Sites at which cerebrospinal fluid is resorbed into the venous blood.

Arcuate fasciculus: A major fiber tract that connects the temporal lobe with regions in the frontal lobe in each hemisphere. The arcuate fasciculus in the left hemisphere is considered the major pathway by which information from the language centers in the temporal lobe reach the frontal lobe for conversion into spoken or written output.

Arteriography: See *angiography.*

Arteriosclerosis: See *atherosclerosis.*

Arteriovenous malformation (AVM): Convoluted collections of weak, thin-walled veins and arteries on the brain's surface or within the brain.

Association cortex: Cortical areas adjacent to sensory or motor cortex. Association cortex is thought to play an important part in integrating motor or sensory information from adjacent cortical areas and input from other regions of the brain.

Association fibers: Nerve fibers connecting adjacent regions of cortex.

Astereognosis (tactile agnosia): Inability to recognize otherwise familiar objects by touch, although the sense of touch is intact.

Astrocytoma: A common, relatively benign glioma.

Ataxia: Clumsiness and incoordination of movements caused by cerebellar damage.

Atherosclerosis (arteriosclerosis): A disease process in which arterial walls become roughened and covered with fatty deposits. These deposits are called atherosclerotic plaque.

Athetosis: Slow, sinuous, writhing, and uncontrollable muscle movements.

Atrophy: Shrinkage and wasting away of tissues.

Attention, alternating: The ability to shift attention from one stimulus to another or from one aspect of a stimulus to another.

Attention, divided: The ability to attend to more than one activity simultaneously.

Attention, selective: The ability to maintain attention on selected stimuli in the presence of competing or distracting stimuli. Sometimes called *focused attention.*

Attention, sustained: The ability to maintain attention on selected stimuli over time.

Auditory cortex: A region of cortex on the top surface of each temporal lobe (the gyrus of Heschl). It has primary responsibility for auditory perception.

Axon: The conducting process of a nerve cell (neuron).

Ballism: See *chorea.*

Basal ganglia: Several nuclei in the diencephalon near the thalamus. They are responsible for regulation of major muscle groups that make postural adjustments and compensate for inertial forces during movement. Depending on who is writing about them, the basal ganglia include the *caudate nucleus, putamen, globus pallidus, subthalamic nucleus,* and *substantia nigra.*

Basilar artery: An artery that connects the two vertebral arteries to the posterior part of the *circle of Willis.* The basilar artery progresses upward on the front surface of the pons and supplies blood to the pons.

Bell's palsy: Ipsilateral paralysis of lower facial muscles caused by compression of the facial nerve (CN 7).

Binswanger's disease: A rare disease caused by multiple infarcts in subcortical white matter.

Biopsy: Removal of a sample of tissue for laboratory analysis.

Brain abscess: A cavity in the brain caused by infection with bacteria, fungi, or parasites.

Brain stem: A stalk-like structure at the base of the brain atop the spinal cord. It contains centers that regulate some vital functions and contains most cranial nerve nuclei. Anatomists divide it into the midbrain (upper), pons (middle), and medulla (lower).

Broca's aphasia: An aphasia syndrome characterized by nonfluent speech, good comprehension, and poor repetition.

Broca's area: A region of cortex just anterior to the lower end of the primary motor cortex. Damage in Broca's areas is said to cause *Broca's aphasia.*

Buccofacial apraxia: Ideomotor apraxia of the oral musculature.

Bulbar: Relating to the brain stem, especially the pons.

Calcarine fissure: A deep groove in the occipital lobe of each hemisphere. It is important because the visual cortex is adjacent to it.

Caloric testing: A diagnostic test in which cold or warm water is introduced into the external auditory canal. Patients with vestibular pathology respond with characteristic patterns of *nystagmus.*

Capgras syndrome: The belief that friends, family, or acquaintances have been abducted and replaced by impostors.

Carotid arteries: There are two external carotid arteries and two internal carotid arteries. The external carotid arteries supply blood to the face. The internal carotid arteries supply blood to the brain via the *circle of Willis.*

Catastrophic reaction: A sudden and intense emotional outburst—usually anger but sometimes crying and, rarely, laughing. Catastrophic reactions usually are a brain-injured patient's response to being pushed beyond his or her limits.

Central fissure: A deep groove that divides each brain hemisphere into roughly equal front and back halves. Sometimes called the fissure of Rolando.

Central nervous system (CNS): The brain, brain stem, cerebellum, and spinal cord.

Cerebellum: A structure that looks like a miniature brain that lies beneath the posterior temporal lobes. It is important in integration and coordination of volitional movements.

Cerebral aqueduct: A long narrow passageway between the third and fourth ventricles. Occlusion of the cerebral aqueduct is a common cause of hydrocephalus (enlarged ventricles). The cerebral aqueduct sometimes is called the aqueduct of Sylvius.

Cerebral arteries: There are three cerebral arteries in each hemisphere. They are called the *anterior, middle,* and *posterior* cerebral arteries, which serve the front, middle, and posterior parts of the hemisphere, respectively.

Cerebral dominance: The belief that one hemisphere has primary responsibility for speech and language. (The left hemisphere in right-handers.)

Cerebral plasticity: The ability of the brain to reassign functions served by one area to a different area, usually in response to brain injury. Cerebral plasticity is greatest in infants and declines steadily with age.

Cerebrospinal fluid (CSF): A clear, colorless fluid that fills the ventricles and surrounds the brain, brain stem, cerebellum, and spinal cord.

Cerebrovascular accident (CVA): Temporary or permanent disruption of brain function due to interruption of its blood supply. Sometimes called *stroke,* or, more recently, *brain attack.*

Cerebrum: What we usually think of as the brain. The two brain hemispheres.

Chorea: A disease that causes quick and forceful involuntary movements *(choreiform movements). Ballism* is an extreme form of chorea, in which the limbs are flung wildly about by the involuntary movements. (The word *ballism* comes from the same root as *ballistic.*)

Choreoathetosis: A combination of choreiform and athetoid movements. (See *chorea* and *athetosis.*)

Choroid plexus: Structures within the ventricles that produce cerebrospinal fluid.

Circle of Willis: A heptagonal arrangement of arteries at the base of the brain that connects the internal carotid arteries and the basilar artery to the cerebral arteries. It is thought to serve as a "safety valve" for occlusions below the circle of Willis.

Circumduction: A characteristic gait of patients with hemiplegia *(circumducted gait).* The patient swings the leg outward from the hip in a semicircular movement without flexing the knee.

Circumlocution: Literally, *talking around* words that an individual is unable to say. Patients with conduction or Wernicke's aphasia often use circumlocution to communicate the sense of words they cannot retrieve.

Cistern: A cavity or space for storage of fluids.

Clasp-knife phenomenon: The tendency of spastic muscles to resist stretching when the examiner first moves the patient's limb and to gradually become less resistant as the examiner continues to move the patient's limb at a constant rate.

Coagulation time: The time it takes for blood to clot. Laboratory tests of coagulation time are useful in treating patients with occlusive vascular disease.

Coherence: The overall unity or point of discourse.

Cohesion: The degree to which words in discourse relate to one another.

Coma: Prolonged loss of consciousness.

Commissural fibers (commissures): Nerve fibers that cross between the brain hemispheres. The corpus callosum is the major commissure in the brain. The anterior and posterior commissures are minor ones.

Commissurotomy: Surgically cutting the corpus callosum.

Computerized tomography (CT scanning): A radiologic test in which a computer constructs cross-sectional images of internal body structures by analyzing information from a series of X-ray exposures made at consecutive horizontal levels of a body part.

Concreteness: Failure to appreciate abstract, indirect, nonliteral meanings of messages, events, or situations.

Conduction aphasia: An aphasia syndrome characterized by fluent speech, fair comprehension, and poor repetition.

Confrontation naming: Naming objects, pictures, color swatches, and so on.

Constructional apraxia: A misnomer. Inability to copy geometric shapes. Usually a disorder of visuospatial perception and integration, rather than a motor-planning disorder.

Constructional impairment: Inability to copy geometric shapes or copy three-dimensional constructions.

Contralateral: On the other side. In neurology, the term usually means *on the other side of the body from the nervous system disease.*

Contrast: Any of several fluids that may be introduced into internal spaces (usually blood vessels) or tissues to make structures easier to see in laboratory imaging studies.

Contrastive stress drill: A treatment for dysarthria and apraxia of speech in which the patient is coached to produce utterances with exaggerated emphatic stress on certain words, as in "Bob hit BILL."

Contrecoup injury: Brain injury on the opposite side of the brain from the impact.

Corpus callosum: The major commissure connecting the brain hemispheres. Almost all neural communication between the hemispheres goes via the corpus callosum.

Cortex: The neuron-rich outer layer of the brain hemispheres. Cortex makes "higher mental processes" (e.g., thinking, reasoning, calculating) possible.

Corticobulbar: Going between the cortex and the brain stem.

Corticopontine: Going between the cortex and the pons.

Corticospinal: Going between the cortex and the spinal cord.

Coup injury: Brain injury at the site of impact.

Cranial nerves: Peripheral nerves that serve muscles and sensory receptors in the head and neck. Most connect with the central nervous system in the brain stem.

Cranial vault: The inside of the skull. It contains the brain and cerebellum. It is divided into compartments by sheets of dura. The two major dural sheets are the *falx cerebri* and the *tentorium cerebelli.*

Creutzfeldt-Jakob disease: A degenerative disease in which brain tissues become soft and spongy *(spongiform encephalopathy).*

Decomposition of movement: Movements that have a jerky, segmented quality, often seen following cerebellar damage. A component of *ataxia.*

Decussate: Cross the midline. Refers to the crossing of pyramidal tracts from one side of the central nervous system to the other, at the medulla.

Delirium: Altered consciousness and mentation. Sometimes called *acute confusional state.*

Dementia: Diffuse impairment of intellect and cognition caused by any of several diseases and conditions.

Dementia, cortical: Dementia caused by pathology that affects the cerebral cortex.

Dementia, mixed: Dementia caused by a combination of cortical and subcortical pathology.

Dementia, subcortical: Dementia caused by pathology affecting the basal ganglia, thalamus, and brain stem.

Dendrite: Short, hair-like receptive processes of a nerve cell (neuron).

Dermatome: A region of skin innervated by a cranial or spinal sensory nerve.

Diagnosis: The act of assigning a label to a disease or condition.

Diaschisis: Disruption of brain function in areas remote from an area of injury but connected to it by nerve pathways.

Diencephalon: A deep central region within the brain hemispheres. Contains the thalamus and basal ganglia. It plays an important part in the regulation and integration of motor activity and sensory experience.

Differential diagnosis: Discriminating a disease or condition from others that may resemble it.

Diffuse axonal injury: Disseminated damage to nerve cell axons caused by *angular acceleration.*

Diplopia: Double vision. Often caused by weakness or paralysis of muscles responsible for moving one eye, which prevents the two eyes from fixating on the same point.

Disability: The effects of a structural or functional abnormality on a skill or ability (e.g., poor ambulation, caused by paralysis). *Disability* was changed to the politically neutral *activity* in the most recent World Health Organization schema. (See *impairment, handicap.*)

Disconnection syndrome: A unique pattern of impairments caused by interruption of fibers in the corpus callosum, which isolates the language-competent hemisphere from the language-incompetent hemisphere.

Distal: Away from the trunk.

Double simultaneous stimulation: Simultaneously stimulating sensory receptors at symmetric points on both sides of the body. Patients with subtle sensory impairments report stimulation only on the unaffected side.

Dressing apraxia: A misnomer. Dressing apraxia is not a true apraxia. It usually is seen in patients with nondominant-hemisphere pathology and is caused by disruptions of body schema, impaired appreciation of the relationship of the body to surrounding space, and, sometimes, neglect.

Dysarthria: Any of several speech abnormalities caused by nervous system damage that affects movement or sensation within body parts involved in speech.

Dyskinesia: Abnormal and involuntary muscle movements, often seen as a consequence of extrapyramidal disease. (See also *tremor, chorea, ballism, dystonia, myoclonus, fasciculations, fibrillations, tics.*)

Dyslexia, deep: A reading impairment in which the individual cannot analyze words phonologically but must depend on whole-word reading to recognize words.

Dyslexia, surface: A reading impairment in which the individual cannot make use of whole-word recognition in reading but must depend on phonologic analysis to recognize words.

Dysmetria: Slow and awkward movements. A component of *ataxia.*

Dystonia: Persisting involuntary contractions of muscles, sometimes called *torsion spasm.*

Echolalia: A tendency to repeat back what is said. A common characteristic of patients with *posterior isolation syndrome.*

Edema: Swelling.

Effectiveness: Whether treatment causes a meaningful change in patients' daily life adequacy.

Efferent: Motor.

Efficacy: Whether treatment causes a significant change in patients' performance on one or more objective measures.

Egocentrism: Inability to view events and situations from another's point of view.

Electroencephalography (EEG): A laboratory test in which the electrical activity of the brain cortex is measured and converted to a pen tracing on a moving strip of paper.

Electromyography (EMG): A procedure in which fine needle electrodes are inserted into muscles and the electrical activity in the muscles is recorded.

Ellipsoidal deformation: Deformation of the restrained skull caused by the impact of a slow-moving object possessing a large surface area.

Embolus: A fragment that travels through a blood vessel. If an embolus lodges and occludes an artery, it causes an embolic stroke.

Emotional lability: Exaggerated emotional responses to stimuli. Unusually wide swings in emotional tone.

Empty speech: Speech that is syntactically correct but conveys little or no overall meaning. Often a result of substituting general words such as *thing* or *stuff* for more specific words.

Encephalopathy: Pathology affecting the brain and meninges.

Epidural: Between the dura mater and the skull.

Evoked cortical potentials: A laboratory procedure in which a computer averages the electrical activity of the brain cortex from many sites on the skull and produces a record of systematic changes in the electrical activity that occur with presentation of auditory, visual, or tactile stimuli.

Extrapyramidal system: That part of the motor system not composed of corticobulbar or corticospinal tracts. Includes the basal ganglia and related structures.

Falx cerebri: A rigid sheet of dura mater that goes from front to back within the longitudinal cerebral fissure. It often is called the *falx* for efficiency.

Familial: Diseases that have a greater than normal occurrence in families but do not have a known genetic inheritance pattern. The exact probability that offspring of parents who have the disease will inherit the disease cannot be calculated. (See also *hereditary.*)

Fasciculations: Involuntary contractions of muscle fibers that are visually obvious.

Fasciculus: A fiber tract that connects regions in different lobes of the brain. The three major fasciculi are the *arcuate fasciculus,* the *uncinate fasciculus,* and the *cingulum.*

Feedback: Information provided contingent on responses. *Incentive feedback* depends on response consequences that have primary reinforcing (or punishing) power. *Information feedback* has no intrinsic reinforcing or punishing power but provides information to an individual about the closeness of responses to a target. See *reinforcement, punishment.*

Festinating gait: Short rapid steps. A common consequence of Parkinson's disease.

Fibrillations: Contractions of a single muscle fiber or small group of fibers that are too small to be seen but are detectable with sensitive instruments.

Fissure: A deep sulcus.

Fluency: When used to classify adults with aphasia, fluency refers to the prosodic or melodic characteristics of speech. Adults with fluent aphasia speak with essentially normal rate, intonation, pauses, and emphatic stress patterns. Adults with nonfluent aphasia speak slowly and with diminished intonation, abnormally placed and excessively long pauses, and diminished variation in emphatic stress. Fluent aphasia is associated with postcentral damage, and nonfluent aphasia is associated with precentral damage.

Focal: Affecting a limited region within the nervous system. The opposite of *diffuse.*

Foramen: An opening. There are several foramina in the skull, through which blood vessels and nerves pass. The major one is the *foramen magnum,* through which the brain stem passes. There are many foramina in the spinal cord, between the vertebrae, through which nerves and blood vessels pass (the intervertebral foramina).

Frontal-lobe dementia: See *Pick's disease.*

Frontal lobes: Make up approximately the anterior one third of the brain. The frontal lobes provide the initial impetus for overt behavior.

Fugue state: A period of disturbed consciousness lasting from minutes to days, in which the patient goes about regular activities of daily living but has no subsequent memory for what happened during the period.

Functional communication: Communication in daily life.

Gag reflex: Coughing or choking when the posterior tongue or pharyngeal walls are touched.

Generalization: Transfer of learned skills, behaviors, or responses from one setting to another.

Generative naming (word fluency, category naming): Providing names according to a category suggested by the examiner. For example, "Tell me all the words you can think of that begin with the letter F" or "Tell me all the vegetables you can think of." (Usually limited to a 1-minute interval.)

Geographic disorientation: Inability to identify one's geographic location, although one recognizes one's personal surroundings. An occasional consequence of right-hemisphere brain damage.

Glial cells: Form the supporting tissue of the brain, which is called *glia.* Most of the cells in the brain are glial cells.

Glioblastoma multiforme: A common, very malignant tumor of glial cells.

Glioma: A tumor that arises in brain glia.

Granulovacuolar degeneration: Neuronal abnormalities seen in Alzheimer's disease and other neurologic diseases and in some normal elderly people. Small fluid-filled cavities appear within nerve cells, and nerve cell function is adversely affected.

Gray matter: Nervous system tissues made up primarily of cell bodies and dendrites. It is actually pinkish-gray in color.

Gyrus: A "hill" on the surface of the brain. (Plural = gyri.)

Gyrus of Heschl: A strip of cortex on the top surface of each temporal lobe. Also known as the *primary auditory cortex.*

Handicap: The effects of a structural or functional abnormality on an individual's ability to carry out daily life roles and responsibilities (e.g., diminished ability to earn a living as a consequence of hemiplegia). *Handicap* was changed to the politically neutral *participation* in the most recent World Health Organization schema. (See *impairment, disability.*)

Hematoma: Accumulation of blood from a hemorrhage.

Hemianopia (Hemianopsia): Blindness in one half of the visual field. *Homonymous hemianopia* is blindness in the same (right or left) half of the visual field in each eye. *Heteronymous hemianopia* is blindness in different halves of the visual field in each eye.

Hemiplegia: Paralysis of an arm and a leg on one side of the body.

Hemorrhage: Bleeding. Accumulation of blood from a hemorrhage is called a *hematoma.*

Hereditary: Diseases that have a known genetic inheritance pattern. The probability that offspring of parents who have the disease will inherit the disease can be calculated, and "family trees" showing inheritance patterns can be constructed.

Herniation: Displacement of brain tissue by swelling or space-occupying lesions such as tumors or brain abscesses.

Heuristic processes: "Top-down" comprehension processes, in which listeners and readers use general knowledge, intuition, and guessing to arrive at the meaning of spoken or printed verbal materials.

Homonymous: The corresponding halves of the visual fields or retinae.

Homunculus: "Little man." A drawing of a human figure showing topographic representation of the motor cortex.

Huntington's disease: A hereditary neurologic disease characterized by progressive chorea and dementia.

Hydrocephalus: Enlargement of the cerebral ventricles. Hydrocephalus usually is caused by obstruction of an intraventricular passageway, but it also can be a result of brain atrophy. The former is called *obstructive hydrocephalus,* and the latter is called *nonobstructive hydrocephalus.*

Hyperesthesia: Abnormal sensitivity to stimulation.

Hypertonia: Abnormally high levels of tension in resting muscles.

Hypesthesia (hypoesthesia): Diminished sensation.

Hypoperfusion: Diminished blood supply to the brain caused by insufficient blood volume or pressure.

Hypotonia: Abnormally low levels of tension in resting muscles.

Ideational apraxia: Inability to carry out movement sequences because of loss of the concept, knowledge, or idea of what the movements are intended to accomplish.

Ideomotor apraxia: Inability to carry out movement sequences because of loss of the ability to organize the motor plans or patterns for the movements.

Impairment: A structural or functional abnormality within an individual (e.g., paralysis.) *Impairment* was changed to the politically neutral *body function and structure* in the most recent World Health Organization schema. (See *disability, handicap.*)

Infarct: Death of tissue caused by loss of blood supply.

Insula: A patch of cortex folded into the lateral fissure, sometimes called the *island of Reil.* The operculum surrounds it.

Integral stimulation: A treatment procedure in which the patient imitates the clinician's model. ("Watch me and do what I do.")

Internal capsule: That section of corticobulbar and corticospinal tracts that lies within the basal ganglia.

Intersystemic reorganization (gestural reorganization): A treatment for apraxia of speech in which patients are taught to execute non-speech movements simultaneously with speech (e.g., gesturing the act of drinking from a glass while saying "Drink some water.").

Intracerebral: Within the brain.

Intrasystemic reorganization: A treatment for apraxia of speech in which the locus of control of speech movements is shifted to another part of the system used to produce speech (e.g., speaking slowly and with exaggerated articulation).

Intraventricular foramen: A short passageway between each lateral ventricle and the third ventricle for movement of cerebrospinal fluid, sometimes called the *foramen of Munro.*

Ipsilateral: On the same side. (See also *contralateral.*)

Ischemia: Lack of oxygen in tissues.

Isolation syndrome: An aphasia syndrome caused by isolation of the central region of the language-dominant hemisphere from the rest of the brain. (See also *anterior isolation syndrome* and *posterior isolation syndrome.*)

Isometric: Pushing against immovable resistance.

Isotonic: Pushing against a movable resistance.

Jargon: Nonsensical utterances, such as *"There's a navy dog flying in the hoghouse this morning,"* in which words are uttered in syntactically legitimate strings, but have no overall meaning. The strings may contain *neologisms.*

Lacunar state: A progressive neurologic disease caused by successive small infarcts in the midbrain and brain stem.

Lateral apertures: Two openings from the fourth ventricle into the subarachnoid space, sometimes called the *foramina of Luschka.*

Lateral cerebral fissure: A deep groove that separates the temporal lobe in each hemisphere from the frontal and parietal lobes, sometimes called the *fissure of Sylvius* or the *fronto-temporo-parietal fissure.*

Lenticular nucleus: The putamen and globus pallidus (basal ganglia).

Limb apraxia: Ideomotor apraxia of the arm and hand. Limb apraxias usually are more severe distally (away from the trunk) than proximally (near the trunk).

Localization: An approach to understanding the functional architecture of the nervous system by relating neurologically damaged patients' symptoms to damaged regions of the nervous system. When damage in a given part of the nervous system consistently causes certain impairments, the impaired function is attributed to the damaged part.

Logorrhea: See *press of speech.*

Longitudinal cerebral fissure: The deep groove at the apex of the cerebrum that separates the hemispheres. (Sometimes it is called the *superior longitudinal fissure* or *interhemispheric fissure.*) (Perhaps it should be called the *superior longitudinal interhemispheric cerebral fissure.*)

Loose training: Generalization training in which stimulus conditions, response requirements, and reinforcement contingencies are permitted to vary to increase generalization from the training environment to other environments.

Lower motor neuron: Another name for the peripheral nervous system.

Lumbar puncture (spinal tap): A procedure in which a needle is inserted into the spinal column and a sample of cerebrospinal fluid is removed and analyzed for the presence of bacteria, viruses, parasites, or abnormalities in its chemical composition.

Lumen: The open passageway in a blood vessel.

Macula: A region in the central retina that provides the greatest visual acuity.

Macular sparing: The presence of a small region of intact vision near the center of a visual field in which a person is otherwise blind. Macular sparing is common when visual field blindness is caused by destruction of the visual cortex in one brain hemisphere.

Magnetic resonance imaging (MRI scanning): A laboratory test that uses a strong magnetic field and a computer to create images of internal structures based on differences in the chemical composition of body tissues.

Manometer: An instrument for measuring breath pressure.

Masked facies: Rigidity of facial muscles, causing fixed, unchanging facial expression. A prominent characteristic of Parkinson's disease.

Median apertures: Two openings from the fourth ventricle into the subarachnoid space, sometimes called the *foramina of Magendi.*

Mediation: Elicitation of one response by another (usually internal) response (e.g., saying the names of letters to oneself while writing complex words).

Medulla: The bottom third of the brain stem. Contains five cranial nerve nuclei plus some centers concerned with hearing and balance. Pyramidal tract fibers decussate (cross the midline) here.

Melodic Intonation Therapy (MIT): A treatment procedure for patients with severe speech production impairments in which melody and exaggerated intonation are used to facilitate speech.

Memory, declarative: What we know about things (e.g., names, faces, places, situations).

Memory, episodic: Memory for personally experienced events.

Memory, long term: (Sometimes called *secondary memory.*) The third stage in some models of memory. It has large (perhaps infinite) capacity, and information in it decays slowly if at all. Considered a repository for our knowledge and sense of self.

Memory, procedural: What we know about how to do things (e.g., make coffee, paint a window).

Memory, prospective: The ability to remember to do things at certain times (remembering to remember).

Memory, retrospective: Memory for past experiences and for knowledge acquired in the past.

Memory, semantic: Stored general knowledge.

Memory, sensory: (Sometimes called *sensory register.*) The first stage in some models of memory, in which the traces of stimuli are briefly stored. The traces decay quickly and cannot be maintained by rehearsal.

Memory, short term: (Sometimes called *primary memory.*) The second stage in some models of memory, in which information can be maintained by rehearsal. Without rehearsal, information decays within a few minutes. Short-term memory has limited capacity. Only a few items of information can be stored there at one time.

Memory, working: A mental space in which processing of information coming from short-term memory or retrieved from long-term memory takes place.

Memory loss, post-traumatic: Loss of memory for a period following brain injury. (Sometimes called *anterograde amnesia.*)

Memory loss, pre-traumatic: Loss of memory for events immediately preceding brain injury. (Sometimes called *retrograde amnesia.*)

Meninges: The membranes between the skull and the brain. The toughest one lines the skull and is called the *dura mater.* (Think of DURable. Also, remember that if protection is the key, it makes sense that nature would put the toughest one on the outside.) The web-like one is the *arachnoid* (think spider). The one on the surface of the brain is the *pia mater.* To keep them in order, think *PAD* (for pia, arachnoid, dura).

Meningioma: A tumor in the meninges.

Mesencephalon (midbrain): A deep brain region that makes up the upper third of the brain stem. Contains several nuclei, including those for cranial nerves that move the eyes.

Metastasis: The process by which a tumor appears at a secondary site from the location of the original tumor.

Monoplegia: Paralysis of one limb.

Motor cortex: A strip of cortex just ahead of the central fissure. It is responsible for initiating most volitional motor activity.

Myasthenia gravis: A neurologic disease caused by damage to the acetylcholine receptors on muscle cells. Characterized by abnormally rapid muscle fatigue with use.

Myelin: Fatty material surrounding the axons of neurons.

Myelogram: A laboratory procedure that permits visualization of the spinal cord. Contrast medium is injected into the subarachnoid space around the spinal cord and a series of X-ray exposures is made to visualize the structure of the spinal cord and surrounding tissues.

Myelopathy: Pathology affecting the spinal cord.

Myoclonus: Fine, rapid, irregular twitching movements caused by contractions of groups of muscle fibers. Usually observable as dimpling or rippling of the skin over the muscle fibers.

Myopathy: Disease of muscle.

Myositis: Inflammation of muscle.

Necrosis: Death of tissue.

Neglect: Inattention to some part of surrounding space. Most often seen as inattention to one half of surrounding space *(hemispatial neglect).* A common consequence of nondominant-hemisphere pathology.

Neologisms: Nonword utterances (e.g., "mandernost") that follow the phonologic conventions of the language. Neologisms often are heard in the speech of adults with severe Wernicke's aphasia or global aphasia.

Neuralgia: Pain caused by inflammation of a nerve.

Neuritic plaques: Neuronal abnormalities seen in Alzheimer's disease and other neurologic diseases and in some normal elderly people. Neuritic plaques are small areas of nerve cell degeneration, primarily occurring in cortical and subcortical brain regions.

Neurofibrillary tangles: Neuronal abnormalities seen in Alzheimer's disease, in other neurologic diseases, and in some normal elderly people. Neurofibrillary tangles are filamentous bodies seen in the nerve cell body, dendrites, axon, and sometimes in synaptic endings.

Neuron: A nerve cell.

Neurotransmitter: Any of several chemical compounds that are involved in transmission of nerve impulses between nerve cells.

Nonaccelaration injury: Brain injury caused when the stationary head is struck by a moving object.

Norms: Any of several statistics that summarize the test performance of a sample of individuals representing a population to which the norms apply. Sample means and standard deviations are the minimum normative statistics needed to relate the performance of an individual to a norm group.

Nucleus: A group of neurons in the brain or spinal cord that are differentiated from surrounding tissue by cell type or by surrounding zones of nerve fibers.

Nystagmus: Rhythmic oscillation of the eyes, sometimes caused by weakness in the muscles that move the eyes and sometimes caused by disturbances of balance and equilibrium.

Occipital lobes: The rearmost portions of the brain hemispheres. The visual cortex is located in the occipital lobes.

Olfactory cortex: A region of cortex on the inferior surface of each frontal lobe. It has principal responsibility for the sense of smell.

Operculum: The patch of cortex surrounding the insula.

Ophthalmoplegia: Paralysis of muscles responsible for eye movements.

Optic chiasm: The point at which the crossing fibers in the human visual system cross. It is located at the base of the brain near the pituitary gland.

Orientation: Awareness of one's surroundings. Orientation is customarily subdivided into orientation for *person, place,* and *time.*

Outcome: The long-term (final) result of treatment.

Palillalia: Involuntary repetition of words and sentences.

Palmar reflex: Sometimes called the *grasp reflex*. A pathologic reflex elicited by stroking the palm of the hand. The hand closes involuntarily and the fingers grasp the object used to stroke the palm.

Palsy: Another word for *paralysis*.

Papilledema: Swelling of the optic disk in the back of the eye, suggesting increased intracranial pressure, inflammation of the optic disk, or ischemia of the optic disk.

Paraphasia: Paraphasias are errors in speaking made by aphasic persons. *Literal (phonemic) paraphasias* are errors in which a speaker substitutes one sound in a word for another, such as saying "spomb" for "comb." *Verbal (semantic) paraphasias* are errors in which a speaker substitutes one word for another, such as saying "cup" for "glass."

Paraplegia: Paralysis of both legs.

Paresis: Muscle weakness.

Paresthesia: Abnormal sensations (e.g., tingling, burning) in the absence of stimulation.

Parietal lobes: The part of the brain hemispheres behind the central fissure and above the lateral fissure. The parietal cortex is important for somesthetic sensation (skin, muscle, joint, and tendon sensation).

Parkinson's disease: A degenerative disease affecting neurons in the midbrain and brain stem.

Passage dependency: The degree to which answering questions that test comprehension of discourse depends on having read or heard the discourse.

Patellar reflex: A normal reflex elicited by tapping the patellar tendon just below the kneecap. The lower leg jerks upward when the patellar tendon is tapped. Diminished patellar reflexes may be a sign of peripheral nerve damage or muscle weakness; exaggerated patellar reflexes may be a sign of upper motor neuron damage.

Percentile: A score that represents the percentage of individuals in a norm group that fall above or below the score. For example, a score that places an individual at the 95th percentile means that 94% of the norm group received lower scores.

Perimetry: A procedure for testing vision in all quadrants of the visual fields with a specialized instrument called a *perimeter*.

Peripheral nervous system (PNS): Consists of the cranial nerves and spinal nerves. The peripheral nervous system is sometimes called the *lower motor neuron*.

Perseveration: Repetition of a response when it is no longer appropriate, as when a patient calls a *comb* a "comb," but continues to call subsequent objects "comb."

Persistent vegetative state: A condition in which the individual has sleep-wake cycles but makes no purposeful responses to the environment.

Pharyngeal flap: A surgical procedure for alleviating hypernasality.

Phonetic contrast: Drills in which a patient produces a series of sounds, syllables, or words that systematically change by a single articulatory feature.

Phonetic derivation: A treatment procedure in which a new speech sound is obtained by modifying a sound the patient can produce.

Phonetic dissolution: Distortion of speech sounds caused by articulatory breakdown. Sometimes resembles literal paraphasia, but literal paraphasia typically is characterized by substitution of one correctly articulated sound for another, whereas phonetic dissolution is characterized by distortions of sounds.

Phonetic placement: A treatment procedure in which drawings, models, or physical positioning are used to help a patient place the articulators in position for making a sound.

Phrenology: A nineteenth century pseudoscience in which personal attributes were said to be related to head shape and contours.

Pick's disease (frontal-lobe dementia): A progressive degenerative disease affecting the brain cortex. It is characterized by the presence of *Pick bodies* (dense globular formations within nerve cells) and *enlarged neurons* in the brain. Pick's disease is an important cause of cortical dementia.

Plantar reflex: Sometimes called the *plantar extensor* or *Babinski* reflex. A pathologic reflex elicited by forcefully stroking the sole of the foot, causing the toes to bend upward and fan out. The *plantar flexor* reflex, in which the toes bend downward and do not fan, is the normal response to this stimulation.

Plaque (arteriosclerotic plaque, atherosclerotic plaque): Fatty deposits on the inner walls of arteries.

-plegia: A suffix denoting *paralysis*.

Pons: The middle third of the brain stem. Contains three cranial nerve nuclei plus some nuclei concerned with balance and hearing.

Positron emission tomography (PET): A laboratory procedure in which the metabolic activity of the brain is measured by introducing a metabolically active compound (usually glucose) tagged with a mildly radioactive element and measuring the regions in which the compound concentrates.

Posterior horn cells: Spinal sensory nerves, located in the posterolateral part of the spinal cord.

Post-traumatic memory loss: See *memory loss, post-traumatic.*

Pragmatics: Language in use.

Premotor cortex: A strip of cortex in the posterior frontal lobes said to be important for planning volitional movements.

Press of speech (logorrhea): Excessive verbosity. Patients with mild to moderate Wernicke's or conduction aphasia are most likely to exhibit press of speech.

Pre-traumatic memory loss: See *memory loss, pre-traumatic.*

Progressive approximation: A treatment procedure in which a new response is created by stepwise modification of an existing response.

Progressive supranuclear palsy (PSP): A progressive disease characterized by degeneration of brain stem neurons, causing increasingly severe motor impairments, especially in muscles served by cranial nerves.

Projection fibers: Nerve fiber tracts that connect the brain, brain stem, and spinal cord. They can be either motor (efferent) or sensory (afferent).

Proprioception: The ability to tell the position of the head and limbs without seeing them.

Prosody: The melodic characteristics of speech—rate, intonation, and stress patterns.

Prosopagnosia: Inability to recognize faces.

Prospective research: Research in which the design is established prior to subject intake, and subject intake and experimental procedures are defined in advance.

Proximal: Near the trunk.

Pseudobulbar affect: Exaggerated emotional responses to minimally emotional stimuli. Often an early, but usually transitory, consequence of brain damage.

Pure word deafness: An auditory impairment in which the individual loses the ability to comprehend spoken verbal materials despite intact hearing but retains the ability to recognize nonverbal auditory stimuli.

Pyramidal system: The neural system that is responsible for initiating most volitional movement. It is made up of the motor neurons in the motor cortex together with projection fibers, which connect the motor cortex to the brain stem and spinal cord. It is sometimes called the upper motor neuron.

Quadrantanopsia: Blindness in less than half of the visual field in each eye. (See also *hemianopia.*)

Quadriplegia: Paralysis of both arms and both legs.

Reduplicative paramnesia: The belief that two or more identical persons, places, or things exist in different locations. An occasional consequence of right-hemisphere brain damage.

Reflex: A spontaneous and uncontrollable movement in response to stimulation. The two major categories of reflexes are *superficial reflexes,* which are elicited by touching, stroking, or brushing the surface of body parts, and *deep reflexes,* which are elicited by tapping or suddenly stretching muscles or tendons. (See also *gag reflex, swallow reflex, plantar reflex, palmar reflex, sucking reflex, patellar reflex.*)

Regional cerebral blood flow (rCBF): A laboratory procedure for measuring blood flow by introducing mildly radioactive substances into the bloodstream and analyzing their concentration by means of sensitive detectors and a computer.

Reinforcement: Positive reinforcement *is delivering positive consequences following desired behaviors to increase their frequency.* Negative reinforcement *is removing negative consequences following desired behaviors to increase their frequency.*

Responsive naming: Providing names in response to questions such as "What do you drink coffee from?" or requests such as "Tell me what you use for digging a hole."

Retention span: The amount of information that can be held in primary memory at one time. (From four to ten items for most normal adults.)

Reticular formation: Structures in the central core of the brain stem that regulate the individual's overall level of consciousness.

Retrospective research: Research in which information about subjects is gathered from preexisting records.

Rigidity: Resistance of muscles to movement in any direction. A prominent characteristic of Parkinson's disease.

Scanning speech: The slow, regular, and monotonous speech of persons with cerebellar ataxia.

Scripts: (Sometimes called *schemata.*) Mental representations of familiar daily life routines or situations, such as eating in a restaurant, going to a party, or shopping for groceries.

Sedimentation rate: The rate at which blood cells sink in a liquid. Sedimentation rate is an indicator of clotting potential.

Seizure: Episodes of disturbed consciousness caused by abnormal patterns of neuronal discharge in the brain. In *generalized seizures* (convulsions, tonic-clonic seizures, *gran mal seizures*) the patient loses consciousness, with spasmodic contractions of most muscle groups. In *partial seizures* (*focal* seizures) the patient does not lose consciousness and only some muscle groups are affected by spasmodic contractions. In *absence seizures* (*petit mal* seizures) the patient does not lose consciousness and does not experience spasmodic muscle contractions but does not respond purposefully to stimulation.

Sequential modification: Generalization training in which stimulus conditions, response requirements, and reinforcement contingencies gradually are changed to resemble a target environment to increase generalization from the training environment to the target environment.

Sign: An objective indicator of illness or disease observed by an examiner. (See *symptom.*)

Social validation: A procedure for evaluating the clinical significance of changes created by a treatment program, in which the effects of treatment on an individual's daily life performance are evaluated.

Somatosensory cortex: A strip of cortex just behind the central fissure. It is responsible for skin, muscle, joint, and tendon sensation.

Somesthetic sensation: Sensation from the skin, muscles, joints, and tendons.

Spastic catch: A sudden increase in muscle tension when spastic muscles are quickly stretched by the examiner.

Spasticity: Abnormally high levels of tension in resting muscles caused by upper motor neuron damage.

Spinal nerves: Peripheral nerves that supply muscles and sensory receptors in the trunk and limbs. Motor nerves have their cell bodies in the anterolateral part of the spinal cord (anterior horn cells), and sensory nerves have their cell bodies in the posterolateral part (posterior horn cells).

Stenosis: Narrowing, as of an artery.

Steppage gait: A characteristic gait of patients with paralysis of muscles in the front of the lower leg, causing the foot to hang down as the patient walks. The patient lifts the legs abnormally high so that the toes clear the ground.

Stereognosis: The ability to identify objects by touch.

Stereotypies, verbal: Repetitive, noncommunicative utterances made by brain-injured patients (e.g., *me-me-me, wuna-wuna-wuna*). Often one indicator of severe aphasia.

Stridor: Audible inhalation.

Stroke: Temporary or permanent disruption of brain function due to interruption of its blood supply. Sometimes called *cerebrovascular accident* (CVA) or *brain attack.*

Subarachnoid: Between the arachnoid and the pia mater.

Subclavian arteries: Two large arteries branching off from the aorta. The vertebral arteries originate at the subclavian arteries.

Subdural: Between the dura mater and the arachnoid.

Sucking reflex: A pathologic reflex elicited by touching or stroking on or near the lips, causing the lips to make involuntary sucking movements.

Sulcus: A "valley" on the surface of the brain. (Plural = sulci.) (See also *fissure.*)

Swallow reflex: Swallowing when the posterior tongue or pharyngeal walls are touched.

Symptom: Indicators of illness or disease experienced by the patient. (See *sign.*)

Synapse: The point at which an axon of one nerve cell meets the dendrite of another, where transmission of nerve impulses takes place by means of chemicals called neurotransmitters.

Syncope: Fainting.

Telegraphic speech: Speech in which function words are left out. (See *agrammatism.*)

Temporal lobes: Make up approximately the bottom third of each hemisphere, beneath the lateral cerebral fissure. The left temporal lobe plays an important role in language and audition.

Tentorium cerebelli: A rigid sheet of dura that separates the cerebellum from the base of the brain. It is often called *the tentorium* for efficiency. Neurologists sometimes use the terms *supratentorial* and *subtentorial* to describe vertical locations in the cranial vault.

Testing the limits: Deviating from standard test procedures to determine the underlying reasons for a patient's deficient performance on a test.

Thalamus: A pair of egg-shaped nuclei in the diencephalon. They are important for integration of sensory information and for regulating motor behavior, and they may regulate the overall activity of the cortex.

Theory of mind: The ability to appreciate others' state of knowledge.

Thrombosis: Accumulation of a plug of material at a specific site in a blood vessel. If it grows large enough to occlude a cerebral artery, it causes a thrombotic stroke.

Tic douloureux: Shooting, lance-like pains associated with inflammation of the trigeminal nerve *(trigeminal neuralgia).*

Tics: Stereotypic repetitive movements such as blinking, coughing, or sniffing. Tics usually are not related to nervous system pathology.

Tongue-anchor test: Pushing out the cheeks with impounded air while protruding the tongue through closed lips.

Topographic impairment (topologic disorientation): A state of confusion regarding surrounding space and how one relates to it. A frequent consequence of right-hemisphere brain damage.

Torsion spasm: See *dystonia.*

Toxemia: Inflammation or poisoning of brain tissue by foreign substances.

Transcortical aphasia—mixed: An aphasia syndrome characterized by profound comprehension impairment, little or no functional language, but good repetition.

Transcortical motor aphasia (anterior isolation syndrome): An aphasia syndrome characterized by good comprehension, sparse speech output, and good repetition.

Transcortical sensory aphasia (posterior isolation syndrome): An aphasia syndrome characterized by poor comprehension, fluent but echolalic speech, and good repetition.

Transcranial Doppler ultrasound: A laboratory test in which sound waves are transmitted into the head and a computer measures blood pressure and flow by analyzing changes in the frequency of the reflected sound waves.

Transient ischemic attack (TIA): A temporary disruption of cerebral circulation that causes a transient disturbance of motor, sensory, or mental functions.

Translational trauma: Brain damage caused by acceleration of the head by outside forces.

Tremor: Cyclic, small amplitude involuntary movements, usually more severe in distal (away from the trunk) muscles than in proximal (near the trunk) muscles.

Trigeminal neuralgia: See *tic douloureux.*

Trismus: Excessive and uncontrollable contraction of the muscles of mastication.

Upper motor neuron: Another name for the pyramidal system.

Validity: The degree to which a test actually measures what it purports to measure. *Content validity* is an indicator of how well the items in a test represent the domain of concern. *Construct validity* is an indicator of how well the content of a test relates to an established model, theory, or concept of the skill, process, or structure to which the test relates.

Vasospasm: Constriction of arteries by contraction of muscles in the arterial wall.

Ventricles (cerebral ventricles): Fluid-filled cavities within the brain. There are four of them—two *lateral ventricles,* a *third ventricle,* and a *fourth ventricle.*

Verbal apraxia (apraxia of speech): Disruption of the motor plans for speech articulation. Verbal apraxia often accompanies Broca's aphasia. (Also see *apraxia.*)

Vertebrae: Bony plates surrounding the spinal cord. From top to bottom they are classified into *cervical, thoracic, lumbar,* and *sacral* divisions.

Vertebral arteries: Two arteries that begin at the subclavian arteries and progress upward on the front side of the medulla. They supply blood to the medulla and, via the basilar artery, to the posterior part of the circle of Willis.

Vestibular-reticular system: A diffuse neural system. It is responsible for balance and orientation of the body in space and for general states of attention and alertness.

Visual cortex: A region of cortex in each occipital lobe. It has principal responsibility for visual perception.

Wernicke's aphasia: An aphasia syndrome characterized by fluent but empty speech, poor comprehension, and poor repetition.

Wernicke's area: A region of cortex in the vicinity of the temporo-parietal-occipital junction. Damage in Wernicke's areas is said to cause *Wernicke's aphasia.*

Wernicke's encephalopathy: A neurologic disease caused by thiamine deficiency and usually associated with alcoholism.

White matter: Nervous system tissues made up primarily of nerve axons. It is white because of the presence of *myelin.*

Word fluency: See *generative naming.*

Responses to Thought Questions

CHAPTER ONE

Response to Question 1-1: Mrs. Redmond's impairments are likely to be less severe than those of Mr. Johnson.

- She is younger. Her arterial system is likely to be in better health than that of Mr. Johnson, and her nervous system is likely to be physiologically more resilient than that of Mr. Johnson.

- Her stroke was in the watershed region of the left hemisphere. Collateral circulation from the posterior cerebral artery may provide an alternative to that previously supplied by the middle cerebral artery.

- The arteries in the watershed region are small in diameter and serve small cortical areas, compared with arteries in the more central regions of the hemisphere. Consequently, the volume of brain tissue affected by Mrs. Redmond's stroke is likely to be less than the volume of brain tissue affected by Mr. Johnson's stroke.

Mrs. Redmond should experience greater neurologic recovery than Mr. Johnson, and her recovery should progress at a faster rate than that of Mr. Johnson, for the reasons enumerated above, which speak to the rate of recovery from nervous system injury as well as to the initial severity of symptoms.

Response to Question 1-2: This is a classic scenario for cerebral hemorrhage. Cerebral hemorrhages tend to occur in hypertensive patients and often occur during periods of exertion, which causes blood pressure to increase, puts pressure on arterial walls, and adds to the risk of bleeding. The delayed onset of Mr. Carillo's symptoms also is consistent with cerebral hemorrhage. Symptoms of hemorrhage often develop slowly, appearing only after enough bleeding has occurred to increase intracranial pressure (unless the hemorrhage is a massive one, in which severe headache and coma occur quickly).

Response to Question 1-3: These patients complain of leg weakness and loss of sensation because the primary motor cortex for the leg, located high on the convexity of the primary motor cortex, and the primary sensory cortex for the leg, high on the primary somatosensory cortex, are pressed against the falx cerebri. The pressure causes the patient's symptoms. The patient's symptoms will affect the leg contralateral to the side on which the motor and sensory cortices are being pressed against the falx cerebri. This usually suggests a mass lesion (e.g., tumor, abscess) in the brain hemisphere contralateral to the side of the patient's symptoms. The mass lesion presses against brain tissue, squeezing it against the inner surface of the skull and displacing brain tissue from regions of high pressure to regions of low pressure—in this case across the falx cerebri into the other side of the cranial vault.

Response to Question 1-4: Harry's symptoms—excruciating pain caused by stimulation of nerves in the face—may suggest trigeminal neuralgia *(tic douloureux)*. Tic douloureux is characterized by momentary episodes of intense, excruciating pain following sensory stimulation of receptors in the cheek, nose, or mouth with heat, cold, touch, or movement. The sudden appearance of Harry's symptoms and their intensity suggest inflammation of the maxillary branch of the trigeminal nerve. Harry saw a neurologist, who concluded that Harry's symptoms were related to trigeminal neuralgia and prescribed an anti-inflammatory medication. Harry's symptoms resolved the day after he began taking the medication. (Harry also transferred his dental care to Dr. Luck.)

Response to Question 1-5: Those who discovered and publicized this phenomenon attribute it to differences in traffic patterns between the United States and England. In the United States vehicle drivers sit on the left side of the vehicle. If they drive with the window open, outside air blows across the left side of the face. In England vehicle drivers sit on the right side of the vehicle and air from an open window blows across the right side of the face. It is known that exposure to cold sometimes leads to inflammation of the facial nerve, causing it to swell. Combining this information leads to the conclusion that the difference in laterality between the two countries is related to driving habits. (If this hypothesis is true, then one would expect that northern regions of the two countries should show a greater disparity in laterality than warmer regions, if the culprit is indeed cold air, but as far as I can determine, no one has addressed this possibility.)

CHAPTER TWO

Response to Question 2-1: The events described here represent a typical scenario, in which a patient seen in the first few hours after a stroke presents a somewhat confusing picture in terms of the probable location, extent, and (sometimes) etiology of the patient's symptoms. The probability is high that this patient has had a stroke in the left hemisphere, probably embolic (because of his history of heart disease). The finding of mild hemiparesis and Wernicke's aphasia are somewhat inconsistent because one ordinarily wouldn't expect a patient with Wernicke's aphasia (and temporal lobe injury) to be hemiparetic. It is important to remember that stroke patients seen in the first few hours (and sometimes days) after stroke may exhibit signs that do not point to the location of the stroke and sometimes may not accurately indicate its nature (occlusion vs. hemorrhage, thrombus vs. embolus). Also remember that one often sees signs that are caused by the generalized immediate consequences of brain injury—swelling, neurotransmitter release, diaschisis—that may confuse one's attempts at localization in the first few days after onset. The co-occurrence of hemiparesis and Wernicke's aphasia is fairly common in the first few hours or days post-injury.

One might be tempted to hypothesize that this man's neurologic signs either (a) require two lesions (one in the temporal lobe and one near the motor cortex) or (b) require a large lesion that extends to the vicinity of the motor cortex. There is a problem with each of these hypotheses. It would be highly unusual for two strokes to occur simultaneously or in such rapid succession to generate the two lesions suggested by (a), and it's unlikely that either could be old "silent" strokes because each would generate symptoms that would be likely to send the patient to his physician. The problem with (b) is that the massive lesion envisioned would generate very severe impairments (global aphasia) rather than the relatively mild symptoms exhibited by this patient.

However, there is a more troublesome inconsistency in this report. One would not expect left hemianopia to occur together with the other signs, all of which point to damage in the left hemisphere. I can think of two possible explanations:

1. The neurologist made a mistake, and it was really a right hemianopia (these things do happen).
2. The hemianopia was the result of an old "silent" lesion in the right hemisphere.

Note that the patient's arm was weaker than his leg. This points to damage low in the hemisphere. If the leg were weaker than the arm, one would suspect damage high in the hemisphere. Can you see why?

Response to Question 2-2: This patient apparently understands the task—he repeats three "words" according to instructions, but the "words" are not real words. That means that a test of memory for words cannot depend on the patient's saying the words, so I would see if I could circumvent the patient's output problem by giving him an alternative way of responding. I'd try the test again, but instead of asking the patient to say the words back to me, I would ask him to choose the words I said from an array of printed words. If that worked, I would give him three new words to remember and subsequently test his memory for the words by asking him to choose them from an array of printed words.

If the patient could not choose the words I said from an array of printed words, I would ask him to choose them from an array containing pictures representing the test words plus several foils. If that worked, I would give him three new words to remember and test his memory for the words by asking him to choose the pictures representing the words from a new array.

If the patient could not choose words I said from an array of printed words nor from an array of pictures (a word recognition/comprehension impairment), I might try to circumvent the patient's comprehension impairment by showing him drawings of the three stimulus items, asking him to remember them, and subsequently testing him with an array of pictures.

Response to Question 2-3: That the patient's symptoms are localized to one side of the body (hemianesthesia) suggests central nervous system pathology. The sudden onset of symptoms and their presence on awakening suggest an acute event such as stroke as the cause of the symptoms. However, the absence of other signs of central nervous system pathology (e.g., motor impairments; speech, language, or cognitive impairments; visuospatial impairments) makes a central nervous system etiology implausible. If a central nervous system source for the patient's symptoms is eliminated, then pathology affecting the peripheral nervous system becomes a candidate. However, peripheral neuropathy rarely, if ever, creates symptoms that affect all of one side of the body, leaving the other side asymptomatic. A typical pattern for peripheral neuropathy is for symptoms to appear distally (in hands and feet) and progress proximally (toward the trunk) because the longest fibers tend to be the first ones affected by peripheral neuropathy. Most peripheral neuropathies develop slowly, over days and weeks, rather than abruptly, as in this case. Finally, the patient's failure to report vibration when bony structures near the midline, but on the left, are stimulated seems unusual, because if sensitivity to vibration on the right side were intact, the patient should sense vibratory stimulation on the left side of the midline via bone conduction to sensory receptors on the right side. This patient's symptoms do not match patterns that would be expected, based on the structure of the nervous system. The probability that their source is functional rather than organic seems high.

Response to Question 2-4: Patients with loss of sensation and position sense and patients with vestibular abnormalities typically are more stable when standing with eyes open than when standing with eyes closed because they use visual information to compensate for the lack of positional information from the legs or the vestibular system. When these patients close their eyes they lose this compensatory information and their unsteadiness increases, usually dramatically (a phenomenon called *Romberg's sign*). Patients with cerebellar ataxia are as unsteady with eyes open as with eyes closed because their unsteadiness arises from inability to maintain constant levels of muscle tension and inability to quickly adjust muscle tension to subtle changes in posture—impairments that are not alleviated by the presence of visual feedback.

Response to Question 2-5: Fred's symptoms are consistent with widespread impairment of peripheral nervous system motor and sensory functions. The rapid development of Fred's symptoms and his otherwise good health make it unlikely that his symptoms are related to vascular disturbance or slowly progressive diseases such as multiple sclerosis. The widespread involvement of peripheral motor and sensory functions rule out focal disturbances such as might be generated by stroke or head injury. That Fred's friend is apparently well rules out the Mexican food as the source of Fred's symptoms. The most likely culprits appear to be the oysters that Fred consumed, and the physician quickly focused on that likelihood because he knew that shellfish sometimes become toxic to humans during the summer months. This happens because the shellfish consume several varieties of plankton that contain toxic chemicals. The shellfish create antitoxins, which in humans disrupt the chemistry of motor and sensory neurons, causing generalized weakness and sensory loss that, unchecked, may lead to respiratory failure and death.

In Fred's case, the physician induced vomiting and hospitalized him overnight. Fred's symptoms gradually resolved and he was discharged the next morning, still slightly weak but otherwise healthy and with a marked aversion to oysters.

CHAPTER THREE

Response to Question 3-1: *What I would do next:* I would say, "I'm pleased to meet you, Mrs. Olson. I'll come back another time and we can talk again," or something to that effect, and leave. I would see little to be gained by more attempts to get her to respond. I then would talk with the patient's nurse to find out if this is a typical behavior pattern and to find out if there are times of the day in which the patient is more alert and

responsive. When the patient's medical record becomes available I would review it. I would look in progress notes for evidence of Mrs. Olson's alertness, responsiveness, and orientation. I would read the physician's report of Mrs. Olson's medical history, signs, and symptoms, and I would look through the doctor's orders to see if Mrs. Olson is on any medications that might explain her lethargy and somnolence.

I would put a note such as the following in the Progress Notes: "I saw Mrs. Olson at bedside this day. She opened her eyes and attended when touched, but did not respond to my verbal requests. Assessment of speech, language, and cognition awaits her improved alertness and responsiveness. I will see her at bedside daily to monitor her progress and will schedule more extensive testing when her alertness and responsiveness permit." I would cross-reference it with an entry in the Doctor's Orders, such as: "See speech pathology preliminary report in Progress Notes."

Potential reasons for Mrs. Olson's unresponsiveness: (1) Mrs. Olson is only 1 day into recovery from a probable right-hemisphere stroke. She may be experiencing general effects of brain injury (e.g., brain swelling, reduction in cerebral blood flow, diaschisis) that diminish her responsiveness and alertness. Such general effects often are present in the first few days following moderate to severe brain injury from strokes. (2) Mrs. Olson may be depressed. Sometimes patients are so traumatized by their personal catastrophe that they withdraw behaviorally and emotionally. (3) Mrs. Olson may be receiving medications that depress her level of responsiveness and alertness (not highly probable because physicians do not routinely prescribe sedative or tranquilizing drugs for patients who are in the early post-onset phase of stroke recovery).

Response to Question 3-2: The only situation in which a brain-injured adult's performance (or anyone else's) on a small number of test items is likely to be as accurate as their performance on a large number is when a patient's responses are extremely homogeneous, such as when all responses are correct or when all responses are errors. When responses are extremely homogenous the results of testing will be equivalent, regardless of the number of items in the test. As performance becomes less homogeneous, the accuracy with which a small number of test items represents the brain-injured adult's true performance level usually declines.

An exception might be when a patient's performance is very symmetric across time. What symmetry means in this context is that a patient who misses 20% of test items always misses every 5th item, and a patient who misses 50% of test items always misses every 2nd item. Under these conditions, one would need five items in a test to specify the true performance of a patient who misses 20% of test items and would need only two items to specify the true performance of a patient who misses 50% of test items.

A brain-injured adult's performance, however, never is this orderly. For most, performance fluctuates unpredictably across test items. A patient who misses 25% of test items may miss the first two questions, get the next eight right, miss one, get seven right, miss two, and so on. For this reason, brain-injured adults' performances rarely match their overall error percentage in any small block of items and may approximate their true performance levels only over relatively large blocks of items (10 or more).

Some brain-injured adults have difficulty "tuning in" to new tasks in a test situation. Their responses to initial test items are inaccurate, delayed, and/or distorted but improve as the test continues, provided that the characteristics of test stimuli and the response requirements do not change. If brain-injured adults with "tuning-in" problems are tested with only a few items, their average performance is worse than it would be if more items were administered. Someone who did not get "tuned in" until the 6th item would produce only error scores if tested with a 5-item test, but would get 50% correct if tested with a 10-item test. (Presumably the last 5 items would all be correct. In practice, usually there is more gradual

improvement in performance from initial test items to later ones.)

Other brain-injured adults seem to develop "noise buildup" or "fatigue" across test items. Their responses to initial test items are prompt and accurate, but as the test progresses their performance deteriorates. These persons' performances look better on a short test than on a long one because the test ends before the noise buildup or fatigue sets in.

It is important to understand that when a brain-injured adult's test performance is affected by processing abnormalities such as tuning-in problems or noise buildup, the test may not be a valid measure of whatever it is the test is designed to measure. Suppose a clinician were to administer a 20-item written spelling test to a brain-injured patient with a tuning-in problem. (The words in the test are approximately equal in frequency of occurrence and spelling difficulty.) The patient misses the first 4 items, gets the next item correct, misses the next 2, and gets the remaining 13 correct. The patient's overall score is 70% correct. Has the clinician tested the patient's knowledge of how to spell the tested words? Probably not, because the patient's performance looks suspiciously like a tuning-in problem. The clinician could test this hypothesis by retesting with the same words in inverted order, putting the first words last and the last words first. If a tuning-in problem were responsible for the patient's performance, the patient will miss items that he previously spelled correctly and will spell correctly items that he had previously missed.

The point is that the test performance of a brain-injured adult often represents some combination of impaired component skills and general information-processing abnormalities, behavioral tendencies, or both. It is important to separate these influences to ensure that a brain-injured adult's test performance represents competence in the skill targeted by the test (e.g., spelling, arithmetic, sentence comprehension) and not the character of the brain-injured adult's information processing or behavioral tendencies. (Lezak's comments in this chapter on *testing the limits* relate to this issue.)

Response to Question 3-3: The test contains 10 items, which ordinarily would be sufficient for a screening test, provided the items were homogeneous. Unfortunately for potential users of this test, these items are not homogeneous. Frequency of occurrence varies widely across test items, from *the* (frequency approximately 1 per 15 words) to *perambulator* (frequency less than 1 per 1 million words). Part of speech also varies across test items. There are 3 nouns, 2 pronouns, 1 verb, 2 adjectives, 1 adverb, and 1 article in the test. Phonologic complexity also varies across test items, from multisyllabic phonologically complex words (perambulator, umbrella, seventy-two) to single-syllable words. The level of abstractness also varies across test items, from concrete words that can be visualized (cat, umbrella) to abstract words that can't be visualized (its, slowly). All of these variables have been shown to affect brain-injured adults' performances in various language tests; consequently, heterogeneity among test items on these variables is likely to lead to differences in performance among patients who are sensitive to different variables. Patients with phonologic encoding problems or patients with speech motor programming problems will miss phonologically complex items. Patients who are sensitive to word frequency effects will miss low-frequency items. Patients who have problems with "little words" in English will miss articles and perhaps pronouns and adverbs. Patients who have difficulty with abstract material will miss more abstract words.

Response to Question 3-4: Mr. Chambers appears to be an impulsive responder. He interrupts the clinician and unnecessarily repeats what the clinician says. His inappropriate verbalizations disrupt the flow of the session and may compromise Mr. Chambers's performance in the task—he talks when he should be listening and so is likely to misunderstand, misinterpret, or flat-out miss what the clinician says.

Some potential reasons for Mr. Chambers's behavior include: (1) He is anxious and threatened by the test situation. He reacts by verbalizing excessively. (2) He is trying to compensate for impaired comprehension and retention by "jumping the gun" when he feels that he's losing the sense of what the clinician is saying. (3) Mr. Chambers's impulsive responding is caused by his brain injury. (4) Mr. Chambers was an impulsive responder before his injury, and what we see here is simply a continuation (or exaggeration) of his pre-injury personality. (5) Some combination of (1) through (4).

What to do next? I'd try telling Mr. Chambers "wait until I'm finished before you say anything," reminding him if necessary as the session progressed. If that didn't work, I'd interject a nonverbal cue to indicate when he should respond—hold up my hand, palm out as I give an instruction or command, and point to him when it's time for him to respond. If that didn't work, I'd end the task, engage Mr. Chambers in a short interval of social conversation to get him relaxed and settled, then try the task again, incorporating gestural cues to signal him when to respond. If that didn't work, I'd switch to a task that I knew would be very easy for him and use that task to train him to respond at the appropriate time and without excessive verbalizations. When I had an appropriate response pattern firmly established, I'd go back to the original task, expecting that the new response pattern would generalize to that task.

CHAPTER FOUR

Response to Question 4-1: The absence of paralysis suggests that the primary motor cortex in the left and right hemispheres is not affected by neuropathology, nor are descending corticospinal tract fibers. (This is an unusual phenomenon—hemiparesis or hemiplegia almost always accompanies limb apraxia.) Neuropathology causing unilateral limb apraxia almost always is a sign of damage in the anterior corpus callosum, which interrupts fiber tracts that connect the premotor cortex in the language-competent hemisphere with the motor cortex in the non-language-competent hemisphere. For right-handers this means that fibers crossing from the left hemisphere premotor cortex to the right hemisphere motor cortex have been affected. As a result, the left hand (controlled by the motor cortex in the right hemisphere) does not have access either to the motor plans set up by the left hemisphere or to the sense of the spoken commands used to test for limb apraxia. Consequently, if a right-hander exhibits unilateral limb apraxia, the left hand will be the apraxic hand. The most reasonable explanation for unilateral apraxia of the right hand and arm is that the patient is right-hemisphere dominant for language (left-handed).

Response to Question 4-2: It is possible, but highly unlikely. Right-handed patients who exhibit alexia without agraphia almost always have right homonymous hemianopia because of destruction of the left-hemisphere visual cortex. (Destruction of visual pathways from the right-hemisphere visual cortex isolates the language areas in the left hemisphere from the remaining visual cortex, creating the alexia.) Alexia without agraphia in the absence of hemianopia would, I believe, require two lesions—one that cuts the crossing fibers in the posterior corpus callosum and another that undercuts the language region (Wernicke's area) in the left temporal lobe so as to cut its connections to the left-hemisphere visual cortex without either destroying the visual cortex or extending deep enough into the temporal lobe to impinge on the optic radiations going back to the visual cortex. Pathology in the posterior corpus callosum implicates the posterior cerebral artery. Pathology near Wernicke's area in the left temporal lobe implicates the posterior branch of the middle cerebral artery. It would be unusual to see simultaneous strokes in both locations. It also would be unusual to see a patient with a lesion undercutting Wernicke's area who is not aphasic because undercutting Wernicke's area should have the same effect as destroying Wernicke's area.

Response to Question 4-3: *Transcortical motor aphasia:* Hemiparesis—leg greater than arm—because of involvement of upper regions of motor cortex. Anterior disconnection syndrome because the patient may have difficulty verbalizing about objects palpated out of sight with the hand contralateral to the language-dominant hemisphere. Limb apraxia, perhaps unilateral, because of damage in the anterior corpus callosum. Behavioral inertia—lack of responsiveness—because of frontal lobe damage. *Transcortical sensory aphasia:* Contralateral somatosensory impairment because of involvement of the parietal sensory cortex. Astereognosis because of involvement of parietal sensory association cortex. Visual field blindness (most likely a contralateral inferior field deficit) because of involvement of the upper optic radiations. Diminished awareness of impairments, which frequently is seen in patients with posterior brain injury.

Response to Question 4-4: Mr. Johnson's stroke (posterior branch, LMCA) implicates temporal and temporo-parietal regions of his left brain hemisphere. Ms. Redmond's stroke (posterior watershed region, LMCA) implicates parietal and parieto-occipital regions of her left brain hemisphere. Because both patients' strokes were posterior to the central fissure I would expect them to exhibit fluent aphasia syndromes. I would expect Mr. Johnson to exhibit aphasia that is consistent with a diagnosis of Wernicke's aphasia (fluent speech, poor repetition, poor comprehension, verbal paraphasias, and perhaps some literal paraphasias). I would expect Ms. Redmond to exhibit impairments consistent with a diagnosis of transcortical sensory aphasia (fluent speech, poor comprehension, good repetition).

Because both are in the immediate post-stroke period, I would expect that the focal signs (aphasia) might be complicated by the diffuse immediate effects of brain injury. However, I would expect some differences in the nature of these effects because of the location of each patient's brain injury and because of potential differences in severity. I would expect that the diffuse effects of Ms. Redmond's injury may be less severe than the diffuse effects of Mr. Johnson's injury because watershed occlusions, being localized primarily in the brain cortex, tend to produce less brain swelling and other immediate physiologic effects than occlusions nearer the origin of an artery, which tend to involve deep penetrating arteries as well as those in and near the cortex.

I also would expect to see differences in the nature of the diffuse symptoms generated by Mr. Johnson's and Ms. Redmond's injuries. Because Ms. Redmond's injury is high in the parietal lobe I would expect some diminished tactile sensation in her right hand, but would not expect weakness or visual field impairments. Because Mr. Johnson's injury is in the temporal or temporo-parietal region, I would not be surprised by contralateral loss of vision in part or all of his right-side visual field (which would mean that the damage extended deep enough into the temporal or temporo-parietal regions to damage the optic radiations). If the damage were confined to the cortex and immediate subcortex but extended back into the visual association areas, I might expect Mr. Johnson to complain of nonspecific visual impairment, but wouldn't be surprised if subsequent testing revealed no "hard" evidence of visual field blindness or diminished visual acuity. However, I would expect moderate to severe reading impairment from damage in the left-hemisphere visual association area. I would not expect either patient to be hemiplegic, although Mr. Johnson might have some weakness in his right hand and arm, but probably not his leg, caused by the diffuse effects of his stroke.

Because there are likely to be less severe diffuse effects of brain injury with watershed injuries, I might expect Ms. Redmond's "spontaneous" neurologic recovery (attributable to resolution of these effects) to be less than Mr. Johnson's. However, in terms of these patients' chronic levels of impairment, Ms. Redmond's prognosis is more favorable because watershed injuries tend to do less damage than injuries nearer the center of an artery's distribution. I would expect the symptoms related to the diffuse effects of brain injury to largely disappear within the first week or two for Ms. Redmond, whereas they might persist (although gradually resolving) for a month or so for Mr. Johnson. Ms. Redmond may have another slight advantage in terms of prognosis because she is 12 years younger than Mr. Johnson, and younger brains tend to heal better than older brains.

CHAPTER FIVE

Response to Question 5-1: The disparate sign is Mr. Portofino's poor reading comprehension. Ordinarily we would expect a patient with Broca's aphasia to have reasonably good auditory comprehension, and reading comprehension also should be relatively well preserved. (Poor oral reading would be expected, reflecting the patient's problems with motor aspects of speech production.) I can think of two reasons for Mr. Portofino's poor reading comprehension. The most likely reason is that the patient's comprehension of printed material was poor before his stroke occurred. A less likely reason is the presence of two lesions, one in the posterior inferior frontal lobe, which created the Broca's aphasia and the hemiplegia, and another in the posterior temporal lobe, which disrupted (but did not completely destroy) communication between the visual cortices and Wernicke's area. (This was perhaps a previous small temporal-lobe stroke that Mr. Portofino did not notice because he didn't do much reading or that he chose to ignore.) However, I would expect at least some partial right-side visual field blindness from a temporal-lobe stroke in such a location. The most likely explanation is poor reading skills before the stroke. (A clinician probably would know of a patient's poor reading skills in advance. Clinicians routinely gather information about a patient's previous reading, writing, spelling, and arithmetic skills before formal assessment begins by asking such questions as, "How far did you go in school?" "How did you do in school?" "Were you a good speller?" "Were you good at arithmetic?" "Did you do much reading before your stroke?")

Response to Question 5-2: Ms. Aldeberan's pattern of performance suggests a visual perceptual problem—errors tend to be visual. Ms. Aldeberan appears to do better on longer words, perhaps because longer words provide more context. Also, the words *tomorrow, mother,* and *newspaper,* which she reads correctly, are not words with visually similar alternatives that might lead the patient with visual-perceptual problems astray. I would expect an aphasic patient to make more semantic errors than visual errors in an oral reading task such as the one in this example—*home* for *house, today* for *tomorrow, father* for *mother,* and so on. So Ms. Aldeberan's performance is somewhat unusual for an aphasic person. Be that as it may, visual errors such as those committed by Ms. Aldeberan implicate the posterior regions of the brain (visual cortex, visual associations areas, connecting pathways), so I would expect her to exhibit a fluent aphasia. It probably is not Wernicke's aphasia because of the absence of semantic reading errors. It is more likely to be mild (anomic) aphasia.

Response to Question 5-3: Ms. Smith's performance on Part F is better than her performance on Part E. Most aphasic persons do better on Part E than on Part F. How to explain Ms. Smith's "unusual" performance? A fatigue or tuning-out problem can't explain it because we would expect fatigue and tuning out to affect Part F more than Part E. An attentional problem also doesn't fit with Ms. Smith's performance because we wouldn't expect fluctuations in attention to coincide so neatly with changes in test items. Let's look at the commands in Parts E and F to see what characteristics change between Part E and Part F. The commands in Part E are syntactically simpler than those in Part F, but that should lead to poorer performance in Part F on Ms. Smith's part. The commands in Part E are longer than most of the commands in Part F. Hmm! Perhaps we're seeing the results of a retention-span problem for Ms. Smith. That possibility seems strengthened by Ms. Smith's performance in Part F—her errors occur on the longer commands, and she tends to miss the final elements in the commands. She also misses preponderantly final items in Parts D and E, which fits our hypothesis. But why doesn't she miss only the final ele-

ments in the commands in Part E? Perhaps overloading Ms. Smith's retention span generated interference that affected earlier parts of the commands. I'd go with a retention-span explanation for Ms. Smith's performance. I might do some follow-up testing to test the hypothesis in more detail. (It's not all that unusual to see patients who do better on Part F of the *Token Test* than on Part E. And it's usually a retention-span problem.)

Response to Question 5-4: *Mrs. Bloom:* Mrs. Bloom probably is aphasic. The evidence is several verbal paraphasias—*cat* for *dog, sitter* for *sofa, cleaned* for *messed, rug* for *floor.*

Some other fairly typical aphasic speech responses: false starts perhaps indicating word-retrieval failure ("the mother is gonna . . . trying to get him out of there" and "those ones there. . . . children . . . boys and girls"), indefinite words without referents ("got into it," "he's hiding," "those ones there"), and incomplete sentences ("the rest of the birthday cake").

The presence of verbal paraphasias and fluent speech suggests Wernicke's aphasia. Mrs. Bloom's major speech deviations are inaccurate and slightly off-the-mark words, suggestive of word-retrieval failure. The other deviations probably are close enough to normal not to be a problem for Mrs. Bloom in daily life interactions. However, her speech deviations are likely to prove annoying to Mrs. Bloom and to her listeners.

Mr. Jones: Mr. Jones's slow speech rate and telegraphic speech are definite indicators of Broca's aphasia. Mr. Jones's major speech deviations are extremely low speech rate, long pauses, the presence of nonword filler, use of the word *and* as a filler and continuant, and telegraphic speech, with utterances averaging about three words in length. He probably can communicate reasonably well in daily life, although with greatly reduced efficiency. His slow speech rate may cause listeners to become impatient and may compromise Mr. Jones's daily life communicative competence.

Response to Question 5-5: The absence of telegraphic writing, the presence of function words, and the overall good syntax of this sample suggest that the patient is not experiencing Broca's aphasia. The absence of semantic paraphasias, the absence of indications of word-retrieval failures, and the overall cohesion and coherence of the sample suggest that the patient is not experiencing Wernicke's aphasia. The patient's spelling errors do not fit what one would expect from a patient with conduction aphasia—we don't see letter substitutions and transpositions of syllables (phonemic paraphasias). We also can eliminate other categories of aphasia based on the nature of the patient's spelling errors, which do not resemble those likely to be made by individuals with aphasia. The patient's spelling errors primarily affect high-frequency words and words whose spelling matches their pronunciation *(is, sink, the, son, back, get, water)*. Although the patient misspells such "easy" words, he spells correctly many less common ("hard") words whose spellings do not match their pronunciation *(although, soaking, young, daughter, reaching, raised)*. The patient also irregularizes a regularly spelled word *(knot* for *not)*. I'd say this sample represents some sort of functional problem—for example, hysteria, psychopathology, or malingering.

CHAPTER SIX

Response to Question 6-1: Strict *peaks* or *valleys* approaches to selecting treatment tasks risk violating three principles that I believe are important to effective treatment of adults with communicative impairments.

- Treatment tasks should be difficult enough to challenge the patient but not so difficult that they overwhelm the patient.
- Treatment should be directed toward mental processes that account for a patient's performance in a task or in a collection of tasks.
- Treatment should target skills that will enhance the patient's daily life communicative competence.

Task Difficulty. When a patient's peak performances represent minimal impairments, treating the peaks may create treatment tasks in which

the patient is not challenged, leading the clinician to treat where no treatment is needed—focusing on impairments so slight as to have minimal effects on the patient's daily life communicative competence. If I were to use a *treat the peaks* approach, I would have to establish upper performance limits for each task beyond which I would not select a task for treatment. These limits might be related either to "normal" performance (for example, the 80th percentile for normal adults) or to the performance of a normative group of brain-injured patients (for example, the 90th percentile for aphasic adults).

When the *valleys* in a patient's test performance represent tasks in which a patient's performance is severely impaired, selecting treatment tasks to represent the valleys will lead to treatment tasks in which error responses predominate, leading to deteriorating performance in which errors generate more errors, lack of progress, and high levels of patient frustration. The exception might be a patient whose overall performance represents normality or mild impairment, with a few valleys that represent moderate impairment. For these patients, treating the valleys may lead to treatment with tasks that challenge but do not overwhelm them.

Treating Underlying Processes. Both *peaks* and *valleys* approaches run the risk of enticing clinicians to *train to the test*—that is, to select treatment tasks that mimic the tests that led to selection of the treatment tasks. Suppose a patient's peak on a test battery was a confrontation-naming subtest. A clinician who followed a strict *treat the peaks* approach might focus treatment on confrontation-naming drills, without considering the relevance of naming to the patient's communicative needs and without considering whether training naming addresses any underlying cognitive processes. Both *peaks* and *valleys* approaches may lead a clinician into a fragmented approach to treatment because a clinician may select treatment tasks based only on their relative level of difficulty for the patient, with no consideration of how the patient's test-to-test pattern of performance may point to impairments in mental processes that underlie performance on several tests.

Enhancing Patients' Daily Life Competence. Strict use of a *treat the peaks* or *treat the valleys* approach fails to take into account the daily life importance of performances sampled by the tests used to select treatment activities and fails to consider the needs and wishes of individual patients and their caregivers.

Response to Question 6-2: I would reply as follows:

- Surface similarity between treatment tasks and daily life communicative interactions is no guarantee of generalization from clinic treatment to a patient's daily life environment.

- Forcing treatment activities to mimic daily life communicative interactions may lead to inefficiency and limit the effectiveness of treatment by directing treatment away from mental processes that may support a wide range of daily life communicative skills.

- The effectiveness of treatment is not indicated by how closely treatment activities resemble actual daily life communicative interactions but by outcome measures that document the degree to which a patient's daily life communication changes concurrent with treatment.

I would suggest to the administrator that the focus of the directive be on measuring outcome using measures that predict daily life communicative competence, rather than on the form of treatment activities.

Response to Question 6-3: Clearly the clinician's repeated attempts to instruct the patient in the task are not succeeding. Perhaps the patient doesn't comprehend the clinician's instructions. Perhaps the patient is perseverating. Perhaps the patient doesn't understand the concept of "opposite." The signs of trouble are there early in the interaction, and the clinician should have heeded them and taken a different tack. After the second failure (when the patient responds "white as snow") I would simplify the task. I might make up some cards on which I

print a stimulus word on one line and print an antonym and two or three foils on another line. I might underline the antonym on some of the cards and use those cards to demonstrate the task—I'd say the stimulus word, then point to the underlined antonym, saying something like "and this word means the opposite of ——." Then I'd try a few trials in which I said a stimulus word and had the patient point to the underlined antonym. Then I'd try a few trials in which I used cards on which the antonym was not underlined. If the patient could do this task, I would eliminate the printed stimulus word and have the patient choose antonyms from my spoken word by pointing to the appropriate word on the card. The point is, when instructions fail, I'd try simplifying the task and use demonstration plus instruction to train the task.

It seems to me that there is a larger issue present here. I'd question the appropriateness of this task to this patient. If the patient's comprehension impairment is so severe that he or she cannot understand the instructions for the task (which seems likely), I don't see the relevance to the patient's needs of drilling the patient to produce antonyms. With this patient I'd probably be working on comprehension, not on producing antonyms.

I'm also puzzled regarding the clinician's purpose in working on antonym production. Working on an arcane skill such as producing antonyms suggests that the clinician's intent is to reorganize the patient's semantic representations or to stimulate or revitalize the patient's semantic processing skills. However, the patient's responses suggest that the patient's semantic representations and semantic processes are in reasonably good condition—the phrases the patient produces are normal semantic associations. I would focus treatment on other issues. If the patient's problem is with understanding the concept of *opposite* and I felt it important to teach that concept—which I think unlikely—I'd teach it nonverbally, rather than with antonyms.

Response to Question 6-4: Several aspects of this interaction deserve comment. The clinician persists with a confrontation-naming drill in the face of four consecutive unacceptable responses by the patient. (That the responses are *unacceptable* is clear from the clinician's feedback. The patient's responses are not necessarily *wrong*.) There seem to me two potential reasons for the patient's failures at confrontation naming in this series: (1) The patient may not understand the task, although this seems unlikely because the patient gives semantically related words on each trial or (2) the patient cannot retrieve and say the target words but gets semantically related words instead. This seems likely to me.

I would question why the clinician insists on an exact match between stimuli and the patient's responses because it seems likely that producing semantically related words when retrieval goes awry might permit the patient to communicate reasonably well in daily life, where such substitutions might work quite well to get the patient's meaning across to listeners. I would also wish to evaluate the patient's word-retrieval in connected speech—sometimes patients who have word-retrieval problems in confrontation-naming drills do considerably better in connected speech.

I don't put much faith in confrontation-naming drills as an effective treatment procedure. I'd probably choose to treat word retrieval with more naturalistic materials. I might have the patient provide missing words in sentences or in short samples of narrative discourse in which semantic and syntactic constraints limit the number of reasonable choices for missing words. I might use story retelling as a treatment procedure because I would expect that having heard the words in the story might enhance the patient's word retrieval in the retellings.

I also see several procedural faults in this clinician's treatment of the patient's unacceptable responses. The clinician does not acknowledge that the patient's responses are semantically related to the target responses. He or she should. The clinician deviates from the purpose of the drill (word retrieval) and strays into word repe-

tition when the patient does not respond appropriately. (The clinician's task is not to *correct* but to *stimulate*.) I would not ask the patient to repeat my production of word names after the patient fails to produce them on confrontation. That's not the point of the drill, and repetition is unlikely to have any effect on the patient's word retrieval. I might try providing some cues (e.g., the first sound or a rhyming word) to see what kinds of cues facilitated the patient's performance. I certainly would not permit a string of five consecutive unacceptable responses without intervening (e.g., explaining, cueing, changing the stimulus or response requirements). The clinician and the patient are getting nowhere in this sample. It's the clinician's fault, and it's the clinician's responsibility to do something to get the treatment session on track.

CHAPTER SEVEN

Response to Question 7-1: I would guess that Mr. Murphy's poor performance on yes-no questions relates to problems in producing understandable yes-no responses. Perhaps he is severely apraxic and does not have the motor skills to produce *yes* and *no*. I would know if this were likely by his performance on other tests of speech production. However, even if Mr. Murphy were severely apraxic, I would expect him to be able to indicate *yes* and *no* by gestures (head nods, head shakes, hand gestures such as thumbs up or thumbs down). In my experience few apraxic patients are so severely apraxic that they cannot indicate *yes* and *no* by some gestural means. Perhaps Mr. Murphy confuses *yes* and *no*. I would know if this were likely by his test performance—whether he indicated dissatisfaction with his responses to yes-no questions by gestures, body language, or facial expressions. It's not uncommon for aphasic patients to confuse *yes* and *no*, but when they do, they usually signal their confusion by indicating, "I know the answer, but I can't tell whether to say *yes* or *no*."

If Mr. Murphy does not have reliable yes-no responses, I would see two possibilities in treatment: (1) Work around the problem. Use materials that do not require yes-no responses. (2) Find a way to give Mr. Murphy reliable yes-no responses. The first alternative, I think, would not be practical from Mr. Murphy's point of view because he will need dependable yes-no responses in many daily life situations. Therefore, I would be inclined to find a way for Mr. Murphy to answer yes-no questions reliably. I'd try training him with a simple task in which the *yes* and *no* responses were very obvious. (For instance, I would show him cards on which pairs of simple geometric symbols were printed. If the symbols in a pair were the same, the appropriate response would be *yes,* and if they were not the same, the appropriate response would be *no.*) I'd start with natural responses—the words *yes* and *no* if Mr. Murphy could produce them, and head nods and head shakes if he could not. If those responses didn't work, I'd try a less natural response (e.g., thumbs up and thumbs down). If that failed, I'd put two cards on the table, on one of which was printed a smiling face and on the other of which was printed a frowning face, and I'd train Mr. Murphy to point to the smiling face to indicate *yes* and to point to the frowning face to indicate *no.*

I'd train Mr. Murphy to use whatever response we chose by starting with strings of consecutive *yes* and *no* trials—say, five trials on which *yes* is appropriate, followed by five trials on which *no* was appropriate, and so on—for several iterations until Mr. Murphy was consistently responding appropriately and changing from *yes* to *no* and vice versa when the sequence changed. Then I'd gradually decrease the length of strings of consecutive *yeses* and *nos* and gradually introduce randomness into the sequences. If I got Mr. Murphy to 100% accuracy with unpredictable sequences of *yes* and *no* trials using a less natural response such as pointing to symbols or thumbs up and thumbs down, I might try to substitute a more natural response (e.g., head nod and head shake or perhaps spoken *yes* and *no*).

Response to Question 7-2: The positive side of Ms. Snyder's response to the "cookie theft" pic-

ture is that she gets the overall theme of the situation and chooses words that relate to that theme. The negatives are (1) severe agrammatism, (2) mispronunciation of content words, and (3) many false starts, filler words, and interjections. Fortunately her mispronunciations are close enough to their targets to make most words intelligible in context. For the time being, I would not work on articulatory accuracy because listeners should be able to decode her off-target productions if given some contextual support, such as knowing the topic of Ms. Snyder's speech. I'd begin by targeting her false starts and filler words and interjections—put her in a structured task such as picture description, instruct her regarding what the objective is (elimination of false starts and filler), have her talk, and signal her when she inserts a false start or a filler. If signaling alone were not effective, I might slow her speaking rate and have her be certain to have a word clearly in mind before she begins an utterance. When she can speak in the structured task with little or no filler, I gradually would loosen the structure—perhaps move on to story retelling or telling about personal experiences—under conditions like those used in the first task. When Ms. Snyder could talk in a variety of contexts without inserting false starts and filler, I then might focus on producing more information by providing more content words and perhaps working on communicating relationships among them, either by a few well-chosen function words or by intonation and gesture. I wouldn't attack Ms. Snyder's agrammatism directly until I felt that she had achieved maximum benefit from treatment that targeted other aspects of her speech. Then I might try training her in the use of a selected list of function words, especially prepositions. (I would not be surprised if her use of function words spontaneously increased as we eliminated filler and false starts and began working on generating more content words and establishing relationships among them.)

Response to Question 7-3: Mrs. Bloom's major speech deviations are slightly off-the-mark words, suggestive of word-retrieval failure. If I were to treat Mrs. Bloom's connected speech, it seems to me that word-retrieval drills may be the most appropriate avenue. I might work on decreasing Mrs. Bloom's production of completely inaccurate words and try to get her to produce words that are "in the ballpark." That way, she will communicate well, although all her words aren't precisely what a "normal" speaker would produce. I might try training Mrs. Bloom to recognize when her words are inaccurate, rather than approximations, and teach her to repair inaccurate words by replacing them with words that approximates what Mrs. Bloom intends. I might train her to "talk around" words that she can't come up with and for which she can't find a word that approximates the word she needs. I'd focus on maximizing Mrs. Bloom's communicative adequacy. I wouldn't worry about whether the words she produces are precisely the ones needed, as long as they are close enough that listeners can follow what she is attempting to communicate.

Mr. Jones's major speech deviations are extremely low speech rate, the presence of many "filler" words, telegraphic speech, and short utterances. The first question I'd ask is whether Mr. Jones is likely to communicate adequately in daily life interactions with his present speech patterns. The answer, I think, is "yes" in terms of communicating essential information. However, his slow speech rate and telegraphic speech in combination are likely to prove burdensome to listeners and are likely to be a source of ongoing frustration to Mr. Jones. Consequently, I might try (first) to increase his speech rate and then see if I can do anything to make his speech less telegraphic. (I'd tackle speech rate first because it probably would be easier to modify than his telegraphic speech, and increasing his speech rate would likely strongly affect listeners' sense of effort as they listened to him.) Because his slow rate is likely the result of motor programming problems, I'd start him off with articulation drills, in which he produced sequences of controlled articulatory complexity, first at a slow rate and then with gradually increasing speech rate. As he got better, I'd increase the articulatory complexity of the materials, dropping speech rate back each time I increased articulatory complexity. I'd try to get him up to a minimum of about 100 words per minute, which I think would make his speech rate pretty tolerable for most listeners. I also might try some work on improving Mr. Jones's syntax by training him to produce more connecting words. However, I've not had much luck with doing this in the past, and I wouldn't expect much success here. I'd still try some trial treatment with this focus. Who knows? I might get lucky.

I also might experiment with decreasing Mr. Jones's use of filler words, but if eliminating fillers simply led to long pauses where the filler words had been, I'd probably back off because Mr. Jones's speech probably would seem more natural with filler words than with an equivalent number of long silent pauses.

Response to Question 7-4: I'd target Mr. Osborne's comprehension of function words. I would stay away from drills with lists of function words—I wouldn't expect such drills to improve his reading comprehension or do much beyond making Mr. Osborne frustrated. Instead I'd use printed cloze exercises to accomplish my objectives. I'd use printed texts in which function words are replaced with blanks. Mr. Osborne's assignment would be to fill in the missing words. I'd begin with simple texts with a small number of function words deleted, and I'd provide Mr. Osborne with a list of the words needed to complete each exercise, plus a few foils as in the following.

> Harry Davis was ____ a hurry. His business meeting in San Diego had lasted ____ hour longer _____ planned and Harry was worried _____ he would miss his flight back ____ Omaha. He stood on the curb ____ front of the hotel. His suitcase was _____ the sidewalk beside him. ____ was raining lightly. He waved frantically _____ the taxicabs as ____ rushed by.

Word list plus foils:

than when that because it by he on out
his to over of an in they beside at

I gradually would add to the list of function words, increase the length and complexity of the cloze texts, and make the choices of which words went into the blanks less obvious. To measure generalization (which I would expect) I periodically would test Mr. Osborne's reading comprehension using passages that Mr. Osborne had not seen previously in which passage comprehension depended on function words.

CHAPTER EIGHT

Response to Question 8-1: Fred's experience strongly indicates cerebral hemorrhage affecting his right hemisphere as the cause of his signs and symptoms. Intense physical exertion is a common precursor to hemorrhagic strokes because physical exertion increases blood pressure, thereby increasing the risk of rupturing a weakened arterial wall. Severe headache is a common early sign of cerebral hemorrhage but is much less common following occlusive stroke. It's hard to predict location, beyond right versus left side, although I'd lean toward surface, rather than deep, based on the presence of exaggerated reflexes, neglect, and hemianopia, which point toward cortical or immediately subcortical involvement. I'd also expect greater effects from an intracerebral hemorrhage—loss of consciousness and vomiting—because of compromised mid-brain functions. Fred's hemorrhage clearly is not in the brain stem. If it were, Fred would be hemiplegic rather than hemiparetic; he probably would be unconscious; and his respiration, heart rate, and other vital functions likely would be affected. I'd expect the physician to order an emergency computed tomography (CT) scan to verify what has happened and to pinpoint the location of the trouble.

That Fred remained conscious and made it to the emergency room and apparently made it through the physician's examination without a worsening of symptoms suggests that the bleeding in Fred's brain has stopped, so the immediate threat of death or progression into coma seems relatively low. However, the next few days will be critical and careful management will be required to stabilize Fred's physiologic condition and get him on the way to recovery.

Assuming that Fred had a cerebral hemorrhage, that the bleeding has stopped, and that surgical intervention (e.g., clipping of an aneurysm) is not needed, I'd guess that Fred might not show a great deal of improvement in the first few weeks but that eventually (anywhere from 2 to 6 weeks) the rate of his recovery may accelerate—a common pattern for hemorrhagic strokes. Fred is a young man. He probably doesn't have generalized vascular disease. Consequently, his brain should be relatively resilient. If he survives the next week or so without another incident, I'd expect very good recovery as the hematoma is resorbed, brain swelling diminishes, and undamaged nerve fiber tracts resume functioning. I'd guess that he might be left with some residual left-sided weakness, but I wouldn't expect his hemianopia or neglect (or other right-hemisphere signs) to persist. I'd expect Fred's recovery to be significantly better than the recovery of a patient with a right-hemisphere occlusive stroke, who is likely to be older with a compromised vascular system and perhaps have other medical problems. A patient with an occlusive stroke may begin the recovery process sooner than Fred, but Fred's eventual level of recovery almost certainly will be better.

Response to Question 8-2: I would expect Ms. Snyder to tend to miss the leftmost stimuli in an array, regardless of the position of the array relative to the midline of the visual space. I would expect the effects of position relative to the midline and position in an array to interact, so that the leftmost items in an array in left hemispace would be most often missed and that the rightmost items in right hemispace would be missed least frequently. In the following diagram, I have indicated the probability that Ms.

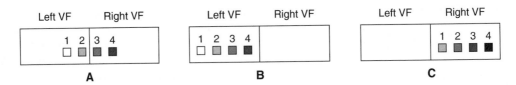

A   B   C

Snyder would identify a square by the density of its shading—the darkest squares are those that I would expect her to report most consistently.

Ms. Snyder is likely to miss squares 1 and 2 in *A* because squares 3 and 4 capture her attention. She is likely to see squares 3 and 4 in *B,* although they are to the left of the midline because there is nothing in right hemispace to capture her attention. However, squares 3 and 4 in *B* might capture her attention, leading her to miss squares 1 and 2, with 1 more likely to be missed than 2. I would expect Ms. Snyder to inconsistently miss squares 1 and 2 in C *(ipsilesional neglect)* for the same reasons, but, because the entire array is in right hemispace, identification of leftward squares should be better than for the array in *B*.

I would guess that many neglect patients might change their performance if given a large number of trials with these three arrays because they eventually would learn that there are always four squares present on each trial. Knowing that, they might verbally cue themselves to find all four and perhaps even count each square as they identified it. If they ended up with less than four squares on a trial, they would know that additional search is necessary, which might lead them to scan visual space (including the left side) more carefully. They also might learn that if they saw nothing, then all the squares must be to the left of where they were looking, which might also lead them to look leftward. If a patient failed to learn such strategies over a large block of trials, I'd worry about the patient's overall cognitive flexibility and adaptability.

Response to Question 8-3: Ms. Glindon seems alert and cooperative but also seems to deny and minimize her impairments. She comprehends and remembers what she has been told

about the reasons for her hospitalization, but what she says suggests that she does not believe what she has been told and that she is unaware of, or refuses to admit, the physical (and perhaps cognitive) effects of her apparent stroke.

I would expect Ms. Glindon to cooperate during testing but perhaps not to try very hard, causing her test performance to underestimate her true potential. Still, I'd do an hour or so of testing to establish baseline performance, track potential recovery, and make preliminary decisions about treatment. I wouldn't expect treatment to be very effective until she gains greater awareness of her impairments and becomes motivated to work on them. I'd probably not put her in a treatment program right away but do some screening testing every 3 or 4 days to track her performance.

Ms. Glindon is only 3 days post-onset of her stroke. It is possible that her awareness of her impairments may increase as she recovers. If she remains in the hospital, I'd do a daily bedside screening to see if her awareness of her impairments improves. If it did, I might schedule a few 30-minute trial treatment sessions to evaluate her response to treatment. If she's discharged from the hospital soon, I would recommend that she return in a few weeks for re-evaluation. If her denial resolved, it would simplify treatment. If her denial were not to resolve, I'd probably spend a few sessions working on it. If I made progress, I'd move into a full-fledged treatment program. If not, I'd probably discharge her, but I might recommend re-evaluation in another 4 weeks, if she's willing.

Response to Question 8-4: First, I would examine Mr. Blanding's medical records and talk with his physician and other patient-care personnel to get a general sense of his impairments, his apparent cognitive and emotional state, and his on-the-ward behavior and how they have changed since onset. Then I'd interview the patient and whatever family members are available. My objectives would be to get a sense of how the patient and family members feel about Mr. Blanding's situation, their concerns, and their understanding of Mr. Blanding's impairments and to get an impression of how Mr. Blanding and family members interact. I'd also answer questions and provide some general information about what happened to Mr. Blanding and what potential outcomes might be. (Estimated time: 30 minutes.)

I'd try to select tests that had the most potential for indicating (1) whether Mr. Blanding needs treatment and (2) whether he would be likely to profit from it. For (1) I'd try to test general processes that are likely to indicate the level of Mr. Blanding's communicative handicaps in daily life and that are likely to be important in a variety of communicative and cognitive activities. For (2) I'd observe Mr. Blanding in testing to evaluate his attention, retention of instructions and ability to stay on task, interpersonal behaviors, and whether he carries over learning from one task to another. I'd also be looking for signs of perceptual impairments such as neglect and visuospatial impairment. I wouldn't administer a general test battery such as CADL, an aphasia test, or a right-hemisphere test battery (which, according to the instructions, is not available anyway). Instead, I would opt for short tests that specifically target abilities that I would be interested in. To get started, I'd plan to administer tests of the following abilities:

- *Attention.* I'd test sustained, selective, and alternating attention. I wouldn't test divided attention at this time. Divided-attention tasks demand high levels of attention and mental flexibility, and I wouldn't be concerned about it so soon after Mr. Blanding's injury. (Estimated time: 30 minutes.)
- *Memory.* I'd evaluate immediate memory with digit-span and word-list tests of immediate recall. I'd also administer the *Rivermead Behavioral Memory Test* to get a sense of Mr.

Blanding's ability to handle quasi-real-life situations requiring memory for different kinds of material. (Estimated time: 30 minutes.)
- *Abstraction, inferences.* I'd administer several short tests to assess Mr. Blanding's ability to get beyond literal meanings and to make inferences.
  - Two stories and questions from the *Discourse Comprehension Test* (DCT). I'd want to know if Mr. Blanding remembers main ideas better than details (which would mean that he is sensitive to relationships among story elements) and whether his performance on implied information is dramatically worse than his performance on stated information. (If I had time, I might retest him with the DCT questions after giving several unrelated tests to assess his long-term retention of such material.)
  - Five multiple-choice items testing appreciation of idioms and metaphor.
  - Two or three common proverbs, which Mr. Blanding is asked to interpret.
  (Estimated time: 30 minutes.)
- *Judgment, reasoning, and problem-solving*
  - To assess judgment, I'd administer five items such as "Suppose you are sitting in a movie theater and you smell smoke. What would you do?"
  - To assess reasoning, I'd administer five items such as "What would happen if all speed limits on roads and highways were removed?"
  - To assess problem-solving I'd administer five items such as "You get up in the morning and discover that your bedroom light does not come on when you flip the switch. What would you do to find out why?"
  (Estimated time: 20 minutes.)
- *Neglect and visuospatial abilities.* I'd administer the following tests:
  - Line bisection, clock drawing, and scene drawing to assess neglect in drawing tasks
  - Reading aloud compound-words, sentences, and short texts (full-page and two column)

—Copying three-dimensional figures and a few multiple-choice spatial-relations test items

(Estimated time: 20 minutes.)

• *Follow-up and exploration.* In-depth exploration of significant impairments indicated by previous testing to specify their nature and severity. (Estimated time: 30 minutes.)

• *Patient and family feedback and instruction.* An interview with the patient and family members to summarize what I found in my evaluation, make recommendations, and answer questions. (Estimated time: 30 minutes.)

I would not test for some "typical" right-hemisphere-syndrome impairments—prosopagnosia, geographic disorientation, reduplicative paramnesia, anosagnosia—because I don't believe they would address the whether-or-not-to-treat question. I also wouldn't do a formal pragmatics assessment. I'd get a sense of the patient's pragmatics from observing him in testing and interviews and watching him interact with family members. I'd get a sense of whether he denies or minimizes impairments in my interactions with him during testing and the interview.

Response to Question 8-5: Although neither individual should be permitted to drive, a driver with left neglect might be slightly safer driving in England. Many accidents in both countries are associated with turns across oncoming traffic (left turns in the United States and right turns in England). In England oncoming traffic is on the right and in the United States oncoming traffic is on the left. Consequently, a driver with left neglect might be better at making turns across traffic in England than in the United States because in England oncoming traffic would be in the driver's non-neglected visual space.

Many accidents in both countries also are associated with failure to obey traffic control signs (especially stop signs). In England traffic control signs usually are on the left-hand side of the roadway, and in the United States traffic control signs usually are on the right-hand side. Consequently, a driver with neglect would be in greater danger of failing to obey traffic control signs in England

than in the United States because in England the signs are likely to be in left hemispace.

Passing another vehicle on a two-lane roadway would seem less risky for a driver with left neglect in England than in the United States because in England drivers pass on the right and oncoming traffic is on the right, whereas the situation is reversed in the United States. Consequently, drivers with left neglect in England would be more likely than drivers with left neglect in the United States to see oncoming traffic before passing. However, in England the passed vehicle is on the left, whereas in the United States the passed vehicle is on the right. Therefore drivers with left neglect in England might be more likely to sideswipe or cut off the passed vehicle than would drivers in the United States. Cross-traffic would present risks for drivers with left neglect in either country—vehicles coming from the left would be problematic both in England and the United States.

How about risks to pedestrians? In England a pedestrian stepping off the curb into oncoming traffic is to the left of an approaching driver. In the United States a pedestrian stepping off the curb into oncoming traffic is to the right of an approaching driver. Therefore pedestrians stepping off a curb in England would be in greater danger from a driver with left neglect than would pedestrians in the United States. (However, pedestrians who make it to the middle of the roadway and are crossing more traffic would be in greater danger in the United States.)

Drivers with left neglect in England might be more likely to run off the roadway and strike signs, lamp posts, and so forth because they would not see them, whereas drivers with left neglect in the United States might be more likely to cross into opposing traffic, with more serious consequences. However, if drivers with neglect were attracted by non-neglected hemispace, as sometimes happens, the situation would be reversed because they would tend to drift into non-neglected hemispace.

Finally, drivers with neglect in England would be more likely to use seat belts than drivers in the United States because in England the seat belt is on the right prior to use, but in the United States it is on the left. Most vehicle-pedestrian accidents happen when pedestrians step off the curb. Therefore, *pedestrians* with left neglect might be safer in England than in the United States. Do you see why?

CHAPTER NINE

Response to Question 9-1: Mary's case is a classic scenario for subdural hemorrhage. Subdural hemorrhages sometimes occur after relatively minor blows to the head, caused by tearing of the fragile blood vessels that traverse the space between the arachnoid and the dura mater. Mary's symptoms did not develop immediately but began to appear only when the bleeding into the subdural space began to create increased intracranial pressure. Initial headache followed by nausea and vomiting are classic indicators of increasing intracranial pressure. Neck stiffness is also a common complaint of patients with elevated intracranial pressure and usually is an ominous sign. That Mary took aspirin for her headache may have contributed to her worsening condition because aspirin, having anticoagulant properties, may exacerbate bleeding. Mary's husband should get her to a medical facility post-haste.

Subdural hemorrhage, and not epidural hemorrhage or subarachnoid hemorrhage, is the most likely explanation for Mary's symptoms. Epidural hemorrhages are caused by tearing or rupture of blood vessels on the surface of the dura mater. They usually require severe blows to the head because the dura mater is not easily torn. Epidural hemorrhages are most common when the skull is fractured, causing tearing of the dura mater and its blood vessels. Subarachnoid hemorrhages usually are caused by ruptured aneurysms and not by blows to the head. However, the exact cause of Mary's symptoms can be determined only by a careful neurologic examination together with comprehensive laboratory tests (especially spinal tap) and brain imaging tests (especially computer-

ized tomography or magnetic resonance imaging scans). Why might the neurologist order a spinal tap in Mary's case?

Response to Question 9-2: Jerry's head injury clearly would be translational trauma—linear acceleration because he was moving in a straight line when he hit the side of the truck. Because he was wearing a helmet his head injury will be much less severe than if he were not wearing one. However, no helmet can protect its user against acceleration injuries when the head is moving rapidly through space and strikes an unyielding surface. The major benefit of a helmet in such a scenario is to protect against skull fracture and penetrating injuries—something for which the hard shell of a helmet is well designed. Helmets are less adept at protecting against acceleration injuries. The polyfoam liner compresses to cushion the impact of a blow (either from an object hitting the helmet or the helmet hitting an object), but the compression is not sufficient to protect the brain against acceleration injury when the head is moving rapidly through space when it strikes an object. In Jerry's case, we could expect coup (occipital) and perhaps contrecoup (frontal) damage. The amount of contrecoup damage would depend in part on what Jerry's helmeted head hit. If it hit the center of the door, which is primarily sheet metal with no reinforcing frame behind it, the sheet metal might collapse inward, slowing the rate at which Jerry's head decelerated and (perhaps) lessening the amount by which Jerry's head rebounds off the door. If Jerry's head hit the door at a reinforcing (and unyielding) frame member, Jerry's head would stop precipitously and the amount of rebound would be increased, increasing the severity of both coup and contrecoup injuries. (Contrecoup injuries are most likely when the head rebounds from the impact and subsequently snaps back in the direction of the original path.) If Jerry were fortunate enough to hit the truck side window with his helmeted head, he might have even less severe head injuries. However, he then might fracture his neck or spine, depending on where his back hit the frame around the window. In addition to his head injuries, Jerry is likely to incur fractures of limbs, ribs, and, as noted, perhaps neck or spine. Neck or spine fractures are, of course, very dangerous because of the probability of subsequent paralysis or, in the case of neck fractures, the possibility of damaging vital brain stem structures that regulate respiration and other autonomic processes. Without a helmet, Jerry would incur severe, and probably fatal, head injuries.

Response to Question 9-3: If I have 1 hour available, I would plan a half hour for medical record review and for talking with ward personnel about the patient. In the medical record I would, of course, review the patient's history to get a sense of what happened to him in the accident and also to get a sense of his previous life—Had he incurred previous head injuries? Does he have a history of substance abuse? Is there evidence of aggressiveness, antisocial behavior, or other signs of problems with personality in his social history? (This information would be important both for anticipating how to approach the patient and for speculating about his eventual recovery.) I also would pay close attention to progress notes to get a sense of the depth of the patient's "coma"; how his condition changed as he emerged from coma; and what his behavior, communication, and cognition have been in the last day or so. The progress notes also would point to potential management issues such as hyperactivity, aggressiveness, assaultiveness, or the like. I also would check the physician's orders to see what medications have been prescribed—especially antiseizure medications, sedatives, or tranquilizers, which might affect the patient's responsiveness and attention span.

For the remaining half hour, I would see the patient at bedside. A patient at Rancho Los Amigos Scale level 4 who is 2 days out of coma would be unlikely to be ambulatory. He would be likely to be connected to monitors, feeding tubes, catheters, and such. If he were agitated and assaultive he might be restrained. I wouldn't plan to do any formal testing but would focus on getting a sense of the patient's responsiveness, attention to his environment, and general pattern of behavior (e.g., agitated, lethargic, aggressive). I also would do some probing to find out what kinds of stimuli are most effective in eliciting responses and what kinds of stimuli elicit the most purposeful responses (e.g., orientation to source of stimulation, cessation of agitated behavior, vocalization). I'd spend some time simply talking to the patient without attempting to elicit any specific responses, just to get the patient accustomed to me and the sound of my voice. I'd be making notes of my findings to help me plan what to do on my next visit.

As for prognosis, it seems to me, based on the information given, that the patient's prognosis for recovery is fair to good. He was in a coma for 7 days. The literature suggests that patients who are in coma no longer than a week or so are likely to be left with mild to moderate residual impairments when recovery is complete. My prediction for this patient would be made somewhat rosier by the fact that he seems to be progressing rapidly—in 2 days he has moved from comatose to Rancho Los Amigos Scale level 4. I'd say the prospects for substantial recovery are good. Predicting outcome is a real guessing game at this point, but I'd expect this patient to end up with mild to moderate residual impairments. (Of course, if the patient had a history of substance abuse, previous head injuries, or other negative indicators, I'd no doubt be somewhat more pessimistic.)

Response to Question 9-4: The achievement test results suggest that Ron is functioning at reasonably high levels in most basic skills (arithmetic, general knowledge, reading comprehension for sentences). His spelling and paragraph comprehension scores are well below the level of his other test scores, suggesting that he is having problems in those areas. I'd want to gather some additional information that might reflect Ron's potential for accomplishing the kinds of tasks that would be required at school were he to return. Important skills include:

- Listening comprehension for discourse (e.g., lectures)
- Note-taking skills
- Reading comprehension for college-level texts
- Ability to organize and remember information from spoken discourse and printed texts
- Spelling, grammar, and writing skills
- Test-taking ability

I would begin by administering several standardized achievement tests:

- Spelling (to find out if that has improved since the previous test)
- Reading comprehension—narratives (the *Nelson-Denny Reading Test* or another standardized reading test that includes college-level texts)
- Discourse comprehension (the *Discourse Comprehension Test* to get a sense of Ron's comprehension of stated and implied main ideas and details in a controlled environment)

I would need information about Ron's performance in less-structured environments in which he would be expected to obtain and retain information from spoken discourse (lectures) in which listening and note taking are required. I might have Ron watch videotapes of speeches or lectures and take notes on their content (public television programs might provide a source for such videotapes). To see how Ron performs in less-controlled environments, in which he is surrounded by others who may be moving about, whispering, or engaging in other potentially distracting activities, I might arrange for Ron to sit in on a lecture at a local college or community organization, take notes, and bring them to me for review.

I would need information about Ron's ability to comprehend long and sometimes complex college-level printed texts, organize the information, and take organized notes that reflect the important information from the texts. I might have Ron bring in two or three textbooks from his previous college courses, assign reading passages from them, have Ron take notes, and then bring the notes to me for review. I might find

books related to classes Ron has taken but that Ron has not previously read and have Ron read assigned material, take notes, and bring them to me. I would time Ron in at least some of these activities to get a sense of how quickly he gets them done and to help determine whether slow reading and note-taking might prove problematic for Ron when he returns to school.

I would need to know something about Ron's study and test-taking skills. I might prepare examinations on the content of videotapes Ron has watched and made notes from or on the content of printed materials Ron has read and made notes on. I would include multiple-choice, fill-in-the-blanks, and short essay items in the examinations to see how Ron handles each kind of test item.

I would wish to get a sense of Ron's ability to produce written discourse. I might have him write a two-page to three-page report on a topic of interest to get a sense of his spelling and grammar and to evaluate the coherence and relevance of what he writes. I would time at least some of Ron's written discourse production to estimate whether slow rate might be problematic at school.

That's where I would begin. Depending on Ron's performance, I might do some follow-up evaluation in given areas, but I'd guess that the foregoing information would permit me to make recommendations regarding the appropriateness of Ron's return to school and to suggest strategies for enhancing Ron's performance (e.g., that Ron tape record lectures and listen to them a second time, during which Ron reviews and edits his original lecture notes). Depending on the results of my evaluation, I might suggest training-retraining activities to deal with weaknesses that I felt would compromise Ron's success at school. (This could go on forever. But I will stop here.)

CHAPTER TEN
Response to Question 10-1:

1. *How old is your spouse?* This is a good opening question because it asks for readily recallable information and provides a good lead-in for more probing questions to fol-

low. It also provides information that may contribute to a diagnosis because increasing age increases the probability that a person will have Alzheimer's disease.

2. *What physical impairments or health problems does your spouse have at this time?* This question addresses the probability that the signs of the man's suspected dementia are caused by illness or other health problems.

3. *What medications is your spouse taking?* This question addresses the possibility that the signs of the man's suspected dementia are caused by medications.

4. *What significant events have occurred in your spouse's life recently?* This question addresses the probability that the signs of the man's suspected dementia represent his emotional response to a stressful life event (e.g., death, divorce).

5. *What was the first thing you noticed that made you suspect the presence of dementia?* The spouse's response to this question may provide information helpful to differential diagnosis. If the first signs were related to memory and orientation, then a diagnosis of Alzheimer's dementia becomes more probable. Altered personality and emotion (e.g., apathy, impulsivity, declining interest in social activities) may suggest Pick's disease or depression. Motor impairments may suggest subcortical pathology (e.g., Parkinson's disease, Huntington's disease).

6. *What other things have you noticed that made you suspect the presence of dementia?* The spouse's response to this question may help establish a pattern of behavior or a collection of signs that may point toward a diagnosis.

7. *Did the changes that led you to suspect dementia occur gradually (over weeks or months) or within a few days?* The spouse's response to this question may point to an identifiable precipitant (e.g., stroke, stressful life event, pain, illness) that would be inconsistent with a slowly developing dementia such as Alzheimer's dementia.

8. *Have you noticed changes in your spouse's memory (e.g., misplacing things, forgetting conversations, repeating the same story several times)?* This question addresses memory impairment—the typical first sign of Alzheimer's disease. An affirmative response would increase the likelihood of Alzheimer's disease.

9. *Have you noticed changes in your spouse's personality (e.g., worry, irritability, changes in mood, loss of interest)?* This question addresses changes in personality and mood—typical first signs of Pick's disease (and of some subcortical diseases, but motor impairments ordinarily would be obvious and not the first signs of possible dementing illness).

10. *What else have you noticed that you think may be significant?* I would end my questions with a catchall question that invites the person being interviewed to tell me about things that may have been missed in earlier questions or to add more detail to information provided in response to other questions.

I might ask additional questions to follow up on leads provided by the spouse in responding to the other questions.

Response to Question 10-2:

1. What is your name?
2. Say "please put the groceries in the refrigerator."
3. Tell me the days of the week, beginning with Sunday.
4. Point to the ceiling, then point to the floor, and blink three times.
5. Who was the first U.S. President?
6. How old are you?
7. What day of the week is it?
8. What is your phone number?
9. Who is the current U.S. President?
10. Count backward from 20 to 1.
11. How would your uncle's daughter be related to you?
12. What does "a stitch in time saves nine" mean?

Comments: Saying one's name (1) should be highly practiced and automatic—therefore very easy. Repetition and producing automatized sequences (2, 3) also should be among the easiest tasks because they do not make demands on memory, sustained attention, or mental flexibility. Comprehension and short-term retention (4) should be relatively well preserved. (However, delayed recall would be impaired.) Memory for well-learned factual information (5) often is well preserved. Many patients with moderate Alzheimer's dementia have lost track of their age (6) and most are unaware of the current date and sometimes time of day (7). Few patients with moderate Alzheimer's disease remember their phone number (8) or know the name of the current president (9). (Someone who had the same phone number for many years and used it many times a day for those years might retain it because of previous "overlearning.") Tasks requiring mental flexibility and sustained attention (10, 11, 12) likely would be impossible for a person with moderate Alzheimer's dementia. My ranking of these three items is based on my sense of increasing need for sustained attention and mental flexibility across these three items. I would guess that my ranking of this list would approximate the performance of many persons with moderate Alzheimer's dementia, but I wouldn't be surprised if items moved up or down a few levels for individuals. However, I would be very surprised if items moved from the beginning of my list to the end or from the middle of the list to the beginning or end.

Response to Question 10-3:

1. Mild Wernicke's aphasia or anomic aphasia. Early-stage Alzheimer's dementia. (Verbal paraphasias.)
2. Mid-stage Alzheimer's dementia. Possibly right-hemisphere syndrome, but unlikely. (Not doing the task. Inappropriate responses socially.)
3. Conduction aphasia. (Literal paraphasias.)
4. Right-hemisphere syndrome. (Focuses on discrete and incidental elements on right side of drawing—does not respond to central theme.)
5. Unknown. It could be Alzheimer's. It could be right-hemisphere syndrome (denial). It could be anyone with visual perceptual problems.
6. Broca's aphasia. (Agrammatism, slow speech rate, many pauses.)
7. Moderate to severe Wernicke's aphasia. Middle-stage to late-stage Alzheimer's dementia. Can't differentiate with this small sample. (Neologisms.)
8. Mild Wernicke's aphasia, moderate anomic aphasia, early-stage Alzheimer's dementia. Any of the three might say this. (Many verbal paraphasias, repeated but unsuccessful attempts at self-correction.)

CHAPTER ELEVEN

Response to Question 11-1: *History of atrial fibrillations.* Atrial fibrillations increase the probability of embolic stroke, so I would expect this patient's motor speech disorder to be consistent with occlusion of an artery in the brain. Emboli are most common in the cerebral arteries, so I would expect either apraxia of speech or unilateral upper motor neuron dysarthria (which might resolve over time) or perhaps spastic dysarthria if emboli had affected cerebral arteries in both hemispheres. Cardiac emboli usually do not travel into the small-diameter penetrating arteries that serve the basal ganglia, so I would not expect hypokinetic or hyperkinetic dysarthria. Although cardiac emboli in the vertebral-basilar arterial system are less common than emboli in the cerebral arteries, they do occasionally occur but do not usually travel into the small-diameter arteries supplying the pons and medulla. They do, however, occasionally affect cerebellar arteries, so an ataxic dysarthria is possible.

Participation in boxing. I definitely would expect hypokinetic dysarthria. Repeated minor closed-head injury to the brain commonly causes a parkinsonian syndrome—pugilistic parkinsonism, such as that exhibited by Mohammed Ali.

Family history of chorea. Too obvious—it is definitely hyperkinetic dysarthria. (Unless another medical condition also were present, in which case one might see a mixed dysarthria. For example, a stroke might create spastic-hyperkinetic dysarthria.)

Traumatic brain injury. This is a difficult one because traumatic brain injury can damage many different parts of the brain and nervous system. Translational trauma may cause bleeding and swelling in the brain hemispheres and lead to spastic dysarthria (not unilateral upper motor neuron dysarthria because the bleeding and swelling should affect both hemispheres). Diffuse axonal injury could cause damage in axial regions—basal ganglia, brain stem, and cerebellum—which would cause mixed dysarthria—perhaps ataxic-flaccid or even spastic-flaccid-ataxic. If the accident physically damaged structures at the base of the skull, I would expect flaccid dysarthria, ataxic dysarthria, or a mixed flaccid-ataxic dysarthria as a result of damage to the brain stem and cerebellum. If the patient incurred a neck fracture, respiratory support may be compromised because of damage to descending corticospinal tracts.

History of transient ischemic attacks. Dysarthria associated with a history of transient ischemic attacks suggests that stroke is responsible for the patient's dysarthria. If the patient's transient ischemic attacks had created symptoms of cerebral artery involvement (slurred speech, confusion, comprehension impairment), then I would expect apraxia of speech, unilateral upper motor neuron dysarthria, or spastic dysarthria. If the patient's transient ischemic attacks suggested involvement of the vertebral-basilar arteries (hemianopia, clumsiness, gait disturbances), I would expect flaccid or ataxic dysarthria or a mixed flaccid-ataxic dysarthria because of involvement of the brain stem, cerebellum, or both.

Response to Question 11-2: The patient's complaints strongly suggest the presence of Parkinson's disease. Difficulty getting out of chairs, turning over in bed, and "freezing" during walking, in combination, suggest the presence of muscle rigidity. (Difficulty getting out of chairs and turning over in bed, by themselves, do not necessarily suggest extrapyramidal disease. "Freezing" during walking is a classic parkinsonian sign.) Weak voice and hoarseness are common complaints of patients with parkinsonian syndromes. Stuttering-like repetitions also are common complaints. My diagnosis is *Parkinson's disease* and *hypokinetic dysarthria.*

Response to Question 11-3: Differences in speech errors and speaking behavior between persons with the anterior syndrome and persons with the posterior syndrome suggest problems at different stages of speech formulation and production, which would mandate different approaches to treatment. The speech errors of persons with the anterior syndrome appear to be more *motoric* than *mental.* Persons with the anterior syndrome exhibit high levels of muscular effort as they struggle to force the articulators into the appropriate movement patterns. Their articulatory movements are slow, clumsy, and effortful, and their attempts at self-correction are slow and labored. Persons with the anterior syndrome behave as if they aware of misarticulations while they are in the act of producing them. They sometimes stop in the middle of a syllable or word and attempt to correct an error. Their self-correction efforts tend to focus on a single sound or syllable, suggesting that they know exactly which sounds are in error. They often insert a neutral vowel between syllables and words. These behaviors suggest immediate, on-line awareness of errors.

The speech errors of persons with the posterior syndrome appear to be more *mental* than *motoric.* Persons with the posterior syndrome speak fluently with little evidence of muscular effort. Their attempts at self-correction are fluent and effortless, although not always successful. Persons with the posterior syndrome behave as if they must hear what they have said before they can attempt repairs. Their self-correction behaviors tend not to target specific sounds but typically consist of repeated attempts at a multisyllabic word or phrase with no particular focus on specific sounds. Their shotgun approach to self-correction suggests that they may not appreciate exactly which sounds are in error. Articulatory errors in successive repair attempts often occur at different locations and represent different kinds of errors (e.g., substitutions, transpositions).

The problem for persons with the *anterior syndrome* seems to be that the speech muscles are not following orders—the orders are correct but execution is flawed. The problem for persons with the *posterior syndrome* seems to be that the speech muscles are following orders. The orders, however, are incorrect.

It seems to me that the speech impairments of persons with the anterior syndrome may represent problems organizing and executing speech movements, whereas the speech impairments of persons with the posterior syndrome may represent problems retrieving and/or retaining the phonologic images of words and, perhaps, in getting the neural representations of those images to the premotor cortex for execution. Persons with the anterior syndrome work very hard at getting their articulators to do what they want them to do and are irritated, rather than surprised, by their speech errors. Individuals with the posterior syndrome have no problem getting the words out but are repeatedly surprised by what they say. (Most, however, have a general sense that phonologically complex material is difficult for them. They often precede an attempt at phonologically complex material with comments such as "Oh boy! This will be a tough one!" It is interesting that the comments almost always are fluent, effortless, and phonologically correct.)

It seems to me that treatment procedures such as phonetic placement, phonetic derivation, articulation drills, and reorganization are appropriate when a patient's problems relate to the motoric aspects of speech (the anterior syndrome) but are not appropriate for persons with the posterior syndrome, whose problems relate to phonologic retrieval, retention, or encoding. I agree in general with those who assert that the speech characteristics of "posterior apraxia of speech" may be appropriately called *literal paraphasia* and that they represent problems in phonologic retention, retrieval, and transmission, rather than a motoric impairment. It seems to me that "posterior apraxia of speech" is a part of the syndrome of *conduction aphasia*. For such patients I would work on their aphasia in addition to their speech production. I would work on *auditory comprehension* (which almost always is impaired in conduction aphasia) and perhaps on word retrieval. I might include *repetition drills* in which patients had to delay their responses to words and phrases to build up their short-term retention of phonologic information. I might include *oral reading* drills in which I had a patient underline words they thought might be difficult and then help them devise strategies to produce them. If a patient showed indications of limited retention span (and many patients with conduction aphasia do) I might do some work on *short-term retention* of digits or word lists—especially word lists containing phonologically complex words.

Response to Question 11-4: I doubt that Darley, Aronson, and Brown ever published a formal definition for *islands of error-free speech.* In their writings they use descriptors such as *fluent* and *well articulated.* Although they have not, as far as I know, defined what they meant by *fluent,* contemporary usage at the time used *fluency* to refer to the prosodic characteristics of speech—*rate, timing, intonation,* and *emphatic stress.* My guess is that Darley, Aronson, and Brown had these characteristics in mind when they used the word *fluent.*

Substituting *normal rate, timing, intonation,* and *emphatic stress* for *fluent* yields a more specific label—*islands of well-articulated speech with normal rate, timing, intonation, and emphatic stress.* The new label does a fairly good job of differentiating apraxia of speech from the dysarthrias, except for hyperkinetic dysarthria because some individuals with hyperkinetic dysarthria may speak fluently and without articulatory errors between incidents of involuntary movement. Some individuals with ataxic dysarthria may have intervals of relatively well-articulated speech but with abnormal intonation and emphatic stress patterns, making the *islands* label inappropriate for their speech patterns. Individuals representing other dysarthria types (spastic, flaccid, hypokinetic) typically do not experience intervals of well-articulated speech or intervals of speech with normal intonation and stress patterns, making the *islands* label clearly not appropriate for their speech patterns.

My definition of *islands of error-free speech* is: *intervals during which speech is correctly articulated and spoken with normal rate and in which timing, intonation, and stress patterns are normal*. This definition doesn't separate the phenomenon seen in apraxia of speech from the intervals of error-free speech experienced by some individuals with hyperkinetic dysarthria, but that's not much of an issue because the movement disorders experienced by individuals with hyperkinetic dysarthria clearly identify them as not having apraxia of speech.

Response to Question 11-5: The patient's normal neurologic examination and the absence of weakness in oral, pharyngeal, and laryngeal muscles and normal range of movement in those muscles rule out pathology in upper or lower motor neurons. The patient's normal articulation and resonance also suggest that upper and lower motor neurons are functioning adequately. The absence of gait disturbance, dysmetria, and scanning speech and the patient's normal articulation argue against cerebellar pathology. This leaves the extrapyramidal system as a potential location for neuropathology. The patient's speech abnormality does not represent either classic hypokinetic dysarthria or classic hyperkinetic dysarthria. The patient's runaway *voice loudness* resembles, in some respects, Parkinson's disease patients' runaway *speech rate*. Patients with Parkinson's disease often speak at a normal rate as they begin to talk, but their rate increases as they continue speaking until they are speaking extremely rapidly—so rapidly that their articulators can no longer keep up and their articulation becomes blurred and indistinct. This patient, it seems to me, exhibits a similar phenomenon, except that vocal loudness, rather than speech rate, gets out of control. I would guess that this patient had damage or neurochemical abnormalities in his basal ganglia, perhaps related to his exposure to toxic chemicals in the pesticides he handled during his work.

Another alternative might be that this patient's speech abnormality is psychogenic, but this explanation appears less likely. This patient's speech abnormality doesn't fit what one typically sees in psychogenic voice disorders, which tend to show up as aphonia and hoarseness. This patient's speech abnormality developed gradually. Psychogenic disorders tend to develop rapidly, over hours to a few days, and often in response to a present or an anticipated life stress.

I might suggest that the neurologist try a trial regimen of treatment with an antiparkinsonian medication to see if medication eliminated the patient's abnormal voice. If the patient's symptoms were controlled by the medication, it would support a diagnosis of extrapyramidal system pathology. (However, it still would be possible that the effects of the medications represented placebo effects. That possibility could be eliminated only by a placebo phase before treatment with antiparkinsonian medications.)

Bibliography

Adamovich, B. (1990, June). *A comparison of FIM evaluations by nurses and speech pathologists.* Paper presented at the Clinical Aphasiology Conference, Santa Fe, NM.

Adamovich, B. B., & Brooks, R. A. (1981). A diagnostic protocol to assess the communication deficits of patients with right hemisphere damage. In R. H. Brookshire (Ed.), *Clinical Aphasiology Conference proceedings* (pp. 244-253). Minneapolis, MN: BRK Publishers.

Adamovich, B. B., & Henderson, J. (1992). *Scales of cognitive ability for traumatic brain injury.* Chicago: Riverside.

Adams, J. H., Graham, D. I., Scott, G., & associates. (1980). Brain damage in fatal non-missile head injury. *Journal of Clinical Pathology, 33,* 1132-1145.

Adams, M. J., & Collins, A. (1979). A schema-theoretic view of reading. In R. O. Freedle (Ed.), *New directions in discourse processing.* Norwood, NJ: Ablex.

Adams, R. D., & Victor, M. (1981). *Principles of neurology* (2nd ed.). New York: McGraw-Hill.

Agranowitz, A., Boone, D., Ruff, M., & associates. (1954). Group therapy as a method of retraining aphasics. *Quarterly Journal of Speech, 40,* 170-182.

Albert, M. L. (1973). A simple test of visual neglect. *Neurology, 23,* 658-664.

Albert, M. L., Feldman, R., & Willis, A. (1974). The subcortical dementia of progressive supranuclear palsy. *Journal of Neurology, Neurosurgery, and Psychiatry, 37,* 121-130.

Albert, M. L., Goodglass, H., Helm, N. A., & associates. (1981). *Clinical aspects of dysphasia.* New York: Springer-Verlag.

Alexander, M. P., & Lo Verme, S. R. (1980). Aphasia after left hemisphere intracerebral hemorrhage. *Neurology, 30,* 193-202.

Alexander, M. P., Naeser, M. A., & Palumbo, C. (1987). Correlations of subcortical CT lesion sites and aphasia profiles. *Brain, 110,* 961-991.

Alfano, D. P. (1994). Recovery of function following brain injury. In M. A. J. Finlayson & S. H. Garner (Eds.), *Brain injury rehabilitation: Clinical considerations* (pp. 34-56). Baltimore: Williams & Wilkins.

Allen-Burge, R., Stevens, A. B., & Burgio, L. D. (1999). Effective behavioral intervention for decreasing dementia-related challenging behavior in nursing homes. *International Journal of Geriatric Psychology, 14,* 213-228.

American Psychiatric Association. (1994). *Diagnostic and statistical manual of mental disorders* (Rev. 4th ed.). Washington DC: American Psychiatric Association.

American Speech-Language-Hearing Association. (1994). *Functional assessment of communication skills for adults: Project update.* Bethesda, MD: American Speech-Language-Hearing Association.

Aminoff, M. J., Greenberg, D. A., & Simon, R. P. (1996). *Clinical neurology* (3rd ed.). Stamford, CT: Appleton & Lange.

Andrews, P. J. D., Piper, I. R., Dearden, N. M., & associates. (1990). Secondary insults during intrahosptial transport of head injured patients. *Lancet, 1,* 327-330.

Annegers, J. F., Grabow, J. D., Kurland, L. T., & associates. (1980). The incidence, causes, and secular trends of head trauma in Olmsted County, Minnesota. *Neurology, 30,* 912-919.

Ansell, B. J., & Keenan, J. E. (1989). The Western neurosensory stimulation profile: A tool for assessing slow-to-recover head-injured patients. *Archives of Physical Medicine and Rehabilitation, 70,* 104-108.

Appell, J., Kertesz, A., & Fishman, M. (1982). A study of language functioning in Alzheimer patients. *Brain and Language, 17,* 73-81.

Arguin, M., & Bub, D. (1993). Modulation of the directional attention deficit in visual neglect by hemispatial factors. *Brain and Cognition, 22,* 148-160.

Armus, S. R., Brookshire, R. H., & Nicholas, L. E. (1989). Aphasic and non-brain-damaged adults' knowledge of scripts for common situations. *Brain and Language, 36,* 518-528.

Aronson, M., Shatin, L., & Cook, J. C. (1956). Sociopsychotherapeutic approach to the treatment of aphasic patients. *Journal of Speech and Hearing Disorders, 21,* 352-364.

Arthur, G. (1947). *A point scale of intelligence tests.* New York: The Psychological Corporation.

Aten, J., Caliguiri, M., & Holland, A. (1982). The efficacy of functional communication therapy for chronic aphasic patients. *Journal of Speech and Hearing Disorders, 47,* 93-96.

Aten, J. L., & Lyon, J. (1978). Measures of PICA subtest variance: A preliminary assessment of their value as predictors of language recovery in aphasia. In R. H. Brookshire (Ed.), *Clinical Aphasiology Conference proceedings* (pp. 106-116). Minneapolis, MN: BRK Publishers.

Backus, O., & Dunn, H. (1952). The use of a group structure in speech therapy. *Journal of Speech and Hearing Disorders, 17,* 116-122.

Baddeley, A., Harris, J., Sunderland, A., & associates. (1987). Closed head injury and memory. In H. S. Levin, J. Grafman, & H. M. Eisenberg (Eds.), *Neurobehavioral recovery from head injury* (pp. 295-317). New York: Oxford University Press.

Baddeley, A. D. (1986). *Working memory.* London: Oxford University Press.

Barber, J. B., & Webster, J. C. (1974). Head injuries: A review of 150 cases. *Journal of the National Medical Association, 66,* 201-204.

Barco, D. P., Crossen, B., Bolesta, M. M., & associates. (1991). Training awareness and compensation in postacute head injury rehabilitation. In J. S. Kreutzer & P. H. Wehman (Eds.), *Cognitive rehabilitation for persons with traumatic brain injury: A functional approach* (pp. 129-146). Baltimore: Paul H. Brookes.

Barlow, D. H., & Herson, M. (1984). *Single-case experimental designs: Strategies for studying behavior change* (2nd ed.). New York: Pergamon Press.

Barton, M., Maruszewski, M., & Urrea, D. (1969). Variation of stimulus context and its effect on word finding ability in aphasics. *Cortex, 5,* 351-365.

Basso, A., Capitani, E., & Vignolo, L. A. (1979). Influence of rehabilitation on language skills in aphasic patients: A controlled study. *Archives of Neurology, 36,* 190-196.

Basso, A., Lecours, A. R., Morashini, S., & associates. (1985). Anatomo-clinical correlations of the aphasias as defined through computerized tomography: Exceptions. *Brain and Language, 26,* 201-229.

Bayles, K. A. (1994). Management of neurogenic communication disorders associated with dementia. In R. Chapey (Ed.), *Language intervention strategies in adult aphasia* (3rd ed., pp. 535-545). Baltimore: Williams & Wilkins.

Bayles, K. A., Boone, D. R., Tomoeda, C. K., & associates. (1989). Differentiating Alzheimer's patients from the normal elderly and stroke patients with aphasia. *Journal of Speech and Hearing Disorders, 54,* 74-87.

Bayles, K. A., Kaszniak, A. W., & Tomoeda, C. (1987). *Communication and cognition in normal aging and dementia.* Boston: College-Hill.

Bayles, K. A., & Tomoeda, C. (1991). *Arizona battery for communication disorders of dementia* (Research ed.). Tucson, AZ: Canyonlands Publishing.

Benson, D. F. (1979a). *Aphasia, alexia, and agraphia.* New York: Churchill-Livingstone.

Benson, D. F. (1979b). Aphasia. In K. M. Heilman & E. Valenstein (Eds.) *Clinical neuropsychology* (pp. 22-58). New York: Oxford Unversity Press.

Benton, A. L. (1974). *The revised visual retention test* (4th ed.). New York: Psychological Corporation.

Benton, A. L. (1992). *The revised visual retention test* (5th ed.). San Antonio: The Psychological Corporation.

Benton, A. L., Smith, K. C., & Lang, M. (1972). Stimulus characteristics and object naming in aphasic patients. *Journal of Communication Disorders, 5,* 19-24.

Beukelman, D. R., & Yorkston, K. (1977). A communication system for the severely dysarthric speaker with an intact language system. *Journal of Speech and Hearing Disorders, 62,* 265-270.

Bever, T. G., Garrett, M. F., & Hurtig, R. (1973). The interaction of perceptual processes and ambiguous sentences. *Memory and Cognition, 1,* 277-286.

Bisiach, E. (1966). Perceptual factors in the pathogenesis of anomia. *Cortex, 2,* 90-95.

Bisiach, E., Capitani, E., Luzzati, C., & associates. (1981). The brain and conscious representation of reality. *Neuropsychologia, 19,* 545-551.

Blackman, D. K., Hoover, M., & Pinkston, E. M. (1976). Increasing participation in social interactions of the institutionalized elderly. *The Gerontologist, 16,* 69-76.

Blessed, G., Tomlinson, B. E., & Roth, M. (1968). The association between quantitative measures of dementia and senile change in the cerebral gray matter of elderly subjects. *British Journal of Psychiatry, 114,* 791-811.

Blonder, L. X., Bowers, D., & Heilman, K. M. (1991). The role of the right hemisphere in emotional communication. *Brain, 114,* 1115-1127.

Bloom, L. M. (1962). A rationale for group treatment of aphasic patients. *Journal of Speech and Hearing Disorders, 27,* 11-16.

Bloom, R. L., Borod, J. C., Obler, L. K., & associates. (1992). Impact of emotional content on discourse production in patients with unilateral brain damage. *Brain and Language, 42,* 153-164.

Bluestone, C. D., Musgrave, R. H., McWilliams, B. J., & associates. (1968). Teflon injection pharyngoplasty. *Cleft Palate Journal, 5,* 19-26.

Boll, T. J. (1994). Neurologically impaired adults. In F. E. Miltersen & S. M. Turner (Eds.), *Diagnostic interviewing* (2nd ed., pp. 345-372). New York: Plenum.

Bond, M. R. (1976). Assessment of the psychosocial outcome of severe head injury. *Acta Neurochirurgica, 34,* 57-70.

Bonin, G. von. (1962). Anatomical asymmetries of the cerebral hemisphere. In V. B. Mountcastle (Ed.), *Interhemispheric relationships and cerebral dominance* (pp. 122-135). Baltimore, MD: Johns Hopkins Press.

Boning, R. A. (1990). *Specific skill series* (4th ed.). New York: Macmillan/McGraw-Hill.

Borkowski, J. G., Benton, A. L., & Spreen, O. (1967). Word fluency and brain damage. *Neuropsychologia, 5,* 135-140.

Bourgeois, M. S. (1990). Enhancing conversational skills in patients with Alzheimer's disease using a prosthetic memory aid. *Journal of Applied Behavior Analysis, 23,* 31-64.

Bourgeois, M. S. (1991). Communication treatment for adults with dementia. *Journal of Speech Language and Hearing Research, 34,* 831-844.

Bourgeois, M. S. (1992). Evaluating memory wallets in conversations with persons with dementia. *Journal of Speech Language and Hearing Research, 35,* 1344-1357.

Bower, G. H., Black, J. B., & Turner, T. J. (1979). Scripts in memory for texts. *Cognitive Psychology, 11,* 177-220.

Bowers, S. A., & Marshall L. F. (1980). Outcome in 200 consecutive cases of severe head injury treated in San Diego County: A prospective analysis. *Neurosurgery, 6,* 237-242.

Breyden, M. P., & Ley, R. G. (1983). Right hemispheric involvement in imagery. In E. Perecman (Ed.), *Cognitive processing in the right hemisphere* (pp. 111-123). New York: Academic Press.

Brink, T. L., Yesavage, J. A., Lum, O., & associates. (1982). Screening tests for geriatric depression. *Clinical Gerontologist, 1,* 37-44.

Brismar, B., Engstrom, A., & Rydberg, U. (1983). Head injury and intoxication: A diagnostic and therapeutic dilemma. *Acta Chirugica Scandinavia, 149,* 11-14.

Brooks, D. N. (1984). Cognitive deficits after head injury. In D. N. Brooks (Ed.), *Closed head injury: Psychological, social, and family consequences* (pp. 44-73). New York: Oxford University Press.

Brooks, N. (1989). Closed head trauma: Assessing the common cognitive processes. In M. Lezak (Ed.), *Assessment of the behavioral consequences of head trauma* (pp. 61-86). New York: A.R. Liss.

Brookshire, R. H. (1972). Effects of task difficulty on naming performance of aphasic subjects. *Journal of Speech and Hearing Research, 15,* 551-558.

Brookshire, R. H. (1973). Consequences in speech pathology: Incentive and feedback functions. *Journal of Communication Disorders, 6,* 1-5.

Brookshire, R. H. (1975). Effects of prompting on spontaneous naming of pictures by aphasic subjects. *Journal of the Canadian Speech and Hearing Association, Autumn,* 63-71.

Brookshire, R. H. (1976). Effects of task difficulty on sentence comprehension performance of aphasic subjects. *Journal of Communication Disorders, 9,* 167-173.

Brookshire, R. H. (1978). Auditory comprehension and aphasia. In D. F. Johns (Ed.), *Clinical management of neurogenic communicative disorders* (pp. 103-128). Boston: Little, Brown and Company.

Brookshire, R. H., Krueger, K., Nicholas, L., & associates. (1977). Analysis of clinician-patient interactions in aphasia treatment. In R. H. Brookshire (Ed.), *Clinical Aphasiology Conference proceedings* (pp. 181-187). Minneapolis, MN: BRK Publishers.

Brookshire, R. H., & Nicholas, L. E. (1984). Comprehension of directly and indirectly stated main ideas and details in discourse by brain-damaged and non-brain-damaged listeners. *Brain and Language, 21,* 21-36.

Brookshire, R. H., & Nicholas, L. E. (1985). Consistency of the effects of rate of speech on brain-damaged subjects' comprehension of information in narrative discourse. In R. H. Brookshire (Ed.), *Clinical aphasiology: Vol. 15* (pp. 262-271). Minneapolis, MN: BRK Publishers.

Brookshire, R. H., & Nicholas, L. E. (1993). *The discourse comprehension test.* Minneapolis, MN: BRK Publishers.

Brookshire, R. H., & Nicholas, L. E. (1995). Performance deviations in the connected speech of adults with no brain damage and adults with aphasia. *American Journal of Speech-Language Pathology, 4,* 118-123.

Brookshire, R. H., Nicholas, L. E., & Krueger, K. M. (1978). Sampling of speech pathology treatment activities: An evaluation of momentary and interval sampling procedures. *Journal of Speech and Hearing Research, 21,* 652-667.

Brookshire, R., Nicholas, L., Redmond, K., & associates. (1979). Effects of clinician behaviors on acceptability of patients' responses in aphasia treatment sessions. *Journal of Communication Disorders, 12,* 369-384.

Brown, J. I., Fischco, V. V., & Hanna, G. (1993). *The Nelson-Denny reading test.* Chicago: Riverside.

Brown, J. W. (1972). *Aphasia, apraxia, and agnosia: Clinical and theoretical aspects.* Springfield, IL: Charles C. Thomas.

Brownell, H., & Friedman, O. (2001). Discourse ability in patients with unilateral left and right hemisphere brain damage. In R. S. Berndt (Ed.), *Handbook of neuropsychology* (2nd ed., pp. 189-203). New York: Elsevier.

Brownell, H., Griffin, R., Winner, E., & associates. (2000). Cerebral lateralization and theory of mind. In S. Baron-Cohen, G. Tager-Flusberg, & D. J. Cohen (Eds.), *Understanding other minds* (2nd ed., pp. 306-333). New York: Oxford University Press.

Brownell, H., Pincus, D., Blum, D., & associates. (1997). The effects of right-hemisphere brain damage on patients' use of terms of personal reference. *Brain and Language, 57,* 60-79.

Brownell, H., Potter, H. H., Bihrle, A. M., & associates. (1986). Influence of deficits in right-brain-damaged patients. *Brain and Language, 27,* 310-321.

Brownell, H. H. (1988). The neuropsychology of narrative comprehension. *Aphasiology, 2,* 247-250.

Brust, J. C., Shafer, S. Q., Richter, R. W., & associates. (1976). Aphasia in acute stroke. *Stroke, 7,* 167-174.

Bryan, K. L. (1989). *The right hemisphere language battery.* Leicester, GB: Far Communications.

Buckingham, H. W. (1979). Explanation in apraxia with consequences for the concept of apraxia of speech. *Brain and Language, 8,* 202-226.

Buckingham, H. W. (1992). Phonological production deficits in conduction aphasia. In S. E. Kohn (Ed.), *Conduction aphasia* (pp. 76-116). Hillsdale, NJ: Earlbaum.

Busch, C., & Brookshire, R. H. (1982). *Aphasic adults' auditory comprehension of yes-no questions.* Unpublished manuscript.

Butfield, E., & Zangwill, O. L. (1946). Re-education in aphasia: A review of 70 cases. *Journal of Neurology, Neurosurgery and Psychiatry, 9,* 75-79.

Butters, N., Granholm, E., Salmon, D. P., & associates. (1987). Episodic and semantic memory: A comparison of amnesic and disoriented patients. *Journal of Clinical and Experimental Neuropsychology, 9,* 479-497.

Cancelliere, A. E. B., & Kertesz, A. (1990). Lesion localization in acquired deficits of emotional expression and comprehension. *Brain and Cognition, 13,* 133-147.

Candelise, L., Landi., G., Orazio, E. N., & associates. (1985). Prognostic significance of hyperglycemia in acute stroke. *Archives of Neurology, 42,* 409-426.

Canter, G. J. (1973). *Dysarthria, apraxia of speech, and literal paraphasia: Three distinct varieties of articulatory behaviors in the adult with brain damage.* Paper presented at the annual convention of the American Speech and Hearing Association, Detroit.

Caplan, D. (1987). *Neurolinguistics and linguistic aphasiology.* New York: Cambridge University Press.

Caplan, D., Baker, C., & DeHaut, F. (1985). Syntactic determinants of sentence comprehension in aphasia. *Cognition, 21,* 117-125.

Caplan, L. R. (1988). *Stroke.* CIBA Clinical Symposia, Summit, NJ: CIBA Pharmaceutical Company.

Caplan, L. R. (1993). *Stroke: A clinical approach.* Boston: Butterworth-Heinemann.

Cappa, S. F., Cavalotti, G., Guidotti, M., & associates. (1983). Subcortical aphasia: Two clinical CT-scan correlation studies. *Cortex, 19,* 227-242.

Cappa, S. F., Cavalotti, G., & Vignolo, L. (1981). Phonemic and lexical errors in fluent aphasia: Correlation with lesion site. *Neuropsychologia, 19,* 171-177.

Cappa, S. F., & Vignolo, L. A. (1979). "Transcortical" features of aphasia following left thalamic hemorrhage. *Cortex, 15,* 121-130.

Caramazza, A., & Zurif, E. B. (1976). Dissociation of algorithmic and heuristic processes in language comprehension: Evidence from aphasia. *Brain and Language, 3,* 572-582.

Carlsson, G. S., Svardsudd, K., & Welin, L. (1987). Long term effects of head injuries sustained during life in three male populations. *Journal of Neuropsychology, 67,* 197-205.

Caronna, J., & Levy, D. (1983). Clinical predictors of outcome in ischemic stroke. In H. J. M. Barnett (Ed.), *Neurologic clinics: Cerebrovascular disease* (pp. 103-117). Philadelphia: W.B. Saunders.

Carrow-Woodfolk, E. (1999). *Test for auditory comprehension of language* (3rd ed.). Austin, TX: Pro-Ed.

Cartensen, L. L., & Erickson, R. J. (1986). Enhancing the social environments of elderly nursing home residents: Are high rates of interaction enough? *Journal of Applied Behavior Analysis, 19,* 349-355.

Carver, R. P. (1973). Reading as reasoning: Implications for measurement. In W. H. MacGinitie (Ed.), *Assessment problems in reading* (pp. 173-195). Newark, DE: International Reading Association.

Celesia, G. G., & Wanamaker, W. M. (1972). Psychiatric disturbances in Parkinson's disease. *Diseases of the Nervous System, 33,* 577-583.

Centers for Disease Control and Prevention. (1997). *Traumatic brain injury: Colorado, Missouri, Oklahoma, and Utah, 1990-1993* (MMWR Report #46, pp. 8-11).

Cermak, L. S. (1975). Imagery as an aid to retrieval in alcoholic Korsakoff's patients. *Cortex, 11,* 163-169.

Chall, J. S. (1983). *Stages of reading development.* New York: McGraw-Hill.

Chapey, R. (1994). *Language intervention strategies in adult aphasia* (3rd ed.). Baltimore: Williams & Wilkins.

Cherney, L. R., Halper, A. S., & Miller, T. K. (1991). Treatment of communication problems. In A. S. Halper, L. R. Cherney, & T. K. Miller (Eds.), *Clinical management of communication problems in adults with traumatic brain injury* (pp. 57-131). Gaithersburg, MD: Aspen.

Cicone, M., Wapner, W., & Gardner, H. (1980). Sensitivity to emotional expressions and situations in organic patients. *Brain and Language, 16,* 145-158.

Clarefield, A. M. (1988). The reversible dementia: Do they reverse? *Annals of Internal Medicine, 109,* 472-478.

Clark, H. H., & Haviland, S. E. (1977). Comprehension and the given-new contract. In R. O. Freedle (Ed.), *Discourse comprehension and production* (pp. 1-40). Norwood, NJ: Ablex.

Clarke, L., & Witter, K. (1990). Nature and efficacy of communication management in Alzheimer's disease. In R. Lubinski (Ed.), *Dementia and communication* (pp. 238-256). Philadelphia: B.C. Decker.

Cohn, R., Neumann, M. S., & Wood, N. H. (1977). Prosopagnosia: A clinicopathological study. *Annals of Neurology, 1,* 177-182.

Collins, M. (1991). *Global aphasia.* San Diego: College-Hill Press.

Colsher, P. L., Cooper, W. E., & Graff-Radford, N. (1987). Intonational variability in the speech of right-hemisphere damaged patients. *Brain and Language, 32,* 379-383.

Corbin, M. L. (1951). Group speech therapy for motor aphasia and dysarthria. *Journal of Speech and Hearing Disorders, 16,* 21-34.

Corkin, S. H., Hurt, R. W., Twitchell, T. E., and associates. (1987). Consequences of penetrating and nonpenetrating head injury: Posttraumatic amnesia, and lasting effects on cognition. In H. S. Levin, J. Grafman, & H. M. Eisenberg (Eds.), *Neurobehavioral recovery from head injury* (pp. 318-329). New York: Oxford University Press.

Corlew, M. M., & Nation, J. E. (1975). Characteristics of visual stimuli and naming performance in aphasic adults. *Cortex, 11,* 186-191.

Correia, L., Brookshire, R. H., & Nicholas, L. E. (1990). Aphasic and non-brain-damaged adults' descriptions of aphasia test pictures and gender-biased pictures. *Journal of Speech and Hearing Disorders, 55,* 713-720.

Corsini, R. J., & Renck, R. (1992). *The verbal reasoning test.* Tucson, AZ: NCS Pearson.

Courville, C.B. (1937). *Pathology of the central nervous system.* Mountain View, CA: Pacific.

Coyne, M. L., & Hoskins, L. (1997). Improving eating behaviors in dementia using behavioral strategies. *Clinical Nursing Research, 6,* 275-290.

Craik, F. I., & Lockhart, R. S. (1972). Levels of processing: A framework for memory research. *Journal of Verbal Learning and Verbal Behavior, 11,* 671-684.

Crary, M. A., Haak, M. J., & Malinsky, A. E. (1989). Preliminary psychometric evaluation of an acute aphasia screening protocol. *Aphasiology, 2,* 67-78.

Crary, M. A., & Rothi, L. J. G. (1989). Predicting the Western aphasia battery aphasia quotient. *Journal of Speech and Hearing Disorders, 54,* 163-166.

Croft, C. B., Shprintzen, R. J., & Rakoff, S. J. (1981). Patterns of velopharyngeal valving in normal and cleft palate subjects: A multi-view videofluoroscopic and nasendoscopic study. *Laryngoscope, 91,* 265-271.

Culton, G. L. (1969). Spontaneous recovery from aphasia. *Journal of Speech and Hearing Research, 12,* 825-832.

Cummings, J. L. (1983). Cortical dementias. In D. F. Benson & D. Blumer (Eds.), *Psychiatric aspects of neurologic disease* (pp. 235-247). New York: Grune & Stratton.

Cummings, J. L. (1990). Clinical diagnosis of Alzheimer's disease. In J. L. Cummings & B. L. Miller (Eds.), *Alzheimer's disease: Treatment and long-term management* (pp. 3-20). New York: Dekker.

Cummings, J. L., & Benson, D. F. (1983). *Dementia: A clinical approach.* Boston: Butterworth.

Cummings, J. L., & Benson, D. F. (1984). Subcortical dementia: Review of an emerging concept. *Archives of Neurology, 41,* 874-879.

Cummings, J. L., & Benson, D. F. (1992). *Dementia: A clinical approach* (2nd ed.). Boston: Butterworth-Heinemann.

Dabul, B. (2000). *The apraxia battery for adults* (2nd ed.). Austin, TX: Pro-Ed.

Dabul, B., & Bollier, B. (1976). Therapeutic approaches to apraxia. *Journal of Speech and Hearing Disorders, 41,* 268-276.

Dale, E., & Chall, J. S. (1948). A formula for predicting readability. *Educational Research Bulletin, 27,* 11-20.

Dalston, R., Warren, D. W., & Dalston, E. T. (1990). The modified tongue-anchor technique as a screening test for velopharyngeal inadequacy: A reassessment. *Journal of Speech and Hearing Disorders, 55,* 510.

Damasio, A. R. (1985). Disorders of complex visual processing: Agnosias, achromatopsia, Baliut's syndrome, and related difficulties of orientation and construction. In M. M. Mesulum (Ed.), *Principles of behavioral neurology* (pp. 259-288). Philadelphia: F.A. Davis.

Damasio, A. R., & Damasio, H. (1983). Localization of lesions in achromatopsia and prosopagnosia. In A. Kertesz (Ed.), *Localization in neuropsychology* (pp. 417-428). New York: Academic Press.

Darley, F. L. (1969). *The classification of output disturbance in neurologic communication disorders.* Paper presented at the American Speech and Hearing Association Convention, Chicago.

Darley, F. L. (1982). *Aphasia.* Philadelphia: W.B. Saunders.

Darley, F. L., Aronson, A. E., & Brown, J. R. (1975). *Motor speech disorders.* Philadelphia, W.B. Saunders.

Davis, G. A. (1993). *A survey of adult aphasia and related language disorders* (2nd ed.). Englewood Cliffs, NJ: Prentice-Hall.

Davis, G. A., & Wilcox, M. J. (1985). *Adult aphasia rehabilitation: Language pragmatics.* San Diego, CA: College-Hill.

Deaton, A. V. (1991). Group interventions for cognitive rehabilitation: Increasing the challenges. In J. S. Kreutzer & P. H. Wehman (Eds.), *Cognitive rehabilitation for persons with traumatic brain injury: A functional approach* (pp. 178-190). Baltimore: Paul H. Brookes.

DeKosky, S. T., Heilman, K. M., Bowers, D., & associates. (1980). Recognition and discrimination of emotional faces and pictures. *Brain and Language, 9,* 206-214.

Delis, D. C., Kramer, J., & Kaplan, E. (1988). *California proverb test.* Lexington, MA: Boston Neuropsychological Foundation.

Delis, D. C., Kramer, J. H., Kaplan, E., & associates. (1987). *The California verbal learning test: Adult version.* San Antonio, TX: The Psychological Corporation.

DeRenzi, E., & Ferrari, C. (1978). The reporter's test: A sensitive test to detect expressive disturbances in aphasics. *Cortex, 14,* 279-283.

DeRenzi, E., Pieszuro, A., & Vignolo, L. A. (1966). Oral apraxia and aphasia. *Cortex, 2,* 50-73.

DeRenzi, E., & Vignolo, L. A. (1962). The token test: A sensitive test to detect receptive disturbances in aphasics. *Brain, 85,* 665-678.

Deutsch, S. E. (1981). Oral form identification as a measure of cortical sensory dysfunction in apraxia of speech and aphasia. *Journal of Communication Disorders, 14,* 65-71.

Deutsch, S. E. (1984). Prediction of site of lesion from speech apraxic error patterns. In J. C. Rosenbek, M. R. McNeil, & A. E. Aronson (Eds.), *Apraxia of speech, physiology, acoustics, linguistics, management* (pp. 113-134). San Diego: College-Hill.

Dewitt, L. D., Grek, A. J., Buonanno, F. S., & associates. (1985). MRI and the study of aphasia. *Neurology, 35,* 861-865.

Diggs, C. C., & Basili, A. G. (1987). Verbal expression of right CVA patients. *Brain and Language, 30,* 130-147.

Diller, L., & Weinberg, J. (1977). Differential aspects of attention in brain-damaged persons. *Perceptual and Motor Skills, 35,* 71-81.

Disimoni, F. (1989). *The comprehensive apraxia test.* Dalton, PA: Praxis House Publishers.

Disimoni, F., Keith, R., & Darley, F. (1980). Prediction of PICA overall scores by short versions of the test. *Journal of Speech and Hearing Research, 25,* 511-576.

Disimoni, F., Keith, R., Holt, D., & associates. (1975). Practicality of shortening the PICA. *Journal of Speech and Hearing Research, 18,* 491-497.

Doyle, P., Goldstein, H., & Bourgeois, M. (1987). Experimental analysis of syntax training in Broca's aphasia: A generalization and social validation study. *Journal of Speech and Hearing Disorders, 52,* 143-155.

Duffy, J. R. (1987). Slowly progressive aphasia. In R. H. Brookshire (Ed.), *Clinical aphasiology* (pp. 349-356). Minneapolis, MN: BRK Publishers.

Duffy, J. R. (1995). *Motor speech disorders: Substrates, differential diagnosis, and management.* St. Louis, MO: Mosby.

Duffy, J. R., Keith, R. L., Shane, H., and associates. (1976). Performance of normal (non-brain-injured) adults on the Porch index of communicative ability. In R. H. Brookshire (Ed.), *Clinical Aphasiology Conference proceedings* (pp. 32-42). Minneapolis, MN: BRK Publishers.

Dunlop, J. M., & Marquardt, T. P. (1977). Linguistic and articulatory aspects of single word production in apraxia of speech. *Cortex, 13,* 17-29.

Dunn, L. M., & Dunn, L. M. (1981). *Peabody picture vocabulary test* (Rev. ed.). Circle Pines, MN: American Guidence Service.

Dworkin, J. P., & Johns, D. F. (1980). Management of velopharyngeal incompetence in dysarthria: A review. *Clinical Otolaryngology, 5,* 61-74.

Eastwood, M. R., Lautenschlaeger, E., & Corbin, S. (1983). A comparison of clinical methods for assessing dementia. *Journal of the American Geriatrics Society, 31,* 342-347.

Eisenberg, H. M., & Weiner, R. L. (1987). Input variables: How information from the acute injury can be used to characterize groups of patients for studies of outcome. In H. S. Levin, J. Grafman, & H. M. Eisenberg (Eds.), *Neurobehavioral recovery from head injury* (pp. 13-29). New York: Oxford University Press.

Eisenson, J. (1964). Aphasia: A point of view as to the nature of the disorder and factors that determine prognosis for recovery. *Neurology, 4,* 287-295.

Eisenson, J. (1974). *Examining for aphasia.* New York: The Psychological Corporation.

Elman, R. J. (1999). Introduction to group treatment of neurogenic communication disorders. In R. J. Elman (Ed.), *Group treatment of neurogenic communication disorders: The expert clinician's approach* (pp. 3-7). Boston: Butterworth-Heinemann.

Elman, R. J., & Bernstein-Ellis, E. (1995). What is functional? *American Journal of Speech-Language Pathology, 4,* 115-117.

Elman, R. J., & Bernstein-Ellis, E. (1999). The efficacy of group communication treatment in adults with chronic aphasia. *Journal of Speech, Language, and Hearing Research, 42,* 411-419.

Erlich, J. S., & Sipes, A. L. (1985). Group treatment of communication skills for head trauma patients. *Cognitive Rehabilitation, 3,* 32-37.

Evans, D. A., Funkenstein, H. H., Albert, M. A., & associates. (1989). Prevalence of Alzheimer's disease in a community population of older persons: Higher than previously reported. *Journal of the American Medical Association, 262,* 2552-2556.

Evans, R. W., Palsane, M. N., & Carrere, S. (1987). Type A behavior and occupational stress: A cross-cultural study of blue-collar workers. *Journal of Personality and Social Psychology, 36,* 1213-1220.

Ewert, J., Levin, H. S., Watson, M. C., & associates. (1989). Procedural memory during posttraumatic amnesia in survivors of severe closed head injury. *Archives of Neurology, 46,* 911-916.

Faber, M. M., & Aten, F. L. (1979). Verbal performance in aphasic patients in response to intact and altered pictorial stimuli. In R. H. Brookshire (Ed.), *Clinical Aphasiology Conference proceedings* (pp. 177-186). Minneapolis, MN: BRK Publishers.

Ferro, J. M., Kertesz, A., & Black, S. E. (1987). Subcortical neglect: Quantification, anatomy, and recovery. *Neurology, 37,* 1487-1492.

Filley, C. M., Cranberg, L. D., Alexander, M. P., & associates. (1987). Neurobehavioral outcome after closed head injury in childhood and adolescence. *Archives of Neurology, 44,* 194-198.

Finlayson, M. A. J., & Garner, S. H. (1994). Challenges in rehabilitation of individuals with acquired brain injury. In M. Allen, M. A. J. Finlayson, & S. H. Garner (Eds.), *Brain injury rehabilitation: Clinical considerations* (pp. 3-10). Baltimore: Williams & Wilkins.

Fitch-West, J., & Sands, E. S. (1987). *Bedside evaluation screening test.* Rockville, MD: Aspen.

Flesch, R. F. (1948). A new readability yardstick. *Journal of Applied Psychology, 32,* 221-223.

Folstein, M. F., Folstein, S. E., & McHugh, P. R. (1975). "Minimental state." *Journal of Psychiatric Research, 12,* 189-198.

Foss, D. J., & Jenkins, C. M. (1973). Some affects of context on the comprehension of ambiguous sentences. *Journal of Verbal Learning and Verbal Behavior, 12,* 577-589.

Fox, D. R., & Johns, D. F. (1970). Predicting velopharyngeal closure with a modified tongue-anchor technique. *Journal of Speech and Hearing Disorders, 35,* 248.

Friedman, A. & Polson, M. C. (1981). The hemispheres as independent processing systems: Limited capacity processing and cerebral specialization. *Journal of Experimental Psychology: Human Perception and Performance, 7,* 1031-1058.

Friedman, W. A. (1983). *Head injuries.* CIBA Clinical Symposia, Summit, NJ: CIBA Pharmaceutical Company.

Froeschels, E. (1943). A contribution to pathology and therapy of dysarthria due to certain cortical lesions. *Journal of Speech and Hearing Disorders, 8,* 301-321.

Froeschels, E. (1952). Chewing method as therapy. *Archives of Otolaryngology, 61,* 427-435.

Fromm, D., & Holland, A. L. (1989). Functional communication in Alzheimer's disease. *Journal of Speech and Hearing Disorders, 54,* 535-540.

Gaddes, W. H., & Crockett, D. J. (1973). *The Spreen-Benton aphasia test: Normative data as a measure of normal language development* (Research monograph #25). Victoria, British Columbia, Canada: Neuropsychology Laboratory, University of Victoria.

Gainotti, G. (1991). Frontal lobe damage and disorders of affect and personality. In M. Swash & J. Oxbury (Eds.), *Clinical neurology* (pp. 71-81). Edinburgh: Churchill-Livingstone.

Gainotti, G., & Tiacci, C. (1970). Patterns of drawing disability in left and right hemisphere patients. *Neuropsychologia, 8,* 379-384.

Gao, S., Hendrie, M. B., Hall, K. S., & associates. (1998). The relationships between age, sex, and the incidence of dementia and Alzheimer disease. *Archives of General Psychiatry, 55,* 809-815.

Gardiner, B. J., & Brookshire, R. H. (1972). Effects of unisensory and multisensory presentation of stimuli upon naming by aphasic subjects. *Language and Speech, 15,* 342-357.

Gardner, H., Albert, M. L., & Weintraub, S. (1975). Comprehending a word: The influence of speed and redundancy on auditory comprehension in aphasia. *Cortex, 11,* 155-162.

Gardner, H., Brownell, H. H., Wapner, W., & associates. (1983). Missing the point: The role of right hemisphere in the processing of complex linguistic materials. In E. Perecman (Ed.), *Cognitive processing in the right hemisphere* (pp. 169-192). New York: Academic Press.

Garner, S. H., & Valadka, A. B. (1994). Medical management and principles of head injury rehabilitation. In M. A. J. Finlayson & S. H. Garner (Eds.), *Brain injury rehabilitation: Clinical considerations* (pp. 83-101). Baltimore: Williams & Wilkins.

Gates, W. H., MacGinitie, R. K., Maria, K., & associates. (2000). *Gates-MacGinitie reading tests.* Chicago: Riverside.

Gauthier, L., Dehaut, F., & Joanette, Y. (1989). The Bells Test: A quantitiative and qualitative test for visual neglect. *International Journal of Clinical Neuropsychology. 11,* 49-54.

German, D. J. (1990). *Test of adolescent/adult word finding.* Austin, TX: Pro-Ed.

Geschwind, N. (1975). The apraxias: Neural mechanisms of disorders of learned movement. *American Scientist, 63,* 188-195.

Geschwind, N., Quadfasel, F. A., & Segarra, J. (1968). Isolation of the speech area. *Neuropsychologia, 6,* 327-340.

Gilchrist, E., & Wilkinson, M. (1979). Some factors determining prognosis in young people with severe head injuries. *Archives of Neurology, 36,* 355-359.

Giles, G. M., & Clark-Wilson, J. (1993). *Brain injury rehabilitation: A neurofunctional approach.* London: Chapman & Hall.

Gleason, J. B., Goodglass, H., Green, E., & associates. (1975). The retrieval of syntax in Broca's aphasia. *Brain and Language, 2,* 451-471.

Glisky, E. L., & Schacter, D. L. (1986). Remediation of organic memory disorders: Current status and future prospects. *Journal of Head Trauma Rehabilitation, 1,* 54-63.

Gloag, D. (1985). Rehabilitation after head injury: Cognitive problems. *British Medical Journal, 290,* 834-837.

Glonig, I., Glonig, K., Haub, C., & associates. (1969). Comparison of verbal behavior in right-handed and non-right-handed patients with anatomically verified lesion of one hemisphere. *Cortex, 5,* 43-52.

Glonig, K., Trappl, R., Heiss, W. D., & associates. (1976). Prognosis and speech therapy in aphasia. In Y. Lebrun & R. Hoops (Eds.), *Recovery in aphasics* (pp. 57-64). Atlantic Highlands, NJ: Humanities Press.

Glosser, G., & Deser, T. (1990). Patterns of discourse production among neurological patients with fluent language disorders. *Brain and Language, 40,* 67-88.

Glosser, G., & Goodglass, H. (1990). Disorders in executive control functions among aphasic and other brain-damaged patients. *Journal of Clinical and Experimental Neuropyschology, 12,* 485-501.

Glosser, G., Wiener, M., & Kaplan, E. (1988). Variations in aphasic language behaviors. *Journal of Speech and Hearing Research, 53,* 115-124.

Godfrey, H., & Knight, R. (1985). Cognitive rehabilitation of memory functioning in amnesic alcoholics. *Journal of Consulting and Clinical Psychology, 43,* 555-557.

Goldman-Eisler, F. (1968). *Psycholinguistics: Experiments in spontaneous speech.* New York: Academic Press.

Goldstein, K. (1948). *Language and language disturbances.* New York: Grune & Stratton.

Golper, L. A. C., & Cherney, L. (1999). Back to basics: Assessment practices with neurogenic communication disorders. *Neurophysiology and Neurogenic Speech and Language Disorders, 9,* 3-8.

Golper, L. A. C., Thorpe, P., Tompkins, C., & associates. (1980). Connected language sampling: An expanded index of aphasic language behavior. In R. H. Brookshire (Ed.), *Clinical Aphasiology Conference proceedings,* (pp. 174-186). Minneapolis, MN: BRK Publishers.

Gonzalez, J., & Aronson, A. (1970). Palatal lift prosthesis for treatment of anatomic and neurologic palatopharyngeal insufficiency. *Cleft Palate Journal, 7,* 91-104.

Goodglass, H. (1993). *Understanding aphasia.* San Diego, CA: Academic Press.

Goodglass, H., Blumstein, S. E., Gleason, J. B., & associates. (1979). The effect of syntactic encoding on sentence comprehension in aphasia. *Brain and Language, 7,* 201-209.

Goodglass, H., & Kaplan, E. (1972, 1983). *The Boston diagnostic aphasia examination.* Philadelphia: Lea & Febiger.

Goodglass, H., & Kaplan, E. (1983). *The assessment of aphasia and related disorders* (2nd ed.). Philadelphia: Lea & Febiger.

Goodglass, H., Kaplan, E., & Barresi, B. (2001). *The assessment of aphasia and related disorders* (3rd ed.). Philadelphia: Lippincott Williams & Wilkins.

Goodglass, H., Kaplan, E., & Barresi, B. (2001a). *The Boston diagnostic aphasia examination* (3rd ed.). Philadelphia: Lippincott Williams & Wilkins.

Goodglass, H., Kaplan, E., Weintraub, S., & associates. (1976). The tip of the tongue phenomenon in aphasia. *Cortex, 12,* 145-153.

Goodglass, H., Klein, B., Carey, P., & associates. (1966). Specific semantic word categories in aphasia. *Cortex, 2,* 74-89.

Goodglass, H., & Quadfasel, F. (1954). Language laterality in left-handed aphasics. *Brain, 77,* 523-528.

Goodglass, H., & Stuss, D. T. (1979). Naming to picture versus description in three aphasia subgroups. *Cortex, 15,* 199-211.

Gordon, W. A., Ruckdeschel-Hibbard, M., Egelko, S., & associates. (1984). *Evaluation of the deficits associated with right brain damage: Normative data on the Institute of Rehabilitation Medicine test battery.* New York: Department of Behavioral Sciences, N.Y.U. Medical Center.

Gorham, D. R. (1956). A proverbs test for clinical and experiemental use. *Psychological Reports, 2,* 1-12.

Gouvier, W. D., Blandon, P. D., LaPorte, K. K., & associates. (1987). Reliability and validity of the Disability Rating Scale and the Levels of Cognitive Functioning Scale in monitoring recovery from severe head injury. *Archives of Physical Medicine and Rehabilitation, 68,* 94-97.

Grafman, J., & Salazar, A. (1987). Methodological considerations relevant to the comparison of recovery from penetrating and closed head injuries. In H. S. Levin, J. Grafman, & H. M. Eisenberg (Eds.), *Neurobehavioral recovery from head injury* (pp. 43-54). New York: Oxford.

Graham, D. I., Adams, J. H., & Doyle, D. (1978). Ischemic brain damage in fatal non-missile head injuries. *Journal of Neurological Science, 39,* 213.

Graham, R. K., & Kendall, B. S. (1960). The memory for designs test: Revised general manual. *Perceptual and Motor Skills, 11*(Monograph Suppl. 2-VIII), 147-188.

Grant, D. A., & Berg, E. A. (1948). A behavioral analysis of degree of reinforcement and ease of shifting to new responses in a Weigl-type card sorting problem. *Journal of Experimental Psychology, 38,* 404-411.

Gray, L., Hoyt, P., Mogil, S., & associates. (1977). A comparison of clinical tests of yes/no questions in aphasia. In R. H. Brookshire (Ed.), *Clinical Aphasiology Conference proceedings* (pp. 265-268). Minneapolis, MN: BRK Publishers.

Greenberg, D. A., Aminoff, M. J., & Simon, R. P. (1993). *Clinical neurology* (2nd ed.). Norwalk, CT: Appleton & Lange.

Gronwall, D. M. A. (1977). Paced auditory serial addition task: A measure of recovery from concussion. *Perceptual and Motor Skills, 44,* 367-373.

Guerrero, J., Thurman, D. J., & Sniezek, J. E. (2000). Emergency department visits associated with traumatic brain injury: United States, 1995-1996. *Brain Injury, 14,* 181-186.

Guilford, A. M., & Hawk, A. M. (1968). A comparative study of form identification in neurologically impaired and normal subjects. In A. Smith (Ed.), *Speech and hearing science research reports* (pp. 34-37). Ann Arbor, MI: University of Michigan.

Gunning, R. (1952). *The technique of clear writing.* New York: McGraw-Hill.

Haas, J., Cope, D. N., & Hall, K. (1987). Premorbid prevalence of poor academic performance in severe head injury. *Journal of Neurology, Neurosurgery, and Psychiatry, 50,* 52-56.

Hachinski, V. C., Lassen, N. A., & Marshall, J. (1974). Multi-infarct dementia: A cause of mental deterioration in the elderly. *Lancet, 2,* 207-210.

Hageman, C. (1997). Flaccid dysarthria. In M. R. McNeil (Ed.), *Clinical management of sensorimotor speech disorders* (pp. 193-215). New York: Thieme.

Hagen, C., & Malkamus, D. (1979). *Interaction strategies for language disorders secondary to head trauma.* Paper presented at the annual convention of the American Speech-Language-Hearing Association, Atlanta, GA.

Hall, K., Cope, N., & Rappoport, M. (1985). The Glasgow Outcome Scale and the Disability Rating Scale: Comparative usefulness in following recovery in traumatic head injury. *Archives of Physical Medicine and Rehabilitation, 66,* 35-37.

Halliday, M. A. K, & Hasan, R. (1976). *Cohesion in English.* New York: Longman.

Halligan, P. W., Manning, L., & Marshal, J. C. (1991). Hemispheric activation via spatiomotor cueing in visual neglect: A case study. *Neuropsychologia, 29,* 165-176.

Halper, A. S., Cherney, L. R., Burns, M. S. & associates. (1996). *Clinical management of right hemisphere dysfunction* (2nd ed.). Rockville, MD: Aspen.

Halpern, H. (1965). Effect of stimulus variables on dysphasic verbal errors. *Perceptual and Motor Skills, 21,* 291-298.

Hammill, D. D. (1985). *Detroit Test of Learning Aptitudes.* Austin, TX: Pro-Ed.

Hand, C. R., Burns, M. O., & Ireland, E. (1979). Treatment of hypertonicity in muscles of lip retraction. *Biofeedback and Self Regulation, 4,* 171-176.

Hannay, H. J., Levin, H. S., & Grossman, R. G. (1979). Impaired recognition memory after head injury. *Cortex, 15,* 269-283.

Happe, F., Brownell, H., & Winner, E. (1999). Acquired "theory of mind" impairments following stroke. *Cognition, 70,* 211-240.

Hardy, J. C., Rembolt, R. R., Spreisterbach, D. C., & associates. (1961). Surgical management of palatal paresis and speech problems in cerebral palsy. *Journal of Speech and Hearing Disorders, 26,* 320-327.

Hart, T., & Hayden, M. E. (1986). The ecological validity of neuropsychological assessment and remediation. In B. P. Uzzell & Y. Gross (Eds.), *Clinical neuropsychology of intervention* (pp. 21-50). Boston: Martinus Nijhoff.

Harvey, A. M., Johns, R. J., McKusick, V. A., & associates. (1988). *The principles and practice of medicine* (19th ed.). Norwalk, CT: Appleton & Lange.

Haskins, S. (1976). A treatment procedure for writing disorders. In R. H. Brookshire (Ed.), *Clinical Aphasiology Conference proceedings* (pp. 192-199). Minneapolis, MN: BRK Publishers.

Hayes, D. P. (1989). *Guide to the lexical analysis of texts.* (Tech. Rep. Series 89-96). Ithaca, NY: Cornell University Department of Sociology.

Heard, K., & Watson, T. (1999). Reducing wandering by persons with dementia using differential reinforcement. *Journal of Applied Behavior Analysis, 32,* 381-384.

Heath, P. D., Kennedy, P., & Kapur, N. (1983). Slowly progressive aphasia without generalized dementia. *Annals of Neurology, 13,* 687-688.

Hecaen, H., & Angelergues, D. (1962). Agnosia for faces. *Archives of Neurology, 7,* 92-100.

Hecaen, H., & Assal, G. (1970). A comparison of constructive deficits following left and right hemisphere lesions. *Neuropsychologia, 8,* 289-303.

Hedera, P., & Whitehouse, P. (1995). Neurotransmitters in neurodegeneration. In D. Calne (Ed.), *Neurodegenerative diseases* (pp. 97-117). Philadelphia: W.B. Saunders.

Heilman, K. M., Schwartz, H. D., & Watson, R.T. (1978). Hypo-arousal in patients with the neglect syndrome and emotional indifference. *Neurology, 28,* 229-232.

Helm, N. (1979). Management of pallilalia with a pacing board. *Journal of Speech and Hearing Disorders, 44,* 350-353.

Helm, N. A., & Barresi, B. (1980). Voluntary control of involuntary utterances: A treatment approach for severe aphasia. In R. H. Brookshire (Ed.), *Clinical Aphasiology Conference proceedings* (pp. 308-315). Minneapolis, MN: BRK Publishers.

Helm-Estabrooks, N., & Hotz, G. (1991). *Brief test of head injury.* Chicago: Riverside.

Helm-Estabrooks, N. A. (1981). "Show me the . . . whatever": Some variables affecting auditory comprehension scores of aphasic patients. In R. H. Brookshire (Ed.), *Clinical Aphasiology Conference proceedings* (pp. 105-107). Minneapolis, MN: BRK Publishers.

Helm-Estabrooks, N. A. (1982). *Helm elicited language program for syntax stimulation (HELPSS).* Chicago: Riverside.

Hier, D., Hagenlocker, K., & Shindler, A. G. (1985). Language disintegration in dementia: Effects of etiology and severity. *Brain and Language, 25,* 117-133.

Hillbom, M., & Holm, L. (1986). Contribution of traumatic head injury to neuropsychological deficits in alcoholics. *Journal of Neurology, Neurosurgery, and Psychiatry, 49,* 1348-1353.

Hixon, T. J. (1987). *Respiratory function in speech and song.* San Diego, CA: College-Hill.

Hixon, T. J., Hawley, J. L., & Wilson, J. L. (1982). An around-the-house device for the clinical determination of respiratory driving pressure. *Journal of Speech and Hearing Disorders, 47,* 413-415.

Holland, A. L. (1977). Some practical considerations in aphasia rehabilitation. In M. Sullivan & M. S. Kommers (Eds.), *Rationale for adult aphasia therapy* (pp. 167-180). Omaha: University of Nebraska Medical Center.

Holland, A. L. (1980). *Communicative abilities in daily living.* Baltimore: University Park Press.

Holland, A. L. (1996). Treatment efficacy: Aphasia. *Journal of Speech and Hearing Research, 30,* S27-S36.

Holland, A. L., & Beeson, P. M. (1999). Aphasia groups: The Arizona experience. In R. Elman (Ed.), *Group treatment of neurogenic communication disorders: The expert clinician's approach* (pp. 77-84). Boston: Butterworth-Heinemann.

Holland, A. L., Frattali, C. M., & Fromm, D. (1998). *Communication activities in daily living* (2nd ed.). Austin, TX: Pro-Ed.

Holland, A. L., & Ross, R. (1999). The power of aphasia groups. In R. J. Elman (Ed.), *Group treatment of neurogenic communication disorders: The expert clinician's approach* (pp. 115-120). Boston: Butterworth-Heinemann.

Holtzapple, P., Pohlman, K., LaPointe, L. L., & associates. (1989). Does SPICA mean PICA? *Clinical Aphasiology, 18,* 131-144.

Hooper, H. E. (1983). *The Hooper Visual Organization Test.* Los Angeles: Western Psychological Services.

Horner, J., Massey, E. W., Woodruff, W. W., & associates. (1989). Task-dependent neglect: Computed tomography size and locus correlations. *Journal of Neurological Rehabilitation, 3,* 7-13.

Howard, D., & Hatfield, F. M. (1987). *Aphasia therapy: Historical and contemporary issues.* Hillsdale, NJ: Lawrence Erlbaum.

Humphrey, M., & Oddy, M. (1981). Return to work after head injury. A review of postwar studies. *Injury, 12,* 107-114.

Hussian, R. A. (1988). Modification of behaviors in dementia via stimulus manipulation. *Clinical Gerontologist, 8,* 37-43.

Jackson, J. H. (1874). On the anatomical and physiological localization of movements in the brain. *Lancet, 1,* 162-165.

Jennett, B. (1976). Assessment of the severity of head injury. *Journal of Neurology, Neurosurgery, and Psychiatry, 39,* 647-655.

Jennett, B., & Bond, M. (1975). Assessment of outcome after severe brain damage: A practical scale. *Lancet, 1,* 480-484.

Jennett, B., & Teasdale, G. (1981). *Management of head injuries.* Philadelphia: F.A. Davis Company.

Jennett, B., Teasdale, G., Braakman, R., & associates. (1976). Predicting outcome in individual patients after severe head injury. *Lancet, 1,* 878-881.

Jennett, B., Teasdale, G., Braakman, R., & associates. (1979). Prognosis of patients with severe head injury. *Neurosurgery, 4,* 283-289.

Jennett, B., Teasdale, G., Galbraith, S., & associates (1977). Severe head injuries in three countries. *Journal of Neurology, Neurosurgery, and Psychiatry, 40,* 291-298.

Jerger, J., Weikers, N., Sharbrough, F., & associates. (1969). Bilateral lesions of the temporal lobe: A case study. *Acta Otolaryngologica, 258,* 1-51.

Joanette, Y., Brouchon, M., Gauthier, I., & associates. (1986). Pointing with the left versus right hand in left visual field neglect. *Neuropsychologia, 24,* 391-396.

Joanette, Y., & Goulet, P. (1994). Right hemisphere and verbal communication: Conceptual, methodological, and clinical issues. *Clinical Aphasiology, 22,* 1-23.

Joanette, Y., Lecours, A. R., Lepage, Y., & associates. (1983). Language in right-handers with right-hemisphere lesions: A preliminary study including anatomical, genetic, and social factors. *Brain and Language, 20,* 217-248.

Johns, D. (Ed.). (1985). *Clinical management of neurogenic communication disorders.* Boston: Little, Brown and Company.

Johns, D. F., & Darley, F. L. (1970). Phonemic variability in apraxia of speech. *Journal of Speech and Hearing Research, 13,* 556-583.

Jorm, A. F., Korten, A. E., & Henderson, A. S. (1987). The prevalence of dementia: A quantitative integration of the literature. *Acta Psychologica Scandinavia, 76,* 465-479.

Kagan, A., Black, S. E., Duchan, J. F., & associates. (2001). Training volunteers as conversation partners using supported conversation for adults with aphasia: A controlled trial. *Journal of Speech, Language, and Hearing Research, 44,* 624-638.

Kagan, A., & Cohen-Schneider, R. (1999). Groups in the introductory program at the Pat Arato Aphasia Center. In R. Elman (Ed.), *Group treatment of neurogenic communication disorders: The expert clinician's approach.* Boston: Butterworth-Heinemann.

Kagan, A., & Dailey, G. F. (1993). Functional is not enough: Training conversation partners for aphasic adults. In A. L. Holland & M. M. Forbes (Eds.), *Aphasia treatment: World perspectives* (pp. 199-225). San Diego: Singular.

Kahneman, D. (1973). *Attention and effort.* Englewood Cliffs, NJ: Prentice-Hall.

Kaplan, E., Goodglass, H., & Weintraub, S. (2001). *The Boston naming test.* Philadelphia: Lippincott Williams & Wilkins.

Katsuki-Nakamura, J., Brookshire, R. H., & Nicholas, L. E. (1988). Comprehension of monologues and dialogues by aphasic listeners. *Journal of Speech and Hearing Research, 53,* 408-415.

Katz, D. I. (1992). Recovery following severe head injuries. *Journal of Head Trauma Rehabilitation, 7,* 1-15.

Katz, D. I., & Alexander, M. P. (1994). Traumatic brain injury. In D. C. Good & J. R. Couch (Eds.), *Handbook of neurorehabilitation* (pp. 493-549). New York: Dekker.

Katz, R. C., & Nagy, V. T. (1983). A computerized approach for improving word recognition in chronic aphasic adults. In R. H. Brookshire (Ed.), *Clinical Aphasiology 1983 Conference proceedings* (pp. 65-72). Minneapolis, MN: BRK Publishers.

Katz, R. C., & Nagy, V. T. (1984). An intelligent computer-based task for chronic aphasic patients. In R. H. Brookshire (Ed.), *Clinical Aphasiology 1984 Conference proceedings* (pp. 159-165). Minneapolis, MN: BRK Publishers.

Katz, R. C., Wertz, R. T., Davidoff, M., & associates. (1989). A computer program to improve written confrontation naming in aphasia. In T. E. Prescott (Ed.), *Clinical Aphasiology 1988 Conference proceedings* (pp. 321-338). Austin, TX: Pro-Ed.

Kay, D., & Bergmann, K. (1980). Epidemiology of mental disorders among the aged in the community. In J. Birren & R. Sloan (Eds.), *Handbook of mental health and aging* (pp. 34-66). Englewood Cliffs, NJ: Prentice-Hall.

Kay, T., & Silver, S. M. (1989). Closed head trauma: Assessment for rehabilitation. In M. Lezak (Ed.), *Assessment of the behavioral consequences of head trauma* (pp. 145-170). New York: A.R. Liss.

Kazdin, A. E. (1982). *Single-case research designs: Methods for clinical and applied settings.* New York: Oxford University Press.

Kearns, K. (1994). Group therapy for aphasia: Theoretical and practical considerations. In R. Chapey (Ed.), *Language intervention strategies in adult aphasia* (3rd ed., pp. 304-321). Baltimore: Williams & Wilkins.

Kearns, K., & Hubbard, D. J. (1977). A comparison of auditory comprehension tasks in aphasia. In R.H. Brookshire (Ed.), *Clinical Aphasiology Conference proceedings* (pp. 32-45). Minneapolis, MN: BRK Publishers.

Kearns, K. P., & Salmon S. J. (1984). An experimental analysis of auxiliary and copula verb generalization in aphasia. *Journal of Speech and Hearing Disorders, 49,* 152-163.

Kearns, K. P., & Simmons, N. N. (1985). Group therapy for aphasia: A survey of V.A. Medical Centers. In R.H. Brookshire (Ed.), *Clinical Aphasiology Conference proceedings* (pp. 176-183). Minneapolis, MN: BRK Publishers.

Kearns, K. P., & Simmons, N. N. (1988). Motor speech disorders: The dysarthrias and apraxia of speech. In N. J. Lass, L. V. McReynolds, J. L. Northern, & associates (Eds.), *Handbook of speech-language pathology and audiology* (pp. 434-448). Philadelphia: B.C. Decker.

Keefe, K. A. (1995). Applying basic neuroscience to aphasia therapy: What the animals are telling us. *American Journal of Speech-Language Pathology, 4,* 88-93.

Keenan, J. S., & Brassell, E. G. (1975). *Aphasia language performance scales.* Murfreesboro, TN: Pinnacle Press.

Kempler, D., Curtiss, S., & Jackson, C. (1987). Syntactic preservation in Alzheimer's disease. *Journal of Speech and Hearing Research, 30,* 343-350.

Kennedy, M., Strand, E., Burton, W., & associates. (1994). Analysis of first-encounter conversations of right-hemisphere-damaged adults. *Clinical Aphasiology, 22,* 67-80.

Kerr, T. A., Kay, D. W. K., & Lassman, L. P. (1971). Characteristics of patients, type of accident, and mortality in a consecutive series of head injuries admitted to a neurosurgical unit. *Journal of Preventative and Social Medicine, 25,* 179-185.

Kertesz, A. (1979). *Aphasia and associated disorders: Taxonomy, localization, and recovery.* New York: Grune & Stratton.

Kertesz, A. (1982). *Western aphasia battery.* New York: Grune and Stratton.

Kertesz, A., & McCabe, P. (1977). Recovery patterns and prognosis in aphasia. *Brain, 100,* 1-18.

Kertesz, A., & Munoz, D. (2000). Differences between Pick disease and Alzheimer disease in clinical appearance and rate of cognitive decline. *Archives of Neurology, 57,* 225-232.

Kimelman, M. D. Z., & McNeil, M. R. (1987). An investigation of emphatic stress comprehension in aphasia: A replication. *Journal of Speech and Hearing Research, 30,* 295-300.

Kimura, D. (1963). Right temporal lobe damage. *Archives of Neurology, 8,* 264-271.

Kintsch, W. (1974). *The representation of meaning in memory.* Hillsdale, NJ: Lawrence Erlbaum.

Kirshner, H. S., Tanridag, O., Thurman, L., & associates. (1987). Progressive aphasia without dementia: Two cases with focal spongiform degeneration. *Annals of Neurology, 22,* 527-533.

Klare, G. R. (1984). Readability. In P. D. Pearson (Ed.), *Handbook of reading research* (pp. 681-744). New York: Longman.

Knopman, D., Selnes, O. A., Niccum, N., & associates. (1983). A longitudinal study of speech fluency in aphasia: CT correlates of recovery and persistent nonfluency. *Neurology (Cleveland), 33,* 1170-1178.

Knopman, D. S., Selnes, O. A., Niccum, N., & associates. (1984). Recovery of naming in aphasia: Relationship to fluency, comprehension, and CT findings. *Neurology, 34,* 1461-1470.

Kokmen, E., Beard, M., Offord, K., & associates. (1989). Prevalence of medically diagnosed dementia in a defined Unites States Population: Rochester, Minnesota, January 1, 1975. *Neurology, 39,* 773-776.

Kratchowill, T. R. (1978). *Single-subject research: Strategies for evaluating change.* New York: Academic Press.

Kraus, J. F. (1993). Epidemiology of head injury. In P. R. Cooper (Ed.), *Head injury* (3rd ed., pp. 1-25). Baltimore: Williams & Wilkins.

Kreindler, A., Gheorghita, N., & Voinescu, I. (1971). Analysis of verbal reception of a complex order with three elements in aphasics. *Brain, 94,* 375-386.

Kremin, H. (1993). Therapeutic approaches to naming disorders. In M. Paradis (Ed.), *Foundations of aphasia rehabilitation* (pp. 261-292). New York: Pergamon.

Kreutzer, J. S., & Wehman, P. H. (Eds.) (1991). *Cognitive rehabilitation for persons with traumatic brain injury: A functional approach.* Baltimore: Brookes.

Lackner, J. R., & Garrett, M. F. (1972). Resolving ambiguity: Effects of biasing context in the unattended ear. *Cognition, 1,* 359-372.

Lambrecht, K., & Marshall, R. (1983). Comprehension in severe aphasia: A second look. In R. H. Brookshire (Ed.), *Clinical Aphasiology Conference proceedings* (pp. 186-192). Minneapolis, MN: BRK Publishers.

Langfitt, T. W. (1978). Measuring outcome from head injuries. *Journal of Neurosurgery, 48,* 673-678.

LaPointe, L. L. (1991). Base-10 response form (revised manual). San Diego: Singular. (Previously published as LaPointe, L. L. [1977]. Base-10 programmed stimulation: Task specification, scoring, and plotting performance in aphasia therapy. *Journal of Speech and Hearing Disorders, 42,* 90-105.)

LaPointe, L. L., Holtzapple, P., & Graham, L. F. (1985). The relationship among two measures of auditory comprehension and daily living communication skills. In R. H. Brookshire (Ed.), *Clinical Aphasiology Conference proceedings* (pp. 38-46). Minneapolis, MN: BRK Publishers.

LaPointe, L. L., & Horner, J. (1979). *Reading comprehension battery for aphasia.* Austin, TX: Pro-Ed.

LaPointe, L. L., & Horner, J. (1998). *Reading comprehension battery for aphasia* (2nd ed.). Austin, TX: Pro-Ed.

LaPointe, L. L., & Johns, D. F. (1975). Some phonemic characteristics in apraxia of speech. *Journal of Communication Disorders, 8,* 259-269.

Larimore, H. W. (1970). *Some verbal and nonverbal factors associated with apraxia of speech.* Unpublished doctoral dissertation, University of Denver.

Lee, L. (1971). *Northwestern syntax screening test.* Evanston, IL: The Northwestern University Press.

Lees, A. (1990). Progressive supranuclear palsy. In J. Cummings (Ed.), *Subcortical dementia* (pp. 123-131). New York: Oxford.

Lenneberg, E. (1967). *Biological foundations of language.* New York: Wiley.

Lesser, R. (1976). Verbal and non-verbal memory components in the token test. *Neuropsychologia, 14,* 79-85.

Levin, B. E., Tomer, R., & Rey, G. J. (1992). Cognitive impairments in Parkinson's disease. *Neurologic Clinics, 10,* 471-481.

Levin, H. S., Benton, A. L., & Grossman, R. G. (1982). *Neurobehavioral consequences of closed head injury.* New York: Oxford University Press.

Levin, H. S., Grossman, R. G., Rose, J. E., & Teasdale, G. (1979). Long term neuropsychological outcome of closed head injury. *Journal of Neurosurgery, 50,* 412-422.

Levin, H. S., O'Donnell, V. M., & Grossman, R. G. (1979). The Galveston orientation and amnesia test: A practical scale to assess cognition after head injury. *Journal of Nervous and Mental Disorders, 167,* 675-684.

Lewelt, W., Jenkins, L. W., & Miller, J. D. (1982). Effects of experimental fluid-percussion injury of the brain on cerebral reactivity to hypoxia and hypercapnia. *Journal of Neurosurgery, 56,* 332-355.

Lewinsohn, P. M., Danaher, B. G., & Kikel, S. (1977). Visual imagery as a mnemonic aid for brain-injured persons. *Journal of Consulting and Clinical Psychology, 45,* 717-723.

Lewy, R., Cole, R., & Wepman, J. (1965). Teflon injection in the correction of velopharyngeal insufficiency. *Annals of Otology, Rhinology, & Laryngology, 78,* 874.

Ley, R. G., & Bryden, M. P. (1979). Hemispheric differences in processing emotions and faces. *Brain and Language, 7,* 127-138.

Lezak, M. D. (1983). *Neuropyschological assessment* (2nd ed.). New York: Oxford University Press.

Lezak, M. D. (1995). *Neuropsychological assessment* (3rd ed.). New York: Oxford University Press.

Li, E. C., & Williams, S. E. (1990). The effects of grammatical class and cue type on cueing responsiveness in aphasia. *Brain and Language, 38,* 48-60.

Lichtheim, L. (1885). On aphasia. *Brain, 7,* 433-484.

Liepmann, H. (1900). Das krankheitsbild der apraxia. *Monatschreift f. Psychiatrie u Neuroligie, 7,* 11-18.

Liles, B. Z., & Brookshire, R. H. (1975). The effects of pause time on auditory comprehension of aphasic subjects. *Journal of Communication Disorders, 8,* 221-236.

Lincoln, N., & Ellis, P. (1980). A shortened version of the PICA. *British Journal of Communication Disorders, 15,* 183-187.

Lincoln, N. B., Mulley, G. P., Jones, A. C., & associates. (1984). Effectiveness of speech therapy for aphasic stroke patients: A randomized controlled trial. *Lancet, 2,* 1197-1200.

Linebaugh, C., & Lehner, L. (1977). Cueing hierarchies and word retrieval: A therapy program. In R. H. Brookshire (Ed.), *Clinical Aphasiology Conference proceedings* (pp. 19-31). Minneapolis, MN: BRK Publishers.

Linebaugh, C. W. (1983). Treatment of anomic aphasia. In W. H. Perkins (Ed.), *Language handicaps in adults* (pp. 35-43). New York: Thieme-Stratton.

Liss, J., Kuehn, D., & Hinkel, K. (1994). Direct training of velopharyngeal musculature. *National Center for Voice and Speech: Progress Report, 6,* 43-52.

Livingstone, M. G., & Livingstone, H. M. (1985). The Glasgow assessment schedule: Clinical and research assessment of head injury outcome. *International Rehabilitation Medicine, 7,* 145-149.

Lomas, J., Pickard, L., Bester, S., & associates. (1989). The communicative effectiveness index: Development and psychometric evaluation of a functional communication measure for adult aphasia. *Journal of Speech and Hearing Disorders, 54,* 113-124.

Longstreth, W. T., Koepsell, T. D., Nelson, L. M., & associates. (1992). Prognosis: Keystone of clinical neurology. In R. W. Evans, D. S. Baskin, & F. M. Yatsu (Eds.), *Prognosis of neurological disorders* (pp. 19-44). New York: Oxford University Press.

Love, R. J., & Webb, W. J. (1977). The efficacy of cueing techniques in Broca's aphasia. *Journal of Speech and Hearing Disorders, 42,* 170-178.

Luria, A. R. (1965). Neuropsychological analysis of focal brain lesions. In B. B. Wolman (Ed.), *Handbook of clinical psychology* (pp. 42-58). New York: McGraw-Hill.

Luria, A. R. (1966). *Human brain and psychological processes.* New York: Harper & Row.

Luria, A. R. (1970). *Traumatic aphasia.* The Hague, Netherlands: Mouton.

Lyon, J. G. (1989). Communicative partners: Their value in reestablishing communication with aphasic adults. In T. Prescott (Ed.), *Clinical aphasiology, 18,* 11-18.

Lyon, J. G. (1992). Communication use and participation in life for adults with aphasia in natural settings: The scope of the problem. *American Journal of Speech-Language Pathology, 1,* 7-14.

Mace, N., & Rabins, P. (1991). *The 36-hour day.* Baltimore: Johns Hopkins University Press.

Mackay, D. G. (1966). To end ambiguous sentences. *Perception and Psychophysics, 1,* 426-436.

Macniven, E. (1994). Factors affecting head injury rehabilitation outcome: Premorbid and clinical parameters. In M. A. J. Finlayson & S. H. Garner (Eds.), *Brain injury rehabilitation: Clinical considerations* (pp. 57-82). Baltimore: Williams & Wilkins.

Mahurin, R. K., & Pirozzolo, F. J. (1986). Chronometric analysis: Clinical applications in aging and dementia. *Developmental Neuropsychology, 2,* 345-362.

Major, B. J., & Wilson, K. J. (1985). *Computerized reading for aphasics.* San Diego, CA: College-Hill.

Marion, D. W., Darby, J., & Yonas, H. (1991). Acute regional cerebral blood flow changes caused by severe head injuries. *Journal of Neurosurgery, 74,* 407-414.

Markwardt, F. C. Jr. (1989). *The Peabody individual achievement test—Revised.* Circle Pines, MN: American Guidance Service.

Marshall, J. C., & Newcombe, F. (1973). Patterns of paralexia: A psycholinguistic approach. *Journal of Psycholinguistic Research, 2,* 175-199.

Marshall, R. C. (1976). Word retrieval behavior of aphasic adults. *Journal of Speech and Hearing Disorders, 41,* 444-451.

Marshall, R. C., & Phillips, D. S. (1983). Prognosis for improved verbal communication in aphasic stroke patients. *Archives of Physical Medicine and Rehabilitation, 64,* 597-600.

Martin, R., & Feher, E. (1990). The consequences of reduced memory span for the comprehension of semantic versus syntactic information. *Brain and Language, 38,* 1-20.

Martino, A. A., Pizzamiglio, L., & Razzano, C. (1976). A new version of the Token Test for aphasics: A concrete objects form. *Journal of Communication Disorders, 9,* 1-5.

Massengill, R., Quinn, G. W., Pickrell, K. L., & associates. (1968). Therapeutic exercise and pharyngeal flap. *Cleft Palate Journal, 5,* 44-52.

McDonald, S. (1993). Viewing the brain sideways? Frontal versus right hemisphere explanations of nonaphasic language disorders. *Aphasiology, 7,* 535-549.

McFie, J., & Zangwill, O. L. (1960). Visual construction disabilities associated with lesions of the left cerebral hemisphere. *Brain, 83,* 243-260.

McKeever, W. F., & Dixon, M. F. (1981). Right-hemisphere superiority for discriminating memorized from unmemorized faces: Affective imagery, sex, and perceived emotionality effects. *Brain and Language, 12,* 246-260.

McNeil, M., Odell, K., & Tseng, C. H. (1990). Toward the integration of resource allocation into a general model of aphasia. In T. Prescott (Ed.), *Clinical aphasiology* (pp. 21-39). Austin, TX: Pro-Ed.

McNeil, M. R., & Kimelman, M. D. Z. (1986). Toward an integrative information-processing structure of auditory comprehension and processing in adult aphasia. *Seminars in Speech and Language, 7,* 123-146.

McNeil, M. R., & Prescott, T. E. (1978). *Revised token test.* Baltimore: University Park Press.

McNeil, M. R., Robin, D. A., & Schmidt, R. A. (1997). Apraxia of speech: Definition, differentiation, and treatment. In M. R. McNeil (Ed.), *Clinical management of sensorimotor speech disorders* (pp. 311-344). New York: Thieme.

Meadows, J. C. (1974). The anatomical basis of prosopagnosia. *Journal of Neurology, Neurosurgery, and Psychiatry, 37,* 489-501.

Mendez, M. F., Selwood, A., Mastri, A. R., & associates. (1993). Pick's disease versus Alzheimer's disease: A comparison of clinical characteristics. *Neurology, 43,* 289-292.

Mesulam, M. M. (1982). A cortical network for directed attention and unilateral neglect. *Annals of Neurology, 10,* 309-325.

Metter, E. J., Riege, W. H., Hanson, W. R., & associates. (1983). Comparisons of metabolic rates, language and memory in subcortical aphasias. *Brain and Language, 19,* 33-47.

Metter, E. J., Riege, W. H., Hanson, W. R., & associates. (1984). Correlations of glucose metabolism and structural damage to language function in aphasia. *Brain and Language, 21,* 187-207.

Meyer, B. J. F. (1975). *The organization of prose and its effects on memory.* Amsterdam: North-Holland.

Meyer, B. J. F., & McConkie, G. W. (1973). What is recalled after hearing a passage? *Journal of Educational Psychology, 65,* 109-117.

Miceli, G., Silveri, M. C., Nocentini, U., & associates. (1988). Patterns of dissociation in comprehension and production of nouns and verbs. *Aphasiology, 2,* 351-358.

Miller, J. D., Sweet, R. G., Narayan, R., & associates. (1978). Early insults in the injured brain. *Journal of the American Medical Association, 240,* 439-442.

Mills, R. H., Knox, A. W., Juola, J. F., & associates. (1979). Cognitive loci of impairments of picture naming by aphasic subjects. *Journal of Speech and Hearing Research, 22,* 73-87.

Milner, B. (1971). Interhemispheric differences in the localization of psychological processes in man. *British Medical Bulletin, 27,* 272-277. (Reported in Lezak, 1995.)

Milner, B. (1975). Psychological aspects of focal epilepsy and its neurosurgical management. *Advances in Neurology, 8,* 299-321.

Miniami, R. T., Kaplan, E. N., Wu, G., & associates. (1975). Velopharyngeal incompetency without overt cleft palate. *Plastic and Reconstructive Surgery, 55,* 573-587.

Mohr, J. P., Pessin, M. S., Finkelstein, S., & associates. (1978). Broca aphasia: Pathologic and clinical aspects. *Neurology, 28,* 311-324.

Mohr, J. P., Walters, W. C., & Duncan, G. W. (1975). Thalamic hemorrhage and aphasia. *Brain and Language, 2,* 3-17.

Moll, K. L. (1968). Speech characteristics of individuals with cleft lip and palate. In D. C. Spriesterbach & D. Sherman (Eds.), *Cleft palate and communication.* New York: Academic Press.

Molloy, R., Brownell, H. H., & Gardner, H. (1990). Discourse comprehension by right-hemisphere stroke patients: Deficits of prediction and revision. In Y. Joanette & H. Brownell (Eds.), *Discourse ability and brain damage: Theoretical and empirical perspectives* (pp. 113-130). New York: Springer-Verlag.

Murdoch, B. E. (1990). *Acquired Speech and Language Disorders.* New York: Chapman & Hall.

Murray, J., Marquardt, T. P., Richardson, A., & associates. (1984). Differential diagnosis of aphasia and dementia from aphasia test battery scores. *Journal of Neurological Communication Disorders, 1,* 33-39.

Myers, P. S. (1979). Profiles of communication deficits in patients with right cerebral hemisphere damage: Implications for diagnosis and treatment. In R. H. Brookshire (Ed.), *Clinical Aphasiology Conference proceedings* (pp. 38-46). Minneapolis, MN: BRK Publishers.

Myers, P. S. (1991). Inference failure: The underlying impairment in right hemisphere communication disorders. In T. E. Prescott (Ed.), *Clinical aphasiology: Volume 20* (pp. 167-180). Austin, TX: Pro-Ed.

Myers, P. S. (1994). Communication disorders associated with right-hemisphere brain damage. In R. Chapey (Ed.), *Language intervention strategies in adult aphasia* (3rd ed., pp. 513-534). Baltimore: Williams & Wilkins.

Myers, P. S. (1999). *Right hemisphere damage: Disorders of communication and cognition.* San Diego, CA: Singular.

Myers, P. S., & Mackisack, E. L. (1990). Right hemisphere syndrome. In L. L. LaPointe (Ed.), *Aphasia and related neurogenic language disorders* (pp. 177-195). New York: Thieme.

Naeser, M. A., Alexander, M. P., Helm-Estabrooks, N., & associates. (1982). Aphasia with predominantly subcortical lesion sites: Description of three capsular putamenal aphasia syndromes. *Archives of Neurology, 39,* 2-14.

Naeser, M. A., & Borod, J. C. (1986). Aphasia in left-handers. *Neurology, 36,* 471-488.

Naeser, M. A., Hayward, R. W., Laughlin, S. A., Becker, J. M. T., & associates. (1981). Quantitative CT scan studies in aphasia: II. Comparison of right and left hemispheres. *Brain and Language, 12,* 165-189.

Naeser, M. A., Hayward, R. W., Laughlin, S. A., & Zatz, L. M. (1981). Quantitative CT scan studies in aphasia: I. Infarct size and CT numbers. *Brain and Language, 12,* 140-164.

Naeser, M. A., Palumbo, C. L., Helm-Estabrooks, N., & associates. (1989). Severe nonfluency in aphasia: Role of the medial subcallosal fasciculus and other white matter pathways in recovery of spontaneous speech. *Brain, 112,* 1-38.

Navia, B. A., Jordan, B. D., & Price, R. W. (1986). The AIDS demential complex: Clinical features. *Annals of Neurology, 19,* 517-524.

Neary, D., Snoden, J. S., Northern, B., & associates. (1988). Dementia of frontal lobe type. *Journal of Neurology, Neurosurgery, and Psychiatry, 44,* 409-411.

Netsell, R., & Cleeland, C. (1973). Modification of lip hypotonia in dysarthria using EMG feedback. *Journal of Speech and Hearing Disorders, 38,* 131-140.

Netsell, R., & Hixon, T. J. (1978). A noninvasive method for clinically estimating subglottal air pressure. *Journal of Speech and Hearing Disorders, 43,* 326-330.

Netsell, R., & Rosenbek, J. C. (1985). Treating the dysarthrias. In J. K. Darby (Ed.), *Speech and language evaluation in neurology: Adult disorders* (pp. 87-101). New York: Grune & Stratton.

Newcombe, F. (1969). *Missile wounds of the brain.* London: Oxford University Press.

Nicholas, L. E., & Brookshire, R. H. (1983). Syntactic simplification and context: Effects on sentence comprehension by aphasic adults. In R. H. Brookshire (Ed.), *Clinical Aphasiology Conference proceedings* (pp. 166-172). Minneapolis, MN: BRK Publishers.

Nicholas, L. E., & Brookshire, R. H. (1986). Consistency of the effects of rate of speech on brain-damaged adults' comprehension of narrative discourse. *Journal of Speech and Hearing Research, 29,* 462-470.

Nicholas, L. E., & Brookshire, R. H. (1987). Error analysis and passage dependecy of test items from a standardized test of multiple-sentence reading comprehension for aphasic and non-brain-damaged adults. *Journal of Speech and Hearing Disorders, 52,* 358-366.

Nicholas, L. E., & Brookshire, R. H. (1993). A system for quantifying the informativeness and efficiency of the connected speech of adults with aphasia. *Journal of Speech and Hearing Research, 36,* 338-350.

Nicholas, L. E., & Brookshire, R. H. (1995a). Presence, completeness, and accuracy of main concepts in the connected speech of non-brain-damaged adults and adults with aphasia. *Journal of Speech and Hearing Research, 38,* 145-156.

Nicholas, L. E., & Brookshire, R. H. (1995b). Comprehension of spoken narrative discourse by adults with aphasia, right-hemisphere brain damage, or traumatic brain injury. *American Journal of Speech-Language Pathology, 4,* 69-81.

Nicholas, L. E., Brookshire, R. H., MacLennan, D. L., & associates. (1989). Revised administration and scoring procedures for the Boston Naming Test and norms for non-brain-damaged adults. *Aphasiology, 3,* 569-580.

Nicholas, L. E., MacLennan, D. L., & Brookshire, R. H. (1986). Validity of multiple-sentence reading comprehension tests for aphasic adults. *Journal of Speech and Hearing Disorders, 51,* 82-87.

Nicholas, M., Obler, L. K., Albert, M. L., & associates. (1985). Empty speech in Alzheimers disease and fluent aphasia. *Journal of Speech and Hearing Research, 28,* 405-410.

Noll, D. J., & Lass, N. D. (1972). *Use of the Token Test with children: Two contrasting socioeconomic groups.* Paper presented at the American Speech and Hearing Association Convention, San Francisco (November).

Nolte, J. (1993). *The human brain* (3rd ed.). St. Louis: Mosby.

Norman, D. A., & Bobrow, D. G. (1975). On data-limited and resource-limited processes. *Cognitive Psychology, 7,* 44-64.

Ogden, J. A. (1985). Contralateral neglect of constructed images in right and left brain-damaged patients. *Neuropsychologia, 23,* 273-277.

Ojemann, G. A. (1975). Language and the thalamus: Object naming and recall during and after thalamic stimulation. *Brain and Language, 2,* 101-120.

Ommaya, A. K., Grubb, R. L., & Naumann, R. A. (1971). Coup and contrecoup injury: Observations on the mechanics of visible brain injuries in the rhesus monkey. *Journal of Neurosurgery, 35,* 503-507.

Orgass, B., & Poeck, K. (1966). Clinical validation of a new test for aphasia: An experimental study of the Token Test. *Cortex, 2,* 222-243.

Osgood, C., & Miron, M. (1963). *Approaches to the study of aphasia.* Chicago: University Park Press.

Pang, D. (1989). Physics and pathophysiology of closed head injury. In M. Lezak (Ed.), *Assessment of the behavioral consequences of head trauma* (pp. 1-19). New York: A.R. Liss.

Parente, R., & DiCesare, A. (1991). Retraining memory: Theory, evaluation, and applications. In J. S. Kreutzer & P. H. Wehman (Eds.), *Cognitive rehabilitation for persons with traumatic brain injury: A functional approach* (pp. 147-162). Baltimore: Brookes.

Parkhurst, B. G. (1970). *The effects of time altered speech stimuli on the performance of right hemiplegic adult aphasics.* Paper presented at the annual convention of the American Speech and Hearing Association, New York.

Parkin, H. J. (1982). Residual learning capability in organic amnesia. *Cortex, 18,* 417-440.

Parr, S. (1992). Everyday reading and writing practices of normal adults: Implications for aphasia assessment. *Aphasiology, 6,* 273-283.

Pashek, G. V., & Brookshire, R. H. (1982). Effects of rate of speech and linguistic stress on auditory paragraph comprehension by aphasic individuals. *Journal of Speech and Hearing Research, 25,* 377-382.

Pasternak, K. F., & LaPointe, L. L. (1982). *Aphasic-nonaphasic performance on the Reading Comprehension Battery for Aphasia (RCBA).* Paper presented to the annual convention of the American Speech Language and Hearing Association, Toronto.

Pease, D. M., & Goodglass, H. (1978). The effects of cueing on picture naming in aphasia. *Cortex, 14,* 178-189.

Penfield, W., & Roberts, L. (1959). *Speech and brain mechanisms.* Princeton, NJ: Princeton University Press.

Pierce, R. (1989). Linguistic context and aphasia treatment. In R. Pierce & M. J. Wilcox (Eds.), *Seminars in speech and language: Pragmatics of aphasia.* New York: Thieme.

Pimental, P. A., & Kingsbury, N. A. (1989). *Mini inventory of right brain injury.* Austin, TX: Pro-Ed.

Pincus, J., & Tucker, G. (1985). *Behavioral neurology.* New York: Oxford University Press.

Podraza, B. L., & Darley, F. L. (1977). Effect of auditory prestimulation on naming in aphasia. *Journal of Speech and Hearing Research, 20,* 669-683.

Poeck, K. (1983). What do we mean by "aphasic syndromes?" A neurologist's view. *Brain and Language, 20,* 79-89.

Poeck, K., Huber, W., & Willmes, K. (1989). Outcome of intensive language rehabilitation in aphasia. *Journal of Speech and Hearing Disorders, 54,* 471-479.

Polinko, P. R. (1985). Working with the family: The acute phase. In M. Ylvisaker (Ed.), *Head injury rehabilitation: Children and adolescents* (pp. 87-101). San Diego: College-Hill.

Poppelreuter, W. (1917). *Die psychischen schodigringen durch kopfschuss im kriege. 1914/1916.* Leipzig: Verlag von Leopold Voss.

Porch, B. E. (1967, 1981a). *Porch Index of Communicative Ability.* Palo Alto, CA: Consulting Psychologists Press.

Porch, B. E. (1981b). Therapy subsequent to the PICA. In R. Chapey (Ed.), *Language intervention strategies in adult aphasia* (2nd ed., pp. 283-296). Baltimore: Williams & Wilkins.

Porch, B. E., & Callaghan, S. (1981). Making predictions about recovery: Is there HOAP? In R. H. Brookshire (Ed.), *Clinical Aphasiology Conference proceedings* (pp. 187-200). Minneapolis, MN: BRK Publishers.

Porch, B. E., Collins, M., Wertz, R. T., & associates. (1980). Statistical prediction of change in aphasia. *Journal of Speech and Hearing Research, 12,* 312-321.

Posner, M. I., Walker, J. A., Friederich, F. A., & associates. (1987). How do the parietal lobes direct covert attention? *Neuropsychologia, 25,* 135-145.

Povlishock, J. T., Becker, D. P., Sullivan, H. G., & associates. (1978). Vascular permeability alterations to horseradish peroxidase in experimental brain injury. *Brain Research, 153,* 233-239.

Powell, J., Martindale, A., & Kulp, S. (1975). An evaluation of time-sampling measures of behavior. *Journal of Applied Behavior Analysis, 8,* 463-469.

Powers, G. L., & Starr, C. D. (1974). The effects of muscle exercise on velopharyngeal gap and nasality. *Cleft Palate Journal, 11,* 28-40.

Price, R. W., & Perry, S. (1994). *HIV, AIDS, and the brain.* New York: Raven Press.

Prigitano, G., Fordyce, D., Zeiner, H., & associates. (1984). Neuropsychological rehabilitation after closed head injury in young adults. *Journal of Neurology, Neurosurgery, and Psychiatry, 47,* 505-513.

Prins, R. S., Snow, C. E., & Wagenaar, E. (1978). Recovery from aphasia: Spontaneous speech versus language comprehension. *Brain and Language, 6,* 192-211.

Prutting, C. A., & Kirchner, D. M. (1987). A clinical appraisal of the pragmatic aspects of language. *Journal of Speech and Hearing Disorders, 52,* 105-119.

Quatrocchi-Tubin, S., & Jason, L. A. (1980). Enhancing social interactions and activity among the elderly through stimulus control. *Journal of Applied Behavior Analysis, 13,* 159-163.

Rabins, P. V., Mace, N. L., & Lucas, M. J. (1982). The impact of dementia on the family. *Journal of the American Medical Association, 248,* 333-336.

Rader, M. A., & Ellis, D. W. (1994). The sensory stimulation assessment measure (SSAM): A tool for early evaluation of brain-injured patients. *Brain Injury, 4,* 309-321.

Rafal, R. D., & Posner, M. I. (1987). Deficits in human spatial attention following thalamic lesions. *Proceedings of the National Academy of Science, 7349-7353.*

Rappoport, M., Hall, K. M., Hopkins, K., & associates. (1982). Disability rating scale for severe head trauma: Coma to community. *Archives of Physical Medicine and Rehabilitation, 63,* 118-123.

Raven, J. C. (1960). *The standard progressive matrices.* New York: The Psychological Corporation.

Raven, J. C. (1965). *The coloured progressive matrices.* New York: The Psychological Corporation.

Reisberg, B., Ferris, S. H., DeLeon, M. J., & associates. (1982). The global deterioration scale for assessment of primary degenerative dementia. *American Journal of Psychiatry, 139,* 1136-1139.

Reitan, R. M., & Wolfson, D. (1993). *The Halstead-Reitan neuropsychological test battery: Theory and clinical interpretation.* Tucson, AZ: Neuropsychology Press.

Repp, A. C., Dietz, D., Boles, S. M., & associates. (1976). Differences among common methods for calculating interobserver agreement. *Journal of Applied Behavior Analysis, 9,* 109-113.

Rey, A. (1941). Psychological examination of traumatic encephalopathy. *Archives de Psycholgie, 28,* 286-340; sections translated by J. Corwin & F. W. Bylsma. (1993). *The clinical neuropsychologist* (pp. 4-9).

Rey, A. (1964). *L'examen clinque en psychologie.* Paris: Presses Universitaires de France. (Reported in Lezak, 1995.)

Ripich, D. N., & Terrell, B. Y. (1988). Patterns of discourse cohesion and coherence in Alzheimer's disease. *Journal of Speech and Hearing Disorders, 53,* 8-15.

Ripich, D. N., & Ziol, E. (1998). Dementia: A review for the speech-language pathologists. In A. F. Johnson & B. H. Jacobson (Eds.), *Medical speech-language pathology: A practitioner's guide* (pp. 467-494). New York: Thieme.

Rivers, D. L. & Love, R. J. (1980). Language performance on visual processing tasks in right hemisphere lesion cases. *Brain and Language, 10,* 348-366.

Rizzo, M., & Robin, D. A. (1990). Simultanagnosia: A defect of sustained attention yields insights on visual information processing, *Neurology, 40,* 447-455.

Robertson, I. (1990). Does computerized cognitive rehabilitation work? A review. *Aphasiology, 4,* 381-405.

Robey, R. R. (1998). A meta-analysis of clinical outcomes in the treatment of aphasia. *Journal of Speech, Language, and Hearing Research, 41,* 172-187.

Robey, R. R., Schultz, M. C., Crawford, A. B., & associates. (1999). Single-subject clinical outcome research: Designs, data, effect sizes, and analyses. *Aphasiology, 13,* 445-473.

Robin, D., & Scheinberg, S. (1990). Subcortical lesions and aphasia. *Journal of Speech and Hearing Disorders, 55,* 90-100.

Robin, D. A., Tranel, D., & Damasio, H. (1990). Auditory perception of temporal and spectral events in patients with focal left and right cerebral lesions. *Brain and Language, 39,* 539-555.

Robertson, I., & North, N. (1993). Active and passive activation of left limbs: Influence on visual and sensory neglect. *Neuropsychologia, 31,* 293-300.

Rochford, G., & Williams, M. (1965). Studies in the development and breakdown in the use of names, IV: The effects of word frequency. *Journal of Neurology, Neurosurgery, and Psychiatry, 28,* 407-413.

Rosenbek, J. C. (1978). Treating apraxia of speech. In D. F. Johns (Ed.), *Clinical management of neurogenic communication disorders* (pp. 191-241). Boston: Little, Brown and Company.

Rosenbek, J. C., Collins, M. J., & Wertz, R. T. (1976). Intersystemic reorganization for apraxia of speech. In R. H. Brookshire (Ed.), *Clinical Aphasiology Conference proceedings* (pp. 255-260). Minneapolis, MN: BRK Publishers.

Rosenbek, J. C., & LaPointe, L. L. (1978). The dysarthrias: Description, diagnosis, and treatment. In D. F. Johns (Ed.), *Clinical management of neurogenic communication disorders* (pp. 251-310). Boston: Little, Brown and Company.

Rosenbek, J. C. & LaPointe, L. L. (1985). The dysarthrias: Description, diagnosis, and treatment. In D. F. Johns (Ed.), *Clinical management of neurogenic communication disorders* (2nd ed., pp. 97-152). Boston: Little, Brown and Company.

Rosenbek, J. C., LaPointe, L. L., & Wertz, R. T. (1989). *Aphasia: A clinical approach.* Boston: Little, Brown and Company.

Rosenbek, J. C., Lemme, M. L., Ahern, M. B., & associates. (1973). A treatment for apraxia of speech in adults. *Journal of Speech and Hearing Disorders, 38,* 462-472.

Rosenbek, J. C., & Wertz, R. T. (1972). Treatment of apraxia of speech in adults. In R. T. Wertz & M. Collins (Eds.), *Clinical Aphasiology Conference proceedings* (pp. 191-198). Madison, WI: Veterans Administration Medical Center.

Rosenbek, J. C., Wertz, R. T., & Darley, F. L. (1973). Oral sensation and perception in apraxia of speech and aphasia. *Journal of Speech and Hearing Research, 16,* 22-36.

Rosenshine, B. V. (1980). Skill hierarchies in reading comprehension. In R. J. Spino, B. C. Bruce, & W. F. Brewer (Eds.), *Theoretical issues in reading comprehension* (pp. 535-554). Hillsdale, NJ: Lawrence Erlbaum.

Rosenthal, M., Griffith, E., Bond, M., & associates. (1990). *Rehabilitation of the adult and child with traumatic brain injury.* Philadelphia: F.A. Davis.

Ross, D. G. (1996). *Ross information processing assessment* (2nd ed.). Austin, TX: Pro-Ed.

Rowley, G., & Fielding, K. (1991). Reliability and accuracy of the Glasgow Coma Scale with experienced and inexperienced users. *Lancet, 2,* 535-538.

Rubens, A. B. (1977). The role of changes within the central nervous system during recovery from aphasia. In M. Sullivan & M. S. Kommers (Eds.), *Rationale for adult aphasia therapy* (pp. 28-43). Lincoln, NE: University of Nebraska Medical Center.

Rubow, R. T., Rosenbek, J. C., Collins, M. J., & associates. (1984). Reduction of hemifacial spasm in dysarthria following EMG feedback. *Journal of Speech and Hearing Disorders, 49,* 26-33.

Ruesch, J. (1944). Intellectual impairment in head injuries. *American Journal of Psychiatry, 100,* 480-496.

Russell, W. R. (1971). *The traumatic amnesias.* New York: Oxford University Press.

Russell, W. R., & Espir, M. L. E. (1961). *Traumatic aphasia.* London: Oxford University Press.

Russell, W. R,. & Nathan, P. W. (1946). Traumatic amnesia. *Brain, 69,* 183-187.

Rutherford, W. H. (1977). Diagnosis of alcohol ingestion in mild head injuries. *Lancet, 1,* 1021-1023.

Rutter, M. (1981). Psychological sequelae of brain damage in children. *American Journal of Psychiatry, 183,* 1533-1549.

Saint-Cyr, J. A., & Taylor, A. E., (1992). The mobilization of procedural learning: The "key signature" of the basal ganglia. In L. R. Squire & N. Butters (Eds.), *Neuropsychology of memory* (2nd ed.) (pp. 126-134). New York: Guilford Press.

Salvatore, A. P., Strait, M., & Brookshire, R. H. (1978). Effects of patient characteristics on delivery of Token Test commands by experienced and inexperienced examiners. *Journal of Communication Disorders, 11,* 325-334.

Sands, E., Sarno, M. T., & Shankweiler, D. (1969). Long term assessment of language function in aphasia due to stroke. *Archives of Physical Medicine and Rehabilitation, 50,* 202-207.

Sarno, M. T. (1969). *The functional communication profile.* New York: NYU Medical Center Monograph Department.

Sarno, M. T., & Levita, E. (1971). Natural course of recovery in severe aphasia. *Archives of Physical Medicine and Rehabilitation, 52,* 175-178.

Sarno, M. T., Silverman, M., & Sands, E. (1970). Speech therapy and language recovery in severe aphasia. *Journal of Speech and Hearing Research, 13,* 607-623.

Sbordone, R. J. (1990). Psychotherapeutic treatment of the client with traumatic brain injury: a conceptual model. In J. S. Kreutzer, & P. H. Wehman, (eds), *Community integration following traumatic brain injury* (pp. 144-145). Baltimore: Paul H. Brookes.

Sbordone, R. J. (1991). Overcoming obstacles in cognitive rehabilitation of persons with severe traumatic brain injury. In J. S. Kreutzer & P. H. Wehman (Eds.), *Cognitive rehabilitation for persons with traumatic brain injury: A functional approach* (pp. 105-115). Baltimore: Brookes.

Schacter, D., Rich, S., & Stampp, A. (1985). Remediation of memory disorders: Experimental evaluation of the spaced-retrieval technique. *Journal of Clinical and Experimental Neuropsychology, 7,* 79-96.

Schacter, D. L., & Glisky, E. L. (1986). Memory remediation: Restorations, alleviation, and the acquisition of domain-specific knowledge. In Y. Gross & B. P. Uzzell (Eds.), *Clinical neuropsychology of intervention* (pp. 257-282). Boston: Martinus Nijhoff.

Schenkenberg, T., Bradford, T. C., & Ajax, E. T. (1980). Line bisection and unilateral visual neglect in patients with neurologic impairment. *Neurology, 30,* 509-517.

Schuell, H. M. (1957). A short examination for aphasia. *Neurology, 7,* 625-634.

Schuell, H. M. (1965, 1972). *The Minnesota test for differential diagnosis of aphasia.* Minneapolis, MN: University of Minnesota Press.

Schuell, H. M., & Jenkins, J. J. (1961). Reduction of vocabulary in aphasia. *Brain, 84,* 243-261.

Schuell, H. M., Jenkins, J. J., & Jimenez-Pabon, E. (1965). *Aphasia in adults.* New York: Harper and Row.

Schuell, H. M., Jenkins, J. J., & Landis, L. (1961). Relationship between auditory comprehension and word frequency in aphasia. *Journal of Speech and Hearing Research, 4,* 30-36.

Segatore, M., & Way, C. (1992). The Glasgow Coma Scale: Time for a change. *Heart and Lung, 21,* 548-557.

Selnes, O. A., Knopman, D. S., Niccum, N., & associates. (1983). Computed tomographic scan correlates of auditory comprehension deficits in aphasia: A prospective recovery study. *Annals of Neurology, 13,* 558-566.

Selnes, O. A., Knopman, D. S., Niccum, N., & associates. (1985). The critical role of Wernicke's area in sentence repetition. *Annals of Neurology, 17,* 549-557.

Seron, X., Deloche, G., Moulard, G., & Rousselle, M. (1980). A computer-based therapy for the treatment of aphasic subjects with writing disorders. *Journal of Speech and Hearing Disorders, 45,* 45-58.

Shallice, T. (1982). Specific impairments of planning. *Philosophical Transactions of the Royal Society of London, 298,* 199-209.

Shallice, T., & Warrington, E. K. (1970). Independent functioning of the verbal memory stores: A neuropsychological study. *Quarterly Journal of Experimental Psychology, 22,* 261-273.

Shankweiler, D., & Harris, K. S. (1966). An experimental approach to the problem of articulation in aphasia. *Cortex, 2,* 277-292.

Shapiro, B. E., & Danly, M. (1985). The role of the right hemisphere in the control of speech prosody in propositional and affective contexts. *Brain and Language, 25,* 19-36.

Shatz, P., & Chute, D. L. (1995). Predicting level of independence following moderate and severe traumatic brain injury. *Archives of Clinical Neuropsychology, 11,* 444-445.

Sheehan, V. (1945). Rehabilitation of aphasia in an army hospital. *Journal of Speech Disorders, 11,* 148-154.

Sheikh, J. I., & Yesavage, J. A. (1986). The Geriatric Depression Scale (GDS): Recent evidence and development of a shorter version. *Clinical Gerontologist, 5,* 165-173.

Shewan, C. M. (1988). The Shewan sponataneous language analysis system (SSLA) for aphasic adults: Description, reliability, and validity. *Journal of Communication Disorders, 21,* 103-138.

Shewan, C. M., & Canter, G. J. (1971). Effects of vocabulary, syntax, and sentence length on auditory comprehension in aphasic patients. *Cortex, 7,* 209-226.

Shewan, C. M., & Kertesz, A. (1980). Reliability and validity characteristics of the Western Aphasia Battery (WAB). *Journal of Speech and Hearing Disorders, 45,* 308-324.

Shewan, C. M., & Kertesz, A. (1984). Effects of speech and language treatment on recovery from aphasia. *Brain and Language, 23,* 272-299.

Silverman, F. H. (1983). Dysarthria: Communication augmentation systems for adults without speech. In W. H. Perkins (Ed.), *Dysarthria and apraxia* (pp. 115-121). New York: Thieme-Stratton.

Skelly, M. (1979). *Amer-Ind gestural code based on universal American Indian hand talk.* New York: Elsevier.

Sklar, M. (1973). *The Sklar aphasia scale.* Los Angeles: Western Psychological Services.

Smith, A. (1972). *Diagnosis, intelligence, and rehabilitation of chronic aphasics. Final report.* Ann Arbor, MI: University of Michigan Press.

Snow, P., Douglas, J., & Ponsford, J. (1995). Discourse assessment following traumatic brain injury: A pilot study examining some demographic and methodological issues. *Aphasiology, 9,* 365-380.

Sohlberg, M. M., & Mateer, C. A. (1989). *Introduction to cognitive rehabilitation: Theory and practice.* New York: Gulford.

Sparks, R., Helm, N. A., & Albert, M. L. (1974). Aphasia rehabilitation resulting from melodic intonation therapy. *Cortex, 10,* 303-316.

Sparks, R., & Holland, A. L. (1976). Method: Melodic intonation therapy for aphasia. *Journal of Speech and Hearing Disorders, 41,* 287-297.

Spector, A., Orrell, M., Davies, S., & associates. (2000). Reality orientation for dementia. *Cochrane Database of Systematic Reviews, 2,* CD0001119.

Spreen, O., & Benton, A. L. (1977). *Neurosensory center comprehensive examination for aphasia.* Victoria, BC: Neuropsychology Laboratory, University of Victoria.

Square, P. A., Darley, F. L., & Sommers, R. K. (1982). An analysis of the production errors made by pure apractic speakers with differing loci of lesions. In R. H. Brookshire (Ed.), *Clinical Aphasiology Conference proceedings* (pp. 245-249). Minneapolis, MN: BRK Publishers.

Square, P. A., & Weidner, W. E. (1976). *Oral sensory perception in adults demonstrating apraxia of speech.* Paper presented to the American Speech and Hearing Association, Houston, Texas.

Stachowiak, F. J., Huber, W., Poeck, K., & associates. (1977). Text comprehension in aphasia. *Brain and Language, 4,* 177-195.

Stanczak, D. E., White, J. G., Gouview, W. D., & associates. (1984). Assessment of level of consciousness following severe neurological insult. *Journal of Neurosurgery, 60,* 955-60.

Stanton, K., Yorkston, K. M., Talley-Kenyon, V., & associates. (1981). Language utilization in teaching reading to left neglect patients. In R. H. Brookshire (Ed.), *Clinical Aphasiology Conference proceedings* (pp. 262-271). Minneapolis, MN: BRK Publishers.

State University of New York at Buffalo Research Foundation. (1993). *Guide for the use of the uniform data set for medical rehabilitation: Functional independence measure.* Buffalo: State University of New York.

Stedman's Medical Dictionary. (1990). Baltimore, MD: Williams & Wilkins.

Steele, J. C., Richardson, J. D., & Olszewski, J. (1964). Progressive supranuclear palsy. *Archives of Neurology, 10,* 333-359.

Stimley, M. A., & Noll, J. D. (1991). The effects of semantic and phonemic prestimulation cues on picture naming in aphasia. *Brain and Language, 41,* 496-509.

Stoicheff, M. L. (1960). Motivating instructions and language performance of dysphasic subjects. *Journal of Speech and Hearing Research, 3,* 75-85.

Stokes, G. (1990). Controlling disruptive and demanding behaviors. In G. Stokes, & F. Goudie (Eds.), *Working with dementia* (pp. 158-173). London: Winslow Press.

Stokes, T. F., & Baer, D. M. (1977). An implied technology of generalization. *Journal of Applied Behavior Analysis, 10,* 349-367.

Sunderland, A., Harris, J. E., & Baddeley, A. D. (1983). Do laboratory tests predict everyday memory? *Journal of Verbal Learning and Verbal Behavior, 22,* 341-357.

Swindell, C. S., Holland, A. L., & Fromm, D. (1984). Classification of aphasia: WAB type versus clinical impression. In R. H. Brookshire (Ed.), *Clinical Aphasiology Conference proceedings* (pp. 48-54). Minneapolis, MN: BRK Publishers.

Teasdale, G., & Jennett, B. (1974). Assessment of coma and impaired consciousness. *Lancet, 2,* 81-84.

Teasdale, G., & Jennett, B. (1976). Assessment and prognosis of coma after head injury. *Acta Neurochirugica, 34,* 45-55.

Teasdale, G., & Mendelow, D. (1984). Pathophysiology of head injuries. In D. N. Brooks (Ed.), *Closed head injury: Psychological, social, and family consequences* (pp. 4-36). Oxford: Oxford University Press.

Teng, E. L., & Chui, H. (1987). The modified Mini-Mental State (3MS) Examination. *Journal of Clinical Psychiatry, 48,* 314-318.

Terman, L. M., & Merrill, M. A. (1973). *Stanford-Binet intelligence scale.* Boston: Houghton-Mifflin.

Thompson, C., & Byrne, M. (1984). Across setting generalization of social conventions in aphasia. In R. H. Brookshire (Ed.), *Clincial Aphasiology Conference proceedings* (pp. 132-144). Minneapolis, MN: BRK Publishers.

Thompson, C., Holmberg, M., & Baer, D. M. (1974). A brief report on a comparison of two time-sampling methods. *Journal of Applied Behavior Analysis, 7,* 623-626.

Thompson, R. S., Rivara, F. P., & Thompson, D. C. (1989). A case control study of the effectiveness of bicycle safety helmets. *New England Journal of Medicine, 320,* 1362-1367.

Thurman, D. J., Alverson, C. A., Dunn, K. A., & associates. (1999). Traumatic brain injury in the United States: A public health perspective. *Journal of Head Trauma Rehabilitation, 14,* 602-615.

Thurman, D. J., & Guerrero, J. (1999). Trends in hospitalization associated with traumatic brain injury. *Journal of the American Medical Association, 282,* 954-957.

Thurstone, L. L. (1944). *A factorial study of perception.* Chicago: University of Chicago Press.

Tombaugh, T. N., & Hurley, A. M. (1997). The 60-item Boston Naming Test: Norms for cognitively intact adults aged 25 to 88 years. *Journal of Clinical and Experimental Neuropsychology, 19,* 922-932.

Tombaugh, T. N., McDowell, I., Kristjansson, B., & associates. (1996). Mini-Mental State Examination (MMSE) and the modified MMSE (3MS): A psychometric comparison and normative data. *Psychological Assessment, 8,* 48-59.

Tomlinson, B. E., & Henderson, G. (1976). Some quantitative cerebral findings in normal and demented old people. In R. Terry & S. Gerskor (Eds.), *Neurobiology of aging.* New York: Raven.

Tompkins, C. A. (1995). *Right hemisphere communication disorders: Theory and management.* San Diego, CA: Singular.

Tompkins, C. A., Baumgaertner, A., Lehman, M. T. & associates. (1997). Suppression and discourse comprehension in right brain-damaged adults: A preliminary report. *Aphasiology, 11,* 505-519.

Tompkins, C. A., & Flowers, C. R. (1985). Perception of emotional intonation by brain-damaged adults: The influence of task processing levels. *Journal of Speech and Hearing Research, 28,* 527-538.

Tompkins, C. A., & Lehman, M. T. (1998). Interpreting intended meanings after right hemisphere brain damage: An analysis of evidence, potential accounts, and clinical implications. *Topics in Stroke Rehabilitation, 51,* 29-47.

Tompkins, C. A., Lehman, M. T., Baumgaertner, A., & associates. (1996). Suppression and discourse comprehension in right brain-damaged adults: Inferential ambiguity processing. *Brain and Language, 55,* 172-175.

Tompkins, C. A., Lehman-Blake, M. T., Baumgaertner, A., & associates. (2001). Mechanisms of discourse comprehension impairment after right hemisphere brain damage: Suppression in referential ambiguity resolution. *Journal of Speech, Language, and Hearing Research, 44,* 400-415.

Tow, P. M. (1955). *Personality changes following frontal leucotomy.* London: Oxford University Press.

Trost, J. E., & Canter, G. J. (1974). Apraxia of speech in patients with Broca's aphasia: A study of phoneme production accuracy and error patterns. *Brain and Language, 1,* 63-79.

Trupe, E. H. (1984). Reliability of rating spontaneous speech in the Western Aphasia Battery: Implications for classification. In R. H. Brookshire (Ed.), *Clinical Aphasiology Conference proceedings* (pp. 55-69). Minneapolis, MN: BRK Publishers.

Tucker, D. M., & Frederick, S. L. (1989). Emotion and brain lateralization. In H. Wagner & A. Manstead (Eds.), *Handbook of social psychophysiology* (pp. 27-70). New York: Wiley.

Tueth, M. J. (1995). How to manage depression and psychosis in Alzheimer's disease. *Geriatrics, 50,* 43-49.

Tuiman, J. J. (1974). Determining the passage dependency of comprehension test questions on five major tests. *Reading Research Quarterly, 2,* 206-233.

Tulving, E. (1972). Episodic and semantic memory. In E. Tulving & W. Donaldson (Eds.), *Organization of memory.* New York: Academic Press.

Tulving, E. (1983). *Elements of episodic memory.* Oxford: Clarendon Press.

Tweedy, J. R., & Shulman, P. D. (1982). Toward a functional classification of naming impairments. *Brain and Language, 15,* 193-206.

Ulatowska, H. K., Doyel, A. W., Freedman-Stern, R. F., & associates. (1983). Production of procedural discourse in aphasia. *Brain and Language, 18,* 315-341.

Uzzell, B. P., Dolinskas, C. A., Wiser, R. F., & associates. (1987). Influence of lesions detected by computed tomography on outcome and neuropsycholgical recovery after severe head injury. *Neurosurgery, 20,* 396-402.

Vaccaro, F. J. (1988). Application of operant procedures in a group of institutionalized aggressive geriatric patients. *Psychology and Aging, 3,* 22-28.

Vallar, G., & Baddeley, A. D. (1984). Phonological short-term store, phonological processing, and sentence processing: A neuropsychological case study. *Cognitive Neuropsychology, 1,* 121-142.

Vallar, G., & Perani, D. (1986). The anatomy of unilateral neglect after right-hemisphere stroke: A clinical/CT scan correlation study in man. *Neuropsychologia, 24,* 609-622.

Van Buskirk, C. (1955). Prognostic value of sensory deficit in rehabilitation of hemiplegics. *Neurology, 6,* 407-411.

VanDemark, A. A., Lemmer, E. C., & Drake, M. L. (1982). Measurement of reading comprehension in aphasia with the RCBA. *Journal of Speech and Hearing Research, 47,* 288-291.

Van Houten, R., Rolider, A., Malenfant, L., & associates. (1994). Prevention of brain injuries by improving safety-related behaviors. In M. A. J. Finlayson & S. H. Garner (Eds.), *Brain injury rehabilitation: Clinical considerations* (pp. 313-331). Baltimore: Williams & Wilkins.

Van Zomeren, A. H., Brouwer, W. H., & Deelman, B. G. (1984). Attentional deficits: The riddles of selectivity, speed, and alertness. In N. Brooks (Ed.), *Closed head injury: Psychological, social, and family consequences* (pp. 74-107). Oxford: Oxford University Press.

Verfaelli, M., Bauer, R. H., & Bowers, D. (1991). Autonomic and behavioral evidence of implicit memory in amnesia. *Brain and Cognition, 15,* 10-25.

Veterans Administration. (1972). Veterans Adminstration cooperative study group on antihypertensive agents: Effects of treatment on morbidity in hypertension III: Influence of age, diastolic pressure, and prior cardiovascular disease; further analysis of side effects. *Circulation, 45,* 991-1004.

Vignolo, L. A. (1964). Evolution of aphasia and language rehabilitation: A retrospective study. *Cortex, 1,* 344-367.

Vignolo, L. A., Frediani, F., Boccardi, F. E., & associates. (1986). Unexpected CT scan findings in global aphasia. *Cortex, 22,* 55-70.

Wagenaar, E., Snow, C. E., & Prins, R. S. (1975). Spontaneous speech of aphasic patients: A psycholinguistic analysis. *Brain and Language, 2,* 281-303.

Waller, M. R., & Darley, F. L. (1978). The influence of context on the auditory comprehension of paragraphs in aphasic subjects. *Journal of Speech and Hearing Research, 21,* 732-745.

Walker-Baston, D., Curtis, S., Smith, P., & associates. (1999). An alternative model for treatment of aphasia: The Lifelink approach. In R. Elman (Ed.), *Group treatment of neurogenic communication disorders: The expert clinician's approach* (pp. 67-75). Boston: Butterworth-Heinemann.

Walsh, K. W. (1985). *Understanding brain damage.* Edinburgh: Churchill-Livingstone.

Warren, R. L. (1992). Functional outcome: An introduction. *Clinical Aphasiology, 21,* 59-65.

Warrington, E. K., & James, M. (1967). Disorders of visual perception in patients with localized cerebral lesions. *Neuropsychologica, 5,* 253-266.

Warrington, E. K., & Shallice, T. (1969). The selective impairment of auditory-verbal short-term memory. *Brain, 92,* 885-896.

Watson, R. T., & Heilman, K. M. (1979). Thalamic neglect. *Neurology, 29,* 690-694.

Waxman, S. (2000). *Correlative neuroanatomy* (24th ed.). New York: McGraw-Hill.

Webb, W. G. (1990). Acquired dyslexias. In L. L. LaPointe (Ed.), *Aphasia and related language disorders* (pp. 130-146). New York: Thieme.

Wechsler, D. (1981). *Wechsler adult intelligence scale—Revised.* New York: The Psychological Corporation.

Wechsler, D. (1987). *Wechsler memory scale—Revised manual.* San Antonio, TX: The Psychological Corporation.

Wegner, M. L., Brookshire, R. H., & Nicholas, L. E. (1984). Comprehension of main ideas and details in coherent and noncoherent discourse by aphasic and nonaphasic listeners. *Brain and Language, 21,* 37-51.

Weidner, W. E., & Jinks, A. F. (1983). The effects of single versus combined cue presentations on picture naming by aphasic adults. *Journal of Speech and Hearing Disorders, 16,* 111-121.

Weigl, E. (1968). On the problem of cortical syndromes: Experimental studies. In M. L. Simmell (Ed.), *The reach of mind* (pp. 143-159). New York: Springer.

Weigel-Crump, C., & Koenigsknecht, R. A. (1973). Tapping the lexical store of the adult aphasic: Analysis of improvement made in word retrieval skills. *Cortex, 9,* 411-418.

Weiner, F. (1983). *Aphasia I: Noun association.* Baltimore: University Park Press.

Weisenburg, T. H., & McBride, K. E. (1935). *Aphasia.* New York: Commonwealth Fund.

Wener, D. L., & Duffy, J. R. (1983). An investigation of the sensitivity of the Reporter's Test to expressive language disturbances (abstract). In R. H. Brookshire (Ed.), *Clinical Aphasiology Conference proceedings* (pp. 15-17). Minneapolis, MN: BRK Publishers.

Wepman, J. M. (1951). *Recovery from aphasia.* New York: Ronald Press.

Wertz, R. T., Collins, M., Weiss, D., & associates. (1981). Veterans Administration cooperative study on aphasia: A comparison of individual and group treatment. *Journal of Speech and Hearing Research, 24,* 580-594.

Wertz, R. T., Deal, J. L., Holland, A. L., & associates. (1986). Comments on an uncontrolled aphasia no treatment trial. *Asha, J 28,* 31.

Wertz, R. T., Deal, J. L., & Robinson, A. J. (1984). Classifying the aphasias: A comparison of the Boston Diagnostic Aphasia Examination and the Western Aphasia Battery. In R. H. Brookshire (Ed.), *Clinical Aphasiology Conference proceedings* (pp. 40-47). Minneapolis, MN: BRK Publishers.

Wertz, R. T., Dronkers, N. F., & Hume, J. L. (1993). PICA intra-subtests variability and prognosis for improvement in aphasia. In M. L. Lemme (Ed.), *Clinical aphasiology, vol. 21,* (pp. 207-211). Austin, TX: Pro-Ed.

Wertz, R. T., Keith, R. L., & Custer, D. D. (1971). *Normal and aphasic behavior on a measure of auditory input and a measure of verbal output.* Paper presented at the annual convention of the American Speech and Hearing Association, Chicago.

Wertz, R. T., LaPointe, L. L., & Rosenbek, J. C. (1984). *Apraxia of speech in adults: The disorder and its management.* Orlando, FL: Grune & Stratton.

Wertz, R. T., Weiss, D., Aten, J., & associates (1986). A comparison of clinic, home, and deferred language treatment for aphasia: A VA cooperative study. *Archives of Neurology, 43,* 653-658.

West, J. F. (1981). Group treatment for aphasia: Panel discussion. In R. H. Brookshire (Ed.), *Clinical Aphasiology: Conference proceedings 1981* (pp. 151-152). Minneapolis, MN: BRK Publishers.

West, J. F., & Kaufman, G. A. (1972). *Some effects of redundancy on the auditory comprehension of adult aphasics.* Paper presented at the annual convention of the American Speech and Hearing Association, San Francisco.

White, L. R., Cartwright, W. S., Cornoni-Huntley, J., & associates. (1986). Geriatric epidemiology. *Annual Review of Gerontology and Geriatrics, 6,* 215-311.

Whitely, A. M., & Warrington, E. K. (1977). Prosopagnosia: A clinical, psychological, and anatomical study of three patients. *Journal of Neurology, Neurosurgery, and Psychiatry, 40,* 395-403.

Wilkinson, G. (1993). *The wide range achievement test* (3rd ed.). Wilmington, DE: Wide Range.

Willanger, R., Danielson, U. T., & Ankerhaus, J. (1981). Visual neglect in right-sided apoplectic lesions. *Acta Neurologica Scandinavia, 64,* 310-326.

Williams, S. E., & Canter, G. J. (1982). The influence of situational context on naming performance in aphasic syndromes. *Brain and Language, 17,* 92-106.

Wilson, B. (1981). Teaching a patient to remember people's names after removal of a left temporal tumor. *Behavioral Psychotherapy, 9,* 338-344.

Wilson, B. A., Cockburn, J., & Baddeley, A. (1985). *The Rivermead behavioural memory test.* Suffolk, England: Thames Valley Test Company.

Wilson, B. A., Cockburn, J., & Baddeley, A. (1999). *The Rivermead behavioural memory test—Extended.* Suffolk, England: Thames Valley Test Company.

Wilson, B. A., Cockburn, J., & Halligan, P. (1987). *Behavioral inattention test.* Suffolk, England: Thames Valley Test Company.

Wilson, J. A., Pentland, B., Currie, C. T., & associates. (1987). The functional effects of head injury in the elderly. *Brain Injury, 1,* 183-188.

Winner, E., Brownell, H., Happe, F., & associates. (1998). Distinguishing lies from jokes: Theory of mind deficits and discourse interpretation in right hemisphere brain-damaged patients. *Brain and Language, 62,* 89-106.

Woodcock, R. W., & Johnson, M. B. (1989). *Woodcock-Johnson psycho-educational battery—Revised.* Allen, TX: DLM Teaching Resources.

World Health Organization. (1980). *International classification of impairments, disabilities, and handicaps.* Geneva: World Health Organization.

World Health Organization. (2000). *International classification of impairments, disabilities, and handicaps 2—Prefinal draft.* Geneva: World Health Organization.

Wyke, M., & Holgate, D. (1973). Colour naming defects in dysphasic patients: A qualitative analysis. *Neurolopsychologia, 11,* 451-461.

Ylvisaker, M., & Urbanczyk, B. (1994). Assessment and treatment of speech, swallowing, and communication disorders following traumatic brain injury. In M. A. J. Finlayson & S. H. Garner (Eds.), *Brain injury rehabilitation: Clinical considerations* (pp. 157-186). Baltimore: Williams & Wilkins.

Ylvisaker, M. S., & Holland, A. L. (1985). Coaching, self-coaching, and rehabilitation of head injury. In D. F. Johns (Ed.), *Clinical management of neurogenic communication disorders* (pp. 243-357). Boston: Little, Brown and Company.

Yorkston, K. M. (1981). Treatment of right hemisphere damaged patients: A panel presentation. In R. H. Brookshire (Ed.), *Clinical Aphasiology Conference proceedings* (pp. 281-283). Minneapolis, MN: BRK Publishers.

Yorkston, K. M., & Beukelman, D. R. (1980). An analysis of connected speech samples of aphasic and normal speakers. *Journal of Speech and Hearing Disorders, 45,* 27-36.

Yorkston, K. M., & Beukelman, D. R. (1981). *Assessment of intelligibility of dysarthric speech.* Tigard, OR: C.C. Publications.

Yorkston, K. M., Beulkelman, D. R., & Bell, K. R. (1988). *Clinical management of dysarthric speakers.* San Diego: College-Hill.

Yorkston, K. M., Dowden, P. A., Beukelman, D. R., & associates. (1986). *A phoneme identification task as a measure of perceived articulatory adequacy.* Paper presented at the third biennial Clinical Dysarthria Conference, Tucson, AZ.

Yorkston, K. M., Marshall, R. C., & Butler, M. (1977). Imposed delay of response: Effects on aphasics' auditory comprehension of visually and nonvisually cued material. *Perceptual and Motor Skills, 44,* 647-655.

Yules, R. B., & Chase, R. A. (1969). A training method for reduction of hypernasality in speech. *Plastic and Reconstructive Surgery, 43,* 180-185.

Index